FOURTH EDITION

Joint Range of Motion
AND
Muscle Length Testing

NANCY BERRYMAN REESE, PT, PhD, MHSA

Professor and Chairperson
Department of Physical Therapy
University of Central Arkansas
Conway, Arkansas

WILLIAM D. BANDY, PT, PhD, SCS

Professor
Department of Physical Therapy
University of Central Arkansas
Conway, Arkansas

ELSEVIER

ELSEVIER

3251 Riverport Lane
St. Louis, Missouri 63043

JOINT RANGE OF MOTION AND MUSCLE LENGTH TESTING,
FOURTH EDITION

ISBN: 978-0-323-83187-1

Previous editions copyrighted 2002, 2010 and 2017

Sr. Content Strategist: Lauren Willis
Sr. Content Development Specialist: Malvika Shah
Publishing Services Manager: Deepthi Unni
Project Manager: Sindhuraj Thulasingam
Design Direction: Renee Duenow

Working together
to grow libraries in
developing countries

www.elsevier.com • www.bookaid.org

Printed in India

Last digit is the print number: 9 8 7 6 5 4 3 2 1

To our parents,
Steve *(1927–) and* Geneva *(1921–2009)* Berryman
and
Dick *(1927–2017) and* Betty *(1930–2010)* Bandy,
whose love and guidance have sustained us throughout our lives.

"My son, keep your father's commands and do not forsake your mother's teaching.
Bind them upon your heart forever; fasten them around your neck.
When you walk, they will guide you; when you sleep, they will watch over you;
when you awake, they will speak to you.
For these commands are a lamp, this teaching is a light."
Proverbs 6:20–23a (NIV)

CONTRIBUTORS

CHAD LAIRAMORE, PT, PhD
Associate Professor and Associate Dean
College of Health and Behavioral Sciences
University of Central Arkansas
Conway, Arkansas

LEAH LOWE, DPT, PhD, PCS
Associate Professor
Department of Physical Therapy
University of Central Arkansas
Conway, Arkansas

JACQUIE RAINEY, DrPH, MCHES
Professor
Department of Health Sciences
University of Central Arkansas
Conway, Arkansas

CHARLOTTE YATES, PhD, PT, PCS
Professor
Department of Physical Therapy
University of Central Arkansas
Conway, Arkansas
Physical Therapist
Department of Physical Therapy
Arkansas Children's Hospital
Little Rock, Arkansas

PREFACE

The fourth edition of *Joint Range of Motion and Muscle Length Testing* has been updated to include the latest research on the reliability and validity of clinical methods of measuring joint range of motion. Additional and updated values for range of motion and minimal detectable change have been added to those chapters where information was available. New techniques for measuring range of motion have also been added, including instructions for the use of a smartphone and flexirule to measure motion where appropriate. The latest studies reporting "normal" range of motion for the joints of the spine and extremities have been added to the extensive tables in Appendix B.

Nancy Berryman Reese

William D. Bandy

ACKNOWLEDGMENTS

We are grateful to so many individuals who helped bring this project to fruition. Our current and former colleagues, Dr. Chad Lairamore, Dr. Leah Lowe, and Dr. Charlotte Yates were critical to the completion of this edition of *Joint Range of Motion and Muscle Length Testing*, particularly Chapters 8, 10, and 16. Their clinical expertise, knowledge of current research, and stellar work on this project have elevated the level of this edition of the text. Dr. Jacquie Rainey, provided statistical expertise for the project.

New photographs for the fourth edition were taken by John Sykes of Little Rock, Arkansas. He was creative, efficient, and wonderful to work with. Thanks to our great models for the fourth edition: Dylan Alexander, Michael Crye, Mackenzie Dear, MaryClaire Guanzon, Amanda Okolo, Nicole Reese, Maddie Stout, and Erin Wodward.

Models in the previous three editions included Michael Adkins, Jamie Bandy, Brooke Bridges, Rachel Cloud, Brandon Chandler, Sherry Holmes, Rachel Laden, Trigg Ross, and Blake Wagner (first edition); Amanda Ball, Nick Barnes, Jennie Baumberger, Miles Butler, McKinney Davis, Rose Dickinson, Regenia Eliano, Steve Forbush, Suzanna Garrison, Neil Hattlestad, Miller McVay, Dr. Myla Quiben, Elizabeth Reese, William Upton, Wendy Wheeler, and Anna Yates (second edition); and Meredith Grubbs, Matt Lincoln, Regis Mawire, Reid Parnell, Andrea Thomas, and Nancy Vo (third edition).

As with any task of this magnitude, revising a book is much too large for any two people to do alone. Several individuals, including Joshua Armstrong, Mackenzie Dear, and Haley Downey, helped with research and editing on the fourth edition. In addition, we remain grateful to the following graduate assistants who assisted with previous editions: Jenny Hood, Stacey Ihler, Danyelle Lusby, Vicki Readnour, and Amanda Whitehead (first edition); Amanda Ball, Carrie Blankenship, Marie Charton, Shannon Craig, Mieke Corbitt, Emily Devan, Chandra Hargis-McClug, Kristen Hook, Paige Kibbey, and Tegan Miller (second edition); and Jordan Chadwick, Brittany Clark, Kayleigh Lewellyn, Emily Noble, Rachel Roberts, Stephanie Sharum, Brandon McKinney, and Andrea Thomas (third edition). We are indebted to Shannon Justice, who wrote most of the scripts for the videos as part of a class project. And, of course, we could never have completed this work without the able assistance of the editorial staff at Elsevier, most notably Malvika Shah, Lauren Willis, Sindhuraj Thulasingam, and Ellen Wurm-Cutter. Thanks guys!

As always, our most important thanks go to those who provided us with emotional support during the completion of this project. We both have been blessed to work with a talented and dedicated group of faculty and staff in the Department of Physical Therapy and in the office of the Dean of Health and Behavioral Sciences at the University of Central Arkansas. We are continuously grateful for their support and encouragement and for their tolerance of missed deadlines in the name of "the book." Finally, our largest debt of gratitude goes to our families: to Nancy's husband, David, and daughters, Elizabeth and Nicole; and to Bill's wife, Beth, and daughters, Melissa and Jamie. We continue to take on big projects, and our families continue to provide unlimited support, love, and tolerance. We are truly humbled that God has blessed us with such wonderful families.

Nancy Berryman Reese
William D. Bandy

CONTENTS

VIDEO CONTENTS

To access the videos, visit Elsevier eBooks+ (eBooks.Health.Elsevier.com).

Chapter 8: Measurement of Range of Motion of the Thoracic and Lumbar Spine

Chapter 9: Measurement of Range of Motion of the Cervical Spine and Temporomandibular Joint

SECTION

I

INTRODUCTION

MEASUREMENT of RANGE of MOTION and MUSCLE LENGTH: BACKGROUND, HISTORY, and BASIC PRINCIPLES

Nancy Berryman Reese and William D. Bandy

Historically, early reports on procedures for the examination of range of motion (ROM) suggested using visual approximation.[1] In fact, as late as the 1960s, the initial edition (1965) of a text for measuring joint ROM published by the American Academy of Orthopaedic Surgeons (AAOS)[2] suggested that visual estimation is as good as, or better than, goniometric measurement. This opinion was shared by Rowe,[3] who suggested that visual estimation was especially important when bony landmarks were difficult to see or to palpate. In contrast, Moore[4] and Salter[5] stated that goniometer measurements are more reliable than visual estimates.

Disagreement exists among studies that have objectively examined the value of visual estimation compared with the goniometer. Studies by both Awan et al.[6] and Hayes et al.[7] reported that little difference existed between visual inspection and a goniometer for the measurement of shoulder ROM. However, upon further examination of the reliability coefficients, intrarater reliability ranged from 0.59 to 0.71 for visual inspection and from 0.53 to 0.71 for the use of the goniometer. In other words, the testers who collected the data were not all that accurate, irrespective of whether or not a goniometer was used. Williams and Callaghan[8] also reported that no significant difference existed between visual estimation and the goniometer in the measurement of shoulder flexion. However, the design of this study, in which three testers measured one subject twice while the subject held the arm elevated, calls into question the rigor of this investigation.

In contrast, Watkins et al.[9] reported that reliability of the measurement of knee flexion was greater when a goniometer rather than visual estimation was used. Two studies in which the lead author was Youdas[10,11] reported that the use of instruments to examine the ankle and the cervical spine resulted in more accurate measurements than were obtained through visual estimation. In a systematic review of the interrater reliability of measurements of passive upper extremity motion, van de Pol et al.[12] reported,

"In general, measuring passive physiological range of motion using instruments, such as goniometers or inclinometers, resulted in higher reliability than using vision." Given the research suggesting objective measurement is more accurate than visual examination for the measurement of joint ROM, and the demand for data documenting improved patient outcomes, accurate and standardized measurements are of utmost importance.

The purpose of this chapter is to lay the groundwork for standardized measurement of ROM and muscle length. To this end, the chapter specifies the difference between joint ROM and muscle length and presents basic but important information on kinematics (including the definitions of arthrokinematics and osteokinematics). Additionally, background information and the history of a variety of measurement techniques, related both to joint ROM and to muscle length testing, are provided. Finally, suggested procedures for standardized measurement are presented. After reading this chapter, the reader will have gained general information on the measurement of ROM and muscle length, which serves as the basis for performance of the more specific measurement techniques presented in subsequent chapters.

JOINT RANGE OF MOTION VS MUSCLE LENGTH

Joint ROM is an integral part of human movement. In order for an individual to move efficiently and with minimal effort, full ROM across the joints is imperative. In addition, appropriate ROM allows the joints to adapt more easily to stresses imposed on the body and decreases the potential for injury. Full ROM across a joint is dependent on two components: joint ROM and muscle length.[13] Joint ROM, the motion available at any single joint, is influenced by associated bony structure and physiologic characteristics of the connective tissue surrounding the joint. Important connective tissue that limits joint ROM includes ligaments and joint capsules.[14]

Muscle length refers to the ability of a muscle crossing the joint to lengthen, allowing one joint or a series of joints to move through the available ROM. The terms muscle length and flexibility often are used synonymously to describe the ability of a muscle to be lengthened to the end of the ROM. In this book, the term muscle length is used to refer to the end of the range of the muscle across the joint.[13]

According to Kendall et al.[15] "For muscles that pass over one joint only, the range of motion and range of muscle length will measure the same. ... For muscles that pass over two or more joints, the normal range of muscle length will be less than the total range of motion of the joints over which the muscle passes." Therefore, if the goal is to measure joint ROM of a joint in which a two-joint muscle is involved, the second joint should be placed in a shortened position. If the goal is to measure muscle length, the muscle should be placed in an elongated position across all joints affected, and a measurement should be taken.[15]

An example that illustrates the difference between ROM and range of muscle length is the measurement of knee flexion. To measure knee flexion joint motion, the hip should be flexed (the patient is supine) to put the rectus femoris muscle in a shortened position and to allow full joint motion at the knee (illustrated in Chapter 12, Figs. 12.8–12.11). When muscle length of the rectus femoris muscle (a two-joint muscle) is measured, the patient is placed in the prone position, which extends the hip and lengthens the rectus femoris muscle (described in Chapter 14, Figs. 14.13–14.15).

KINEMATICS

Neumann[16] defines kinematics as "a branch of mechanics that describes the motion of a body without regard to the forces or torques that may produce the motion." In other words, kinematics describes human movement and ignores the cause of the motion (e.g., forces, momentum, energy). This description of motion may include movement of the center of gravity of the body or movement of the extremities, or it may pertain to motion specific to one joint. Kinematics can be subcategorized into specific movements, referred to as arthrokinematics and osteokinematics. To more fully understand kinematics as it relates to measurement of range of joint motion and muscle length, clarification of the terms arthrokinematics and osteokinematics is necessary.

Arthrokinematics

Arthrokinematics refers to actual movements of the joint surfaces in relation to one another. In addition to movement of the lever arm of the bone during ROM activities, the articulating ends of the bone roll, slide (or glide), or spin on each other. Roll is a rotary motion that occurs when new points on one joint surface come in contact with new points on a second joint surface. Slide is a translatory motion that occurs when one joint surface glides across a second surface, so that the same point on one surface is continually in contact with new points on the second surface. A rolling surface usually occurs with a concurrent, oppositely directed slide. Spinning occurs during joint rotation when the longitudinal axis of long bones interacts at a right angle to the articular joint surface. An example is medial and lateral rotation of the shoulder joint when the humerus is abducted to 90 degrees.[16] Although arthrokinematic motion is vital for normal ROM, this textbook does not address the measurement or grading of this type of motion.

Osteokinematics

The quality and degree of motion actually observed in the bony lever arm is called osteokinematic motion. Osteokinematic motion is movement of the whole bone that results from rolling and sliding (arthrokinematics) between the articulating surfaces that compose the joint measured.[16] For example, when the arm is raised overhead, the bony lever arm (the humerus) moving overhead is the osteokinematic motion. However, for this motion to occur, the head of the humerus must roll and slide on the glenoid fossa (arthrokinematic motion). In most cases, osteokinematic motion is the actual motion that is measured; this type of motion is the focus of this textbook.

Osteokinematic descriptions of movement follow a generalized system that is based on definitions of planes of movement around axes of rotation. For effective discussion of planes of motion and axes of movement, a reference point is required, a point referred to as the anatomical position. This reference point (anatomical position) is defined as "standing erect with the head, toes, and palms of the hands facing forward and with the fingers extended."[17] When ROM at a joint is measured, the starting position is typically the anatomical position. Figs. 1.1–1.4 all show the model standing in the anatomical position.

Osteokinematic movement may be described as occurring in one of three imaginary planes of the body, arranged perpendicular to each other, with the axes of each plane intersecting the center of gravity of the body. These imaginary planes are referred to as the cardinal planes of the body. It should be emphasized that human motion is not limited to movement in these cardinal planes, but that this system of planes of movement around axes of rotation provides a simple method for describing ROM and muscle length.[16]

Sagittal Plane

The sagittal plane is a vertical plane that divides the body into right and left sides (Fig. 1.1). Photographically, this is a side view. Joint movement in the sagittal plane occurs around a line perpendicular to the plane that is referred to as the medial-lateral axis. The osteokinematic motions that occur in the sagittal plane are flexion and extension[16] (Fig. 1.2). *Gray's Anatomy* defines flexion as occurring "when the angle between two bones is decreased."[18] In other words, during flexion, two bony levers move around the joint axis so that the two levers approach each other. Flexion at the ankle is given a special term, with approximation of the plantar surface of the foot and the leg in the sagittal plane referred to as plantarflexion.

Extension is the opposite of flexion. It occurs when the two bony levers move away from each other, and it is defined as "the act of straightening a limb," which "occurs when the angle between the bones is increased."[18] Hyperextension is defined as extension beyond the normal anatomical ROM. Dorsiflexion of the foot at the ankle in the sagittal plane is the opposite of plantarflexion.

Frontal Plane

The frontal (or coronal) plane is a vertical plane that divides the body into anterior (ventral, or front) and posterior (dorsal, or back) halves (Fig. 1.3). Photographically, this is a front view. Joint movement in the frontal plane occurs around a line perpendicular to the plane that is referred to as the anterior–posterior axis. The osteokinematic motions that occur in the frontal plane consist of abduction, adduction, and lateral flexion of the spine[16] (see Fig. 1.2). Abduction is defined as occurring "when a limb is moved away from the midsagittal plane, or

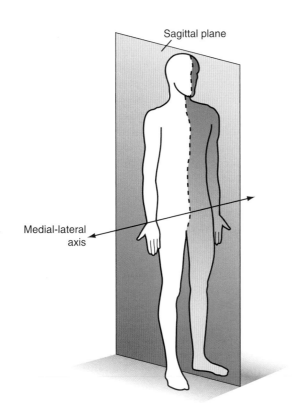

Fig. 1.1 Sagittal plane; note that model is standing in anatomical position.

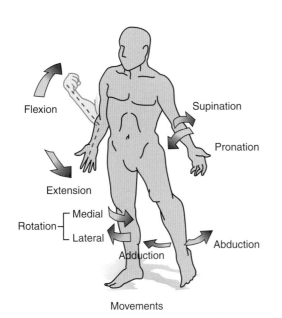

Fig. 1.2 Osteokinematic motions; note that model is standing in anatomical position.

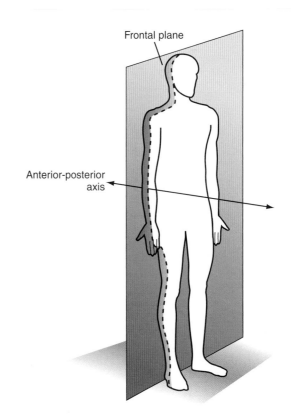

Fig. 1.3 Frontal plane; note that model is standing in anatomical position.

when the fingers or toes are moved away from the median longitudinal axis of the hand or foot."[18] Abduction of the wrist is often referred to as radial deviation. The median longitudinal axis of the hand is the third metacarpal, and for the foot, this axis is the second metatarsal. An exception to this definition is abduction that takes place at the carpometacarpal (CMC) joint of the thumb, which is defined as "that action by which the thumb is elevated anterior to the palm."[18] Therefore, abduction at the CMC joint actually takes place in the sagittal plane.

Adduction is the opposite of abduction and "occurs when a limb is moved toward or beyond the midsagittal plane, or when the fingers or toes are moved toward the median longitudinal axis of the hand or foot."[18] Adduction of the wrist is often referred to as ulnar deviation. At the CMC joint of the thumb, adduction is moving the thumb posteriorly toward the palm (sagittal plane movement).

Transverse Plane

The transverse plane is a horizontal plane that divides the body into upper (superior or cranial) and lower (inferior or caudal) halves (Fig. 1.4). Photographically, this is a view from the top of the head. Joint movement in the transverse plane occurs around a line perpendicular to the plane (a line running from cranial to caudal) that

is referred to as the longitudinal (or long) axis. The osteokinematic motions that occur in the transverse plane include medial rotation, lateral rotation, pronation, and supination[16] (see Fig. 1.2).

Rotation "is a form of movement in which a bone moves around a central axis without undergoing any other displacement."[18] Medial (or internal) rotation refers to rotation toward the body's midline, and lateral (or external) rotation refers to rotation away from the body's midline. Pronation is defined as medial rotation of the forearm that occurs when the segment is turned in a way that causes the palm of the hand to face posteriorly (in relation to anatomical position). Supination is lateral rotation of the forearm that occurs when the segment is turned so that the palm of the hand faces anteriorly (related to anatomical position).

Special Case: Oblique Axis at the Foot and Ankle

Motions that occur at the talocrural, subtalar, and midtarsal joints do not take place around the previously described cardinal axes. Explanations describe motion at these joints as occurring around oblique axes that lie at angles to all three cardinal planes.[16,19,20] These so-called triplanar axes run in an anteromedial-to-posterolateral direction and allow motion in all three planes simultaneously (Fig. 1.5). The motions thus produced have been termed pronation (a combination of dorsiflexion, abduction, and eversion) and supination (a combination of plantarflexion, adduction, and inversion).[16,19,20]

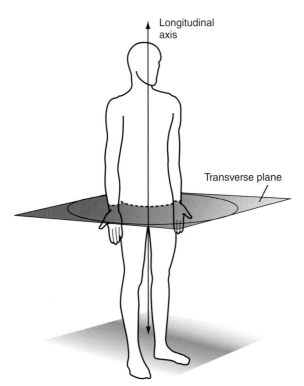

Fig. 1.4   Transverse plane; note the model is standing in anatomical position.

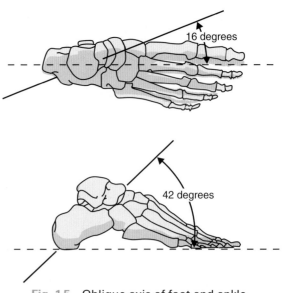

Fig. 1.5   Oblique axis of foot and ankle.

HISTORY OF INSTRUMENTS USED TO MEASURE RANGE OF MOTION AND MUSCLE LENGTH

Universal Goniometer

The inspiration for the universal goniometer appears to have been devices used to measure ROM that were developed in France early in the 1900s.[21] Initial publications describing the use of goniometers apparently are contained in the French medical literature, and descriptions of goniometric use did not appear in the American or British literature until the second decade of the 20th century.[22,23] With the advent of each of the World Wars came an increased interest in and use of the goniometer.[4] Although many variations and specialized designs of the goniometer have been developed over the years,[23–31] today's universal goniometer remains little changed from the instrument described in 1920 by Clark.[32] The universal goniometer has been used frequently for measurement of joints of the upper extremity,[33,34] lower extremity,[35–37] and spine.[11,38–40]

Measurement Techniques

Although reliable goniometers were available for measuring joint ROM early in the 20th century, examiners did not agree on correct procedures for performing goniometric measurements. In 1920, Clark[32] attempted to alleviate this problem by providing some standards for examining and recording joint ROM using the universal goniometer. He described a standardized starting position for measurement that was identical to the anatomical position currently used, with the exception of the position of the ankle, which Clark[32] described as fully plantarflexed. Additionally, Clark[32] provided values for normal ROM of joints of the spine and extremities, although the source and method of measurement on which these values were based were not stated. However, no description of techniques for patient positioning and goniometer placement was included in Clark's recommendations.[32] Numerous other individuals and groups have proposed methods for measuring and recording joint ROM using the universal goniometer.[2,4,27,28,41–44]

The most widely accepted techniques appear to be those published by the AAOS,[2,45] which were based on work done by Cave and Roberts.[42] These techniques, which are cited more often than the techniques of any other group in studies involving measurement of ROM, were developed by a committee of the AAOS in the early 1960s. The pamphlet containing the original techniques was sent to members of the AAOS in 1961, and subsequently to orthopedic societies in Australia, Great Britain, Canada, New Zealand, and South Africa. Following multiple revisions, the techniques were published in booklet form by the AAOS in 1965[2] and gained the approval of orthopedic societies in all countries to which the original pamphlet was sent. The most recent version of the AAOS techniques was published in 1994 by Greene and Heckman.[45]

Although the AAOS techniques[45] provide illustrations to aid in the measurement of ROM, specific landmarks for alignment of the goniometer during measurement are not provided. Instructions consist primarily of line drawings of a subject in what is termed the "zero starting position," with limits of normal ROM indicated in some but not all cases. These norms are based, for the most part, on studies of adults, with small sample sizes and no accompanying reliability data. The reliability of techniques used to measure joint motion is not discussed.

Efforts have been made and continue to be made to refine the techniques of goniometry used to measure ROM of the joints. Several groups of investigators have examined the reliability of currently used techniques (see Chapters 7, 10, and 15), and, in some cases, recommendations have been made as to preferred techniques for measuring a particular joint motion, based on reliability studies. However, the most reliable techniques for measuring motion at most joints in the body are yet to be determined, and much additional work remains to be done in this area.

Methods of Documentation

Currently, the most widely accepted method of recording ROM information is based on a system of measurement known as the 0–180 system. This system defines the anatomical position as the 0-degree starting position of all joints except the forearm, which is fully supinated. Thus neutral extension at each joint is recorded as 0 degrees, and as the joint flexes, motion progresses toward 180 degrees. The 0–180 system, which was first described in 1923 by Silver,[28] has been endorsed by the AAOS[2,45] and the American Medical Association (AMA)[46] as well as in the physical therapy literature.[4] Descriptions of how to document ROM using the 0–180 method are provided later in this chapter.

Other measurement systems have been used as a basis for recording ROM, but these methods are rarely used today. In 1920, Clark[32] described a system for recording ROM that was based on the idea that neutral extension at each joint is recorded as 180 degrees, movement toward flexion approaches 0 degrees, and movement toward extension past neutral also approaches 0 degrees.[32] According to this 180–0 system, the shoulder position that would be indicated as 145-degree flexion according to the 0–180 system would be designated as 35-degree flexion in the 180–0 system. A second system that has been used in the past but is not in common use today is based on a full 360-degree circle, in which the 0-degree position of each joint is full flexion, neutral extension is recorded as 180 degrees, and motions toward extension past neutral approach 360 degrees.[44,47]

Other Measurement Devices

Although the universal goniometer remains the most widely used instrument in the measurement of joint motion, limitations in the application of this device to some joints have led to the development of specialized devices for measuring joint motion. Most of these devices are designed to measure motion at only one joint, or at most a few joints, although some are capable of more widespread application. Examples of highly specialized devices for measuring joint ROM include Therabite (Atos Medical AB, Hörby, Sweden), for measuring motion of the temporomandibular joint, and specialized devices for measuring motion of the shoulder,[27,48–50] forearm,[25,36,51,52] wrist,[26,51–55] hand,[56] spine,[57–64] hip,[27,65–67] knee, and foot and ankle.[68–74]

Some of the more specialized devices used to measure joint ROM are adaptable for measuring motion at several joints. Examples of such devices include the inclinometer (also called the bubble goniometer, the pendulum goniometer, and the gravity goniometer), Smartphone, flexicurve, and the electrogoniometer, as well as various types of radiographic, photographic, and video recording equipment, including highly sophisticated motion analysis systems.[75,76] Of these specialized devices, the inclinometer is probably the most widely used because of its portability and relatively low cost.

Inclinometer

In the early 1930s, Fox and van Breeman[77] reported that they measured ROM using an instrument called the pendulum goniometer, which consisted of a circular scale, "to the center of which is attached a weighted pointer at one end so that it remains vertical while the scale rotates around it." Early studies reported use of a pendulum goniometer to measure ROM of the upper and lower extremities.[4,78,79]

In 1955, Leighton[80] introduced a similar instrument, referred to as the "Leighton flexometer," which consisted of a 360-degree dial and a weighted pointer mounted in a case. The dial and pointer operated freely, with movement controlled by gravity. The device was strapped to the segment being measured, the dial was locked at the extreme of motion, and the arc of movement was registered by the pointer. Leighton's study[80] was one of the first to use the device to attempt to provide normative data on ROM and muscle length in 30 joints of the extremities and trunk in a group of 16-year-old males. More recently, Ekstrand et al.[81] used a modification of the Leighton flexometer to measure ROM of the hip, knee, and ankle.

Schenker[82] introduced the fluid goniometer (bubble goniometer) in 1956. The fluid goniometer contains a 360-degree scale with a fluid-filled circular tube containing a small air bubble. Strapping the device to the segment being measured and moving the segment causes the scale to rotate while the bubble remains stationary, thereby indicating the ROM in the scale. The fluid goniometer has been used to measure the shoulder,[83] knee,[84] elbow,[85] ankle,[71] and cervical spine.[86]

Loebl[87] was the first to use the term inclinometer to describe the wide range of measuring instruments that rely on the principle of gravity. In general, these instruments are calibrated or referenced on the basis of gravity and contain a sensor to detect movement. Inclinometers may contain an electrolytic tilt sensor, mercury, gas bubble liquid, or a pendulum. Inclinometers may be labeled for how the instrument works (gravity goniometer, bubble goniometer, digital inclinometer), as well as for the manufacturer that developed the measurement tool (Myrin goniometer [LIC Reha Care, Sweden], Rangiometer [Maker, Inc.], CROM and BROM [Performance Attainment Associates, Lindstrom, Minn.]).[14,88–91]

Most recently, inclinometer applications have been developed for smartphones, and their use for measuring joint range of motion is becoming increasingly popular. These applications are easily accessible and are inexpensive in comparison to digital inclinometers. Several groups have investigated the reliability of applications such as the iGoniometer,[92] the Simple Goniometer,[93] DrGoniometer,[94–96] and other smartphone applications.[97] The majority of these studies reported high levels of reliability for the smartphone inclinometer applications.

Smartphone

Most recently, inclinometer applications have been developed for Smartphones, and their use for measuring joint ROM is becoming increasingly popular. By equipping Smartphones with sensors and software programs that allow the phone to act as an inclinometer, the device can be used to quantify ROM of several joints. In addition, adding the ROM application (app) to the Smartphone is inexpensive and those who use the Smartphone indicate using the device is easy to use and requires minimal training.[98]

As early as 2011, several groups have investigated the Smartphone application for the reliable measurement of the extremities.[92–97,99] More recently, as early as 2016, the Smartphone has been used to measure the reliability of movements in the lumbar spine[100], and as early as 2018, for measurement of the cervical spine.[101] The majority of these studies reported high levels of reliability for the Smartphone inclinometer applications.

Flexicurve

The Flexicurve or draughtsman's flexible curve is a bendable ruler made out of wire covered in plastic (Fig. 1.19). Use of this device to capture lumbar curvature angles and assess lumbar flexion and extension was first proposed in the late 1950s.[60] Since that time, the use of the Flexicurve has also been expanded to assessing thoracic range of motion in the sagittal place.[58,63] While the Flexicurve is easily accessible, inexpensive, and provides angles similar to radiographic assessments, it's use has been limited in the clinical setting because the curvature must be traced onto paper and the angles calculated after the assessment which results in increased time requirements for the clinician.

Electrogoniometer

Electrogoniometers, which convert angular motion of the joint into an electric signal, first appeared in the 1950s.[102] The basic principle of this type of goniometer has been modified to produce a variety of styles of electrogoniometer that are currently in use. Some electrogoniometers are designed to measure motion at a single joint, such as the elbow[103] or the hip,[104] whereas others are designed to measure motion at a variety of joints.[36,105–107] Designs range from fairly cumbersome devices to more compact, portable systems. Although many electrogoniometers are capable of measuring motion in several planes simultaneously, the cost of these devices and the skill required for application have resulted in electrogoniometers being used primarily in research applications.

Photography and Video Recording Equipment

Still photography has been used to measure joint ROM for decades[108,109] and remains in use today.[7,57,110] Although still photography has been reported to be more accurate than standard methods of goniometry in measuring ROM of the elbow joint[111] and shoulder,[7] measuring ROM with the use of still photography may require more time and effort than is practical in a normal clinical situation. More recently, photography has been incorporated into smartphone and computer applications for measuring joint range of motion[76,110,112–118] and is thus likely to become more commonly used as a method of assessing range of motion, particularly as telehealth becomes more commonplace.

Video recording techniques also have been used to measure joint ROM.[68,98,101–106] Although many motion analysis systems are commercially available, the examination of joint ROM using video recording equipment, such as motion analysis systems, remains generally confined to the research arena because of the prohibitive cost and decreased portability of such equipment.

Radiographic Equipment

The gold standard against which all other techniques of measuring joint ROM are compared is radiographic measurement of joint motion. Radiographic techniques have been used to study the amount and type of motion that is occurring at various joints, as well as to examine the validity of goniometry.[119–128] However, the routine use of radiographic techniques for the measurement of joint motion is not recommended because of the health risks associated with repeated exposure to radiation and because of the high costs involved.

MEASUREMENT METHODS OF MUSCLE LENGTH

A review of the literature indicates that muscle length is measured primarily through two methods. The first method uses traditional composite tests, which consist of measuring movement across more than one muscle or more than one joint.[129] Frequently used composite tests include the sit-and-reach test (Fig. 1.6), Apley's scratch test (Fig. 1.7), the shoulder-lift test (Fig. 1.8), and the

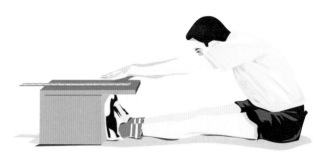

Fig. 1.6   Sit-and-reach test: Composite muscle length test for lower extremity.

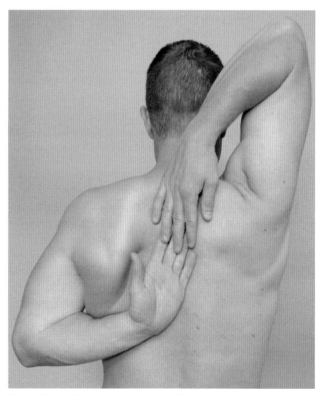

Fig. 1.7   Apley's scratch test: Composite muscle length test for upper extremity. (From Magee DJ. *Orthopedic Physical Assessment.* ed. 6, Philadelphia: Saunders; 2014.)

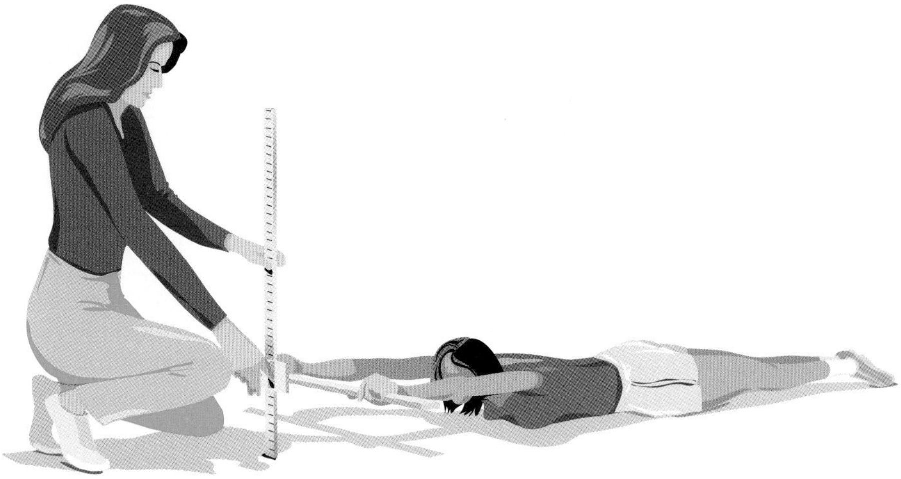

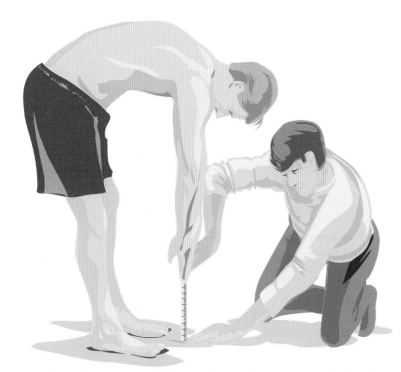

Fig. 1.8   Shoulder-lift test: Composite muscle length test for upper extremity.

Fig. 1.9   Fingertip-to-floor test: Composite muscle length test for lumbar spine.

fingertip-to-floor test (Fig. 1.9). The second method is direct measurement of muscle length, in which excursion between adjacent segments of one joint is involved.[130]

Composite Method

Examination of muscle length originated in the physical education literature and can be traced back to the 1940s, when a large number of veterans returned from World War II with limited movement capabilities.[131] Following World War II, great emphasis was placed on physical fitness testing, with flexibility being one component that was measured. In 1941, Cureton[132] published a "14-Item Motor Fitness Test" that contained four measures of flexibility. These flexibility measurements

consisted of composite tests involving flexion and extension of the entire length of the body.

Interest in the importance of examining muscle length was heightened when Kraus[133] reported that lack of flexibility and lack of strength were major factors in the high incidence of back pain in the United States. Testing by Kraus,[133] who used strength testing and composite flexibility tests, indicated that American children were minimally fit and significantly less fit than European children, leading to the further increase in the use of fitness testing.

In the 1970s, the American Alliance for Health, Physical Education, Recreation, and Dance (AAHPERD) built on the work of these fitness pioneers and developed language to describe health-related physical fitness. Health-related physical fitness consists of qualities that "have been formed to contribute to one's general health by reducing the risk of cardiovascular disease, problems associated with obesity, and chronic back problems."[131] Health-related fitness consists of five categories that should be examined: aerobic endurance, muscular endurance, muscular strength, body composition, and flexibility. The AAHPERD developed a standardized health-related fitness test battery, referred to as the "Physical Best Assessment Program." Included in this program is the composite flexibility test, referred to as the sit-and-reach test[131] (described later in this text in Chapter 8). The American College of Sports Medicine[134] recommends a flexibility examination consisting of the "sit-and-reach test or goniometer measurements of isolated joints" as part of a suggested comprehensive health fitness evaluation.

Direct Measurement

Not only is flexibility one of the five specific components of health-related physical fitness defined by the AAHPERD, but research indicates that flexibility is highly specific to each muscle involved. It does not exist as a general characteristic but is specific to the joint and muscle in question.[129,130,135] This research has shown that it is possible to have ideal muscle length in one muscle crossing a joint and poor flexibility at another joint in the body. Harris[129] suggested that "there is no evidence that flexibility exists as a single general characteristic of the human body. Thus no one composite test can give a satisfactory index of the flexibility characteristics of an individual."

Hubley-Kozey[130] suggested that composite tests do not provide accurate measurements of flexibility because these tests assess combinations of movements across several joints and involving several muscles. The author continues by indicating that composite tests are of questionable accuracy owing to difficulty in determining which muscles actually are being examined and to the complexity of the movement. In conclusion, Hubley-Kozey[130] suggests that composite tests "serve as gross approximations for flexibility, at best."

On the basis of information provided by authors such as Harris[129] and Hubley-Kozey,[130] composite measurement does not appear to be the appropriate measurement technique for muscle length. Therefore, in this text, every effort is made to provide only direct measurement of flexibility in describing techniques for upper (see Chapter 6) and lower (see Chapter 14) extremity muscle length testing.

PROCEDURES FOR MEASUREMENT

Instrumentation

Three primary types of instruments will be employed in this text in the measurement of ROM and muscle length. These instruments include linear forms of measurement such as the tape measure, the universal goniometer variations of this measurement tool and the inclinometer and its variations. A description of each type of instrument and activities that will help the student become familiar with each instrument are presented in this section.

Tape Measure

One of the simplest tools for measuring ROM and muscle length is the tape measure (or ruler) (Fig. 1.10). Tape measures can be made of cloth or metal. They can possess a centimeter scale, an inch scale, or both. The tape measure is easy to use and is readily available in most clinics. One negative aspect related to use of the tape measure is that most systems used for rating ROM and muscle length impairment rely on measurement in degrees.

Further Exploration: Familiarization With the Tape Measure

The activities in Box 1.1 are designed to help the reader become familiar with a simple tape measure and attain proficiency in manipulating the device and reading the scale correctly. Make sure several different styles of tape measures are examined and that the features of each are compared.

Universal Goniometer

The universal goniometer is produced in a variety of forms and sizes (Fig. 1.11). Most commonly, the universal goniometer is made of either metal or clear plastic and consists of a central protractor portion on which are mounted two arms of varying lengths. The protractor portion of the goniometer may be either a full circle or a half circle, both of which are calibrated in degrees. Although the scales of some goniometers are marked in gradations of 2.5 or 5 degrees, for optimal accuracy the scale should be marked at 1-degree intervals. Many goniometers are marked with a line that runs from the

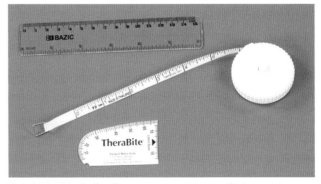

Fig. 1.10   Tools for linear measurement: Ruler, tape measure, Therabite.

BOX 1.1	FEATURES OF THE TAPE MEASURE

1. Is the tape measure cloth or metal?
2. Does the tape measure retract into a receptacle, or is the tape measure free-standing?
3. Is the tape measure marked in centimeters on one side and inches on the other?
4. Is the zero point at the very tip of the tape measure, or is the zero point indented *from the tip* of the tape measure?

5. For practice: From a sitting position, cross one leg over the other. Palpate the following anatomical landmarks on your own crossed leg: medial malleolus and tibial tubercle. Using a tape measure, measure the distance between these two landmarks three times, removing the tape measure between each measurement. Did you get the exact same measurement each time? Be honest!

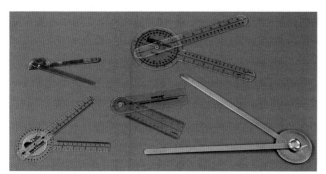

Fig. 1.11 Various styles and sizes of universal goniometers.

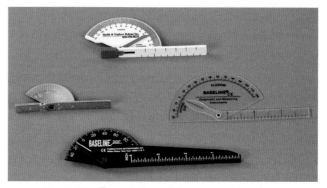

Fig. 1.13 Two styles of finger goniometers.

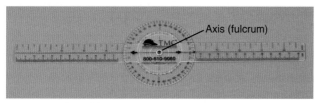

Fig. 1.12 Plastic universal goniometer with full circle protractor. Stationary arm, moving arm, and axis are labeled. Scale of goniometer is marked in increments of 1 degree.

0-degree to the 180-degree mark on the protractor. This line represents the base line of the protractor and serves as a reference point for measurements. One of the two arms of the goniometer is an extension of the protractor (the stationary arm); the other arm is riveted to, and can move independently of, the protractor (the moving arm) (Fig. 1.12). The central rivet, which attaches the moving arm to the protractor, functions as the axis, or fulcrum, of the goniometer.

If the goniometer is made of metal, the end of the moving arm that is in contact with the protractor (the proximal end) should be tapered to a point on its end or should contain a cutout so that the degree indicators on the protractor scale can be viewed (see Fig. 1.11). This concern is not relevant with a plastic goniometer because the scale can be viewed easily through the plastic arm. The arms of a plastic goniometer generally are calibrated along their length in centimeters or inches

for convenience when linear measurements are needed. Additionally, a prominent line extends from the axis of the goniometer down the midline of each arm, providing a landmark on the goniometer that can be maintained in line with bony landmarks on the body during goniometric measurements (see Fig. 1.12).

Many modifications of the basic design for the universal goniometer exist. One of the most common, and one that is used in this text, is the finger goniometer. The finger goniometer is basically a scaled-down version of the universal goniometer, with some modifications so that it fits the finger joints more precisely (Fig. 1.13). The finger goniometer is designed to be used over the dorsum of the finger joints, and many styles have broad arms that lie flat against the dorsal surfaces of the metacarpals or phalanges when the goniometer is in place. Some styles of finger goniometer are limited as to the amount of extension that can be measured because of a physical block built into the goniometer at 30 degrees of extension.

Further Exploration: Familiarization With the Universal Goniometer

The activities in Box 1.2 are designed to help the reader become familiar with a goniometer and attain proficiency in manipulating the device and reading the scale correctly. Select a goniometer and locate the parts and features listed in Box 1.2. Make sure several different styles of goniometers are examined and the features of each are compared.

BOX 1.2   FEATURES OF THE GONIOMETER

Protractor

1. Is the protractor a half or a full circle?
2. Is the protractor marked in 1-, 2.5-, or 5-degree increments?
3. Is a single scale marked on the protractor, or is more than one scale present?
4. If more than one scale is present, are the scales marked in the same direction, or in opposite directions?
5. Locate the base line of the protractor (line extending between the 0-degree mark and the 180-degree mark). The base line is the reference from which measurements are made.

Stationary Arm

1. Locate the line that extends from the protractor of the goniometer down the midline of the stationary arm. This is an extension of the protractor's base line.
2. Are markings visible along the length of the stationary arm? If so, are the markings in centimeters or in inches?

Moving Arm

1. If the goniometer is metal, is a tapered end or a cutout present on the proximal end of the moving arm?
2. If the goniometer is plastic, is the length of the arm marked in centimeters or in inches?

3. Locate the prominent line along the midline of the arm.
4. Holding the goniometer so that the stationary arm is in your right hand and the moving arm is in your left hand, move the moving arm to different positions and read the scale of the goniometer. The reading is taken at the point where the midline of the proximal end of the free arm crosses the scale of the protractor.
5. If more than one scale is present on the protractor, move the moving arm and read first one and then the other scale. Note how the scales relate to each other.
6. Position the moving arm at your estimation of various angles (e.g., 45 degrees, 60 degrees, 90 degrees), and then read the scale of the goniometer to see how close your estimate was. If more than one scale is present on the goniometer, note the reading from each scale, and examine the relationship between the two scales.
7. Reverse the goniometer so that the stationary arm is in your left hand and the moving arm is in your right hand. Repeat steps 4, 5, and 6 while holding the goniometer in this position. Note any differences in how the scale must be read.

Inclinometer

An inclinometer consists of a circular, fluid-filled disc with a bubble or weighted needle that indicates the number of degrees on the scale of a protractor. Most inclinometers are calibrated or referenced to gravity, analogous to the principle related to the level used by a carpenter. Because gravity does not change, using gravity as a reference point means that the starting position of the inclinometer can be identified and repeated consistently.

Inclinometers are available in two types: mechanical and electronic. The least expensive of the two is the mechanical, with most inclinometers today consisting of a protractor and a weighted gravity-pendulum indicator that remains in the vertical position to indicate degrees on the protractor (Fig. 1.14).

A second type of mechanical inclinometer is the fluid-level inclinometer, which indicates degrees by alignment of the meniscus (bubble) of the fluid to the protractor. Although it was used in the past, the fluid-level goniometer is not used frequently today; most clinicians who use inclinometers choose to use the weighted gravity-pendulum device.

Electronic inclinometers are more expensive, may have to be connected to computers with special

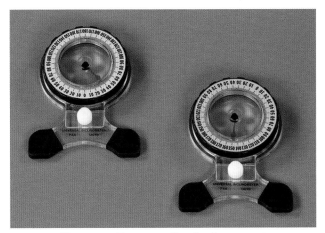

Fig. 1.14 Free-standing inclinometer.

programs and software, and frequently must be calibrated against some horizontal surface between measurements. Given that the mechanical inclinometer is easy to use, inexpensive, and fairly well represented in research in the literature, this textbook presents only information related to the mechanical inclinometer.

The inclinometer can be used in a variety of ways. The inclinometer can be held against the patient during

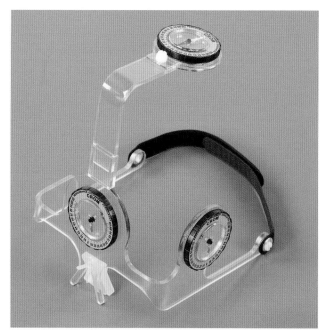

Fig. 1.15 Cervical range of motion (CROM) device; note inclinometers mounted vertically in frontal plane (to measure lateral flexion), vertically in the sagittal plane (to measure flexion and extension), and in the horizontal plane on top of the head (to measure rotation).

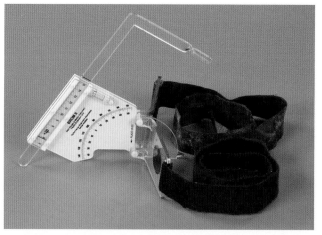

Fig. 1.16 Apparatus for measuring flexion and extension using back range of motion (BROM) device.

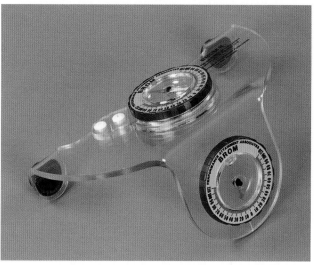

Fig. 1.17 Apparatus for measuring lateral flexion and rotation using back range of motion (BROM) device; note inclinometers mounted vertically (to measure lateral flexion) and horizontally (to measure rotation).

a variety of movements or an inclinometer application can be added to the Smartphone. Additionally, the inclinometer can be mounted to a plastic frame including the cervical range of motion (CROM) device and the back range of motion (BROM) device (both manufactured by Performance Attainment Associates, Lindstrom, Minn.).

CROM

The CROM device consists of a plastic frame that is placed over the patient's head, aligned on the bridge of the nose and on the ears, and secured to the back of the head with straps made of Velcro (Fig. 1.15). Cervical flexion and extension are measured by an inclinometer mounted on the side of the headpiece. An inclinometer mounted on the front of the headpiece is used to measure lateral flexion. Both inclinometers work by force of gravity. To measure cervical rotation, a compass inclinometer is attached to the top of the headpiece in the transverse plane and operated in conjunction with a magnetic yoke. The yoke consists of two padded bars, mounted on the shoulders, that contain magnetic poles.

BROM

The BROM device consists of two plastic frames that are secured to the lumbar spine of the patient by two elastic straps. One frame consists of an L-shaped slide arm that is free to move within a notch of the fixed base unit during flexion and extension; ROM is read from a protractor scale (Fig. 1.16). The second frame has two measurement devices attached to it (Fig. 1.17).

One attachment is a vertically mounted gravity-dependent inclinometer, which measures lateral flexion. The second attachment is a horizontally mounted compass to measure rotation. During measurement of trunk rotation, the device requires a magnetic yoke to be secured to the pelvis.

Further Exploration: Familiarization With the Inclinometer

The activities in Box 1.3 are designed to help the reader become familiar with an inclinometer and attain proficiency in manipulating the device and reading the scale correctly. Make sure several different styles of inclinometers are examined and the features of each are compared. Compare various free-standing inclinometers vs the inclinometers mounted on the CROM and the BROM.

BOX 1.3   FEATURES OF THE INCLINOMETER

1. Is the free-standing inclinometer fixed to a base that is a straight-edge, or is it fixed to a two-point contact base? Can you speculate on the advantage of one base over the other?
2. Is the protractor on the inclinometer immobile, or does it rotate, allowing you to set the zero point?
3. Is the scale of the protractor marked in 1-, 2.5-, or 5-degree increments?
4. Does the scale of the protractor have a 0- to 360-degree scale running in a full circle, or does it have a 0- to 180-degree scale running in the clockwise direction and another 0- to 180-degree scale running in the counterclockwise direction?
5. Is the scale of the protractor indicated by a weighted pointer, by a floating bubble, or by both?

6. Holding the inclinometer vertically in your hand with 0 degrees at the bottom and 180 degrees at the top, tip the inclinometer in a clockwise direction. What happens to the indicator (weighted pointer or bubble)? Read the scale of the inclinometer. Try turning the inclinometer in a counterclockwise direction. What happens? Read the scale of the inclinometer.
7. Place the inclinometer horizontally on a flat surface such as a table. Turn the inclinometer in a clockwise direction. What happens to the indicator (weighted pointer or bubble)? Keeping the inclinometer on the flat surface, turn the inclinometer in a counterclockwise direction. What happens?

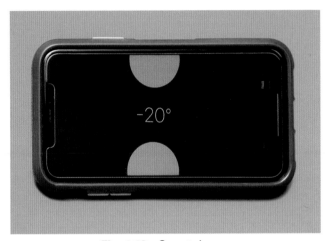

Fig. 1.18   Smartphone.

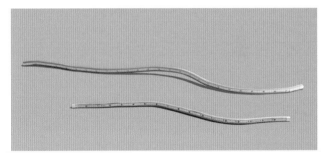

Fig. 1.19   Two sizes of the flexicurve—one for adults and one for children.

Smartphone

An available (most people own a Smartphone) and easy to use device for measuring ROM is the Smartphone. The use of Smartphone devices will vary between each phone type (Fig. 1.18). Studies attaching the Smartphone to the helmet or goggles were not included. The attempt was to present the use of the Smartphone without any additional equipment or attachments as much as possible.

Flexicurve

Originally used by craftsmen and woodworkers to draw a curve, because the flexicurve is adjustable and able and will maintain its shape without external support, the tool is frequently used for measuring the flexion and extension of the spine (Fig. 1.19). As early as 1959, Israel[60] described the use of the Flexicurve technique for measuring spinal curves.

TECHNIQUES FOR MEASURING RANGE OF MOTION AND MUSCLE LENGTH

Regardless of the instrument that is used, the individual who uses the measurement tool must become skilled in its use. Once a level of comfort in handling and reading a measurement device has been attained, the user must become skillful in using the instrument to measure joint ROM and muscle length. Skill in the use of any measurement device comes only after much repeated practice. Practice in using an instrument should continue until the user has established a high level of intrarater reliability (more detailed information on reliability is presented in Chapter 2), that is, repeated measurements taken by the same person on the same subject should be identical or should fall within a small margin of error. Because techniques of measurement differ from joint to joint, each examiner should practice the techniques until all measurements can be performed in a reliable manner.

Many of the steps involved in measuring joint ROM and muscle length are the same, no matter which joint is being measured. These steps provide the basic framework for measurement and are outlined in Box 1.4 and expounded in this section. How the basic steps are

BOX 1.4	PROCEDURES FOR MEASURING JOINT RANGE OF MOTION

1. Determine the type of measurement to be performed (AROM or PROM).
2. Explain the purpose of the procedure to the patient.
3. Position the patient in the preferred patient position for the measurement.
4. Stabilize the proximal joint segment.
5. Instruct the patient in the specific motion that will be measured while moving the patient's distant joint segment passively through the ROM. Determine the end-feel at the end of the PROM.
6. Return the patient's distal joint segment to the starting position.
7. Palpate bony landmarks for measurement device alignment.
8. Align the measurement device with the appropriate bony landmarks.
9. Read the scale of the measurement device and note the reading.
10. Have the patient move actively, or move the patient passively, through the available ROM.
11. Repalpate the bony landmarks and readjust the alignment of the measurement device as necessary.
12. Read the scale of the measurement device and note the reading.
13. Record the patient's ROM. The record should include, at a minimum,
    a. Patient's name and identifying information
    b. Date measurement was taken
    c. Identification of person taking measurement
    d. Type of motion measured (AROM or PROM) and device used
    e. Any alteration from preferred patient position
    f. Readings taken from measurement device at beginning and end of ROM

AROM, Active range of motion; *PROM*, passive range of motion; *ROM*, range of motion.

applied at each joint, such as which landmarks are used for alignment of the instrument or what patient positioning is used, differs from joint to joint. The use of standardized techniques is critical for accurate measurement of joint ROM and muscle length. Without standardized techniques, ROM and muscle length measurements are likely to be unreliable and, thus, of questionable validity.[5,136,137] Specific techniques for measuring ROM at each joint are provided in Chapters 3 through 5 for the upper extremity, Chapters 8 through 9 for the spine and the temporomandibular joint, and Chapters 11 and 13 for the lower extremity. Specific techniques for measuring muscle length are presented in Chapters 6 and 14.

Preparation for Measurement

Before a patient's ROM or muscle length is measured, the examiner should determine whether measurement of active or passive ROM is most appropriate. Both active ROM (AROM), which occurs when a patient moves a joint actively through its available ROM, and passive ROM (PROM), which occurs when the examiner moves the patient's joint through the available ROM, may be used to examine the amount of motion available at a given joint. Although in many cases the examiner will be interested in how much AROM the patient possesses, sometimes PROM may be the motion of interest. For example, a patient with supraspinatus tendinitis may be unwilling to abduct the shoulder more than 75 degrees because of pain, so AROM would be limited to 0–75 degrees. To ensure that the patient is not developing

adhesive capsulitis of the shoulder, the examiner also may wish to measure the amount of passive shoulder abduction that is present. In some instances, the examiner has no choice but to measure PROM because the patient is unable or unwilling to perform AROM. Such cases include measuring ROM in infants, in young children, and in any patient who lacks the motor control to perform active movement at the joint in question. In its *Guides to the Evaluation of Permanent Impairment*,[41] the AMA recommends the measurement and comparison of both AROM and PROM in the evaluation process.

Active and passive ROM may differ widely for a given joint in an individual, particularly if muscle weakness, pain, or related pathologies are present. Studies that have compared AROM and PROM in subjects without pathology have reported that PROM is greater than AROM for most joints.[66,138–141] In many cases, the increase in PROM over AROM is significant. However, PROM is not greater than AROM at all joints. For example, measurements of ankle dorsiflexion ROM tend to be higher when the patient actively dorsiflexes the ankle than when passive motion alone is measured. Because of the variability that exists between AROM and PROM even in pathology-free individuals, care should be taken to document the type of ROM (AROM or PROM) measured in each patient.

Instructing the Patient

Patients should be provided with thorough instructions before any examination technique, including taking ROM and muscle length measurements, is performed.

Measurement of ROM and muscle length, particularly active motion, requires the full cooperation of the patient. As the patient's understanding of the procedure increases, so does the likelihood that the patient will provide his or her best effort during the process.

Before beginning the procedure, describe to the patient exactly what will be taking place and why the measurement must be performed. Show the patient the measurement tool, and explain in laypersons' terms its purpose and how it will be used. Instruct the patient in the position he or she is to assume, again using laypersons' terms and avoiding terms such as supine or prone. Detailed explanations of every step of the procedure should not be provided initially because they will only confuse the patient. A brief, general explanation is best at this point, and additional explanations may be given once the procedure is in progress. An example of initial patient instructions is as follows:

"Ms. Haynes, I need to measure how much you can move your knee. This information will tell me how much progress you are making since your surgery and help me estimate how soon you will be able to be discharged from treatment. I am going to use this instrument, called a goniometer, to measure your movement. I will need you to lie on this table on your back so that I can perform the measurement."

Positioning the Patient: Measuring Joint Range of Motion

Proper positioning of the patient during measurement is critical to accurate measurement. The choice of a preferred patient position for measurement of motion at each joint is based on several criteria. For a position to be considered optimal, all criteria should be met. Although this is not an exhaustive list, the major criteria used in selecting a preferred patient position for measurement of ROM are as follows:

1. **The joint should be placed in the zero starting position.** The zero starting position for almost all joints is the anatomical position of that joint (described previously). The only joint that is not placed in the anatomical position to start is the forearm, which is placed midway between full pronation and full supination (the neutral position of the forearm). When a joint is positioned in the zero starting position, the joint is considered to be at 0-degree ROM.
2. **The joint should be positioned such that the proximal segment of the joint is stabilized most easily.** This positioning allows maximal isolation of the intended motion.
3. **The bony landmarks to be used to align the measurement tool should be palpable and in proper alignment.** In some cases, this necessitates placing more proximal joints out of anatomical position. For example, when flexion of the wrist is measured, the shoulder is abducted to 90 degrees, the elbow flexed

to 90 degrees, and the forearm pronated for placement of the bony landmarks for goniometric alignment in a linear relationship.

4. **The joint to be measured should be free to move through its complete available ROM.** Motion should not be blocked by external objects, such as the examining table, or by internal forces, such as muscle tightness. An example of the latter is positioning the patient in the prone position to measure knee flexion. Because tension in the rectus femoris muscle can limit knee flexion when the hip is extended (patient positioned prone), a better position for this measurement is with the patient supine. Such a position allows free flexion of the hip during knee flexion, thus eliminating potential restriction of knee flexion by rectus femoris tightness.
5. **The patient must be able to assume the position.** In some cases, this criterion cannot be met, and an alternative position must be used. In any instance in which an alternative position is used, the examiner should design the position so that it adheres as closely as possible to the previous four criteria.

The amount of ROM measured may vary significantly, depending on the position in which the patient is placed during the measurement. Two studies have demonstrated a statistically significant difference in the ROM obtained from a joint when the position in which the joint was measured was altered. A significantly higher amount of shoulder abduction was obtained when active or passive shoulder abduction was measured with the patient in the supine, compared with the sitting, position.[142] Similarly, when hip lateral rotation was measured with the patient in both seated and prone positions, significantly more motion was obtained in the prone position.[143] Preferred patient positions are provided for each joint measurement technique described in this text. Whenever a position other than the preferred position is used, careful documentation should be made of the exact position chosen. In this way, techniques used in ROM measurements can be duplicated by others, and more accurate comparisons of measurements taken on separate occasions or by different examiners can be made.

Further Exploration: Preferred Patient Position

The following activities are designed to help the student evaluate and design preferred patient positions for measurement of ROM:

1. Select from the text a technique for the measurement of joint ROM (e.g., shoulder lateral rotation). Apply the criteria listed to the preferred patient position described. How well does the position meet the criteria listed? Repeat this exercise for the techniques of several other motions.
2. Analyze the following scenarios, devising a preferred patient position in each situation. Once your preferred position is complete, apply the criteria

listed. How well does your devised position meet the criteria? Make modifications to your devised position as needed, so that it adheres more closely to the criteria.

A. Mr. Barnes suffered a spinal cord injury 2 years previously, currently has a decubitus ulcer on his sacrum, and is unable to sit or lie supine. How would you alter the preferred patient position for Mr. Barnes to perform the following measurements? (Refer to the techniques in Chapters 3–5 and Chapter 11 for information on the standard method for performing each measurement.)

    i. Shoulder flexion
    ii. Wrist extension
    iii. Forearm pronation
    iv. Hip abduction
    v. Hip lateral rotation

B. Mrs. Kelley is 8 months pregnant and is unable to lie on her right side because of pressure placed by the baby on her inferior vena cava. She is also unable to lie prone. How would you alter the preferred patient position for Mrs. Kelley in order to perform the following measurements? (Refer to the techniques in Chapters 3 and 11 for information on the standard method for performing each measurement.)

    i. Hip extension (consider both right and left sides)
    ii. Shoulder extension (consider both right and left sides)

Positioning the Patient: Measuring Muscle Length

Please note that the preparation for measurement and instructions to the patient are similar, whether one is measuring ROM or is examining muscle length. However, positioning of the patient differs for the two types of measurement. When muscle length is examined, the following guidelines for patient positioning should be followed:

1. **The muscle to be measured should be placed in the fully elongated position.** In measurement of muscle length, the examiner is most concerned about the final, elongated position of the muscle and is not as concerned about measurement from the zero starting position (as would be appropriate for measurement of joint ROM). In some instances, movement is initiated from the zero position to demonstrate to the patient the motion desired, but in most cases, the muscle is placed in the elongated position and the measurement is taken.

2. **As much as possible, the muscle should be isolated across one, or possibly two, joints.** Composite tests that measure movement across three or more joints should not be used. (Refer to the earlier section of this chapter on the history of muscle length testing.)

3. **The bony landmarks to be used to align the measurement tool should be palpable and in proper alignment.** In some cases, this necessitates placing more proximal joints out of anatomical position. For example, when muscle length of the extensor digitorum muscle is measured, the shoulder is abducted to 70–90 degrees, the forearm pronated, and the fingers flexed, to place the bony landmarks for goniometric alignment in a linear relationship.

4. **Motion should not be blocked by external objects such as the support surface or a pillow.**

5. **The patient must be able to assume the position.** In some cases, this criterion cannot be met, and an alternative position must be used. In any instance in which an alternative position is used, the examiner should design the position so that it adheres as closely as possible to the previous four criteria.

Stabilization

Accurate measurement of joint ROM and muscle length requires stabilization of the proximal bony segment of the joint being measured. Failure to provide adequate stabilization will prevent isolation of the intended motion and may allow the patient to substitute motion at another joint for the motion requested. For example, a patient who lacks forearm pronation may abduct and medially rotate the shoulder in an attempt to substitute for the lack of forearm motion. If the examiner fails to stabilize the humerus in an adducted position during measurement of forearm pronation, the patient may perform the substitute motion, and the measurement of forearm pronation would then be inflated falsely. Three separate studies[6,144,145] demonstrated that measurements of shoulder internal rotation with the scapula stabilized yielded significantly different results than when the motion was measured without scapular stabilization.

Lack of sufficient stabilization also may affect the reliability of measurements of ROM or muscle length testing. Ekstrand et al.[81] performed ROM and muscle length testing of selected lower extremity joints in adult male subjects using a modified goniometer and a Leighton flexometer. Standardized testing procedures were employed, and the motions were repeated on two occasions, 2 months apart. On the first occasion, subjects were positioned on a soft padded surface; on the second occasion, measurements were made with the subject positioned on a hard wooden board. Results demonstrated significantly lower intratester variability for both ROM and muscle length measurements when patients were measured while positioned on a hard surface compared with a soft surface.

The ease with which the proximal joint segment is stabilized varies from joint to joint. In some instances, the patient's weight assists in stabilizing the proximal joint segment, but the examiner should always stabilize the proximal segment manually as well. In general, smaller segments, such as the forearm, are easier to stabilize than are larger segments, such as the pelvis. Some motions (e.g., shoulder flexion, hip flexion) cannot be isolated completely[146] and in those cases, the examiner must realize that the motion measured is, at a minimum, a combination of motion at the joint being measured and motion at the next most proximal articulation.

Directions and illustrations for stabilization are provided for each ROM and muscle length testing technique found in this text. The examiner should be very careful to provide the stabilization indicated when performing each measurement technique. Failure to do so could result in inaccurate and unreliable results.

Estimating Range of Motion and Determining End-Feel

Once the patient has been positioned and the proximal joint segment stabilized, the examiner should move the joint passively through the available ROM. This maneuver accomplishes a variety of objectives. First, by movement through the ROM to be measured, the patient is made aware of the exact movement to be performed and can cooperate more fully and accurately with the procedure. Second, a rough estimation of the patient's available ROM can be made by the examiner. Estimating the patient's ROM provides the examiner with a self-check against gross errors in reading the goniometer. For example, if the examiner estimates that the patient has 125 degrees of elbow flexion but reads 55 degrees on the goniometer, then an error in measurement obviously has been made (in this case, the wrong scale on the goniometer has been read). Estimating the patient's ROM before measurement is performed is a particularly valuable technique for the novice examiner because novices are prone to error in reading the measurement device. Finally, moving the patient passively through the ROM allows the examiner to note any limitations to full ROM, such as those caused by pain, muscle tightness, or other reasons.

Clues to the cause of ROM limitations may be obtained by examining the quality of resistance at the end of ROM. Each joint has a characteristic feel to the resistance encountered at the end of normal ROM. Typical end-feels encountered at the end of normal ROM include bony, capsular, muscular, and soft-tissue end-feels.[147,148] These end-feels are described in the activities that follow this section and are defined for each joint in the introductory material for Chapters 3–5 and 11–13. Chapters 6 and 14 describe measurement of muscle length of the upper and lower extremities, respectively. Given that the muscles are placed in the fully elongated position for these measurements, the end-feel is muscular.

Other end-feels are encountered only in situations of joint pathology. These include empty, muscle spasm, and springy block end-feels. Although explanations of these end-feels are beyond the scope of this text, definitions can be found in any basic musculoskeletal examination text.[148,149] Deviation from the expected end-feel when passive ROM is performed at a joint should alert the examiner that further examination of the joint is warranted.

Further Exploration: Identifying End-Feels

Bony End-Feel: Elbow Extension. The bony end-feel occurs when approximation of two bones stops the ROM at a joint. The quality of the resistance felt is very hard and abrupt, and further motion is impossible.
1. Position the subject in the supine or sitting position.
2. Grasp the posterior aspect of the subject's distal humerus in one hand and the anterior aspect of the distal forearm in the other hand.
3. Flex the subject's elbow slightly, then gently return it to the fully extended position, repeating this maneuver several times.
4. While performing the passive movement described in step 3, pay close attention to the feel of the resistance at the point of full elbow extension. The resistance should feel hard and abrupt—a bony end-feel.

Capsular End-Feel: Hip Medial Rotation. The capsular end-feel occurs when the joint capsule and the surrounding noncontractile tissues limit the ROM at a joint. The quality of the resistance felt is firm but not hard. There is a very slight "give" to the movement, as would be felt when a piece of leather is stretched.
1. Position the subject in the sitting position.
2. Place one hand on the subject's knee and the other hand over the subject's medial malleolus.
3. Passively rotate the subject's hip medially by moving the subject's leg laterally (keeping the knee stationary) until firm resistance is felt. From this point, oscillate the subject's leg medially and laterally very slightly without allowing the knee to move.
4. While performing the passive movement described in step 3, pay close attention to the feel of the resistance at the point of full medial rotation of the hip. The resistance should feel firm and leathery—a capsular end-feel.

Muscular End-Feel: Knee Extension With Hip Flexion. The muscular end-feel occurs when muscular tension limits the ROM at a joint. The quality of the resistance felt is firm, although not as firm as with the capsular end-feel, and somewhat springy.
1. Position the subject in the supine position.
2. Place one hand on the anterior aspect of the subject's knee and the other hand on the posterior aspect of the subject's foot, cupping the subject's heel.
3. Flex the subject's hip completely. Then slowly extend the subject's knee until resistance is felt. From this point, gently oscillate the leg into full extension and then into slight flexion.

4. While performing the passive movement described in step 3, pay close attention to the feel of the resistance at the end point of knee extension. The resistance should feel firm and slightly springy—a muscular end-feel.

   Soft-Tissue End-Feel: Knee Flexion
1. Position the subject in the supine position.
2. Place one hand on the anterior aspect of the subject's knee, and grasp the subject's ankle with the other hand.
3. Flex the subject's knee completely (slight hip flexion is allowed during this procedure, but only enough to allow full flexion of the knee) until the subject's calf is stopped by his or her posterior thigh. From this point, oscillate the leg into, and slightly out of, full knee flexion.
4. While performing the passive movement described in step 3, pay close attention to the feel of the resistance at the end point of knee flexion. The resistance, which is caused by compression of the soft tissue of the calf and posterior thigh, should feel mushy or soft—a soft-tissue end-feel.

Palpating Bony Landmarks and Aligning the Measurement Device

Accurate palpation of landmarks and precise alignment of the measurement device with those landmarks are critical to correct measurement of joint ROM and muscle length. Bony landmarks are used for alignment of the measurement device whenever possible because bony structures are more stable and are less subject to change in position caused by factors such as edema or muscle atrophy.

Aligning the Tape Measure

With the tape measure, specific landmarks are established before measurement. These landmarks may be only anatomical, such as the distance between the tip of the chin and the sternal notch. Sometimes an anatomical landmark may be combined with the support surface on which the subject is sitting or lying, such as the perpendicular distance between the tip of the olecranon fossa and the support surface in a subject lying supine with hands clasped behind the head.

Aligning the Goniometer

Three landmarks, as a minimum, are used to align the goniometer. Two landmarks are used to align the arms of the goniometer—one landmark for the stationary arm and one for the moving arm. The stationary arm is generally aligned with the midline of the stationary segment of the joint, while the moving arm is aligned with the midline of the moving segment of the joint. The bony landmarks provided for alignment of the goniometer arms are generally target points on the bones of the stationary and moving joint segments. Although the arms of the goniometer may not actually cross these

bony targets once the instrument is aligned, the examiner should sight the midline of each goniometer arm so that it points directly at the corresponding bony target.

The third bony landmark provides a point for alignment of the fulcrum of the goniometer. The fulcrum of the goniometer is placed over a point that is near the axis of rotation of the joint. However, because the axis of rotation for most joints is not stationary but moves during motion of the joint, the goniometer's fulcrum often will not remain aligned over its corresponding bony landmark throughout the ROM. Because the joint axis is not stationary, **the landmark for alignment of the fulcrum of the goniometer is the least important of the three landmarks for goniometer alignment**. To ensure accurate alignment, priority should be given to alignment of the stationary and moving arms of the goniometer. Once the examiner is satisfied that the goniometer is aligned correctly, a reading should be taken from the scale of the goniometer at the beginning of the ROM (see "Determining and Recording the Range of Motion with the Goniometer," discussed subsequently).

Aligning the Inclinometer

Only one bony landmark per measurement is needed for alignment of the standard inclinometer; therefore, the measurement device is not subject to error in estimating multiple anatomical landmarks for one measurement. An inclinometer with a two-point contact base is preferred because this type of base best maintains contact over convex surfaces of the body. Because of its ease of use, the inclinometer has gained favor for measurement of the spine.

The inclinometer has not been used as frequently as the goniometer to measure the extremities because of difficulties involved in stabilizing the instrument along the different anatomical contours of the body, especially on smaller joints. Additionally, any attempt to strap the inclinometer to the extremity introduces problems of soft-tissue variability, edema, and slippage.

Aligning the Smartphone

Generally, the Smartphone will be located similarly to the inclinometer. Once the bony landmark is located, the "level utility" in the measurement application for the Smartphone is activated. After that activation, the examiner holds the smartphone against the patient until the end ROM is achieved. At that end point, the examiner waits until the degrees of measurement maintain a steady number on the phone application.

Determining and Recording the Range of Motion With the Goniometer

Determination of the patient's ROM is accomplished by comparing the reading taken from the goniometer with the patient in the starting position vs a second reading that is taken once the patient has completed the AROM or PROM. Before this second reading is taken, the goniometer alignment must be rechecked. Bony landmarks must be palpated again at the end of the patient's ROM, and the arms and the fulcrum of the goniometer readjusted as necessary, so that alignment is once again accurate. Failure to confirm accurate goniometer alignment before the instrument is read may result in gross errors in ROM measurement.

When the scale of the goniometer is read, the reading is taken at the point where the midline of the end of the moving arm crosses the scale of the protractor portion of the instrument. Many goniometers are imprinted with more than one scale, and these scales may encircle the protractor portion of the instrument in opposing directions. The examiner must pay careful attention to make sure that the correct scale is being read (see points 4, 5, 6, and 7 under "Moving Arm" in Box 1.2).

After readings have been taken from the goniometer at the beginning and at the end of the patient's movement, the examiner is ready to document the ROM. Several items must be noted in the record of the patient's ROM. These items include the following:

- Patient's name and identifying information
- Date measurement was taken
- Identification of person taking measurement
- Type of motion measured (AROM or PROM)
- Any alteration in patient's position (from preferred patient position) during measurement
- Beginning and ending readings from the goniometer for each motion measured

This information provides sufficient details should any question arise regarding the patient's ROM at a particular joint. Additionally, information regarding the type of motion measured and any alterations in normal procedure allow other examiners to reproduce the technique should someone other than the original examiner need to measure the patient's ROM.

When readings taken from the goniometer are recorded, both the beginning and ending readings should be reported, even if the beginning reading is 0 degrees. The beginning reading tells anyone who needs information from the patient's record where the ROM begins. Two patients may both have 110 degrees of elbow flexion, but the motion in Patient A may start at 0 degrees and progress to 110 degrees of flexion, whereas the motion in Patient B may start at 25 degrees of flexion and progress to 135 degrees. Recording either patient's motion as 110 degrees would not allow anyone examining either patient's record to know where the motion began and where it ended. To avoid confusion on the part of those reading the patient's record, the use of a single number to record the ROM should be avoided (except in certain cases—see "Single Motion Recording Technique," discussed later).

Occasionally, the goniometer will not read 0 degrees at the beginning of the ROM, even when the patient is at the 0-degree starting position for that motion. An example of this phenomenon occurs during the measurement of hip abduction and adduction. At the beginning of these two motions, the alignment of the goniometer is such that the stationary and moving arms of the instrument make a 90-degree angle with each other. Thus at the 0-degree starting position for hip abduction and adduction, the scale of the goniometer reads 90 degrees. This reading is taken as equivalent to 0 degrees, and the reading from the goniometer at the end of the ROM is added to or subtracted from 90 degrees to obtain the ROM. For example, in a patient with 20 degrees of hip adduction, the goniometer would read 90 degrees at the beginning of the ROM and 110 degrees at the end of the ROM. Subtract: 110–90=20. Therefore, the patient's hip adduction ROM is recorded as 0- to 20-degree hip adduction.

Several methods of recording ROM are available. Two methods are presented here, and the reader may choose which method to use. However, in a clinical situation in which multiple individuals are measuring and recording ROM, a standardized method of recording these measurements should be agreed on by all individuals involved. Otherwise, a great deal of confusion is likely to result among those using the patient record as the basis for decision making.

Single Motion Recording Technique

One method of recording joint ROM involves separately documenting the range of each motion at each joint. Thus when ROM at the shoulder is recorded, shoulder flexion is documented separately from shoulder extension, and shoulder lateral rotation is documented separately from shoulder medial rotation. Both beginning and ending readings from the goniometer are recorded for each motion measured. An example of single motion recording of ROM is provided in Fig. 1.20.

Mrs. Stephenson is able to actively move her right shoulder from the 0-degree starting position to 165 degrees in the direction of shoulder flexion and to 35 degrees in the direction of shoulder extension. Her ROM would be documented as in Fig. 1.20.

For some motions, the patient may not be able to attain the 0-degree starting position for the movement. In such cases, the patient is limited in one motion and completely lacks the opposing motion. For example, suppose Mrs. Stephenson is unable to attain the 0-degree starting position for elbow extension but instead lacks 15 degrees of full extension (in other words, her elbow is in 15-degree flexion as she begins the flexion movement). Suppose further that she is able to move from this starting position to 140 degrees of elbow flexion. Mrs. Stephenson's elbow flexion is documented as shown in the chart in Fig. 1.21, since she began the motion at 15 degrees and ended it at 140 degrees. In the case of elbow extension, Mrs. Stephenson has no range of motion because she is unable to attain the 0-degree starting position for the movement.

JOINT RANGE OF MOTION

Patient: _Nicole Stephenson_
Age: _68_

Indicate:
AROM _X_
PROM _____

LEFT   RIGHT

		Date/Examiner's Initials	01/03/09 NBR		
		Shoulder			
		Flexion	0°–165°		
		Extension	0°–35°		
		Abduction			
		Adduction			
		Medial Rotation			
		Lateral Rotation			

Fig. 1.20   JOINT ROM TABLE.

JOINT RANGE OF MOTION

Patient: _Nicole Stephenson_
Age: _68_

Indicate:
AROM _X_
PROM _____

LEFT   RIGHT

		Date/Examiner's Initials	01/03/09 NBR		
		Elbow/Forearm			
		Flexion	15°–140°		
		Extension	–15°		
		Pronation			
		Supination			

Fig. 1.21

Therefore, elbow extension for Mrs. Stephenson is documented as −15 degrees, as shown in Fig. 1.21, indicating that she lacks 15 degrees of attaining the 0-degree starting position for elbow extension. Only in cases in which the patient has no motion in a given direction is a single number used to document ROM.

Now suppose that Mrs. Stephenson's knee ROM is measured, and the examiner discovers that Mrs. Stephenson is able to attain the 0-degree starting position for knee extension. She also can actively move her knee 10 degrees in the direction of extension and 145 degrees in the direction of flexion. In this case, Mrs. Stephenson's knee extension is recorded as 0- to 10-degree knee hyperextension. When the normal amount of extension at a joint is 0 degrees, motion into extension beyond 0 degrees is documented as hyperextension. Use of the term hyperextension reflects that the motion is in excess of the normal amount of extension expected at that joint. In this case, knee flexion is documented as 0- to 145-degree flexion, since the

JOINT RANGE OF MOTION

Patient: _Elizabeth Atchley_
Age: _20_
Indicate:
    AROM _____
    PROM _____

LEFT				RIGHT	
		Date/Examiner's Initials			
		Knee			
		Flexion			
		Extension			

Fig. 1.22

JOINT RANGE OF MOTION

Patient: _David Tamon_
Age: _46_
Indicate:
    AROM _____
    PROM _____

LEFT				RIGHT	
		Date/Examiner's Initials			
		Hip			
		Flexion			
		Extension			
		Abduction			
		Adduction			
		Medial Rotation			
		Lateral Rotation			

Fig. 1.23

starting position for flexion is 0 degrees. Even though Mrs. Stephenson is able to attain more than 0 degrees of extension, the extra motion is not included in the documentation for knee flexion because the flexion movement begins at 0 (Fig. 1.22).

Further Exploration: Documenting Range of Motion Using Single Motion Recording Technique

Using the charts that follow, practice documenting ROM by recording the motion for each of the patients presented below:

1. Ms. Atchley is able to begin from the 0-degree starting position and to actively move her knee 8 degrees in the direction of extension and 140 degrees in the direction of flexion. Record Ms. Atchley's knee flexion and extension ROM (Fig. 1.23).
2. Mr. Taman is unable to attain the 0-degree starting position for hip flexion and extension. He begins the motion of hip flexion with his hip at 12 degrees of flexion and is able to actively move from 3 to 118 degrees of flexion. He is unable to move past 12 degrees of flexion toward the direction of extension. Record Mr. Taman's hip flexion and extension ROM (Fig. 1.24).

JOINT RANGE OF MOTION

Patient: _Nicole Stephenson_
Age: _68_
Indicate:
   AROM _X_
   PROM _____

				LEFT / RIGHT			

LEFT   **RIGHT**

			Date/Examiner's Initials	01/03/09 NBR		
			Knee			
			Flexion	0°–145°		
			Extension	0°–10°		

Fig. 1.24

JOINT RANGE OF MOTION

Patient: _Danielle Lusby_
Age: _32_
Indicate:
   AROM _____
   PROM _____

LEFT   **RIGHT**

			Date/Examiner's Initials			
			Shoulder			
			Flexion			
			Extension			
			Abduction			
			Adduction			
			Medial Rotation			
			Lateral Rotation			

Fig. 1.25

3. Ms. Lusby is unable to abduct her shoulder to 90 degrees. Therefore, the examiner measures Ms. Lusby's shoulder rotation with her shoulder positioned in 45 degrees of abduction. From this position, she is able to attain the 0-degree starting position for shoulder rotation and to actively move her shoulder 60 degrees in the direction of medial rotation and 48 degrees in the direction of lateral rotation. Record Ms. Lusby's shoulder rotation ROM. What notation should be made of Ms. Lusby's altered position for testing (Fig. 1.25)?

A wide variety of forms may be used in recording ROM. Appendix A provides a sampling of forms that can be used in the clinical setting.

Sagittal Frontal Transverse Rotational (SFTR) Recording Technique

A second method of recording joint ROM records all motions that occur together in a given plane. For example, all motions occurring at the shoulder in the sagittal plane are recorded on the same line in the patient's record.

Motions occurring in the frontal plane are then recorded, followed by motions occurring in the transverse plane, and so forth. When motion for each plane of movement is recorded, a sequence of three numbers is used. The first number represents the extreme of motion in one direction, the second number represents the starting position, and the third number represents the extreme of motion in the opposite direction. For each plane of motion, movements are listed in the following order:

Sagittal plane:	Extension/Starting position/Flexion
	Dorsiflexion/Starting position/ Plantarflexion
Frontal plane:	Abduction/Starting position/ Adduction
	Lateral flexion to left/Starting position/Lateral flexion to right
Transverse plane:	Horizontal abduction/Starting position/Horizontal adduction
Rotation:	Lateral rotation/Starting position/ Medial rotation
	Supination/Starting position/ Pronation
	Eversion/Starting position/ Inversion
	Rotation to left/Starting position/ Rotation to right

To use the example of Mrs. Stephenson that was provided previously, under the SFTR system, Mrs. Stephenson's ROM would be documented thus:

- Shoulder S: 35°–0°–165°
- Elbow S: 0°–15°–140°
- Knee S: 10°–0°–145°

The notation for elbow motion indicates that Mrs. Stephenson is unable to move the elbow into extension, and that she begins flexion at 15 degrees of flexion rather than at the 0-degree starting position. In other words, she has a 15-degree elbow flexion contracture.

The chart in Fig. 1.26 shows how Mrs. Stephenson's elbow ROM is documented by the SFTR method.

On some occasions, motion at a joint is measured with the joint in some position other than the anatomical 0-degree starting position. In these cases, the SFTR system allows easy notation of the altered position. For example, if hip rotation is measured with the hip positioned in 90 degrees of flexion, a notation of the hip's position can made in the hip rotation record as follows: Hip R (S90): 32°–0°–28°. The designation (S90) indicates that the hip was positioned at 90 degrees in the sagittal plane when the hip rotation measurement was taken.

Further Exploration: Documenting Range of Motion Using SFTR Recording Technique

Using the information already provided for sample patients, Ms. Atchley, Mr. Taman, and Ms. Lusby, document the ROM of each patient using the SFTR technique in the charts provided in Figs. 1.27–1.29.

Determining and Recording Muscle Length

As indicated previously, in measuring muscle length, the examiner is most concerned about the final, elongated position of the muscle and is not as concerned about measurement from the zero starting position (as would be appropriate for measurement of joint ROM). Therefore for measurement of muscle length, the muscle to be examined is placed in the elongated position, and the measurement is taken using the suggested instrument (as is described in detail in Chapters 6 and 14). This actual measurement is the only information that is documented.

Assume that Mr. Ihler is a 35-year-old weekend tennis player with a diagnosis of patellar tendinitis in the

---

JOINT RANGE OF MOTION

Patient: _Nicole Stephenson_
Age: _68_
Indicate:
  AROM _X_
  PROM _____

LEFT				RIGHT		
			Date/Examiner's Initials	01/03/09 NBR		
			Elbow/Forearm: S	0°–15°–140°		
			Elbow/Forearm: R			

Fig. 1.26

JOINT RANGE OF MOTION

Patient: _Elizabeth Atchley_
Age: _20_
Indicate:
 AROM _____
 PROM _____

LEFT				RIGHT	
		Date/Examiner's Initials			
		Knee: S			

Fig. 1.27

JOINT RANGE OF MOTION

Patient: _David Tamon_
Age: _46_
Indicate:
 AROM _____
 PROM _____

LEFT				RIGHT	
		Date/Examiner's Initials			
		Hip:S			
		Hip:F			
		Hip:R			

Fig. 1.28

JOINT RANGE OF MOTION

Patient: _Danielle Lusby_
Age: _32_
Indicate:
 AROM _____
 PROM _____

LEFT				RIGHT	
		Date/Examiner's Initials			
		Shoulder:S			
		Shoulder:F			
		Shoulder:R			

Fig. 1.29

right knee. Measurement of muscles on his right side indicates 0 degrees for the gastrocnemius, 5 degrees for the soleus, and 40 degrees from full knee extension for the hamstrings (using the passive 90/90 test described later in Chapter 14). Measurement of flexibility on his left side indicates 5 degrees for the gastrocnemius, 10

degrees for the soleus, and 20 degrees from full knee extension for the hamstrings. His muscle length data are documented as in Fig. 1.30.

A wide variety of forms can be used for recording muscle length data. Appendix A provides a sampling of forms that can be used in the clinical setting.

		01/03/09 WDB	Date/Examiner's Initials	01/03/09 WDB		
		5°	**Gastrocnemius**	0°		
		10°	**Soleus**	5°		
		90/90 Passive 20°	**Hamstring - (Indicate test used)**	90/90 Passive 40°		

MUSCLE LENGTH

Patient: _John Ihler_
Age: _35_
Indicate:
AROM _____
PROM __X__

LEFT   **RIGHT**

Fig. 1.30

References

1. Cleveland DE. Diagrams for showing limitation of movements through joints, as used by the Board of Pensions Commissioners for Canada. *Can Med Assoc J.* 1918;8:1070–1076.
2. American Academy of Orthopaedic Surgeons. *Joint Motion: Method of Measuring and Recording.* Chicago: American Academy of Orthopaedic Surgeons; 1965.
3. Rowe CR. Joint measurement in disability evaluation. *Clin Orthop Relat Res.* 1964;32:43–53.
4. Moore ML. The measurement of joint motion; introductory review of the literature. *Phys Ther Rev.* 1949;29:195–205.
5. Salter N. Methods of measurement of muscle and joint function. *J Bone Joint Surg Br.* 1955;37-B:474–491.
6. Awan R, Smith J, Boon AJ. Measuring shoulder internal rotation range of motion: a comparison of 3 techniques. *Arch Phys Med Rehabil.* 2002;83:1229–1234.
7. Hayes K, Walton JR, Szomor ZR, Murrell GA. Reliability of five methods for assessing shoulder range of motion. *Aust J Physiother.* 2001;47:289–294.
8. Williams J, Callaghan M. Comparison of visual estimation and goniometry in determination of a shoulder joint angle. *Physiotherapy.* 1990;76:655–657.
9. Watkins MA, Riddle DL, Lamb RL, Personius WJ. Reliability of goniometric measurements and visual estimates of knee range of motion obtained in a clinical setting. *Phys Ther.* 1991;71:90–96 [discussion 96–97].
10. Youdas JW, Bogard CL, Suman VJ. Reliability of goniometric measurements and visual estimates of ankle joint active range of motion obtained in a clinical setting. *Arch Phys Med Rehabil.* 1993;74:1113–1118.
11. Youdas JW, Carey JR, Garrett TR. Reliability of measurements of cervical spine range of motion–comparison of three methods. *Phys Ther.* 1991;71:98–104 [discussion 105–106].
12. van de Pol RJ, van Trijffel E, Lucas C. Inter-rater reliability for measurement of passive physiological range of motion of upper extremity joints is better if instruments are used: a systematic review. *J Physiother.* 2010;56:7–17.
13. Zachazewski J. *Flexibility for Sports, Sports Physical Therapy.* Norwalk, CT: Appleton & Lange; 1990.
14. Fletcher JP, Bandy WD. Intrarater reliability of CROM measurement of cervical spine active range of motion in persons with and without neck pain. *J Orthop Sports Phys Ther.* 2008;38:640–645.
15. Kendall F, McCreary E, Provance P. *Muscles: Testing and Function.* Baltimore: Elsevier; 1993.
16. Neumann D. *Kinesiology of the Musculoskeletal System: Foundations for Rehabilitation.* St. Louis, MO: Mosby/Elsevier; 2017.
17. Smith L, Weiss E, Lehmkuhl L. *Brunnstrom's Clinical Kinesiology.* Philadelphia: F.A. Davis; 1996.
18. Clemente C. *Gray's Anatomy of the Human Body.* Philadelphia: Lea & Febiger; 1985.
19. Donatelli R, Wolf SL. *The Biomechanics of the Foot and Ankle: Contemporary Perspectives in Rehabilitation.* Philadelphia: Davis; 1996:391.
20. Root ML, Orien WP, Weed JH. *Normal and Abnormal Function of the Foot: Clinical Biomechanics.* Los Angeles: Clinical Biomechanics Corp; 1977:478.
21. Smith DS. Measurement of joint range—an overview. *Clin Rheum Dis.* 1982;8:523–531.
22. Fox RF. Demonstration of the mensuration apparatus in use at the Red Cross clinic for the physical treatment of officers, Great Portland Street, London. *W Proc R Soc Med.* 1917;10:63–68.
23. Gifford H. Instruments for measuring joint movements and deformities in fracture treatment. *Am J Surg.* 1914;28:237–238.
24. Brosseau L, Tousignant M, Budd J, et al. Intratester and intertester reliability and criterion validity of the parallelogram and universal goniometers for active knee flexion in healthy subjects. *Physiother Res Int.* 1997;2:150–166.
25. Clark W. A protractor for measuring rotation of joints. *J Orthop Surg.* 1921;3:154–155.
26. Noer H, Pratt DR. A goniometer designed for the hand. *J Bone Joint Surg Am.* 1958;40-A:1154–1156.
27. Rosen N. A simplified method of measuring amplitude of motion in joints. *J Bone Joint Surg.* 1922;20:570–579.
28. Silver D. Measurement of the range of motion in joints. *J Bone Joint Surg.* 1923;569–578.
29. Wakeley C. A new form of goniometer. *Lancet.* 1918;23:300.
30. Wiechec F, Krusen F. A new method of joint measurement and a review of the literature. *Am J Surg.* 1939;43:659–668.
31. Yang RS. A new goniometer. *Orthop Rev.* 1992;21:877–882.
32. Clark W. A system of joint measurements. *J Orthop Surg.* 1920;2:687–700.
33. Ellis B, Bruton A. A study to compare the reliability of composite finger flexion with goniometry for measurement of range of motion in the hand. *Clin Rehabil.* 2002;16:562–570.
34. Kato M, Echigo A, Ohta H, et al. The accuracy of goniometric measurements of proximal interphalangeal joints in fresh cadavers: comparison between methods of measurement, types of goniometers, and fingers. *J Hand Ther.* 2007;20:12–18. quiz 19.
35. Aalto TJ, Airaksinen O, Härkönen TM, Arokoski JP. Effect of passive stretch on reproducibility of hip range of motion measurements. *Arch Phys Med Rehabil.* 2005;86:549–557.
36. Armstrong AD, MacDermid JC, Chinchalkar S, Stevens RS, King GJ. Reliability of range-of-motion measurement in the elbow and forearm. *J Shoulder Elbow Surg.* 1998;7:573–580.
37. Menadue C, Raymond J, Kilbreath SL, Refshauge KM, Adams R. Reliability of two goniometric methods of measuring active inversion and eversion range of motion at the ankle. *BMC Musculoskelet Disord.* 2006;7:60.
38. Burdett RG, Brown KE, Fall MP. Reliability and validity of four instruments for measuring lumbar spine and pelvic positions. *Phys Ther.* 1986;66:677–684.
39. Nitschke JE, Nattrass CL, Disler PB, Chou MJ, Ooi KT. Reliability of the American Medical Association guides' model for measuring

spinal range of motion. Its implication for whole-person impairment rating. *Spine (Philadelphia, Pa 1976).* 1999;(24):262–268.

40. Pringle RK. Intra-instrument reliability of 4 goniometers. *J Chiropr Med.* 2003;2:91–95.

41. American Medical Association. *Guides to the Evaluation of Permanent Impairment.* Chicago: American Medical Association; 1993:339.

42. Cave E, Roberts S. A method for measuring and recording joint function. *J Bone Joint Surg.* 1936;455–465.

43. Dorinson SM, Wagner ML. An exact technic for clinically measuring and recording joint motion. *Arch Phys Med Rehabil.* 1948;29:468–475.

44. West C. Measurement of joint motion. *Arch Phys Med.* 1945;26:414–425.

45. Greene WB, Heckman JD. *The Clinical Measurement of Joint Motion.* Rosemont, IL: American Academy of Orthopaedic Surgeons; 1994.

46. American Medical Association. *Guides to the Evaluation of Permanent Impairment.* Chicago: American Medical Association; 1995.

47. Mundale MO, Hislop HJ, Rabideau RJ, Kottke FJ. Evaluation of extension of the hip. *Arch Phys Med Rehabil.* 1956;37:75–80.

48. Allander E, Björnsson OJ, Olafsson O, Sigfússon N, Thorsteinsson J. Normal range of joint movements in shoulder, hip, wrist and thumb with special reference to side: a comparison between two populations. *Int J Epidemiol.* 1974;3:253–261.

49. Cadogan A, Laslett M, Hing W, McNair P, Williams M. Reliability of a new hand-held dynamometer in measuring shoulder range of motion and strength. *Man Ther.* 2011;16:97–101.

50. Penning LI, Guldemond NA, de Bie RA, Walenkamp GH. Reproducibility of a 3-dimensional gyroscope in measuring shoulder anteflexion and abduction. *BMC Musculoskelet Disord.* 2012;13:135.

51. Darcus HD, Salter N. The amplitude of pronation and supination with the elbow flexed to a right angle. *J Anat.* 1953;87:169–184.

52. Hewitt D. The range of active motion at the wrist of women. *J Bone Joint Surg.* 1928;10:775–787.

53. Ellis B, Bruton A, Goddard JR. Joint angle measurement: a comparative study of the reliability of goniometry and wire tracing for the hand. *Clin Rehabil.* 1997;11:314–320.

54. Hamilton GF, Lachenbruch PA. Reliability of goniometers in assessing finger joint angle. *Phys Ther.* 1969;49:465–469.

55. Stam HJ, Ardon MS, den Ouden AC, Schreuders TA, Roebroeck ME. The compangle: a new goniometer for joint angle measurements of the hand. A technical note. *Eura Medicophys.* 2006;42:37–40.

56. de Kraker M, Selles RW, Schreuders TA, Stam HJ, Hovius SE. Palmar abduction: reliability of 6 measurement methods in healthy adults. *J Hand Surg Am.* 2009;34:523–530.

57. Burton AK. Regional lumbar sagittal mobility: measurement by flexicurves. *Clin Biomech.* 1986;1:20–26.

58. de Oliveira TS, Candotti CT, La Torre M, et al. Validity and reproducibility of the measurements obtained using the flexicurve instrument to evaluate the angles of thoracic and lumbar curvatures of the spine in the sagittal plane. *Rehab Res Pract.* 2012;2012, 186156.

59. Hart DL, Rose SJ. Reliability of a noninvasive method for measuring the lumbar curve. *J Orthop Sports Phys Ther.* 1986;8:180–184.

60. Israel M. A quantitative method of estimating flexion and extension of the spine; a preliminary report. *Mil Med.* 1959;124:181–186.

61. Stokes IA, Bevins TM, Lunn RA. Back surface curvature and measurement of lumbar spinal motion. *Spine.* 1987;12:355–361.

62. Tillotson KM, Burton AK. Noninvasive measurement of lumbar sagittal mobility an assessment of the flexicurve technique. *Spine.* 1991;16:29–33.

63. Valle MB, Dutra VH, Candotti CT, et al. Validity of flexicurve for the assessment of spinal flexibility in asymptomatic individuals. *Fisioterapia em Moviomento.* 2020;33:1–9.

64. Youdas JW, Suman VJ, Garrett TR. Reliability of measurements of lumbar spine sagittal mobility obtained with the flexible curve. *J Orthop Sports Phys Ther.* 1995;21:13–20.

65. Fairbank JC, Pynsent PB, Phillips H. Quantitative measurements of joint mobility in adolescents. *Ann Rheum Dis.* 1984;43:288–294.

66. Haley ET. Range of hip rotation and torque of hip rotator muscle groups. *Am J Phys Med.* 1953;32:261–270.

67. Pott P, Selley A, Tyson SF. The reliability, responsiveness and clinical utility of the Proximat: a new tool for measuring hip range of movement in children with cerebral palsy. *Physiother Res Int.* 2008;13:223–230.

68. Aström M, Arvidson T. Alignment and joint motion in the normal foot. *J Orthop Sports Phys Ther.* 1995;22:216–222.

69. Brody DM. Running injuries. *Clin Symp.* 1980;32:1–36.

70. Donnery J, Spencer RB. The Biplane Goniometer. A new device for measurement of ankle dorsiflexion. *J Am Podiatr Med Assoc.* 1988;78:348–351.

71. Mann R. *Principles of Examination of the Foot and Ankle, Surgery of the Foot.* St. Louis: Mosby; 1986.

72. Muwanga CL, Dove AF, Plant GR. The measurement of ankle movements—a new method. *Injury.* 1985;16:312–314.

73. Rome K. Ankle joint dorsiflexion measurement studies. A review of the literature. *J Am Podiatr Med Assoc.* 1996;86:205–211.

74. Wilken J, Rao S, Estin M, Saltzman CL, Yack HJ. A new device for assessing ankle dorsiflexion motion: reliability and validity. *J Orthop Sports Phys Ther.* 2011;41:274–280.

75. Meskers CG, Fraterman H, van der Helm FC, Vermeulen HM, Rozing PM. Calibration of the "Flock of Birds" electromagnetic tracking device and its application in shoulder motion studies. *J Biomech.* 1999;32:629–633.

76. Vermeulen HM, Stokdijk M, Eilers PH, Meskers CG, Rozing PM, Vliet Vlieland TP. Measurement of three dimensional shoulder movement patterns with an electromagnetic tracking device in patients with a frozen shoulder. *Ann Rheum Dis.* 2002;61:115–120.

77. Fox R, van Breeman J. *Chronic Rheumatism, Causation, and Treatment.* London: Churchill Livingstone; 1934.

78. Glanville A, Kreeyer G. The maximum amplitude and velocity of joint movements in normal male human adults. *Hum Biol.* 1937;197–201.

79. Hand J. A compact pendulum arthrometer. *J Bone Joint Surg.* 1938;494–497.

80. Leighton JR. An instrument and technic for the measurement of range of joint motion. *Arch Phys Med Rehabil.* 1955;36:571–578.

81. Ekstrand J, Wiktorsson M, Oberg B, Gillquist J. Lower extremity goniometric measurements: a study to determine their reliability. *Arch Phys Med Rehabil.* 1982;63:171–175.

82. Schenker AW. Goniometry; an improved method of joint motion measurement. *N Y State J Med.* 1956;56:539–545.

83. Clark G, Willis L, Fish W, Nichols P. Assessment of movement at the glenohumeral joint. *Orthopaedics.* 1974;55–71.

84. Rheault W, Miller M, Nothnagel P, Straessle J, Urban D. Intertester reliability and concurrent validity of fluid-based and universal goniometers for active knee flexion. *Phys Ther.* 1988;68:1676–1678.

85. Petherick M, Rheault W, Kimble S, Lechner C, Senear V. Concurrent validity and intertester reliability of universal and fluid-based goniometers for active elbow range of motion. *Phys Ther.* 1988;68:966–999.

86. Bennett JG, Bergmanis LE, Carpenter JK, Skowlund HV. Range of motion of the neck. *J Am Phys Ther Assoc.* 1963;43:45–47.

87. Loebl WY. Measurement of spinal posture and range of spinal movement. *Ann Phys Med.* 1967;9:103–110.

88. de Winter AF, Heemskerk MA, Terwee CB, et al. Inter-observer reproducibility of measurements of range of motion in patients with shoulder pain using a digital inclinometer. *BMC Musculoskelet Disord.* 2004;5:18.

89. Kachingwe AF, Phillips BJ. Inter- and intrarater reliability of a back range of motion instrument. *Arch Phys Med Rehabil.* 2005;86:2347–2353.

90. Lea RD, Gerhardt JJ. Range-of-motion measurements. *J Bone Joint Surg Am.* 1995;77:784–798.

91. Lee C, Robbins D, H Robert, et al. Reliability and validity of single inclinometer measurements for thoracic spine range of motion. *Physiother Can.* 2000;73–78.

92. Hambly K, Sibley R, Ockendon M. Level of agreement between a novel smartphone application and a long arm goniometer for the assessment of maximum active knee flexion by an inexperienced tester. *Int J Physiother Rehabil.* 2012;2:1–14.

93. Jones A, Sealey R, Crowe M, Gordon S. Concurrent validity and reliability of the Simple Goniometer iPhone app compared with the Universal Goniometer. *Physiother Theory Pract.* 2014;30:512–516.

94. Ferriero G, Sartorio F, Foti C, Primavera D, Brigatti E, Vercelli S. Reliability of a new application for smartphones (DrGoniometer) for elbow angle measurement. *PMR.* 2011;3:1153–1154.

95. Ferriero G, Vercelli S, Sartorio F, et al. Reliability of a smartphone-based goniometer for knee joint goniometry. *Int J Rehabil Res.* 2013;36:146–151.

96. Otter SJ, Agalliu B, Baer N, et al. The reliability of a smartphone goniometer application compared with a traditional goniometer for measuring first metatarsophalangeal joint dorsiflexion. *J Foot Ankle Res.* 2015;8:30.

97. Shin SH, Ro du H, Lee OS, Oh JH, Kim SH. Within-day reliability of shoulder range of motion measurement with a smartphone. *Man Ther.* 2012;17:298–304.

98. Guidetti L, Placentino U, Baldari C. Reliability and criterion validity of the smartphone inclinometer application to quantify cervical spine mobility. *Clin Spine Surg.* 2017;30:e1359–e1366.

99. Keogh JWL, Cox A, Anderson S, et al. Reliability and validity of clinically accessible smartphone applications to measure joint range of motion: a systematic review. *PLoS One.* 2019;14(5):e0215806. https://doi.org/10.1371/journal.pone.0215806.

100. Pourahmadi MR, Taghipour T, Jannati E, et al. Reliability and validity of an iPhone application for the measurement of lumbar spine flexion and extension range of motion. *Peer J.* 2016;4:2355.

101. Pourahmadi MR, Bagheri R, Taghipour T, et al. A new iPhone application for measuring active craniocervical range of motion in patients with non-specific neck pain: a reliability and validity study. *Spine J.* 2018;18:447–457.

102. Karpovich P, Karpovich G. Electrogoniometer: new device for study of joints in action. *Fed Proc.* 1959;18:79.

103. Morrey BF, Askew LJ, Chao EY. A biomechanical study of normal functional elbow motion. *J Bone Joint Surg Am.* 1981;63:872–877.

104. Ellis MI, Stowe J. The hip. *Clin Rheum Dis.* 1982;8:655–675.

105. Clapper MP, Wolf SL. Comparison of the reliability of the orthoranger and the standard goniometer for assessing active lower extremity range of motion. *Phys Ther.* 1988;68:214–218.

106. Goodwin J, Clark C, Deakes J, Burdon D, Lawrence C. Clinical methods of goniometry: a comparative study. *Disabil Rehabil.* 1992;14:10–15.

107. Nicol A. Measurement of joint motion. *Clin Rehabil.* 1989;1–9.

108. Wilson G, Stasch W. Photographic record of joint motion. *Phys Med.* 1945;26:361–362.

109. Zankel HT. Photogoniometry; a new method of measurement of range of motion of joints. *Arch Phys Med Rehabil.* 1951;32:227–228.

110. Bohannon RW, Tiberio D, Zito M. Selected measures of ankle dorsiflexion range of motion: differences and intercorrelations. *Foot Ankle.* 1989;10:99–103.

111. Fish DR, Wingate L. Sources of goniometric error at the elbow. *Phys Ther.* 1985;65:1666–1670.

112. Hoffmann T, Russell T, Cooke H. Remote measurement via the Internet of upper limb range of motion in people who have had a stroke. *J Telemed Telecare.* 2007;13:401–405.

113. Chiu HY, Su FC, Wang ST, Hsu HY. The motion analysis system and goniometry of the finger joints. *J Hand Surg Br.* 1998;23:788–791.

114. Jordan K, Dziedzic K, Jones PW, Ong BN, Dawes PT. The reliability of the three-dimensional FASTRAK measurement system in measuring cervical spine and shoulder range of motion in healthy subjects. *Rheumatology (Oxford).* 2000;39:382–388.

115. Kebaetse M, McClure P, Pratt NA. Thoracic position effect on shoulder range of motion, strength, and three-dimensional scapular kinematics. *Arch Phys Med Rehabil.* 1999;80:945–950.

116. Melton C, Mullineaux DR, Mattacola CG, Mair SD, Uhl TL. Reliability of video motion-analysis systems to measure amplitude and velocity of shoulder elevation. *J Sport Rehabil.* 2011;20:393–405.

117. Safaee-Rad R, Shwedyk E, Quanbury AO, Cooper JE. Normal functional range of motion of upper limb joints during performance of three feeding activities. *Arch Phys Med Rehabil.* 1990;71:505–509.

118. Van Herp G, Rowe P, Salter P, Paul JP. Three-dimensional lumbar spinal kinematics: a study of range of movement in 100 healthy subjects aged 20 to 60+ years. *Rheumatology (Oxford).* 2000;39:1337–1340.

119. Bailey D. Subtalar joint neutral. *J Am Podiatr Med Assoc.* 1984;74:59–64.

120. Enwemeka CS. Radiographic verification of knee goniometry. *Scand J Rehabil Med.* 1986;18:47–49.

121. Lundberg A, Goldie I, Kalin B, Selvik G. Kinematics of the ankle/foot complex: plantarflexion and dorsiflexion. *Foot Ankle.* 1989;9:194–200.

122. Lundberg A, Svensson OK, Bylund C, Goldie I, Selvik G. Kinematics of the ankle/foot complex—part 2: pronation and supination. *Foot Ankle.* 1989;9:248–253.

123. Lundberg A, Svensson OK, Németh G, Selvik G. The axis of rotation of the ankle joint. *J Bone Joint Surg Br.* 1989;71:94–99.

124. Phillips A, Goubran A, Naim S, Searle D, Mandalia V, Toms A. Reliability of radiographic measurements of knee motion following knee arthroplasty for use in a virtual knee clinic. *Ann R Coll Surg Engl.* 2012;94:506–512.

125. Resch S, Ryd L, Stenström A, Johnsson K, Reynisson K. Measuring hallux valgus: a comparison of conventional radiography and clinical parameters with regard to measurement accuracy. *Foot Ankle Int.* 1995;16:267–270.

126. Stuberg W, Temme J, Kaplan P, Clarke A, Fuchs R. Measurement of tibial torsion and thigh-foot angle using goniometry and computed tomography. *Clin Orthop Relat Res.* 1991;208–212.

127. Tousignant M, Poulin L, Marchand S, Viau A, Place C. The Modified-Modified Schober Test for range of motion assessment of lumbar flexion in patients with low back pain: a study of criterion validity, intra- and inter-rater reliability and minimum metrically detectable change. *Disabil Rehabil.* 2005;27:553–559.

128. Weseley MS, Koval R, Kleiger B. Roentgen measurement of ankle flexion–extension motion. *Clin Orthop Relat Res.* 1969;65:167–174.

129. Harris ML. A factor analytic study of flexibility. *Res Q.* 1969;40:62–70.

130. Hubley-Kozey C. Testing flexibility. In: MacDougall JD, Wenger HA, Green HJ, eds. *Physiological Testing of the High-Performance Athlete.* Champaign, IL: Human Kinetics Books; 1991.

131. Barrow H, Mcgee R, Tritschler K. *Practical Measurement in Physical Education and Sports.* Philadelphia: Lea & Febiger; 1989.

132. Cureton T. Flexibility as an aspect of physical fitness. *Res Q.* 1941;381–383.

133. Kraus S. *Evaluation and Management of Temporomandibular Disorders, Evaluation, Treatment, and Prevention of Musculoskeletal Disorders.* Chaska, MN: The Saunders Group; 2004.

134. American College of Sports Medicine. *Guidelines for Exercise Testing and Prescription.* Indianapolis: ACSM; 2006.

135. Brodie DA, Bird HA, Wright V. Joint laxity in selected athletic populations. *Med Sci Sports Exerc.* 1982;14:190–193.

136. Gajdosik RL, Bohannon RW. Clinical measurement of range of motion. Review of goniometry emphasizing reliability and validity. *Phys Ther.* 1987;67:1867–1872.

137. Pratt AL, Burr N, Stott D. An investigation into the degree of precision achieved by a team of hand therapists and surgeons using hand goniometry with a standardised protocol. *Br J Hand Ther.* 2004;9:116–121.

138. Buell T, Green DR, Risser J. Measurement of the first metatarsophalangeal joint range of motion. *J Am Podiatr Med Assoc.* 1988;78:439–448.

139. Günal I, Köse N, Erdogan O, Göktürk E, Seber S. Normal range of motion of the joints of the upper extremity in male subjects, with special reference to side. *J Bone Joint Surg Am.* 1996;78:1401–1404.

140. Joseph J. Range of movement of the great toe in men. *J Bone Joint Surg.* 1954;450–457.

141. Smith J, Walker J. Knee and elbow range of motion in healthy older individuals. *Phys Occup Ther Geriatr.* 1983;2:31–38.

142. Sabari JS, Maltzev I, Lubarsky D, Liszkay E, Homel P. Goniometric assessment of shoulder range of motion: comparison of testing in supine and sitting positions. *Arch Phys Med Rehabil.* 1998;79:647–651.

143. Simoneau GG, Hoenig KJ, Lepley JE, Papanek PE. Influence of hip position and gender on active hip internal and external rotation. *J Orthop Sports Phys Ther.* 1998;28:158–164.

144. Boon AJ, Smith J. Manual scapular stabilization: its effect on shoulder rotational range of motion. *Arch Phys Med Rehabil.* 2000;81:978–983.

145. Wilk KE, Reinold MM, Macrina LC, et al. Glenohumeral internal rotation measurements differ depending on stabilization techniques. *Sports Health.* 2009;1:131–136.

146. Bohannon RW, Gajdosik RL, LeVeau BF. Relationship of pelvic and thigh motions during unilateral and bilateral hip flexion. *Phys Ther.* 1985;65:1501–1504.

147. Cyriax JH, Coldham M. *Textbook of Orthopaedic Medicine.* London: Baillière Tindall; 1982.

148. Hertling D, Kessler R. *Management of Common Musculoskeletal Disorders.* Philadelphia: Lippincott: Williams & Wilkins; 1996.

149. Magee DJ. *Orthopedic Physical Assessment.* St. Louis, MO: Elsevier: Saunders; 2014.

2

MEASUREMENT of RANGE of MOTION and MUSCLE LENGTH: CLINICAL RELEVANCE

William D. Bandy, Jacquie Rainey, and Nancy Berryman Reese

Chapter 1 introduced the background necessary to measure joint range of motion (ROM) and muscle length using standardized procedures. The purpose of this chapter is to educate the individual who is collecting data on ROM and muscle length regarding the meaning of that information. The clinician must be aware of the strengths and weaknesses of referring to data as "normative." The reader needs to understand both the changes that occur with age and the differences that exist between men and women, as well as among different cultures. In addition, changes that occur as a result of participation in athletic activities are important to understand. Finally, if measurements are not accurate, then the information gained from collected data is literally worthless. The clinician not only must be aware of the need for accurate measurements but also must have an understanding of the reliability and validity of the procedures and instruments that are being used. After reading this chapter, readers should have a better understanding of the clinical relevance of the data collected in measuring ROM and muscle length to better educate their patients and to guide their intervention.

NORMATIVE DATA FOR RANGE OF MOTION AND MUSCLE LENGTH

Numerous individuals and groups have provided "norms" for ROM of the joints of the spine and extremities (see Appendix B). However, the validity of most of these "norms" is suspect for one reason or another. Many individuals and groups who have provided "norms" for ROM have done so without substantiating the source of the "normative" data. For example, the long-used and accepted "norms" for ROM provided by the American Academy of Orthopaedic Surgeons (AAOS)[1] were published without an explanation of how the data were obtained or any description of the population from which the data came. The newest edition of the AAOS joint motion manual repeats many of the 1965 "norms" and provides other normative data that are derived from studies with small or nonrandomized samples.[2] Likewise, the American Medical Association (AMA)[3] does not describe the source for its published "norms" for ROM. Instead of providing unsubstantiated normative data for the various movements, Appendix B attempts to provide "norms" for ROM for movements of the extremities and the spine that are based on available published literature.

FACTORS AFFECTING RANGE OF MOTION

CHANGES IN RANGE OF MOTION WITH AGE

Lower Extremity

Table 2.1 reports ROM of the lower extremity as adults progress in age. A significant decrease in the amount of hip motion (abduction, adduction, medial rotation, and lateral rotation) was reported in male and female subjects aged 60–84 years compared with mean values reported for younger adults.[4,6] Similar results indicating a progressive decrease in hip ROM in 77 male subjects as they aged from 15 to 73 years was reported by Nonaka et al.[8] Macedo and Magee[9] reported statistically significant declines in hip motion (flexion and lateral rotation) with aging in their study of PROM in females aged 18–59 years. McKay et al.[5] reported statistically significant declines in hip active range of motion (medial and lateral rotation) with aging. Anderson and Madigan[10] also reported declines in hip extension range of motion in older adults (age 75–86 years) compared to young adults (age 20–31 years).

However, these reported decreases in ROM in the hip joints of older adults were not substantiated by Roach and Miles,[4] who reported on data from the first National Health and Nutrition Examination Survey (NHANES I). In their analysis of 1313 of the original 1892 subjects (aged 25–74 years) on whom hip and knee ROM measurements were taken as part of NHANES I, Roach and Miles[4] reported that, generally, differences in mean ROM between younger (aged 25–39 years) and older (aged 60–74 years) age groups were small, ranging from 3 to 5 degrees. The only motion of the hip that did appear to decrease in range with aging, according

Table 2.1	CHANGES IN LOWER EXTREMITY RANGE OF MOTION: 25–101 YEARS OF AGE				
HIP	**25–39 YEARS** (Roach and Miles[4])	**40–59 YEARS** (Roach and Miles[4])	**20–59 YEARS** (McKay et al.[5])	**60–84 YEARS** (Walker et al.[6])	**60–101 YEARS** (McKay et al.[5])
Flexion	$122° \pm 12°$	$120° \pm 14°$	$120° \pm 9°$ (M) $123° \pm 10°$ (F)	$111° \pm 12°$	$115° \pm 11°$ (M) $114° \pm 13°$ (F)
Extension	$22° \pm 8°$	$18° \pm 7°$		$-11° \pm 4°$	
Abduction	$44° \pm 11°$	$42° \pm 11°$		$24° \pm 8°$	
Adduction	$26° \pm 4°$ᵃ	$26° \pm 4°$ᵃ		$15° \pm 4°$	
Medial rotation	$33° \pm 7°$	$31° \pm 8°$	$36° \pm 8°$ (M) $40° \pm 9°$ (F)	$22° \pm 6°$	$33° \pm 8°$ (M) $35° \pm 8°$ (F)
Lateral rotation	$34° \pm 8°$	$32° \pm 8°$	$30° \pm 8°$ (M) $27° \pm 8°$ (F)	$32° \pm 6°$	$26° \pm 7°$ (M) $22° \pm 7°$ (F)
KNEE	**25–39 YEARS** (Roach and Miles[4])	**40–59 YEARS** (Roach and Miles[4])	**20–59 YEARS** (McKay et al.[5])	**60–84 YEARS** (Walker et al.[6])	**60–101 YEARS** (McKay et al.[5])
Flexion	$134° \pm 9°$	$132° \pm 11°$	$136° \pm 6°$ (M) $137° \pm 6°$ (F)	$133° \pm 6°$	$133° \pm 7°$ (M) $131° \pm 8°$ (F)
Extension	$-1° \pm 2°$ᵃ	$-1° \pm 2°$ᵃ	$1° \pm 2°$ (M) $2° \pm 3°$ (F)	$-1° \pm 2°$	$-1° \pm 2°$ (M) $1° \pm 2°$ (F)
ANKLE/FOOT	**25–39 YEARS** (Roach and Miles[4])	**40–59 YEARS** (Roach and Miles[4])	**20–59 YEARS** (McKay et al.[5])	**60–84 YEARS** (Walker et al.[6])	**60–101 YEARS** (McKay et al.[5])
Dorsiflexionᵇ	$12° \pm 4°$ᵃ	$12° \pm 4°$ᵃ	$32° \pm 6°$ (M) $29° \pm 6°$ (F)	$10° \pm 5°$	$31° \pm 6°$ (M) $26° \pm 6°$ (F)
Plantarflexionᵃ	$54° \pm 6°$ᵃ	$54° \pm 6°$ᵃ	$56° \pm 8°$ (M) $62° \pm 9°$ (F)	$29° \pm 7°$	$53° \pm 7°$ (M) $57° \pm 7°$ (F)
Inversionᵇ	$36° \pm 4°$ᵃ	$36° \pm 4°$ᵃ		$30° \pm 11°$	
Eversion[7]	$19° \pm 5°$ᵃ	$19° \pm 5°$ᵃ		$13° \pm 6°$	

F, females; *M*, males.
ᵃComponent of supination.
ᵇComponent of pronation.

to Roach and Miles,[4] was hip extension, which showed a greater than 20% decline between the youngest (aged 25–39 years) and oldest (aged 60–74 years) age groups.

The apparent discrepancy in reported results between the study by Walker et al.[6] and the Roach and Miles[4] study may have been due to differences in the age groups studied. The sample population in the Walker et al.[6] study included subjects aged up to 84 years, whereas no subjects over the age of 74 were included in the data reported by Roach and Miles.[4] More recent studies by McKay et al.[5] and Nonaka et al.[8] supported the findings of the Walker et al.[6] group. Additionally in a study that focused on subjects between the ages of 70 and 92 years, James and Parker[11] reported progressive decreases in all lower extremity joint motions with increasing age, with the most pronounced decreases in motion occurring after age 80. The largest changes in ROM occurred with hip abduction and ankle dorsiflexion. Numerous other investigators also have reported declines in ankle ROM with age.[12-16] Such declines appear to be more marked in females[15] and have been correlated with falls, decreased gait speed, and with decreased performance on measures of balance and physical performance.[16-21] One lower extremity joint that does not appear to lose motion with increasing age is the knee, with motion remaining stable well into the ninth decade.[6,22] However, if a loss of knee extension

range of motion occurs, it can be associated with difficulty walking[23] and a loss of knee flexion range of motion is associated with difficulty with sit to stand.[6,20,22]

Although some motions of the lower extremity do not appear to show significant decline until the ninth decade, other lower extremity motions have been reported to decline in range at earlier ages. Decreased ROM of the first metatarsophalangeal joint after age 45 has been reported both for flexion and for extension of that joint.[24] Loss of extension ROM appears to be both more marked and more significant in terms of potential loss of function.[24]

Upper Extremity

Several investigators have reported decreases in shoulder ROM in older adults (Table 2.2). Abduction, lateral rotation, and flexion are the motions of the shoulder most frequently reported to demonstrate statistically significant decline with age.[5,14,26-34] Macedo and Magee[9] reported declines in passive shoulder flexion and abduction range of motion at or very near 10 degrees by the fourth decade in women. McKay et al.[5] demonstrate declines in shoulder active lateral rotation beginning in the age group of 20–59 with further observed declines in ages 60 and above. Other groups generally report such declines as common beginning

Table 2.2 CHANGES IN UPPER EXTREMITY RANGE OF MOTION: 20–101 YEARS OF AGE			
SHOULDER	**20–54 YEARS** (Boone et al.[25])	**20–59 YEARS** (McKay et al.[5])	**60–84 YEARS** (Walker et al.[6])	**60–101 YEARS** (McKay et al.[5])
Flexion	$165° \pm 5°$		$165° \pm 10°$	
Extension	$57° \pm 8°$		$44° \pm 12°$	
Abduction	$183° \pm 9°$		$165° \pm 19°$	
Medial rotation	$67° \pm 4°$	$58° \pm 12°$ (M) $63° \pm 14°$ (F)	$63° \pm 15°$	$57° \pm 11°$ (M) $63° \pm 12°$ (F)
Lateral rotation	$100° \pm 8°$	$83° \pm 13°$ (M) $83° \pm 16°$ (F)	$81° \pm 15°$	$71° \pm 12°$ (M) $72° \pm 14°$ (F)
ELBOW	**20–54 YEARS** (Boone et al.[25])	**20–59 YEARS** (McKay et al.[5])	**60–84 YEARS** (Walker et al.[6])	**60–101 YEARS** (McKay et al.[5])
Flexion	$141° \pm 5°$	$147° \pm 5°$ (M) $149° \pm 5°$ (F)	$144° \pm 10°$	$146° \pm 6°$ (M) $149° \pm 5°$ (F)
Extension	$0° \pm 3°$	$2° \pm 5°$ (M) $4° \pm 5°$ (F)	$-4° \pm 4°$	$-1° \pm 5°$ (M) $0° \pm 5°$ (F)
FOREARM	**20–54 YEARS** (Boone et al.[25])		**60–84 YEARS** (Walker et al.[6])	
Pronation	$75° \pm 5°$		$71° \pm 11°$	
Supination	$81° \pm 4°$		$74° \pm 11°$	
WRIST	**20–54 YEARS** (Boone et al.[25])		**60–84 YEARS** (Walker et al.[6])	
Flexion	$75° \pm 7°$		$64° \pm 10°$	
Extension	$74° \pm 7°$		$63° \pm 8°$	
Abduction (radial deviation)	$21° \pm 4°$		$19° \pm 6°$	
Adduction (ulnar deviation)	$35° \pm 4°$		$26° \pm 7°$	

F, females; *M*, males.

after age 60,[28–31] although this may be because the age ranges studied by these investigators did not include younger subjects. In a community-based study of over 2400 participants, Gill et al. examined active range of motion in the shoulders of males and females aged 20 to over 85 and found statistically significant declines in flexion, abduction, and lateral rotation with increasing age.[34] Shoulder extension has been reported to show a significant decline with age by fewer groups,[9,27] and Walker et al.[6] reported this decrease occurs in older males only. However, few studies investigating ROM changes with aging included measures of shoulder extension. Whether shoulder medial rotation declines with age is less clear. Stubbs et al.[14] reported statistically significant declines in shoulder medial rotation as early as the fourth decade, and McKay et al.[5] report statistically significant declines in shoulder active medial rotation for males after their second decade but no further declines with aging. McIntosh et al.[32] and Fiebert et al.[31] based their reports of declines in shoulder medial rotation on significant differences in measured motion and AAOS norms, although Fiebert did report further declines in medial rotation in subjects aged 90–99 years. Conversely, other investigators reported no significant changes in shoulder medial rotation in subjects as old as 94 years,[9,29] and Barnes et al.[27] reported increases in

shoulder medial rotation with aging in their study of subjects as old as 70 years.

Alterations in elbow and forearm ROM with aging have not been widely studied, although some changes have been reported. Elbow flexion ROM does not appear to change with age.[5,9,14] Passive elbow extension ROM has been reported to decline with age in women,[9] and active elbow extension ROM has been reported to decline after the second decade with men,[5] although the declines reported in both studies were within the range of measurement error. Although some investigators have reported no significant declines in forearm rotation ROM through the sixth decade,[9,14] studies including older subjects have reported declines in both forearm supination[6,35,36] and pronation.[35,36]

As was seen with the elbow and forearm, declines in wrist ROM do not seem to appear until later in life. Macedo and Magee[9] reported no change in all passive motions of the wrist in females up to age 59. Stubbs et al.[14] reported similar findings in males up to age 54 with the exception of wrist ulnar deviation, which was reported to demonstrate significant declines by the mid-1940s in the studied population. Declines in wrist ROM appear to be more common in later years. Statistically significant decreases with increasing age were reported for wrist flexion and wrist extension ROM in a group of

720 subjects in Iceland and Sweden, aged 33–70 years.[26] Klum et al.[37] reported declines in all wrist motions with aging in their study of adults aged 18 to 65. The results of Allander et al.[26] and Klum et al.[37] were substantiated for wrist extension by Walker et al.[6] but only in male subjects.

Lumbar Spine

An investigation by van Adrichem and van der Korst[38] examined the changes that occur as children age from 6 to 18 years. Using a tape measure, the authors measured lumbar flexion in 248 children and reported that as the child became older and progressed to adulthood, flexion ROM increased.

After investigating differences in lumbar ROM in 405 healthy subjects (196 females, 209 males) ranging in age from 16 to 90 years, Troke et al.[39] reported that lumbar ROM declined in a linear fashion as age increased. Declines in ROM were 40%–42% for flexion, 76% for extension, and 43% for lateral flexion. However, the authors reported no change in lumbar rotation with increasing age. Results presented by Troke et al.[39] were supported by several studies[40–45] that examined lumbar ROM across the age span by categorizing subjects into 10-year increments and comparing the amount of lumbar motion in each age group. In one of the earliest studies, Loebl[40] used an inclinometer to measure lumbar flexion and extension in 176 individuals between the ages of 15 and 84 years and reported that a decrease in ROM was "readily demonstrated." Similarly, Moll and Wright[41] used the tape measure technique to measure flexion, extension, and lateral flexion in 237 subjects (aged 18–71 years) and reported that an initial increase in lumbar motion occurred from the age 15-to-24 decade to the age 25-to-34 decade, followed by "a progressive decrease in advancing age."

Sullivan et al.[42] used double inclinometry to measure flexion and extension in 1126 healthy volunteers and reported that "flexion and extension declined as age increased." These results were supported by van Herp et al.,[43] who used a computerized three-dimensional system to examine lumbar flexion, extension, lateral flexion, and rotation in 100 subjects with ages ranging from 20 to 77 years. The authors found a consistent reduction in motion with each decade of life and reported that "a clear trend of reducing motion with age in both male and female is apparent." Also using a computerized system to measure lumbar flexion, extension, lateral flexion, and rotation, McGregor et al.[44] examined 203 subjects. Results indicated that age had "an influence on motion with a gradual reduction seen with each decade."

Trudelle-Jackson et al.[45] divided 766 subjects (mean age 52.13 years ±13) into three groups: young 20–39 years ($n = 126$), middle 40–59 ($n = 412$), and older 60+ ($n = 228$). The groups were measured for lumbar flexion and extension. Results indicated that both lumbar flexion and extension ROM were significantly greater in the young group than in middle and older, and no difference was found between the middle and older groups.

After examining flexion (using a tape measure), extension (using a goniometer), and lateral flexion (using a goniometer) in 172 primarily male subjects (only four subjects were female) between the ages of 20 and 82 years, Fitzgerald et al.[46] reported that lumbar motion decreased across the age span, with the difference being statistically significant at 20-year intervals. In reporting similar results after measuring flexion (with a tape measure), extension (with a goniometer), and lateral flexion (with a goniometer) in 109 females, Einkauf et al.[47] described significant differences between the two youngest decades (ages 20–29 and ages 30–39) and the two oldest decades (ages 60–69 and ages 70–84). Additionally, Einkauf et al.[47] reported that extension showed the greatest decrease in motion with increasing age. Declines in flexion and extension ROM appear to be more marked in older adults (60–85) with persistent low back pain and have been correlated with decreased performance on repeated chair rise and timed up and go tests.[48] Table 2.3 provides information on normative data related to lumbar ROM with increased age derived from the research by Fitzgerald et al.[46] and Einkauf et al.[47]

Table 2.3	NORMATIVE RANGE OF MOTION OF THORACIC AND LUMBAR SPINE USING THE TAPE MEASURE (FLEXION ONLY) AND GONIOMETER (EXTENSION AND LATERAL FLEXION): AGE 40–80+ YEARS									
	SAMPLE SIZE		**FLEXION, CM**		**EXTENSION, DEGREES**		**RIGHT LATERAL FLEXION, DEGREES**		**LEFT LATERAL FLEXION, DEGREES**	
AGE, YEARS	**A**	**B**	**A**	**B**	**A**	**B**	**A**	**B**	**A**	**B**
40–49	16	17	3 (±0.8)	6 (±1.0)	31 (±9)	21 (±8)	27 (±7)	29 (±5)	29 (±5)	28 (±7)
50–59	44	15	3 (±1.0)	6 (±1.0)	27 (±8)	22 (±7)	25 (±6)	31 (±6)	26 (±6)	28 (±5)
60–69	27	16	2 (±0.7)	5 (±1.0)	17 (±8)	19 (±5)	20 (±5)	24 (±8)	20 (±5)	22 (±6)
70–84	9	15	2 (±0.7)	5 (±1.0)	17 (±9)	18 (±4)	18 (±5)	24 (±4)	19 (±6)	20 (±4)

A = Measurement of flexion with use of the Schober technique; all other measurements obtained via goniometer (Fitzgerald et al.[46]).
B = Measurement of flexion with use of the modified Schober; all other measurements obtained via goniometer (Einkauf et al.[47]).

Cervical Spine and Temporomandibular Joint

Although inconsistencies related to the effects of aging on joint ROM in other joints may exist, agreement is noted in the literature that ROM of the cervical spine decreases in aging adults. Using an inclinometer attached by straps to the head and under the chin, Kuhlman[49] compared a group of 20- to 30-year-old subjects ($n=31$) with a group of 70- to 90-year-old individuals ($n=42$) for cervical flexion, extension, lateral flexion (right and left measured separately), and rotation (right and left measured separately). The authors reported that "the elderly group had significantly less motion than the younger group for all six motions measured." The authors reported that the loss of motion was greatest for cervical extension and least for cervical flexion.[49] Furthermore, Peolsson et al.[50] reported similar results to the study by Kuhlman[49] in that the decrease in ROM was most pronounced in extension. These findings are further supported in a study by McKay et al.[5] where the authors demonstrated a more pronounced decline in cervical extension as compared to cervical flexion in older adults (60–101 years) when compared to adults (20–59 years).

In a study of 25 men (mean age 73.32 ± 5.88 years) and 61 women (mean age 73.07 ± 6.16 years), Kalscheur et al.[51] compared the range of cervical flexion, extension, left and right lateral deviation, and left and right rotation in this group to normative data provided by the AAOS.[52] Results indicated that significant decreases in ROM were found with aging compared with established norms for cervical extension, left lateral flexion, and right rotation.

A review of the literature revealed several studies that supported the conclusions reported by Kuhlman.[49] Five studies used the cervical ROM (CROM) device to examine the changes in cervical motion that occur with age. Examining combined flexion/extension, combined right/left lateral flexion, and combined right/left rotation in 90 subjects with an age range of 21–60 years, Nilsson[53] reported that results revealed "significant differences between ROM in different age groups for all directions of movement, in the sense that ROM decreased with increasing age."

After examining change with age in 84 subjects ranging in age from 20 to 69 years, Hole et al.[54] reported that cervical ROM in all planes decreased significantly, and "an individual can be expected to lose about 3.8 degrees and 6.9 degrees in cervical flexion and extension, respectively, per decade." Both Peolsson et al.[50] (101 subjects; aged 25–63 years) and Castro et al.[55] (157 subjects; aged 20–89 years) reported that cervical ROM decreased with increasing age. Wood and Sosnoff[56] (57 subjects; $n=20$ aged 18–30 years, $n=23$ aged 60–74, and $n=14$ aged 75–89) also demonstrated statistically significant decreases in active and passive cervical flexion, extension, and lateral flexion ROM with age. Additionally, those in the old-old group (age 75–89) continued to demonstrate significant losses in cervical extension passive ROM when compared to the young-old group (age 60–74).[56]

Also using CROM to examine cervical flexion, extension, lateral flexion, and rotation in subjects categorized in 10-year increments across eight decades, Youdas et al.[57] examined 337 individuals ranging in age from 11 to 97 years. The authors concluded that males and females should expect a loss of 3 to 5 degrees for all cervical ranges of motion per 10-year increase in age—similar to the amount of loss of motion reported by Hole et al.[54] Table 2.4 provides the only published data on normative ranges of motion related to cervical motion with increased age.

Two studies in which similar three-dimensional devices were used to measure cervical ROM also divided subjects into categories of 10-year intervals. Examining 150 subjects for combined flexion/extension, combined right/left lateral flexion, and combined right/left rotation from age 20 to "older than 60 years," Dvorak et al.[58] reported that ROM decreased as age increased, "with the most dramatic decrease in ROM occurring between the 30–39th and 40–49th decades." Similarly, Trott et al.[59] examined cervical flexion, extension, lateral flexion (right and left measured separately), and rotation (right and left measured separately) in 120 subjects aged 20–59 years and reported that "age had a significant effect on all the primary movements."

Grouping subjects ranging in age from 12 to 79 years into seven groups by age using 10-year increments

Table 2.4	NORMATIVE RANGE OF MOTION OF CERVICAL SPINE USING CERVICAL RANGE OF MOTION DEVICE (CROM): AGE 40–97 (YOUDAS[57])					
AGE, YEARS	FLEXION, DEGREES	EXTENSION, DEGREES	LEFT LATERAL FLEXION, DEGREES	RIGHT LATERAL FLEXION, DEGREES	LEFT ROTATION, DEGREES	RIGHT ROTATION, DEGREES
40–49	50 (±11)	70 (±13)	38 (±9)	40 (±10)	63 (±8)	67 (±8)
50–59	46 (±9)	63 (±13)	35 (±6)	36 (±6)	60 (±9)	61 (±8)
60–69	41 (±8)	61 (±12)	32 (±6)	31 (±8)	58 (±8)	59 (±9)
70–79	39 (±9)	54 (±12)	26 (±8)	27 (±7)	50 (±8)	52 (±10)
80–89	40 (±9)	50 (±13)	23 (±7)	25 (±6)	49 (±10)	50 (±9)
90–97	36 (±10)	53 (±18)	24 (±7)	22 (±8)	49 (±12)	48 (±12)

($n = 70$), Lind et al.[60] reported that radiographic examination indicated that "the motion in all three planes (flexion/extension, lateral flexion, and rotation) decreased with age." This decrease was significant and began in the third decade. Additionally, results reported by Lind et al.[60] were consistent with a report by Kuhlman[49] that "in the sagittal plane, extension motion decreased more than motion in flexion."

An investigation by Mayer et al.[61] was the only study to report that no age-related differences occurred in the measurement of cervical flexion, extension, lateral flexion (right and left measured separately), and rotation (right and left measured separately) when a double-inclinometer method was used. However, a review of the study's procedures indicated that the authors compared the youngest 50% of subjects with the oldest 50% of subjects ($n = 58$). Although the age range of subjects was reported as 17–62 years, no data were provided as to the mean age of each group. Therefore, the mean age of each group compared in this study is unknown, and any conclusions of this study are unclear.

Thurnwald[62] evaluated active ROM of the temporomandibular joint (TMJ) in 100 asymptomatic subjects with calipers. In comparing a group of 50 (25 male, 25 female) subjects aged 17–25 years vs 50 subjects (equal numbers of males and females) aged 50–65 years, the author reported that the older group had a significant decrease in ROM for mandible depression, protraction, right lateral deviation, and left lateral deviation. The author concluded that the TMJ "behaves in a similar manner to other synovial joints with increasing age." Mezitis et al.[63] also compared the effects of age on mouth opening in 1100 healthy adults (500 male, 600 female) between the ages of 18 and 70 years. After dividing subjects into age groups by decade between the ages of 20 and 70, the authors reported that the significantly greatest maximal opening was seen in those of younger age, whereas the significantly smallest maximal opening was recorded in those of older age.

DIFFERENCES IN RANGE OF MOTION BASED ON SEX

Lower Extremity

The amount of ROM present in the joints of males and females appears to differ but not with respect to all joints. However, in almost all cases cited, the greater ROM is found in the female population. Bell and Hoshizaki[64] compared 124 females to 66 males ranging in age from 18 to 88 years for differences in ROM at 17 joint actions at the hip, knee, and ankle and reported that "females have greater range of motion in joint action than their males counterparts throughout life."

In a study of 60 college-age subjects in which the influences of hip position and gender on hip rotation were investigated, females demonstrated a statistically greater range of active hip medial and lateral rotation compared with males.[65] Similar differences between the sexes regarding the range of available hip rotation were reported by James and Parker[11] in a sample of elderly (ages 70–92) males and females, and Sankar et al.[66] reported greater lateral rotation range of motion in females compared with males when studying subjects in the 11- to 17-year-old age group. However, multiple other investigators have reported statistically significant differences only in hip medial rotation between adult males and females. Increased medial, but not lateral, hip rotation in females has been reported by Walker et al.[6] in a study of 60 male and female subjects aged 60–84 years. Likewise, in studies of NCAA Division I athletes[67] and in individuals with symptoms of early osteoarthritis,[68] consistently greater medial, but not lateral, rotation of the hip was found in female as compared to male subjects. Similar results were reported by Svenningsen et al.,[69] who studied 761 Norwegian subjects ranging in age from 4 years to adulthood (the 20s). Other motions of the hip that have been reported as being increased in females compared with males are hip flexion in adolescents,[66,69] adults,[68,69] and elderly females (aged 70–92 years)[11] and hip abduction in children,[69] adolescents,[66,69] and young adults,[69] and hip adduction and extension in adolescents.[66]

Two studies of older adults[6,11] have reported a statistically increased range of knee flexion in female compared with male subjects. However, in one study, the difference did not exceed the interrater error for that measurement.[6] A greater amount of ankle plantarflexion also appears to be present in females compared with males in children[70] and across all adult age groups.[6,11,71,72] Conversely, there appears to be some indication that ankle dorsiflexion ROM becomes significantly greater in males than in females among persons older than 70 years.[71]

Upper Extremity

Some motions of the upper extremity also appear to differ according to sex. Barnes et al.[27] examined 280 subjects between the ages of 4 and 70 years and found that female subjects had a greater shoulder ROM than men at all ages, with the greatest difference occurring in abduction and medial and lateral rotation.[27] Three studies of adults over the age of 60 demonstrated significantly more shoulder flexion in females than in their male counterparts,[6,29,31] and both Fiebert et al.[31] and Walker et al.[6] reported statistically higher amounts of shoulder abduction in females compared with males aged 60 and older. In contrast, two separate studies have reported statistically higher shoulder range of motion in males than in females. In a large community cohort study that involved over 2400 subjects from age 20 to 85+, males were found overall to have more active shoulder abduction and flexion than females.[34] In another study in which shoulder abduction was measured (this one involving 894 subjects over the age of 65), results revealed that females had less shoulder ROM than men.[28] In the sample presented, about 50% of subjects were over the age of 78, and the authors speculated that functional use of the shoulder may have differed between males and females, with older males possessing increased function and therefore increased ROM compared with females.[28]

Greater shoulder rotation in females has been reported by several investigators. Kalscheur et al.[51] examined 86 subjects over the age of 62 years and reported higher shoulder range of motion in females compared with males, including medial and lateral rotation. In a study of 720 adult subjects from Sweden and Iceland,[73] significantly greater ranges of shoulder medial and lateral rotation were reported in females compared with males. These differences in shoulder lateral, but not medial, rotation were substantiated in a group of subjects aged 40–59 years[33], in a group of older subjects[6], and in a large community cohort study.[34] Conversely, two studies involving older subjects reported higher medial, but not lateral, rotation in females compared with males.[31,32]

Differences in elbow and forearm ROM between male and female subjects have been demonstrated in several studies. Three studies examined similar age groups in older adults (55–84 years, 60–84 years, and 62 years and older), and all reported a significantly increased amount of elbow flexion in female compared with male subjects.[6,51,74] Two studies also reported a significantly greater amount of elbow extension in female subjects.[6,36] Studies of younger subjects, adults,[36,75] and children[76] also have demonstrated more elbow flexion range of motion in females than in males, although the differences revealed in the pediatric population were deemed clinically insignificant.[76]

Forearm rotation has been reported to be higher in females than in males at all ages. Two studies, each involving several hundred healthy individuals from young to older adulthood, reported significantly higher amounts of forearm pronation and supination in women compared with men.[35,36] The difference in forearm pronation, but not supination, was substantiated in a study of adults aged 62 and older.[51] The lack of difference in forearm supination between older men and women may be due to a finding demonstrating declines in forearm rotation ROM two decades earlier in females than in males.[35]

Wrist and hand motions also appear to differ in male compared with female subjects. Allander et al.[26] reported significantly higher ranges of wrist flexion and extension in female than in male adults. A study of 750 white adults aged 18–65 years demonstrated significantly increased wrist flexion, extension, radial deviation, and ulnar deviation in female compared with male subjects.[37] Increased wrist extension and adduction (ulnar

deviation) in females, but not increased wrist flexion, were reported in a sample of older adults.[6] In a study of 120 young adults (aged 18–35 years), Mallon et al.[77] demonstrated increased active and passive extension at all joints of the fingers (metacarpophalangeal, proximal interphalangeal, and distal interphalangeal) in female subjects compared with males. In contrast, De Smet et al.[78] reported no significant differences in the range of motion of females and males for the metacarpophalangeal and interphalangeal joints of the thumb.[78] Details of studies undertaken to investigate differences in ROM according to sex are found in Appendix B.

Lumbar Spine

Only two studies have investigated the differences between males and females in ROM of the lumbar spine before adulthood. Using a tape measure to measure flexion and lateral flexion, Haley et al.[79] compared 142 females vs 140 males between the ages of 5 and 9 years and reported that girls were significantly more flexible than boys. Conversely, van Adrichem and van der Korst[38] used a tape measure to measure lumbar flexion in children between the ages of 6 and 18 years and reported that no significant difference was discerned between boys (n = 149) and girls (n = 149).

Differences in lumbar ROM between the sexes in older subjects remain unclear. Macrae and Wright[80] also used a tape measure to measure lumbar flexion but in an older (aged 18–71 years) sample of 195 females and 147 males. The authors reported that regardless of age, males had significantly greater lumbar flexion than females. This result of males possessing greater lumbar flexion (and extension) ROM than females was supported by McGregor et al.[44] (103 males, 100 females; aged 20–70 years) and Troke et al.[39] (196 females, 209 males; aged 16–90 years) for young subjects. However, both of these studies reported that with increased age, no difference in lumbar ROM was noted between the sexes.

Greater flexion in males than in females was supported in a later study by Moll and Wright,[41] who compared the differences between 119 males and 118 females, also using a tape measure. In addition, Moll and Wright[41] reported that males had greater lumbar mobility than females for extension but that females had greater motion for lateral flexion than males. The opposite was reported by Sullivan et al.[42] who, after comparing flexion and extension in 686 males and 440 females between the ages of 15 and 65 years, reported that males had greater flexion ROM than females and that females had greater extension ROM than males. In contrast, when comparing lumbar ROM in 50 males and 50 females ranging in age from 20 to 60 years, van Herp et al.[43] reported "consistently greater flexibility in males than in females throughout the age range" and in all movements.

When examining the differences in lumbar rotation related to sex, Boline et al.[81] compared the amount of lumbar rotation in 14 males with the amount of rotation in 11 females and reported that no significant difference existed between males and females in terms of right and left rotation. This equality of lumbar rotation between the sexes at all ages was supported in the study by Troke et al.[39]

Lumbar Spine—Summary

In summary, no clear answer exists as to which sex has greater lumbar ROM. At all ages, and in both sexes, a wide range of lumbar mobility appears to exist.

Cervical Spine

Lind et al.[60] radiographically examined cervical ROM in 35 male and 35 female subjects. Using three measurement devices (CROM device, radiography, and a computerized tracking system), Ordway et al.[82] examined 20 subjects (11 female, 9 male) for cervical flexion and extension. The authors of both studies reported that no significant differences were found between males and females with any of the measurement devices.

No significant difference between males and females in terms of cervical flexion, extension, lateral flexion, and rotation was reported by Hole et al.[54] (44 males, 40 females; aged 20–69 years) and Peolsson et al.[50] (51 males, 50 females; aged 25–63 years). Similar results were found by Castro et al.[55] with one variation. No significant differences in cervical flexion, extension, lateral flexion, and rotation were found between men and women between the ages of 20 to 69. However, women older than 70 years had significantly greater mobility in all movements of the cervical spine compared with men.

In a study by Kalscheur et al.,[51] 25 men (mean age 73.32 ± 5.88 years) and 61 women (mean age 73.07 ± 6.16 years) were measured for cervical flexion, extension, left and right lateral deviation, and left and right rotation. Women had statistically significant greater ROM only for extension and left lateral flexion.

Mayer et al.[61] used the double-inclinometer method to compare the cervical ROM of 28 males (aged 17–61 years) vs that of 30 females (aged 19–62 years) and reported that, regardless of age, the only sex-specific difference in ROM occurred in cervical extension; the authors reported that females possessed greater ROM than males. No significant sex-related differences were found for cervical flexion, lateral flexion, and rotation.

Using an inclinometer attached to the top of the head with a head adapter and an adjustable headband and cloth chinstrap, Kuhlman[49] reported that "females had higher mean cervical range of motion than males for all cervical motion examined." In actuality, these differences between males and females were statistically significant

only for cervical extension, lateral flexion (right and left), and rotation (right and left); no significant difference related to sex was found for cervical flexion.

Nilsson[53] used the CROM device to compare 59 females vs 31 males with an age range of 20–60 years. Although the author concluded that differences were found between males and females, the results indicated that ROM for lateral flexion (right and left total lateral flexion combined) was the only motion for which females had a statistically greater range than males. Results of statistical analyses comparing males and females in terms of cervical flexion/extension (combined) and rotation (left and right total rotation combined) were not reported. Youdas et al.[57] also used the CROM device, comparing cervical ROM between 171 females and 166 males ranging in age from 11 to 97 years. The authors concluded that across all ages, females had a greater range of motion than males for all cervical motions.

Using a three-dimensional recording of cervical motion made with a computer-integrated electrogoniometric device, Trott et al.[59] examined differences in ROM between 60 males and 60 females. Results of this study revealed "a gender difference in cervical range of motion that was reported at all decades, where women had a larger range of motion in all cardinal planes than men."

Using a measurement device similar to the one used by Trott et al.,[59] Dvorak et al.[58] measured three-dimensional motion of the cervical spine using computer-integrated potentiometers. When comparing cervical ROM in 86 males and 64 females ranging in age from 20 to "older than 60" years, they found that within each decade, females showed a significantly greater range than did males for all cervical motions.

Cervical Spine—Summary

Results of studies that compared the cervical ROM of males with that of females are not as consistent as those of investigations related to changes that occur in cervical ROM with advancing age. However, although reports are inconsistent as to whether a difference exists between the cervical ROM of males vs that of females, a review of the literature indicates that no study has reported that males have a greater cervical ROM than females. In other words, the investigations related to cervical ROM that were reviewed reported that no difference in ROM existed between sexes or that females had a greater ROM than males.

Temporomandibular Joint

In the study by Thurnwald[62] described previously, 50 males were compared with 50 females in terms of temporomandibular (TMJ) ROM. The author reported that males had larger ranges of mandibular depression and right lateral deviation than females, but no differences were found between the sexes in terms of protraction and left lateral deviation. The results of this study were similar to those reported by Agerberg,[83] who reported that maximal opening was significantly greater in males ($n = 102$) than in females ($n = 103$), but no difference between the sexes was evident in terms of lateral movement left and right and protrusions (the mean age of both groups was 20.5 years; range, 18–25 years). The finding that males have greater TMJ motion than females has been supported by other studies. Lewis et al.[84] reported a difference in mandibular opening between groups of 29 asymptomatic males (aged 23–39 years) and 27 asymptomatic females (aged 23–35 years). In addition to examining changes in mouth opening across age, Mezitis et al.[63] compared maximal opening between males and females in the same 1100 healthy adult subjects presented previously. The authors reported that the maximal opening for males was significantly greater than for females. A unique study by Pullinger et al.[85] that examined 21 men and 22 women (mean age, 24.7 years; range, 21–32 years) adjusted the amount of opening for body size. After adjustment, the authors reported that the amount of opening was the same for men and women.

DIFFERENCES IN RANGE OF MOTION BASED ON CULTURE AND RECREATIONAL ACTIVITIES

Differences in ROM among individuals have been attributed both to culture and to occupation. Range of motion of lower extremity joints has been shown to be significantly increased in populations of Chinese and Saudi Arabian subjects compared with British and Scandinavian subjects, respectively.[73,86] All lower extremity joint motions, with the exception of hip adduction, were reported to be significantly greater in a group of 50 Saudi Arabian males when their mean ROMs were compared with those of a group of 105 males of the same age group from Sweden.[87] Higher ranges of hip flexion, abduction, medial rotation, and lateral rotation were reported in a group of 500 Chinese

subjects over the age of 54 years, compared with values for hip ROM in British adults.[86] In both instances in which cultural differences in ROM were noted, the authors were unable to define the cause of the differences. Suppositions between the studies included biologic differences such as capsular laxity; differences in activities of daily living, as many individuals in China and Saudi Arabia squat and kneel routinely during daily activities; and differences in measurement techniques.[83,86]

In a study comparing lumbar flexion and extension range of motion in 619 white individuals to 147 African American individuals (mean age = 52.13 ± 13 years), Trudelle-Jackson et al.[45] examined the differences in range of motion due to race. The authors reported lumbar extension range of motion of the African American group was significantly greater than the white group. No differences in race were found for lumbar flexion range of motion.

Recreational activities also appear to be related to changes in ROM at various joints. Shoulder motion, particularly rotation but also abduction, has been reported as differing from normal values in certain athletes. Tables 2.5 and 2.6 present several studies reporting that when shoulder ROM in the dominant (throwing) arm of baseball players (pitchers and nonpitchers) is compared with that of the nondominant (nonthrowing) arm, lateral rotation is increased and medial rotation is decreased.[88,90–104] Conflicting reports exist regarding whether total range of shoulder rotation is statistically different in the two extremities.[92,97] Increased lateral rotation of the shoulder also was found when the ROM of baseball pitchers was compared with that of nonpitchers[90,91,98,105,106] (Table 2.7).

Similar patterns of difference in shoulder ROM have been reported in racket ball, tennis, and volleyball players.[107–120] A trend toward increased shoulder lateral rotation and decreased shoulder medial rotation in the dominant arm compared with the nondominant arm has been reported. Studies reporting on shoulder ROM in tennis players are presented in Table 2.8, and those reporting on shoulder ROM in volleyball players are presented in Table 2.9.

Table 2.5 **SHOULDER ROM IN BASEBALL PITCHERS (DOMINANT VS NONDOMINANT)**				
STUDY	**SAMPLE SIZE**	**AGE**	**LR AT 90° ABD**	**MR AT 90° ABD**
Borsa et al.[88]	93 Pitchers	25.1 ± 3.3 years	↑	↓
Borsa et al.[89]	34 Pitchers	24.4 ± 3.7 years	↑	↓
Brown et al.[90]	18 Pitchers	$\bar{X} = 27.02 \pm 4.25$ years	↑	↓
Crockett et al.[91]	25 Pitchers	18–35 years	↑	↓
Ellenbecker et al.[92]	46 Pitchers	22.6 ± 2.0 years	↑	↓
Hurd et al.[93]	210 Pitchers	16 ± 1.1 years	↑	↓
Osbahr et al.[94]	19 Pitchers	$\bar{X} = 19.0$ years (18–21 years)	↑	↓
Sethi et al.[95]	37 Pitchers	18–22 years	↑	↓
Sueyoshi et al.[96]	41 Pitchers	14.9 ± 2.6 years	↑	↓
Wilk et al.[97]	122 Pitchers	25.6 ± 4.1 years	↑	↓

ABD, Abduction; *LR,* lateral rotation; *MR,* medial rotation; ↑, significantly increased in dominant arm compared with nondominant arm; ↓, significantly decreased in dominant arm compared with nondominant arm.

Table 2.6 SHOULDER ROM IN BASEBALL PLAYERS (DOMINANT VS NONDOMINANT)				
STUDY	**SAMPLE SIZE**	**AGE**	**LR AT 90° ABD**	**MR AT 90° ABD**
Bigliani et al.[98]	148 baseball players	$\bar{X}$ = 22.8 years (16–28 years)	↑	↓
Baltaci et al.[99]	38 baseball players	18–21 years	↑	↓
Reagan et al.[100]	54 baseball players	18–22 years	↑	↓
Downar and Sauers[101]	27 baseball players	$\bar{X}$ = 20.0 ± 1.6 years	↑	↓
Meister et al.[102]	294 baseball players	8–16 years	↑	↓
Chant et al.[103]	19 baseball players	$\bar{X}$ = 23.4 ± 1.4 years	↑	↓
Schilling et al.[104]	50 baseball players	$\bar{X}$ = 19.3 ± 1.0 years	↑	↓

ABD, Abduction; *LR,* lateral rotation; *MR,* medial rotation; $\bar{X}$, mean; ↑, significantly increased in dominant arm compared with nondominant arm; ↓, significantly decreased in dominant arm compared with nondominant arm.

Table 2.7 SHOULDER ROM—DIFFERENCES BETWEEN PITCHER VS NONPITCHER				
STUDY	**SAMPLE SIZE**	**AGE**	**LR AT 90° ABD**	**MR AT 90° ABD**
Brown et al.[90]	18 pitchers; 23 position players	$\bar{X}$ = 27.02 ± 4.25	↑	No diff
Johnson[105]	32 pitchers; 26 position players	$\bar{X}$ = 20.4 ± 1.4 years (16–28 years)	↑	No diff
Bigliani et al.[99]	72 pitchers; 76 position players	$\bar{X}$ = 20.4	↑	↓
Crockett et al.[91]	25 pitchers; 25 nonathletes	18–35 years	↑	No diff
Dodds et al.[106]	9 pitchers; 9 position players	$\bar{X}$ = 20.9 ± 1.2 years	No diff	No diff

ABD, Abduction; *LR,* lateral rotation; *MR,* medial rotation; *No diff,* no difference between pitchers and nonpitchers, $\bar{X}$, mean; ↑, significantly increased in pitchers compared with nonpitchers; ↓, significantly decreased in pitchers compared with nonpitchers.

Table 2.8 SHOULDER ROM IN TENNIS PLAYERS (DOMINANT VS NONDOMINANT)				
STUDY	**SAMPLE SIZE**	**AGE**	**LR AT 90° ABD**	**MR AT 90° ABD**
Chandler et al.[108]	86 (20 F, 66 M)	15.4 years (12–22 years)	↑	↓
Chinn et al.[109]	30 F	14–31 years	No diff	↓
Chinn et al.[109]	53 M	18–50 years	↑	↓
Ellenbecker et al.[110]	203 (90 F, 113 M)	14–21 years	No diff	↓
		11–17 years		
Ellenbecker et al.[92]	117 M	16.4 ± 1.6 years	No diff	↓
Kibler et al.[111]	39*		↑	↓
Schmidt-Wietnof et al.[112]	27 M	26.5 years (19–33 years)	↑	↓
Chiang et al.[114]	21 F	14.9 ± 1.5 years (12.8–17.4 years)	No diff	↓
Nutt et al.[115]	122 (62 F, 122 M)	11–24 years	↑	↓
Cigercioglu et al.[116]	42 (21 F, 21 M)	11.3 ± 1.2 years (10–14 years)	↑	↓
Gillet et al.[117]	91 M	8–15 years	↑	↓

ABD, Abduction; *LR,* lateral rotation; *MR,* medial rotation; *No diff,* no difference between dominant and nondominant arm; ↑, significantly increased in dominant arm compared with nondominant arm; ↓, significantly decreased in dominant arm compared with nondominant arm.
*20 men and 19 women: statistical analysis showed no difference in ROM between sexes, so data were collapsed into 39.

Table 2.9 SHOULDER ROM IN VOLLEYBALL PLAYERS (DOMINANT VS NONDOMINANT)				
STUDY	**SAMPLE SIZE**	**AGE**	**LR AT 90° ABD**	**MR AT 90° ABD**
Forthomme et al.[120]	66 (32 F, 34 M)	24 ± 5 years	↑	↓
Harput et al.[119]	39 (17 F, 22 M)	16 ± 1.4 years	↑	↓
Saccol et al.[118]	14 F	18.5 ± 1.09 years	↑	↓
	19 M	18.57 ± 1.42 years	No diff	↓

Shoulder ROM in swimmers[113,121,122] and in javelin throwers[123] has been investigated. At this time, the research does not show a consistent pattern of ROM changes in the population of these athletes, as has been reported in baseball and tennis players. However, there is some evidence that both shoulder internal rotation and total ROM is decreased in the dominant, compared with the nondominant, arm in competitive swimmers.[122]

At least seven studies have compared ROM of the lower extremity in dancers and nondancers.[124–130] Results of these studies are presented in Table 2.10.

							PLANTAR	
Table 2.10	**LOWER EXTREMITY RANGE OF MOTION—DANCERS VS NONDANCERS**							
STUDY	**ABDUCTION**	**ADDUCTION**	**EXTENSION**	**FLEXION**	**LR**	**MR**	**FLEXION**	**DORSIFLEXION**
Reid et al.[127]	↑	↓	↑	↑	↑	↓		
Hamilton et al.[125]	↑	↓	–	↑	↑	↓		
Khan et al.[126]	–	–	–	–	↑	↓		
Steinberg et al.[128]	↑	–	↑	No diff	↑	No diff		
Alfuth et al.[129]	↑	No diff	↑	↑	–	–	↑	↑
Cho et al.[130]	–	–	–	–	–	–	↑	↓

LR, Lateral rotation; *MR*, medial rotation; *No diff*, no difference between dancers and nondancers; ↑, significantly increased in dancers compared with nondancers; ↓, significantly decreased in dancers compared with nondancers; –, not measured in the study.

Although results varied across the studies, the dancers consistently showed significantly higher ranges of ankle plantarflexion and several hip motions than nondancers.

FACTORS AFFECTING MUSCLE LENGTH

CHANGES IN MUSCLE LENGTH WITH AGE

Although several previous reports examined changes in ROM with age, studies that investigated muscle length using direct measurement (defined in Chapter 1) are relatively uncommon. Of those studies that examined changes in muscle length using direct measurement, the muscles most commonly examined were the hamstrings. Therefore, this section and the section on changes in muscle length based on sex will report only available information on hamstring muscles.

Youdas et al.[131] measured hamstring muscle flexibility in a large sample of 214 adults (108 women and 106 men) ranging in age from 20 to 79 years. The authors reported no significant changes in hamstring muscle length as age increased.

CHANGES IN MUSCLE LENGTH BASED ON SEX

In the Youdas et al.[131] study previously described, the authors compared hamstring muscle length between 108 females and 106 males. They reported that the female hamstring muscles were significantly more flexible than those of males—by 8 degrees with the straight leg method of measurement and by 10 degrees with the passive knee extension test. Similar results were obtained by Corkery et al.,[132] who examined 47 females and 25 males—all of college age (mean age, 20 years). The authors reported a significant difference between male and female hamstring muscle length, with females having 12 degrees more hamstring flexibility than males when the active knee extension test was used.

RELIABILITY AND VALIDITY

RELIABILITY

The usefulness of a measurement device for the examination of a patient's ROM and muscle length depends on the extent to which the device can be used by the clinician to accurately perform the activity, called reliability. Throughout this text, information is presented on the reliability of the various techniques described. Reliability refers to whether or not the same trait can be measured consistently on repeated measurements. In other words, reliability is "the extent to which measurements are repeatable."[133]

To establish reliability for a measurement device, a test-retest design is frequently used. With the use of a test-retest design, a sample of subjects is measured on two occasions, with all testing variables kept as constant as possible during each test session. For example, if the reliability of the goniometer to measure knee flexion is to be tested, knee flexion ROM would be measured on two (or more) occasions. The goniometer would be considered reliable if the ROM measurements of knee flexion taken on the two occasions were similar.

Frequently, a clinical measurement requires the observation of a human observer, or a rater. Two types of reliability are important when one is dealing with clinical measurement: intrarater reliability and interrater reliability. Intrarater reliability is "the consistency with which one rater assigns scores to a single set of responses on two [or more] separate occasions."[133] To return to the example of measuring knee flexion ROM, a check of intrarater reliability would involve one tester, or rater, who examines knee flexion ROM in 30 individuals on two occasions and compares the results. Information obtained from this study would indicate whether the rater is reliable within (intra-) himself or herself.

Interrater reliability refers to the "consistency of performances among different raters or judges in assigning scores to the same objects or responses... determined when two or more raters judge the performance of one group of subjects at the same point in time."[133]

An example of interrater reliability is seen when two testers, or raters, measure knee flexion ROM on 30 individuals on one occasion and compare the results. Interrater reliability is especially important if more than one clinician is going to be measuring ROM of a particular patient.

Quantification

For quantification of reliability, both the relationship and the agreement between repeated measurements must be examined. Domholdt[133] referred to assessment of the relationship between repeated measurements as assessing relative reliability and examination of the magnitude of the difference between repeated measurements as assessing absolute reliability.

Relative Reliability

Relative reliability "is based on the idea that if a measurement is reliable, individual measurements within a group will maintain their position within the group on repeated measurements."[133] For example, an individual with a large amount of shoulder ROM on an initial measurement compared with a sample would be expected to have a large amount of ROM compared with a sample on subsequent measurements.

The statistic most commonly used to analyze relative reliability of measurement is the correlation coefficient. The assumption is that relative reliability is established if the paired measurements correlate highly. A method commonly used to interpret the correlation coefficient and, therefore, the reliability of the measurement is to examine the strength of the relationship. Correlation coefficients range from −1.0 to +1.0; a perfect positive relationship (+1.0) indicates that a higher value on one variable is associated with a higher value on the second variable.[133]

For correlations to be used as reliability coefficients, the values assume scores between 0 and 1.0. Reliability is rarely perfect; therefore, correlation coefficients of 1.0 are rare. A review of the literature related to the measurement of ROM and muscle length reveals that several authors suggest that in order to achieve acceptable reliability, a correlation of at least 0.80 is necessary.[111,134–137]

The Pearson product-moment correlation (referred to as Pearson's r) has been used traditionally to analyze the strength of the correlation and, hence, its reliability. However, the Pearson correlation is limited because although it is appropriate for measuring the association between two variables (relative reliability), it cannot measure agreement between the two variables (absolute reliability).[133]

Absolute Reliability

The Pearson correlation coefficient provides only information regarding the relative reliability of a measurement.

Information about the variability of a score with repeated measurements that is caused by measurement error also is important in the assessment of reliability of ROM and muscle length tests. Reliability should examine not only the consistency of the rank of the score, but also the degree of similarity between repeated scores. This consistency between scores (also referred to as agreement) is referred to as absolute reliability.[133]

One method that can be used to accommodate the fact that the Pearson correlation does not measure absolute reliability is to supplement the information obtained with the Pearson correlation with follow-up testing. Several tests are used to determine absolute reliability; two of the most common of these are the paired t-test and the standard error of the measurement (SEMm).

The *t*-Test

One way to extend the reliability analysis beyond the Pearson correlation in measuring relative reliability is to conduct a t-test. The t-test is the most basic standard procedure used to compare the difference between group means.[85,132] For example, suppose the goal of a study is to determine whether the measurement of knee flexion ROM using a goniometer is the same for Examiner #1 and Examiner #2 (intertester reliability). Each examiner measures 30 subjects. First, a Pearson correlation can be calculated to determine relative reliability for each tester. Second, each tester can obtain mean scores for each group and can perform a t-test to compare the two groups. If the t-test that is performed to compare the means of the two samples indicates a significant difference, researchers can conclude that the population means are different from one another. This significant difference between the two testers would call into question the intertester reliability. Conversely, if results of the t-test indicate that no significant difference exists, the researcher can assume that any difference between the two examiners occurred by chance and can conclude that agreement exists between the two examiners. For a more detailed discussion of the t-test, the reader is referred to texts written by Carter and Lubinsky[138] and by Portney and Watkins.[139]

Standard Error of the Measurement (SEMm)

A second way to examine for the absolute reliability of a measurement is to calculate the SEMm, defined as "the range in which a single subject's true score could be expected to lie when measurement error is considered."[140] In fact, Rothstein and Echternach[141] suggested that the SEMm is the "ideal statistic for estimating the error associated with reliability."

The SEMm is an estimate of the amount of error that would occur if repeated measurements were taken on the same subjects. Given that it is not practical to take repeated measurements 25 to 30 times to establish the actual SEMm, the value can be estimated from the following formula:

$$SEMm = SD - \sqrt{1-r}$$

where *SD* is the standard deviation, and *r* is the reliability coefficient. The more reliable a measure is, the smaller the errors would be, and the SEMm would be low. As indicated by the formula, the magnitude of the SEMm is directly related to the standard deviation (as the standard deviation decreases, the SEMm decreases) and is indirectly related to the correlation coefficient (as the correlation approaches 1.0, the SEMm approaches 0).[133,139]

The SEMm is based on the standard deviation and has properties similar to those of the standard deviation. Once the SEMm is calculated, it can be concluded that a repeated measurement would fall within 1 SEMm of the mean 68% of the time and within 2 SEMm of the mean 95% of the time. For example, if the mean value of the range of shoulder flexion obtained by an examiner who is measuring 30 individuals is 160 degrees and the SEMm is 2 degrees, then a 95% chance exists that the true value of shoulder flexion would fall between 156 and 164 degrees (2 SEMm above and below the mean). In this example, absolute reliability would be considered very good. If, on the other hand, data collected indicate a mean value of shoulder flexion of 160 degrees and an SEMm of 10 degrees, then a 95% chance exists that the true value of shoulder flexion would fall between 140 and 180 degrees. In this second example, absolute reliability would be in question because the amount of measurement error was so large. Again, both Portney and Watkins[139] and Domholdt[133] are excellent sources of more detailed information on the SEMm, as well as on statistical analysis in general.

Intraclass Correlation Coefficient (ICC)

Portney and Watkins[139] expressed concern about using both a Pearson correlation and a follow-up test because such analyses do not provide a single index by which to describe reliability. When a Pearson correlation and a follow-up test are used, "the scores may be consistent but significantly different, or they may be poorly correlated but not significantly different. How should these results be interpreted?" A correlation analysis that accounts for both absolute and relative reliability is the intraclass correlation coefficient (ICC), considered by some as the preferred correlation coefficient to be used when reliability is examined.[139] The ICC is calculated by using variance estimates obtained from an analysis of variance, thereby reflecting both relative and absolute reliability in one index. Domholdt[133] described the ICC as a "family of coefficients" that allows analysis of reliability with at least six different ICC formulas classified

by the use of two numbers in parentheses. Portney and Watkins[139] described three models of the ICC, with each model expressed in two possible forms (for a total of six), depending on whether the scores collected as part of a study are single ratings or mean ratings.

For a detailed discussion of the three models, the reader is referred to Portney and Watkins[139] For the purpose of this textbook, if "it is important to demonstrate that a particular measurement tool can be used with confidence by all clinicians, then Model 2 should be used. This approach [Model 2] is appropriate for clinical studies and methodological research, to document that a measurement tool has broad application."[139]

The various types of ICCs are classified by using two numbers in parentheses. The first number designates the model (1, 2, 3), and the second number indicates the form. If the form is to use a single measurement, the number is 1; if the form is the mean of more than one measurement, a constant (k) is used. For example, ICC (2, 1) indicates that model 2 is used with single measurement (not mean) scores.[139]

Responsiveness to Change

An instrument's responsiveness to change is important for instruments that are used to measure change over time. The smallest valid change in the score that is not due to random error is the minimal detectable change (MDC).[142] Values for the MDC provide the examiner with the ability to judge whether changes in scores at a later time point are due to actual changes in the patient (client) or are likely to be merely the result of random error from the measurement. Where available, the MDC for measurements of a single examiner are provided for each motion. All of the MCD values provided were calculated at the 95% confidence interval. Therefore, a 95% certainty exists that if the ROM is measured by the same person, changes in ROM measurements that exceed the MDC for the motion are the result of changes in the patient and not measurement error.

VALIDITY

A measurement instrument not only must be reliable, the device also must produce valid results. Domholdt[133] has defined validity as the "appropriateness, meaningfulness, and usefulness of the test scores." In other words, validity deals with whether an instrument is truly measuring what the device is intended to measure.

Several types of validity exist and are described in Box 2.1. For the purpose of determining the validity of measurements obtained with the devices presented in this text, the most appropriate type of validity is concurrent validity (a subcategory of criterion-related validity). For example, the gold standard for measurement of flexion of the spine can be considered the radiological examination. If measurement of flexion of

---

BOX 2.1	TYPES OF MEASUREMENT VALIDITY

Face validity: Indicates that an instrument appears to test what it is supposed to test; the weakest form of measurement validity

Content validity: Indicates that the items that make up an instrument adequately sample the universe of content that defines the variable being measured; most useful with questionnaires and inventories

Criterion-related validity: Indicates that the outcomes of one instrument, the target test, can be used as a substitute measure for an established gold standard criterion test; can be tested as concurrent or predictive validity

Concurrent validity: Establishes validity when two measures are taken at relatively the same time; most often used when the target test is considered more efficient than the gold standard and therefore can be used instead of the gold standard

Predictive validity: Establishes that the outcome of the target test can be used to predict a future criterion score or outcome

Prescriptive validity: Establishes that the interpretation of a measurement is appropriate for determining effective intervention

Construct validity: Establishes the ability of an instrument to measure an abstract construct and the degree to which the instrument reflects the theoretical components of the construct.

From Portney LG, Watkins MP. *Foundations of Clinical Research: Applications to Practice*. ed. 2, Upper Saddle River. NJ: Prentice-Hall; 2000.

the spine obtained with the use of an inclinometer is found to be consistent with the amount of flexion of the spine measured with an X-ray, validity is established, and the inclinometer can be said to measure what it was purported to measure (flexion of the spine). Of course, the validity of the measurement is dependent on the assumption that radiographic analysis of flexion of the spine is an accurate gold standard.

Quantification

Criterion-related validity can be quantified by using correlation coefficients and follow-up tests, as appropriate, similar to those described in the Reliability section of this chapter. The process of interpreting statistical analyses related to validity is the same as that used for interpreting the reliability coefficient.

RELIABILITY AND VALIDITY: CRITERION FOR INCLUSION

Subsequent chapters of this text describe techniques used for the measurement of range of joint motion and length of muscles of the extremities, spine, and TMJ. Additionally, Chapters 7, 10, and 15 present available information regarding the reliability and validity of these measurement techniques. The criterion for inclusion of an article in these chapters was that the study that examined reliability or validity had to provide an analysis of both relative and absolute reliability or validity. For example, if a Pearson correlation was performed (relative reliability) and no follow-up testing was performed for absolute reliability, the study was not included in the chapter, unless an exception for inclusion could be rationalized. Exceptions to this criterion included an

article that was the only study investigating a specific technique and a study that was the original study of a specific technique commonly used in the clinic.

On the other hand, if a Pearson correlation and follow-up analysis or an ICC was used, the study was included in these chapters. However, no interpretive comments are made on reliability or validity related to the information presented in these chapters. As an example, if in providing two indexes for reliability (i.e., a Pearson correlation and a *t*-test), contradictory views are presented, no interpretations are presented to clarify the results. Although presenting both indexes may cause confusion in interpretation of results, "uncertainty based on complete information is preferable to a sense of certainty based on incomplete information."[133]

These chapters on reliability and validity of measurement techniques are presented as a reference for readers who wish to possess the information needed to choose measurement devices and techniques best suited for their own clinical situations. Additionally, it is hoped that gaps in the literature on specific techniques or devices will stimulate much needed additional research in the area of measurement of joint ROM and muscle length.

References

1. American Academy of Orthopaedic Surgeons. *Committee for the Study of Joint Motion., and British Orthopaedic Association. Joint Motion: Method of Measuring and Recording.* Edinburgh: Published for the British Orthopaedic Association by Churchill-Livingstone; 1966:87.
2. Greene WB, Heckman JD. *The Clinical Measurement of Joint Motion.* Rosemont, IL: American Academy of Orthopaedic Surgeons; 1994.
3. American Medical Association. *Guides to the Evaluation of Permanent Impairment.* Chicago: American Medical Association; 1993:339.
4. Roach KE, Miles TP. Normal hip and knee active range of motion: the relationship to age. *Phys Ther.* 1991;71:656–665.

5. McKay MJ, Baldwin JN, Ferreira P, Simic M, Vanicek N, Burns J. Normative reference values for strength and flexibility of 1,000 children and adults. *Neurology.* 2017;88:36–43.

6. Walker JM, Sue D, Miles-Elkousy N, Ford G, Trevelyan H. Active mobility of the extremities in older subjects. *Phys Ther.* 1984;64:919–923.

7. Boone DC, Azen SP. Normal range of motion of joints in male subjects. *J Bone Joint Surg.* 1979;61:756–759.

8. Nonaka H, Mita K, Watakabe M, et al. Age-related changes in the interactive mobility of the hip and knee joints: a geometrical analysis. *Gait Posture.* 2002;15:236–243.

9. Macedo LG, Magee DJ. Effects of age on passive range of motion of selected peripheral joints in healthy adult females. *Physiother Theory Pract.* 2009;25:145–164.

10. Anderson DE, Madigan ML. Healthy older adults have insufficient hip range of motion and plantar flexor strength to walk like healthy young adults. *J Biomech.* 2014;47:1104–1109.

11. James B, Parker AW. Active and passive mobility of lower limb joints in elderly men and women. *Am J Phys Med Rehabil.* 1989;68:162–167.

12. Nitz JC, Choy NL. The relationship between ankle dorsiflexion range, falls and activity level in women aged 40 to 80 years. *N Z J Physiother.* 2004;32:121–125.

13. Nolan M, Nitz J, Choy N, Illing S. Age-related changes in musculoskeletal function, balance, and mobility measures in men aged 30-80years. *Aging Male.* 2010;13:194–201.

14. Stubbs N, Fernandez J, Glenn W. Normative data on joint ranges of motion of 25- to 54-year-old males. *Int J Ind Ergonomics.* 1993;12:265–272.

15. Vandervoort AA, Chesworth BM, Cunningham DA, Paterson DH, Rechnitzer PA, Koval JJ. Age and sex effects on mobility of the human ankle. *J Gerontol.* 1992;47:M17–M21.

16. Hernández-Guillén D, Tolsada-Velasco C, Roig-Casasús S, Costa-Moreno E, Borja-de-Fuentes I, Blasco JM. Association ankle function and balance in community-dwelling older adults. *PLoS One.* 2021;4:16.

17. Mecagni C, Smith JP, Roberts KE, O'Sullivan SB. Balance and ankle range of motion in community-dwelling women aged 64 to 87 years: a correlational study. *Phys Ther.* 2000;80:1004–1011.

18. Menz HB, Morris ME, Lord SR. Foot and ankle risk factors for falls in older people: a prospective study. *J Gerontol A Biol Sci Med Sci.* 2006;61:866–870.

19. Spink MJ, Fotoohabadi MR, Wee E, Hill KD, Lord SR, Menz HB. Foot and ankle strength, range of motion, posture, and deformity are associated with balance and functional ability in older adults. *Arch Phys Med Rehabil.* 2011;92:68–75.

20. Jacob ME, Travison TG, Ward RE, et al. Neuromuscular attributes associated with lower extremity mobility among community-dwelling older adults. *J Gerontol A Biol Sci Med Sci.* 2019;74:544–549.

21. Justine M, Ruzali D, Hazidin E, Said A, Bukry SA, Manaf H. Range of motion, muscle length, and balance performance in older adults with normal, pronated, and supinated feet. *J Phys Ther Sci.* 2016;28:916–922.

22. Fahlman L, Sangeorzan E, Chheda N, Lambright D. Older adults without radiographic knee osteoarthritis: knee alignment and knee range of motion. *Clin Med Insights Arthritis Musculoskelet Disord.* 2014;7:1–11.

23. Beauchamp MK, Leveille SG, Patel KV, et al. What physical attributes underlie self-reported vs. observed ability to walk 400 m in later life? An analysis from the in CHIANTI study. *Am J Phys Med Rehabil.* 2014;93:396–404.

24. Buell T, Green DR, Risser J. Measurement of the first metatarsophalangeal joint range of motion. *J Am Podiatr Med Assoc.* 1988;78:439–448.

25. Boone DC, Azen SP, Lin CM, Spence C, Baron C, Lee L. Reliability of goniometric measurements. *Phys Ther.* 1978;58:1355–1360.

26. Allander E, Björnsson OJ, Olafsson O, Sigfússon N, Thorsteinsson J. Normal range of joint movements in shoulder, hip, wrist and thumb with special reference to side: a comparison between two populations. *Int J Epidemiol.* 1974;3:253–261.

27. Barnes CJ, Van Steyn SJ, Fischer RA. The effects of age, sex, and shoulder dominance on range of motion of the shoulder. *J Shoulder Elbow Surg.* 2001;10:242–246.

28. Bassey EJ, Morgan K, Dallosso HM, Ebrahim SB. Flexibility of the shoulder joint measured as range of abduction in a large representative sample of men and women over 65 years of age. *Eur J Appl Physiol Occup Physiol.* 1989;58:353–360.

29. Desrosiers J, Hébert R, Bravo G, Dutil E. Upper extremity performance test for the elderly (TEMPA): normative data and correlates with sensorimotor parameters. Test d'Evaluation des Membres Supérieurs de Personnes Agées. *Arch Phys Med Rehabil.* 1995;76:1125–1129.

30. Downey P, Fiebert I, Stackpole-Brown I. Shoulder range of motion in persons aged sixty and older. *Phys Ther.* 1991;575.

31. Fiebert IM, Downey PA, Brown JS. Active shoulder range of motion in persons aged 60 years and older. *Phys Occup Ther Geriatr.* 1995;13:115–128.

32. McIntosh L, McKenna K, Gustafsson L. Active and passive shoulder range of motion in healthy older people. *Br J Occup Ther.* 2003;66:318–324.

33. Roy JS, Macdermid JC, Boyd KU, Faber KJ, Drosdowech D, Athwal GS. Rotational strength, range of motion, and function in people with unaffected shoulders from various stages of life. *Sports Med Arthrosc Rehabil Ther Technol.* 2009;1:4.

34. Gill TK, Shanahan EM, Tucker GR, Buchbinder R, Hill CL. Shoulder range of movement in the general population: age and gender stratified normative data using a community-based cohort. *BMC Musculoskelet Disord.* 2020;21:676.

35. Rickert M, Bürger A, Günther CM, Schulz CU. Forearm rotation in healthy adults of all ages and both sexes. *J Shoulder Elbow Surg.* 2008;17:271–275.

36. Zwerus EL, Willigenburg NW, Scholtes VA, Somford MP, Eygendaal D, van den Bekerom MPJ. Normative values and affecting factors for the elbow range of motion. *Shoulder Elbow.* 2019;11:215–244.

37. Klum M, Wolf MB, Hahn P, Leclère FM, Bruckner T, Unglaub F. Normative data on wrist function. *J Hand Surg Am.* 2012;37:2050–2060.

38. van Adrichem JA, van der Korst JK. Assessment of the flexibility of the lumbar spine. A pilot study in children and adolescents. *Scand J Rheumatol.* 1973;2:87–91.

39. Troke M, Moore AP, Maillardet FJ, Hough A, Cheek E. A new, comprehensive normative database of lumbar spine ranges of motion. *Clin Rehabil.* 2001;15:371–379.

40. Loebl WY. Measurement of spinal posture and range of spinal movement. *Ann Phys Med.* 1967;9:103–110.

41. Moll JM, Wright V. Normal range of spinal mobility. An objective clinical study. *Ann Rheum Dis.* 1971;30:381–386.

42. Sullivan MS, Dickinson CE, Troup JD. The influence of age and gender on lumbar spine sagittal plane range of motion. A study of 1126 healthy subjects. *Spine (Phila Pa 1976).* 1994;(19):682–686.

43. Van Herp G, Rowe P, Salter P, Paul JP. Three-dimensional lumbar spinal kinematics: a study of range of movement in 100 healthy subjects aged 20 to 60+ years. *Rheumatology (Oxford).* 2000;39:1337–1340.

44. McGregor AH, McCarthy ID, Hughes SP. Motion characteristics of the lumbar spine in the normal population. *Spine (Phila Pa 1976).* 1995;(20):2421–2428.

45. Trudelle-Jackson E, Fleisher LA, Borman N, Morrow JR, Frierson GM. Lumbar spine flexion and extension extremes of motion in women of different age and racial groups: the WIN study. *Spine (Phila Pa 1976).* 2010;(35):1539–1544.

46. Fitzgerald GK, Wynveen KJ, Rheault W, Rothschild B. Objective assessment with establishment of normal values for lumbar spinal range of motion. *Phys Ther.* 1983;63:1776–1781.

47. Einkauf DK, Gohdes ML, Jensen GM, Jewell MJ. Changes in spinal mobility with increasing age in women. *Phys Ther.* 1987;67:370–375.

48. Coyle PC, Velasco T, Sions JM, et al. Lumbar mobility and performance-based function: an investigation in older adults with and without chronic low back pain. *Pain Med.* 2017;1(18):161–168.

49. Kuhlman KA. Cervical range of motion in the elderly. *Arch Phys Med Rehabil.* 1993;74:1071–1079.

50. Peolsson A, Hedlund R, Ertzgaard S, Oberg B. Intra- and intertester reliability and range of motion of the neck. *Physiother Can.* 2000;233–242.

51. Kalscheur MS, Costello PS, Emery LJ. Gender differences in range of motion in older adults. *Phys Occup Ther Geriatr.* 2004;22:77–89.

52. American Academy of Orthopaedic Surgeons. *Joint Motion: Method of Measuring and Recording.* Chicago: American Academy of Orthopaedic Surgeons; 1965.

53. Nilsson N. Measuring passive cervical motion: a study of reliability. *J Manipulative Physiol Ther.* 1995;18:293–297.

54. Hole DE, Cook JM, Bolton JE. Reliability and concurrent validity of two instruments for measuring cervical range of motion: effects of age and gender. *Man Ther.* 1995;1:36–42.

55. Castro WH, Sautmann A, Schilgen M, Sautmann M. Noninvasive three-dimensional analysis of cervical spine motion in normal subjects in relation to age and sex. An experimental examination. *Spine (Phila Pa 1976).* 2000;(25):443–449.

56. Wood TA, Sosnoff JJ. Age-related differences to neck range of motion and muscle strength: potential risk factors to fall-related traumatic brain injuries. *Aging Clin Exp Res.* 2020;32:2287–2295.

57. Youdas JW, Garrett TR, Suman J, Bogard CL, Hallman HO, Carey JR. Normal range of motion of the cervical spine: an initial goniometric study. *Phys Ther.* 1992;72:770–780.

58. Dvorak J, Antinnes JA, Panjabi M, Loustalot D, Bonomo M. Age and gender related normal motion of the cervical spine. *Spine (Phila Pa 1976).* 1992;(17):S393–S398.

59. Trott PH, Pearcy MJ, Ruston SA, Fulton I, Brien C. Three-dimensional analysis of active cervical motion: the effect of age and gender. *Clin Biomech (Bristol, Avon).* 1996;11:201–206.

60. Lind B, Sihlbom H, Nordwall A, Malchau H. Normal range of motion of the cervical spine. *Arch Phys Med Rehabil.* 1989;70:692–695.

61. Mayer T, Brady S, Bovasso E, Pope P, Gatchel RJ. Noninvasive measurement of cervical tri-planar motion in normal subjects. *Spine (Phila Pa 1976).* 1993;(18):2191–2195.

62. Thurnwald P. The effect of age and gender on normal temporomandibular joint movement. *Physiother Theory Pract.* 1991;209–221.

63. Mezitis M, Rallis G, Zachariades N. The normal range of mouth opening. *J Oral Maxillofac Surg.* 1989;47:1028–1029.

64. Bell RD, Hoshizaki TB. Relationships of age and sex with range of motion of seventeen joint actions in humans. *Can J Appl Sport Sci.* 1981;6:202–206.

65. Simoneau GG, Hoenig KJ, Lepley JE, Papanek PE. Influence of hip position and gender on active hip internal and external rotation. *J Orthop Sports Phys Ther.* 1998;28:158–164.

66. Sankar WN, Laird CT, Baldwin KD. Hip range of motion in children: what is the norm? *J Pediatr Orthop.* 2012;32:399–405.

67. Hogg JA, Schmitz RJ, Nguyen AD, Shultz SJ. Passive hip range-of-motion values across sex and sport. *J Athl Train.* 2018;53:560–567.

68. Holla JFM, Steultjens MPM, van der Leeden M, et al. Determinants of range of joint motion in patients with early symptomatic osteoarthritis of the hip and/or knee: an exploratory study in the CHECK cohort. *Osteoarthr Cartil.* 2011;19:411–419.

69. Svenningsen S, Terjesen T, Auflem M, Berg V. Hip motion related to age and sex. *Acta Orthop Scand.* 1989;60:97–100.

70. Alanen JT, Levola JV, Helenius HY, Kvist MH. Ankle joint complex mobility of children 7 to 14 years old. *J Pediatr Orthop.* 2001;21:731–777.

71. Nigg BM, Fisher V, Allinger TL, Ronsky JR, Engsberg JR. Range of motion of the foot as a function of age. *Foot Ankle.* 1992;13:336–343.

72. Cho KH, Jeon Y, Lee H. Range of motion of the ankle according to pushing force, gender and knee position. *Ann Rehabil Med.* 2016;40:271–278.

73. Ahlberg A, Moussa M, Al-Nahdi M. On geographical variations in the normal range of joint motion. *Clin Orthop Relat Res.* 1988;229–231.

74. Smith J, Walker J. Knee and elbow range of motion in healthy older individuals. *Phys Occup Ther Geriatr.* 1983;31–38.

75. Chapleau J, Canet F, Petit Y, Sandman E, Laflamme GY, Rouleau DM. Demographic and anthropometric factors affecting elbow range of motion in healthy adults. *J Shoulder Elbow Surg.* 2013;22:88–93.

76. Barad JH, Kim RS, Ebramzadeh E, Silva M. Range of motion of the healthy pediatric elbow: cross-sectional study of a large population. *J Pediatr Orthop B.* 2013;22:117–122.

77. Mallon WJ, Brown HR, Nunley JA. Digital ranges of motion: normal values in young adults. *J Hand Surg Am.* 1991;16:882–887.

78. De Smet L, Urlus M, Spriet A, Fabry G. Metacarpophalangeal and interphalangeal flexion: influence of sex and age, relation to ligamentous injury. *Acta Orthop Belg.* 1993;59:357–359.

79. Haley SM, Tada WL, Carmichael EM. Spinal mobility in young children. A normative study. *Phys Ther.* 1986;66:1697–1703.

80. Macrae IF, Wright V. Measurement of back movement. *Ann Rheum Dis.* 1969;28:584–589.

81. Boline PD, Keating JC, Haas M, Anderson AV. Interexaminer reliability and discriminant validity of inclinometric measurement of lumbar rotation in chronic low-back pain patients and subjects without low-back pain. *Spine (Phila Pa 1976).* 1992;(17):335–338.

82. Ordway NR, Seymour R, Donelson RG, Hojnowski L, Lee E, Edwards WT. Cervical sagittal range-of-motion analysis using three methods. Cervical range-of-motion device, 3space, and radiography. *Spine (Phila Pa 1976).* 1997;(22):501–508.

83. Agerberg G. Maximal mandibular movements in young men and women. *Sven Tandlak Tidskr.* 1974;67:81–100.

84. Lewis RP, Buschang PH, Throckmorton GS. Sex differences in mandibular movements during opening and closing. *Am J Orthod Dentofacial Orthop.* 2001;120:294–303.

85. Pullinger AG, Liu SP, Low G, Tay D. Differences between sexes in maximum jaw opening when corrected to body size. *J Oral Rehabil.* 1987;14:291–299.

86. Hoaglund FT, Yau AC, Wong WL. Osteoarthritis of the hip and other joints in southern Chinese in Hong Kong. *J Bone Joint Surg Am.* 1973;55:545–557.

87. Roaas A, Andersson GB. Normal range of motion of the hip, knee and ankle joints in male subjects, 30-40 years of age. *Acta Orthop Scand.* 1982;53:205–208.

88. Borsa PA, Wilk KE, Jacobson JA, et al. Correlation of range of motion and glenohumeral translation in professional baseball pitchers. *Am J Sports Med.* 2005;33:1392–1399.

89. Borsa PA, Dover GC, Wilk KE, Reinold MM. Glenohumeral range of motion and stiffness in professional baseball pitchers. *Med Sci Sports Exerc.* 2006;38:21–26.

90. Brown LP, Niehues SL, Harrah A, Yavorsky P, Hirshman HP. Upper extremity range of motion and isokinetic strength of the internal and external shoulder rotators in major league baseball players. *Am J Sports Med.* 1988;16:577–585.

91. Crockett HC, Gross LB, Wilk KE, et al. Osseous adaptation and range of motion at the glenohumeral joint in professional baseball pitchers. *Am J Sports Med.* 2002;30:20–26.

92. Ellenbecker TS, Roetert EP, Bailie DS, Davies GJ, Brown SW. Glenohumeral joint total rotation range of motion in elite tennis players and baseball pitchers. *Med Sci Sports Exerc.* 2002;34:2052–2056.

93. Hurd WJ, Kaplan KM, ElAttrache NS, Jobe FW, Morrey BF, Kaufman KR. A profile of glenohumeral internal and external rotation motion in the uninjured high school baseball pitcher, part II: strength. *J Athl Train.* 2011;46:289–295.

94. Osbahr DC, Cannon DL, Speer KP. Retroversion of the humerus in the throwing shoulder of college baseball pitchers. *Am J Sports Med.* 2002;30:347–353.

95. Sethi PM, Tibone JE, Lee TQ. Quantitative assessment of glenohumeral translation in baseball players: a comparison of pitchers versus nonpitching athletes. *Am J Sports Med.* 2004;32:1711–1715.

96. Sueyoshi T, Nakatani T, Tsuruta T, Emoto G. Upper extremity range of motion and pitching profile of baseball pitchers in Japan. *Orthop J Sports Med.* 2017;5.

97. Wilk KE, Macrina LC, Fleisig GS, et al. Correlation of glenohumeral internal rotation deficit and total rotational motion to shoulder injuries in professional baseball pitchers. *Am J Sports Med.* 2011;39:329–335.

98. Bigliani LU, Codd TP, Connor PM, Levine WN, Littlefield MA, Hershon SJ. Shoulder motion and laxity in the professional baseball player. *Am J Sports Med.* 1997;25:609–613.

99. Baltaci G, Johnson R, Kohl H. Shoulder range of motion characteristics in collegiate baseball players. *J Sports Med Phys Fitness.* 2001;41:236–242.

100. Reagan KM, Meister K, Horodyski MB, Werner DW, Carruthers C, Wilk K. Humeral retroversion and its relationship to glenohumeral rotation in the shoulder of college baseball players. *Am J Sports Med.* 2002;30:354–360.

101. Downar JM, Sauers EL. Clinical measures of shoulder mobility in the professional baseball player. *J Athl Train.* 2005;40:23–29.

102. Meister K, Day T, Horodyski M, Kaminski TW, Wasik MP, Tillman S. Rotational motion changes in the glenohumeral joint of the adolescent/little league baseball player. *Am J Sports Med.* 2005;33:693–698.

103. Chant CB, Litchfield R, Griffin S, Thain LM. Humeral head retroversion in competitive baseball players and its relationship to glenohumeral rotation range of motion. *J Orthop Sports Phys Ther.* 2007;37:514–520.

104. Schilling DT, Mallace AJ, Elazzi AM. Shoulder range of motion characteristics in division III collegiate softball and baseball players. *Int J Sports Phys Ther.* 2019;14:770–784.

105. Johnson L. Patterns of shoulder flexibility among college baseball players. *J Athl Train.* 1992;27:44–49.

106. Dodds FT, Knotts SS, Penrod MI, Scoggins WA, Conners RT. Shoulder strength and range of motion between collegiate pitchers and position players in baseball. *Int J Exerc Sci.* 2020;13:123–130.

107. Almeida GP, Silveira PF, Rosseto NP, Barbosa G, Ejnisman B, Cohen M. Glenohumeral range of motion in handball players with and without throwing-related shoulder pain. *J Shoulder Elbow Surg.* 2013;22:602–607.

108. Chandler TJ, Kibler WB, Uhl TL, Wooten B, Kiser A, Stone E. Flexibility comparisons of junior elite tennis players to other athletes. *Am J Sports Med.* 1990;18:134–136.

109. Chinn CJ, Priest JD, Kent BE. Upper extremity range of motion, grip strength, and girth in highly skilled tennis players. *Phys Ther.* 1974;54:474–483.

110. Ellenbecker TS, Roetert EP, Piorkowski PA, Schulz DA. Glenohumeral joint internal and external rotation range of motion in elite junior tennis players. *J Orthop Sports Phys Ther.* 1996;24:336–341.

111. Kibler WB, Chandler TJ, Livingston BP, Roetert EP. Shoulder range of motion in elite tennis players. Effect of age and years of tournament play. *Am J Sports Med.* 1996;24:279–285.

112. Schmidt-Wietnof R, Rapp W, Mauch F. Shoulder rotation characteristics in professional tennis players. *Int J Sports Med.* 2004;25:154–158.

113. Bak K, Magnusson SP. Shoulder strength and range of motion in symptomatic and pain-free elite swimmers. *Am J Sports Med.* 1997;25:454–459.

114. Chiang CC, Hsu CC, Chiang JY, Chang WC, Tsai JC. Flexibility of internal and external glenohumeral rotation of junior female tennis players and its correlation with performance ranking. *J Phys Ther Sci.* 2016;28:3296–3299.

115. Nutt C, Mirkovic M, Hill R, Ranson C, Cooper SM. Reference values for glenohumeral joint rotational range of motion in elite tennis players. *Int J Sports Phys Ther.* 2018;13:501–510.

116. Cigercioglu NB, Guney-Deniz H, Unuvar E, Colakoglu F, Baltaci G. Shoulder range of motion, rotator strength, and upper-extremity functional performance in junior tennis players. *J Sport Rehabil.* 2021;30:1129–1137.

117. Gillet B, Begon M, Digger M, Berger-Vachon C, Rogowski I. Shoulder range of motion and strength in young competitive tennis players with and without history of shoulder problems. *Phys Ther Sport.* 2018;31:22–28.

118. Saccol MF, Almeida GPL, de Souza VL. Anatomical glenohumeral internal rotation deficit and symmetric rotational strength in male and female young beach volleyball players. *J Electromyogr Kinesiol.* 2016;26:121–125.

119. Harput G, Guney H, Toprak U, Kaya T, Colakoglu FF, Baltaci G. Shoulder-rotator strength, range of motion, and acromiohumeral distance in asymptomatic adolescent volleyball attackers. *J Athl Train.* 2016;51:733–738.

120. Forthomme B, Wieczorek V, Frisch A, Crielaard JM, Croisier JL. Shoulder pain among high-level volleyball players and preseason features. *Med Sci Sports Exerc.* 2013;45:1852–1860.

121. Beach ML, Whitney SL, Dickoff-Hoffman S. Relationship of shoulder flexibility, strength, and endurance to shoulder pain in competitive swimmers. *J Orthop Sports Phys Ther.* 1992;16:262–268.

122. Riemann BL, Witt J, Davies GJ. Glenohumeral joint rotation range of motion in competitive swimmers. *J Sports Sci.* 2011;29:1191–1199.

123. Herrington L. Glenohumeral joint: internal and external rotation range of motion in javelin throwers. *Br J Sports Med.* 1998;32:226–228.

124. Bennell K, Khan KM, Matthews B, et al. Hip and ankle range of motion and hip muscle strength in young female ballet dancers and controls. *Br J Sports Med.* 1999;33:340–346.

125. Hamilton WG, Hamilton LH, Marshall P, Molnar M. A profile of the musculoskeletal characteristics of elite professional ballet dancers. *Am J Sports Med.* 1992;20:267–273.

126. Khan K, Roberts P, Nattrass C, et al. Hip and ankle range of motion in elite classical ballet dancers and controls. *Clin J Sport Med.* 1997;7:174–179.

127. Reid DC, Burnham RS, Saboe LA, Kushner SF. Lower extremity flexibility patterns in classical ballet dancers and their correlation to lateral hip and knee injuries. *Am J Sports Med.* 1987;15:347–352.

128. Steinberg N, Hershkovitz I, Peleg S, et al. Range of joint movement in female dancers and nondancers aged 8 to 16 years: anatomical and clinical implications. *Am J Sports Med.* 2006;34:814–823.

129. Alfuth M, Luetkecosmann J, Knicker A. Comparison of plantar sensitivity, dynamic balance, and lower extremity joint range of motion between experienced female ballet dancers and female non-dancing athletes: a cross-sectional study. *J Dance Med Sci.* 2021;25:238–248.

130. Cho HJ, KIm S, Jung JY, Kwak DS. Foot and ankle joint movements of dancers and non-dancers: a comparative study. *Sports Biomech.* 2019;18:587–594.

131. Youdas JW, Krause DA, Hollman JH, Harmsen WS, Laskowski E. The influence of gender and age on hamstring muscle length in healthy adults. *J Orthop Sports Phys Ther.* 2005;35:246–252.

132. Corkery M, Briscoe H, Ciccone N. Establishing normal values for lower extremity muscle length in college-age students. *Phys Ther Sport.* 2007;66–74.

133. Domholdt E. *Rehabilitation Research: Principles and Applications.* Philadelphia: WB Saunders; 2004.

134. Currier D. *Elements of Research in Physical Therapy.* Baltimore: Williams & Wilkins; 1984.

135. Elveru RA, Rothstein JM, Lamb RL. Goniometric reliability in a clinical setting. Subtalar and ankle joint measurements. *Phys Ther.* 1988;68:672–677.

136. Landis JR, Koch GG. The measurement of observer agreement for categorical data. *Biometrics.* 1977;33:159–174.

137. Richman T, Madridis L, Prince B. Research methodology and applied statistics, part 3: measurement procedures in research. *Phsyiother Can.* 1980;253–257.

138. Carter R, Lubinsky J. *Rehabilitation Research: Principles and Applications.* St. Louis, MO: Elsevier; 2016.

139. Portney LG, Watkins MP. *R2 Library (Online Service). Foundations of Clinical Research Applications to Practice. Upper Saddle River.* NJ: Pearson/Prentice Hall; 2009.

140. Anastasi A. *Psychological Testing.* New York: Macmillan; 1988.

141. Rothstein J, Echternach J. *Primer on Measurement: An Introductory Guide to Measurement Issues.* Alexandria, VA: American Physical Therapy Association; 1993.

142. Turner D, et al. The minimal detectable change cannot reliably replace the minimal important difference. *J Clin Epidemiol.* 2010;63(1):28–36.

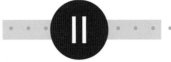

SECTION

II

UPPER EXTREMITY

3

MEASUREMENT of RANGE of MOTION of the SHOULDER

Nancy Berryman Reese

The *shoulder joint complex* is composed of three synovial joints (glenohumeral, acromioclavicular, and sternoclavicular) along with the articulation between the ventral surface of the scapula and the dorsal thorax (herein referred to as the scapulothoracic articulation)[1] (Fig. 3.1). Although other structures, such as the "subacromial joint,"[2] occasionally are included as part of the shoulder joint complex, a more conservative, four-articulation description of the complex is used in this text.[1] In the following sections, anatomy and motion at each articulation will be described separately before the combined motions of the shoulder complex are discussed.

GLENOHUMERAL JOINT

ANATOMY

The glenohumeral joint is classified as a ball-and-socket joint that is formed by the articulation of the rounded humeral head with the anterolaterally facing glenoid fossa of the scapula[3] (see Fig. 3.1). Because the glenoid fossa is shallow and provides only a small articular surface for the head of the humerus, the glenohumeral joint possesses some inherent instability. Reinforcement of the joint is provided by ligamentous (Fig. 3.2) and musculotendinous structures as well as by the fibrocartilaginous glenoid labrum, which is attached to the margin of the glenoid fossa, effectively increasing its depth and adding stability to the joint.[4] Musculotendinous reinforcement of the glenohumeral joint is supplied by the tendons of rotator cuff muscles (subscapularis, supraspinatus, infraspinatus, and teres major) as they cross the anterior, superior, and posterior aspects of the joint capsule, respectively.[5,6] The glenohumeral ligaments consist of superior, middle, and inferior bands, although the distinctness of these ligaments has been questioned.[7] The collective role of the glenohumeral ligaments is to strengthen the anterior and inferior walls of the joint capsule and to provide some limitation to lateral rotation of the shoulder, particularly between 0 and 90 degrees of arm elevation.[8–10]

Additional reinforcement of the superior aspect of the glenohumeral joint is provided by the coracohumeral ligament, which runs from the coracoid process of the scapula to the greater tuberosity of the humerus.[9]

OSTEOKINEMATICS

The relative instability of the glenohumeral joint allows large freedom of movement, permitting placement of the upper extremity in a wide variety of positions for function. The joint has 3 degrees of freedom of movement, allowing the motions of flexion/extension, abduction/adduction, and medial/lateral rotation.

Motion at the glenohumeral joint is limited primarily by muscular and capsuloligamentous structures. Elevation (flexion or abduction) is limited by tension in the inferior glenohumeral ligament and the inferior joint capsule.[10] Extension is limited by the superior and middle glenohumeral ligaments.[2] Glenohumeral rotation is limited by ligamentous structures and by tension in muscles of the rotator cuff. Lateral rotation is limited by tension in the subscapularis muscle, in the antero-inferior joint capsule, and in the coracohumeral, superior and middle glenohumeral, and anterior band of the inferior glenohumeral ligaments.[9,11–13] Medial rotation at the glenohumeral joint is limited by tension in the infraspinatus and teres minor muscles, in the posterior joint capsule, and in the posterior band of the inferior glenohumeral ligament.[11–13]

ARTHROKINEMATICS

At the glenohumeral joint, motion is produced by gliding, rolling, and spinning of the convex head of the humerus against the shallow, concave surface of the glenoid fossa of the scapula. During movement at this joint, the head of the humerus rolls in the same direction in which the distal end of the humerus is moving and glides in the opposite direction. For example, as one moves from 0–90 degrees of flexion, the humeral head rolls superiorly and glides inferiorly. In addition, the head of the humerus spins within the glenoid fossa, particularly during rotational motion of the joint.[14]

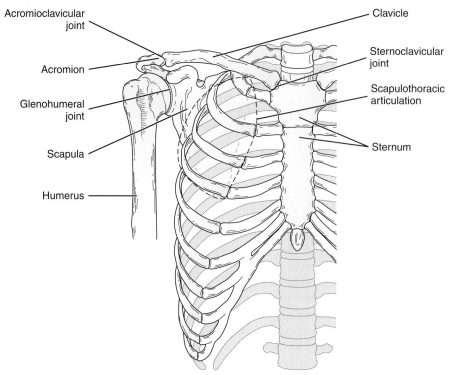

Fig. 3.1 Joints of the shoulder complex.

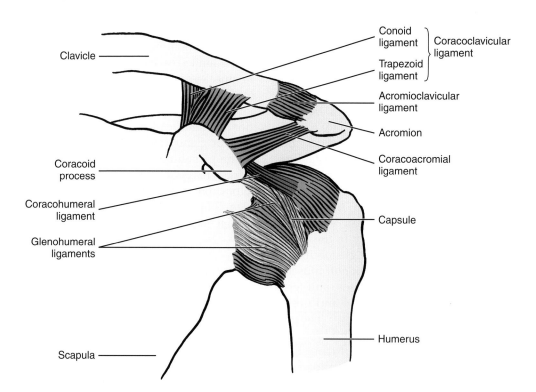

Fig. 3.2 Ligamentous reinforcement of the glenohumeral and acromioclavicular joints.

STERNOCLAVICULAR JOINT

ANATOMY

The sternoclavicular joint, the only synovial articulation between the upper limb and the axial skeleton, is formed by the articulation of the sternal end of the clavicle with the manubrium of the sternum and cartilage of the first rib[3] (Fig. 3.3). No actual bony contact occurs between the clavicle and the sternum. Instead, a thick fibrocartilaginous disc is interposed between the articular surfaces of the two bones, increasing the congruency between them and separating the joint into two completely separate parts.[1,6] Four ligaments provide reinforcement for and limit motion at the sternoclavicular joint: the anterior and posterior sternoclavicular ligaments, the costoclavicular ligament, and the interclavicular ligaments. The anterior and posterior sternoclavicular ligaments are attached laterally to the sternal end of the clavicle and medially to the manubrium of the sternum, and they reinforce the anterior and posterior aspects of the joint capsule, respectively. Further reinforcement of the joint is provided by the costoclavicular ligament, which runs from the inferior aspect of the clavicle to the superior aspect of the first rib. The interclavicular ligament attaches to the sternal end of each clavicle and reinforces the superior aspect of the sternoclavicular joint.[1,3,6]

OSTEOKINEMATICS

Three degrees of freedom of movement are allowed by the structure of the sternoclavicular joint. Because the distal end of the clavicle is attached to the acromion process of the scapula (acromioclavicular joint), all movements of the clavicle are accompanied by movements of the scapula. Motions at the sternoclavicular joint consist of the following:

Elevation/Depression—Defined as superior and inferior movement of the distal end of the clavicle, respectively.

Protraction/Retraction—Anterior/posterior movement of the distal end of the clavicle.
Rotation—A spinning motion of the clavicle around its longitudinal axis.[15,16]

Motions of the sternoclavicular joint are limited by the ligaments that surround the joint and the fibrocartilaginous joint within. The anterior and posterior sternoclavicular ligaments limit protraction and retraction of the clavicle. Elevation of the clavicle is checked by tension in the costoclavicular ligament, and depression is limited by the interclavicular ligament and the articular disc.[6,14]

ARTHROKINEMATICS

During the motions of clavicular elevation and depression, movement occurs between the clavicle and the articular disc. Because the sternal end of the clavicle is convex in a cephalocaudal direction, elevation of the acromial end of the clavicle causes the sternal end to glide inferiorly, and depression causes the sternal end to glide superiorly. Clavicular protraction and retraction occur as motions between the articular disc and the sternum. In this instance, the articular surface on the clavicle is concave, causing the medial and lateral ends of the clavicle to move in the same direction. Thus protraction is accompanied by an anterior glide of the sternal end of the clavicle, while the sternal end glides posteriorly during retraction. Rotary movements of the clavicle result in a spin of the sternal end of the clavicle. Because of the S-shape of the clavicle, posterior rotation at the sternoclavicular joint results in elevation of the lateral end of the clavicle.[1,14,17]

ACROMIOCLAVICULAR JOINT

ANATOMY

The acromioclavicular (AC) joint is classified as a plane synovial joint and is formed by the articulation of the acromial end of the clavicle with the medial border of the

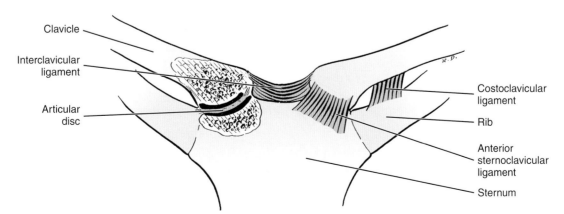

Fig. 3.3   Bony and ligamentous anatomy of the sternoclavicular joint.

acromion process of the scapula (see Fig. 3.2). Both articular surfaces are covered with fibrocartilage, and the joint line formed by the two bones slopes inferiorly and medially, causing the clavicle to tend to override the acromion. This tendency is prevented to a large extent by the strong coracoclavicular ligament that runs from a broad area of origin on the inferior aspect of the clavicle to a tapered insertion on the coracoid process of the scapula.[18,19] The more horizontally oriented fibers of the trapezoid component of this ligament resist medial displacement of the scapula.[20] The other component of the coracoclavicular ligament, the conoid ligament, has fibers that are oriented more vertically. Additional reinforcement of the AC joint is supplied by the AC ligament and by fibers of the deltoid and trapezius muscles, all of which span and reinforce the superior aspect of the joint.[13,19,20]

OSTEOKINEMATICS

The AC joint has been described as having 3 degrees of freedom. Although considerable variation has been noted in the nomenclature used to describe motions that occur at the AC joint,[1,14,16] these motions include rotation around an anterior–posterior axis, winging around a vertical axis, and tilting around a medial-lateral axis.[16] AC motions of rotation, winging, and tilting occur during scapular motions of rotation, abduction/adduction, and elevation/depression, respectively.

ARTHROKINEMATICS

The articular surfaces at the AC joint consist of a slightly convex to relatively flat facet of the clavicle and a slightly convex to relatively flat acromial surface. Because of the irregularity of the joint surfaces and the complexity of movement produced at this joint, arthrokinematics of the AC joint are not well described in the literature.[14,17]

SCAPULOTHORACIC ARTICULATION

ANATOMY

Although the scapula moves on the thorax during motions of the shoulder complex, the articulation between the scapula and the thorax is not a true joint in any sense of the term. However, motion between the scapula and the thorax contributes greatly to full mobility of the shoulder complex. Articulation here occurs between the concave costal surface of the scapula and the convex surface of the posterior thorax (Fig. 3.4).

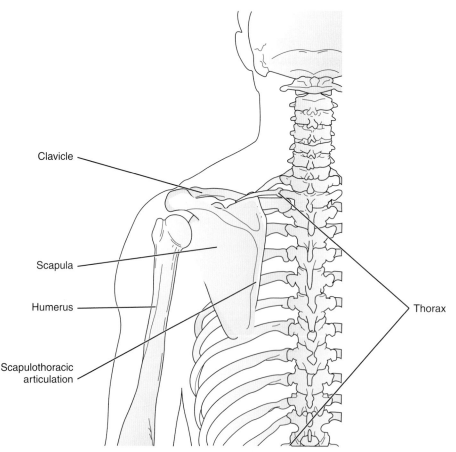

Fig. 3.4 Scapulothoracic articulation (posterior view).

OSTEOKINEMATICS

Movements of the scapula on the thorax result from combined motions of the sternoclavicular and AC joints and are essential for full range of motion (ROM) of the shoulder complex. Motions available at the scapulothoracic articulation include scapular elevation and depression, abduction and adduction, and upward and downward rotation.[14]

ARTHROKINEMATICS

Because the scapular surface is concave and moves on a convex thorax, the scapula moves as a unit, gliding along the thoracic surface as it follows motions of the clavicle.[14]

SHOULDER COMPLEX

Motions of the shoulder joint complex include flexion, extension, abduction, adduction, medial rotation, and lateral rotation. These movements of the shoulder joint contain component motions that occur at all four articulations composing the shoulder complex. For example, elevation of the arm in the frontal plane (shoulder abduction) or the sagittal plane (shoulder flexion) is accomplished by motions that occur at the glenohumeral joint (glenohumeral flexion or abduction), at the sternoclavicular joint (clavicular elevation), at the AC joint (clavicular rotation), and at the scapulothoracic articulation (scapular abduction, elevation, and upward rotation). Elevation of the arm is produced by a combination of humeral and scapular motion, which has been described as occurring in varying ratios of glenohumeral to scapulothoracic motion. Although it is widely accepted that the relative contributions of glenohumeral and scapulothoracic movements vary throughout the range of arm elevation, the overall ratios of glenohumeral to scapulothoracic motion have been reported from as high as 2:1[21] to as low as 1.1:1,[22] with other ratios reported between those values.[23–25] There also is evidence that the ratio of scapulothoracic to glenohumeral motion decreases as the motion progresses from the coronal plane (abduction) to the sagittal plane (flexion).[26] The motion of the scapula is a result of motion that occurs at the AC and sternoclavicular joints, whereas humeral motion is produced at the glenohumeral joint. Because isolated glenohumeral motion does not occur during normal elevation of the arm past the first 30 degrees or so,[21,27] no attempt is made in this text to measure isolated glenohumeral flexion or abduction. Rather, flexion and abduction are measured as shoulder complex motions, allowing full excursion at all involved joints.

LIMITATIONS OF MOTION: SHOULDER JOINT

Because motions involving elevation of the arm are combined motions involving movement at the AC, glenohumeral, and sternoclavicular joints, as well as at the scapulothoracic articulation, shoulder flexion and abduction are limited by anatomical structures located at multiple joints. For example, elevation of the arm may be limited by tension in the costoclavicular ligament,[3] which limits clavicular elevation (necessary for complete elevation of the arm). The same motion may be limited by tension in the inferior glenohumeral ligament, thereby restricting motion at the glenohumeral joint. For a complete description of structures that limit joint motion, refer to the descriptions of osteokinematics for each joint of the shoulder complex. Information regarding normal ranges of motion for all motions of the shoulder is found in Appendix B.

END-FEEL

All motions of the shoulder joint complex are restricted by capsuloligamentous or musculotendinous structures. Thus the normal end-feel for all motions of the normal shoulder joint complex is firm.

CAPSULAR PATTERN

Decreased shoulder ROM should be assessed to determine whether the limitation occurs in a capsular pattern. Capsular involvement should be suspected if shoulder ROM deficits are characterized by lateral rotation that is the most limited, abduction that is also limited but is less than that seen in the limitation of lateral rotation, and medial rotation that is only minimally limited or is not limited at all.[28,29]

RANGE OF MOTION AND FUNCTIONAL ACTIVITY

A number of studies have been published that examined the motion of the shoulder complex during various activities. Both Safaee-Rad et al.[30] and Cooper et al.[31] analyzed upper extremity motion, including motion of the shoulder joint, during various feeding activities. Results from these two studies were fairly similar (Table 3.1), although Cooper et al.[31] combined data from the three feeding activities while Safaee-Rad et al.[30] reported their data separately. Other investigators who have examined shoulder motion during feeding activities have obtained reasonably similar results,[34,36] with the exception of Magermans et al.,[33] who reported their results as based on standards proposed by the International Society of Biomechanics (ISB),[42] making comparison of their

Table 3.1	SHOULDER ROM DURING FUNCTIONAL ACTIVITIES				
FUNCTIONAL ACTIVITY	**ELEVATION**	**PLANE OF ELEVATION***	**MEDIAL ROTATION**	**LATERAL ROTATION**	**COMMENTS**
Comb Hair					
Aizawa et al.[32]	110°	60°			Average maximal joint angle of 20 healthy subjects (10 M, 10 F, aged 18–34 years) during ADL task; ROM measured using an electromagnetic three-dimensional tracking system
Magermans et al.[33,‡]	90° ± 9°	59° ± 14°		70° ± 19°	Average maximal joint angle of 24 healthy female subjects (mean age 36.8 years) used during ADL task; ROM measured using Flock of Birds electromagnetic tracking device
Pearl et al.[34,§]	112° ± 10°	54° ± 27°			Average maximal joint angle of 8 "normal" subjects (aged 20–45 years) during ADL task; ROM measured using a 6° freedom spatial tracking system and electromagnetic sensors pinned to the humerus
van Andel et al.[35,‡]	98° ± 11°	64° ± 13°		81° ± 6°	Average maximal joint angle of 10 healthy adults (6 M, 4 F, mean age 28.5 years) during ADL task; ROM measured using Optotrak motion analysis system
Drink from Cup					
Aizawa et al.[32]	87°	80°			Average maximal joint angle of 20 healthy subjects (10 M, 10 F, aged 18–34 years) during ADL task; ROM measured using an electromagnetic three-dimensional tracking system
Safaee-Rad et al.[30,§]	43° ± 16° / 31° ± 9°	90°[†] / 0°[†]	23° ± 12°		Average maximal joint angle in 10 healthy men (aged 20–29 years) measured using three-dimensional measurement system
van Andel et al.[35,‡]	64° ± 11°	62° ± 8°		59° ± 5°	Average maximal joint angle of 10 healthy adults (6 M, 4 F, mean age 28.5 years) during ADL task; ROM measured using Optotrak motion analysis system
Eat					
Cooper et al.[31,§]	36° (M); 31° (F) / 23° (M); 28° (F)	90°[†] / 0°[†]	22° (M); 28° (F)		Average maximum joint angle in two groups (10 M, 9 F) of healthy adults (aged 18–50 years) measured using video-based three-dimensional measurement system during a combination of 3 feeding tasks
Henmi et al.[36,§]	43° ± 6°	90°[†]			Average maximum joint angle of 5 healthy adults (3 F; 2 M, aged 20–28 years) during ADL task; ROM measured using Vicon three-dimensional motion analysis system
Magermans et al.[33,‡]	74° ± 13°	60° ± 14°		49° ± 14°	Average maximal joint angle of 24 healthy female subjects (mean age 36.8 years) used during ADL task; ROM measured using Flock of Birds electromagnetic tracking device
Pearl et al.[34,§]	52° ± 8°	87° ± 29°			Average maximal joint angle of 8 "normal" subjects (aged 20–45 years) during ADL task; ROM measured using a 6° freedom spatial tracking system and electromagnetic sensors pinned to the humerus
Safaee-Rad et al.[30,§]	35° ± 20° (fork); 36° ± 14° / 17° ± 6° (fork); 22° ± 7° (spoon)	90°[†] / 0°[†]	18° ± 10° (fork); 17° ± 12° (spoon)		Average maximal joint angle in 10 healthy men (aged 20–29 years) measured using three-dimensional measurement system
Pour from Pitcher					
O'Neill et al.[37,§]	74° ± 8°	42° ± 8°			Average joint angle of 10 healthy subjects (unstated age) measured using 3Space Isotrak system
Grasp Top of Steering Wheel					
O'Neill et al.[37,§]	70° ± 8°	90° ± 7°			Average joint angle of 10 healthy subjects (unstated age) measured using 3Space Isotrak system

Table 3.1	SHOULDER ROM DURING FUNCTIONAL ACTIVITIES—cont'd				
FUNCTIONAL ACTIVITY	**ELEVATION**	**PLANE OF ELEVATION***	**MEDIAL ROTATION**	**LATERAL ROTATION**	**COMMENTS**
Hand behind Head					
Matsen et al.[38,§]	118°	13°			Data from single subject (unstated age and sex) measured using electromagnetic sensor pinned to humerus
Namdari et al.[39]				61.3° ± 2.3° dominant arm 56.3° ± 2.2° nondominant arm	20 healthy subjects (18 M, 2 F, aged 26–34 years) used during ADL task; ROM measured using the Polhemus 3Space Fastrak electromagnetic device
O'Neill et al.[37,§]	127° ± 11°	57° ± 16°			Average joint angle of 10 healthy subjects (unstated age) measured using 3Space Isotrak system
Hand to Back Pocket					
Petuskey et al.[40,§]	47° ± 11°	−90°[†]	27° ± 11°		Average maximum joint angle of 28 "normal" children (aged 9–12 years) measured using three-dimensional motion analysis system
van Andel et al.[35,‡]	48° ± 9°	52° ± 12°	102° ± 11°		Average maximal joint angle of 10 healthy adults (6 M, 4 F, mean age 28.5 years) during ADL task; ROM measured using Optotrak motion analysis system
Hand to Forehead					
Mackey et al.[41,§]	105° ± 10° 49° ± 15°	90°[†] 0°[†]			Average maximum joint angle of 10 healthy children (aged 6–12 years) during ADL task; ROM measured using three-dimensional motion analysis system
Hand to Mouth					
Mackey et al.[41,§]	70° ± 10° 46° ± 14°	90°[†] 0°[†]			Average maximum joint angle of 10 healthy children (aged 6–12 years) during ADL task; ROM measured using three-dimensional motion analysis system
O'Neill et al.[37,§]	87° ± 15°	77° ± 11°			Average joint angle of 10 healthy subjects (unstated age) measured using 3Space Isotrak system
Hand to Top of Head					
Petuskey et al.[40,§]	85° ± 17° 36° ± 13°	90°[†] 0°[†]	−32° ± 15°		Average maximum joint angle of 28 "normal" children (aged 9–12 years) measured using three-dimensional motion analysis system
Lift Object/Reach-Head Level/High Shelf					
Mackey et al.[41,§]	94° ± 13° 58° ± 10°	90°[†] 0°[†]			Average maximum joint angle of 10 healthy children (aged 6–12 years) during ADL task; ROM measured using three-dimensional motion analysis system
Matsen et al.[38,§]	93°	66°			Data from single subject (unstated age and sex) measured using electromagnetic sensor pinned to humerus
Namdari et al.[39]				38.1° ± 2.2° soup can dominant arm 41.8° ± 2.6° 1-gallon container dominant arm 32.1° ± 1.7° soup can nondominant arm 41.6° ± 1.6° 1-gallon container nondominant arm	20 healthy subjects (18 M, 2 F) (aged 26–34 years) used during ADL task; ROM measured using the Polhemus 3Space Fastrak electromagnetic device
O'Neill et al.[37,§]	105° ± 7°	61° ± 7°			Average joint angle of 10 healthy subjects (unstated age) measured using 3Space Isotrak system

Continued

Table 3.1   SHOULDER ROM DURING FUNCTIONAL ACTIVITIES—cont'd

FUNCTIONAL ACTIVITY	ELEVATION	PLANE OF ELEVATION*	MEDIAL ROTATION	LATERAL ROTATION	COMMENTS
Lift Object/Reach-Shoulder Level					
Matsen et al.[38,§]	78°	86°			Data from single subject (unstated age and sex) measured using electromagnetic sensor pinned to humerus
Namdari et al.[39]				39.1°±2.1° 1-gallon container dominant arm 33.9°±1.9° soup can dominant arm 38.5°±1.9° 1-gallon container nondominant arm 30.8°±1.2° soup can nondominant arm	20 healthy subjects (18 M, 2 F, aged 26–34 years) used during ADL task; ROM measured using the Polhemus 3Space Fastrak electromagnetic device
O'Neill et al.[37,§]	62°±7°	66°±6°			Average joint angle of 10 healthy subjects (unstated age) measured using 3Space Isotrak system
Perineal Care					
Magermans et al.[33,‡]	35°±10°	−67°±24°	105°±25°		Average maximal joint angle of 24 healthy female subjects (mean age 36.8 years) used during ADL task; ROM measured using Flock of Birds electromagnetic tracking device
Pearl et al.[34,§]	38°±10°	−86°±13°			Average maximal joint angle of 8 "normal" subjects (aged 20–45 years) during ADL task; ROM measured using a 6° freedom spatial tracking system and electromagnetic sensors pinned to the humerus
O'Neill et al.[37,§]	31°±3°	−77°±11°			Average joint angle of 10 healthy subjects (unstated age) measured using 3Space Isotrak system
Reach Up Back					
Pearl et al.[34,§]	56°±13°	−69°±11°			Average maximal joint angle of 8 "normal" subjects (aged 20–45 years) during ADL task; ROM measured using a 6° freedom spatial tracking system and electromagnetic sensors pinned to the humerus
Reach to Receive Change					
Petuskey et al.[35,§]	32°±17° 5°±10°	90°[†] 0°[†]		12°±21°	Average maximum joint angle of 28 "normal" children (aged 9–12 years) measured using three-dimensional motion analysis system
Shampoo Hair					
Henmi et al.[36,§]	64°±9°	90°[†]			Average maximum joint angle of 5 healthy adults (3 F, 2 M, aged 20–28 years) during ADL task; ROM measured using Vicon three-dimensional motion analysis system
Tie Shoes					
O'Neill et al.[37,§]	72°±14° (R) 63°±12° (L)	88°±17° (R) 73°±7° (L)			Average joint angle of 10 healthy subjects (unstated age) measured using 3Space Isotrak system
Tuck in Shirt					
Namdari et al.[39]			88.3°±9.1° dominant arm 86.9°±8.7° nondominant arm		20 healthy subjects (18 M, 2 F, aged 26–34 years) used during ADL task; ROM measured using the Polhemus 3Space Fastrak electromagnetic device
Pearl et al.[34,§]	57°	−54°			Data from single subject (unstated age and sex) measured using electromagnetic sensor pinned to humerus
Wash Axilla					
Magermans et al.[33,‡]	53°±9°	100°±9°		15°±7°	Average maximal joint angle of 24 healthy female subjects (mean age 36.8 years) used during ADL task; ROM measured using Flock of Birds electromagnetic tracking device

		Table 3.1 SHOULDER ROM DURING FUNCTIONAL ACTIVITIES—cont'd			
FUNCTIONAL ACTIVITY	**ELEVATION**	**PLANE OF ELEVATION***	**MEDIAL ROTATION**	**LATERAL ROTATION**	**COMMENTS**
Pearl et al.[34,§]	52° ± 14°	104° ± 12°			Average maximal joint angle of 8 "normal" subjects (aged 20–45 years) during ADL task; ROM measured using a 6° freedom spatial tracking system and electromagnetic sensors pinned to the humerus
Wash Face					
Henmi et al.[36,§]	50° ± 7°	90°[†]			Average maximum joint angle of 5 healthy adults (3 F, 2 M, aged 20–28 years) during ADL task; ROM measured using Vicon three-dimensional motion analysis system
Wash Opposite Shoulder					
Matsen et al.[38,§]	71°	128°			Data from single subject (unstated age and sex) measured using electromagnetic sensor pinned to humerus
O'Neill et a[37,§]	69° ± 11°	124° ± 9°			Average joint angle of 10 healthy subjects (unstated age) measured using 3Space Isotrak system
van Andel et al.[35,‡]	53° ± 3°	102° ± 11°	27° ± 9°		Average maximal joint angle of 10 healthy adults (6 M, 4 F, mean age 28.5 years) during ADL task; ROM measured using Optotrak motion analysis system

*Plane of elevation defines the position of the humerus in the horizontal plane such that shoulder abduction occurs in the 0-degree plane, shoulder flexion occurs in the 90-degree plane, and shoulder extension occurs in the −90-degree plane.
†90° = shoulder flexion; 0° = shoulder abduction; −90° = shoulder extension.
‡Humeral elevation (does not include scapulothoracic motion).
§Shoulder complex motion (glenohumeral and scapulothoracic motion combined).
Vicon Three-Dimensional Motion Analysis System by Vicon Motion Systems and Peak Performance Inc., Oxford, United Kingdom.
3Space Isotrak by Polhemus 3Space, Colchester, Vt.
Flock of Birds electromagnetic tracking device by Ascension Technology Corp, Burlington, Vt.
Optotrak Motion Analysis system by Northern Digital Inc., Ontario, Canada.
ADL, Activities of daily living.

results with results from previous studies impossible. Several subsequent studies have reported their results as based on ISB standards.[35,40] Caution should be used in making comparisons between studies that report data based on ISB standards vs studies that use more conventional descriptions of motion because the results are not likely to be comparable.

When results of studies focusing on shoulder motion are compared during functional activity, the reader must pay close attention to the motion that is being measured. Some investigators measure total motion of the shoulder complex, while others attempt to separate glenohumeral from scapulothoracic and other motions of the joints of this complex. Each of the studies reported in Table 3.1 is labeled as to the type of motion measured.

In 1992, Pearl et al.[34] proposed a system for describing motion of the shoulder that involved using a global positioning diagram in which planes of humeral motion were related to longitude and latitude lines on a globe. As part of this system, these investigators defined the plane of elevation as it corresponds to longitudinal markers on a globe, with the coronal plane (shoulder abduction) being the 0-degree plane, the anterior sagittal plane (shoulder flexion) being the +90-degree plane, and the posterior sagittal plane (shoulder extension) being the −90-degree plane. The angle of elevation was defined as corresponding to latitude markers and as "the angle between the

unelevated and the elevated humerus."[34] Thus an individual positioned in 45 degrees of shoulder abduction would have an angle of elevation of 45 degrees in the 0-degree plane of elevation. Many subsequent groups have reported data on functional shoulder motion using the conventions described by Pearl et al.[34] Both angle of elevation and the plane of elevation data are reported in Table 3.1. For authors who did not report plane of elevation data, shoulder flexion, abduction, and extension were converted to plane of elevation using definitions provided by Pearl et al.[34]

Table 3.1 contains the results of several studies that examined shoulder motion used during a variety of functional activities. Most of the studies from which data were derived were performed in young, healthy adults, although some data were obtained in children. Essentials of the method and study populations used are included in the table. Caution should be used in extrapolating these data to the general population because the sample sizes for all of the studies were small. For more in-depth information on each study, the reader is directed to the reference list at the end of this chapter. Additional information on shoulder range of motion required to perform functional tasks may be found in the review article by Oosterwijk and colleagues.[43] Figs. 3.5–3.7 demonstrate examples of shoulder motion used during selected functional tasks.

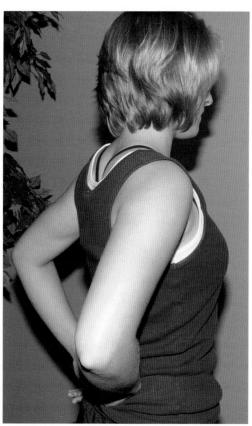

Fig. 3.5   Shoulder motion used when tucking in a shirt.

TECHNIQUES OF MEASUREMENT: SHOULDER FLEXION/EXTENSION

Shoulder flexion is a composite of motions that occur at multiple joints that make up the shoulder complex. Although some texts attempt to isolate the flexion that occurs at the glenohumeral joint and to measure that motion alone, no such attempt to isolate glenohumeral motion is presented in this text because such isolated movement does not occur past the first 30 degrees or so of shoulder flexion in normal motion.

Preferred patient positions for measuring shoulder flexion and extension are supine and prone, respectively, because of the greater stabilization of the spine that occurs in those positions compared with other positions in which flexion and extension can be measured. Measurement of flexion and extension also can be performed with the patient in the standing, sitting, or side-lying position. The American Academy of Orthopaedic Surgeons (AAOS) advocates measuring shoulder flexion and extension with the patient standing but states, "If spine and pelvic motion cannot be controlled, external rotation and elevation should be assessed with the patient supine."[44] Reliability of measurements of shoulder flexion taken with the patient supine is generally greater than for the same measurements taken with the patient in an upright position.[45] When shoulder flexion and extension are measured,

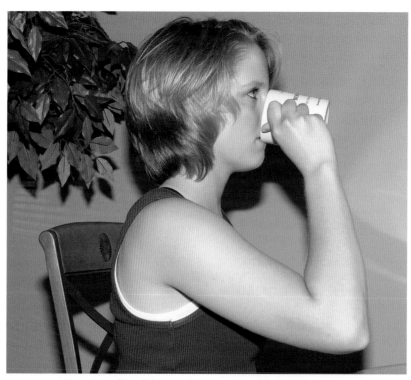

Fig. 3.6   Shoulder motion used to drink from a cup.

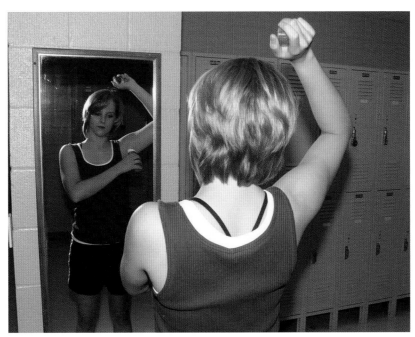

Fig. 3.7   Shoulder motion used to wash the opposite axilla or apply deodorant.

regardless of the position used, care should be taken to prevent extension of the spine in the case of shoulder flexion and flexion of the spine in the case of shoulder extension, which artificially inflate the resulting measurement and increase measurement error.

TECHNIQUES OF MEASUREMENT: SHOULDER ABDUCTION

As is the case for shoulder flexion, shoulder abduction is a composite movement, and no attempt is made in this text to isolate and measure the glenohumeral component of shoulder abduction. In obtaining the full range of shoulder abduction, the patient's glenohumeral joint should be placed in a neutral or, preferably, an externally rotated position. When abduction is attempted with the glenohumeral joint in internal rotation, the greater tuberosity of the humerus impinges upon the acromion, greatly restricting the range of shoulder abduction.[16] Because of issues of stabilization in the spine, shoulder abduction is best measured with the patient in a supine position, although measures of abduction in standing have also demonstrated high reliability.[45] Other positions for measuring abduction include standing, sitting, and prone, with standing being the position advocated by the AAOS.[44] During any measurement of shoulder abduction, regardless of the position used, care should be taken to prevent lateral

flexion of the spine by the patient, because this motion artificially inflates the range of shoulder abduction obtained.[46]

TECHNIQUES OF MEASUREMENT: SHOULDER MEDIAL-LATERAL ROTATION

The AAOS recommends measuring lateral rotation of the shoulder with the patient's shoulder placed in 0 or 90 degrees of abduction; medial rotation is measured with the shoulder in 90 degrees of abduction.[44] Other authors have advocated a slightly abducted position of the shoulder during measurement of medial-lateral rotation.[47] Because studies have demonstrated that range of lateral rotation of the shoulder increases and the range of medial rotation decreases with the amount of shoulder abduction used during the measurement,[14,47–49] standardized techniques for patient positioning should be followed for these as for all other goniometric procedures. In this text, shoulder medial and lateral rotation is measured with the patient positioned in 90 degrees of shoulder abduction. However, some patients with shoulder pathology are unable to attain 90 degrees of shoulder abduction, and in such cases, alternative positioning may be required. When used, such alternative positioning should be clearly documented. Reliability of rotation measurements, whether the shoulder is in 0 or 90 degrees of abduction, appears to be similarly high.[50,51]

Shoulder Flexion (Video 3.1)

Fig. 3.8 Starting position for measurement of shoulder flexion. Bony landmarks for goniometer alignment (lateral aspect of acromion process, lateral midline of thorax, lateral humeral epicondyle) indicated by red line and dots.

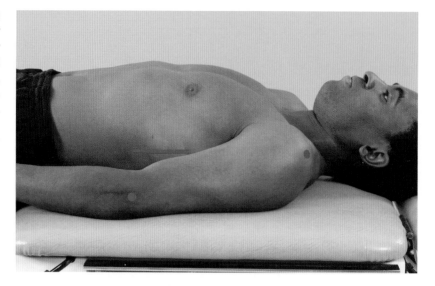

Normal ROM = 160–190 degrees.[49,52–58]

MDC for shoulder flexion goniometry measured by a single examiner = 5–7 degrees in normal and 5–13 degrees in pathological shoulders.[45,58–61]

Patient position	Supine with shoulder in 0-degrees flexion, elbow fully extended, forearm in neutral rotation with palm facing trunk (Fig. 3.8).
Stabilization	Over anterosuperior aspect of ipsilateral shoulder, proximal to humeral head (Fig. 3.9).
Examiner action	After instructing patient in motion desired, flex patient's shoulder through available ROM, avoiding extension of spine. Return limb to starting position. Performing passive movement provides an estimate of ROM and demonstrates to patient exact motion desired (see Fig. 3.9).
Goniometer alignment	Palpate the following bony landmarks (shown in Fig. 3.8) and align goniometer accordingly (Fig. 3.10).
Stationary arm	Lateral midline of thorax.

Fig. 3.9 End of shoulder flexion ROM, showing proper hand placement for stabilizing thorax and flexing shoulder. Bony landmarks for goniometer alignment (lateral midline of thorax, lateral humeral epicondyle) indicated by red line and dot.

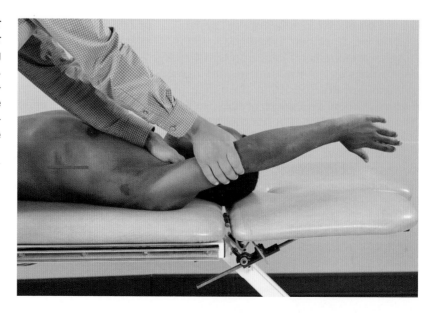

Fig. 3.10 Starting position for measurement of shoulder flexion, demonstrating proper initial alignment of goniometer.

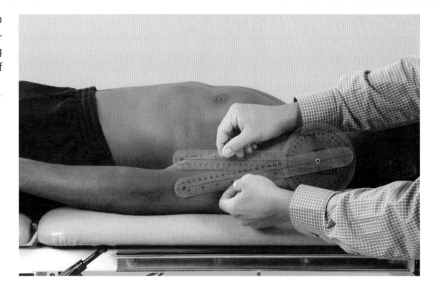

Axis	Midpoint of lateral aspect of acromion process.
Moving arm	Lateral midline of humerus toward lateral humeral epicondyle.
	Read scale of goniometer.
Patient/Examiner action	Perform passive, or have patient perform active, shoulder flexion (Fig. 3.11).
Confirmation of alignment	Repalpate landmarks and confirm proper goniometric alignment at end of ROM, correcting alignment as necessary (see Note). Read scale of goniometer (see Fig. 3.11).
Documentation	Record patient's ROM.
Note	To prevent artificial inflation of ROM measurements, no extension of spine should be allowed during measurement of shoulder flexion.
Alternative patient position	Seated or side-lying; goniometer alignment remains the same. Because of decreased ability to stabilize trunk in these positions, great care must be taken to ensure that stationary arm of goniometer remains aligned with lateral midline of thorax and that extension of spine does not occur. Failure to exercise such care will result in errors of measurement.

Fig. 3.11 End of shoulder flexion ROM, demonstrating proper alignment of goniometer at end of range.

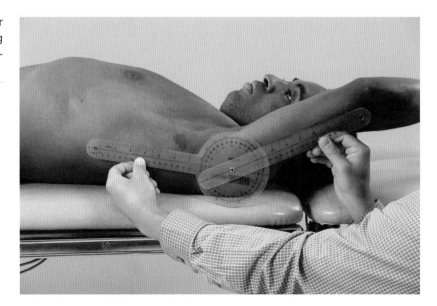

Shoulder Extension (Video 3.2)

Fig. 3.12 Starting position for measurement of shoulder extension. Bony landmarks for goniometer alignment (lateral aspect of acromion process, lateral midline of thorax, lateral humeral epicondyle) indicated by red line and dots.

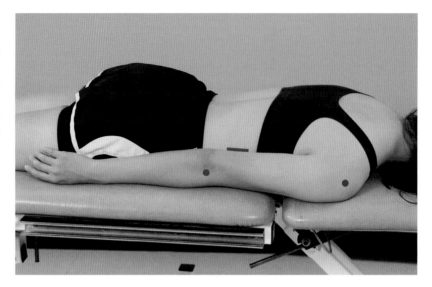

Normal ROM = 60–70 degrees.[49,52,53,58]

MDC for shoulder extension goniometry measured by a single examiner = 11–14 degrees in normal and 14 degrees in pathological shoulders.[45,58]

Patient position	Prone with shoulder in 0-degrees flexion, elbow fully extended, forearm in neutral rotation with palm facing trunk (Fig. 3.12).
Stabilization	Over posterosuperior aspect of ipsilateral shoulder, proximal to humeral head (Fig. 3.13).
Examiner action	After instructing patient in motion desired, extend patient's shoulder through available ROM, avoiding rotation of trunk. Return limb to starting position. Performing passive movement allows an estimate of ROM and demonstrates to patient exact motion desired (see Fig. 3.13).
Goniometer alignment	Palpate the following bony landmarks (shown in Fig. 3.12) and align goniometer accordingly (Fig. 3.14).

Fig. 3.13 End of shoulder extension ROM, showing proper hand placement for stabilizing thorax and extending shoulder. Bony landmarks for goniometer alignment (lateral aspect of acromion process, lateral midline of thorax, lateral humeral epicondyle) indicated by red line and dots.

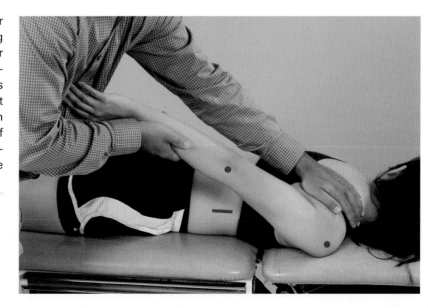

Fig. 3.14 Starting position for measurement of shoulder extension, demonstrating proper initial alignment of goniometer.

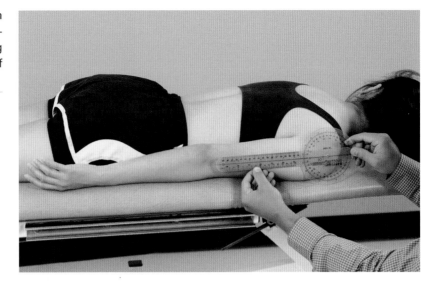

Stationary arm	Lateral midline of thorax.
Axis	Midpoint of lateral aspect of acromion process.
Moving arm	Lateral midline of humerus toward lateral humeral epicondyle.
	Read scale of goniometer.
Patient/Examiner action	Perform passive, or have patient perform active, shoulder extension (Fig. 3.15).
Confirmation of alignment	Repalpate landmarks and confirm proper goniometric alignment at end of ROM, correcting alignment as necessary (see Note). Read scale of goniometer (see Fig. 3.15).
Documentation	Record patient's ROM.
Note	To prevent artificial inflation of ROM measurements, no rotation of spine should be allowed during measurement of shoulder extension.
Alternative patient position	Seated or side-lying; goniometer alignment remains same. Because of decreased ability to stabilize trunk in these positions, great care must be taken to ensure that stationary arm of goniometer remains aligned with lateral midline of thorax and that flexion of spine does not occur. Failure to exercise such care will result in errors of measurement.

Fig. 3.15 End of shoulder extension ROM, demonstrating proper alignment of goniometer at end of range.

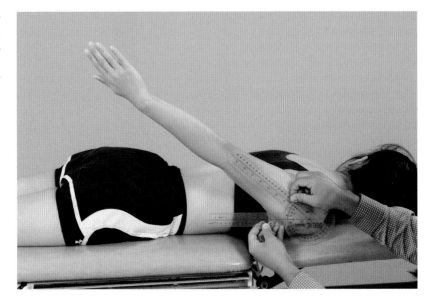

Shoulder Abduction (Video 3.3)

Fig. 3.16 Starting position for measurement of shoulder abduction with patient in the supine position. Bony landmarks for goniometer alignment (anterior aspect of acromion process, midline of sternum, medial humeral epicondyle) indicated by red line and dots.

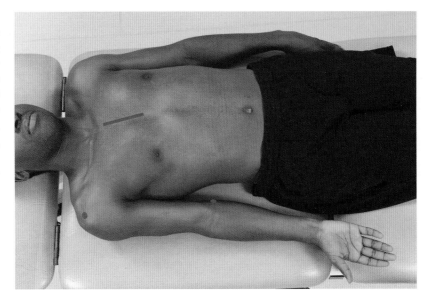

Normal ROM = 165–190 degrees.[49,52,53,56,58,62–64]

MDC for shoulder abduction goniometry measured by a single examiner = 5–16 degrees in normal and 5–18 degrees in pathological shoulders.[45,58,61]

Patient position	Supine with arm at side, upper extremity in anatomical position (Fig. 3.16).
Stabilization	Over superior aspect of ipsilateral shoulder, proximal to humeral head (Fig. 3.17).
Examiner action	After instructing patient in motion desired, abduct patient's shoulder through available ROM, avoiding lateral trunk flexion. Return limb to starting position. Performing passive movement provides an estimate of the ROM and demonstrates to patient exact motion desired (see Fig. 3.17).
Goniometer alignment	Palpate the following bony landmarks (shown in Fig. 3.16) and align goniometer accordingly (Fig. 3.18).

Fig. 3.17 End of shoulder abduction ROM, showing proper hand placement for stabilizing thorax and abducting shoulder. Bony landmarks for goniometer alignment (midline of sternum, medial humeral epicondyle) indicated by red line and dot.

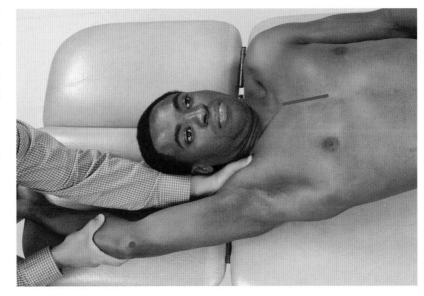

Fig. 3.18 Starting position for measurement of shoulder abduction, demonstrating proper initial alignment of goniometer.

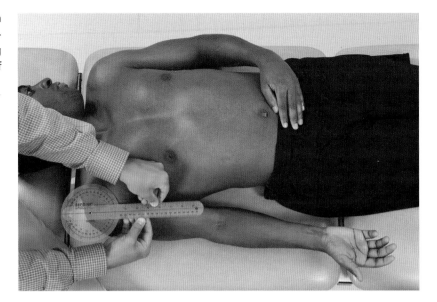

Stationary arm	Parallel to sternum.
Axis	Anterior aspect of acromion process.
Moving arm	Anterior midline of humerus toward medial humeral epicondyle.
	Read scale of goniometer.
Patient/Examiner action	Perform passive, or have patient perform active, shoulder abduction (Fig. 3.19).
Confirmation of alignment	Repalpate landmarks and confirm proper goniometric alignment at end of ROM, correcting alignment as necessary (see Note). Read scale of goniometer (see Fig. 3.19).
Documentation	Record patient's ROM.
Note	To prevent artificial inflation of ROM measurements, no lateral flexion of spine should be allowed during measurement of shoulder abduction.
Alternative patient position	Seated; goniometer is aligned as follows: Stationary arm parallel to spinous process of vertebral column, axis with posterior aspect of acromion, and moving arm along posterior midline of humerus toward lateral humeral epicondyle.

Fig. 3.19 End of shoulder abduction ROM, demonstrating proper alignment of goniometer at end of range.

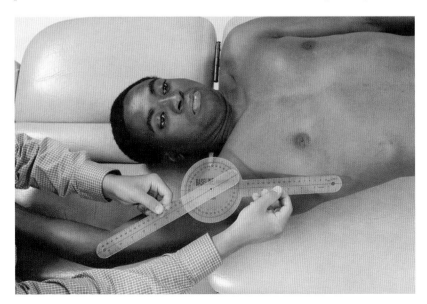

Shoulder Adduction (Video 3.4)

Fig. 3.20 Starting position for measurement of shoulder adduction with patient in the supine position. Bony landmarks for goniometer alignment (anterior aspect of acromion process, midline of sternum, medial humeral epicondyle) indicated by red line and dots.

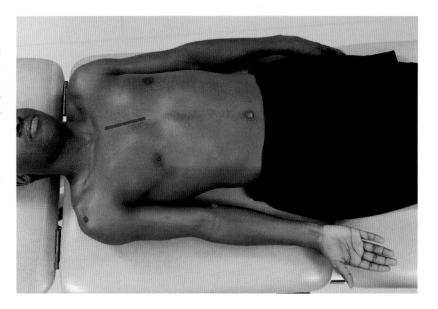

Patient position	Supine with arm at side, upper extremity in anatomical position (Fig. 3.20).
Stabilization	Over superior aspect of ipsilateral shoulder, proximal to humeral head (Fig. 3.21).
Examiner action	After instructing patient in motion desired, adduct patient's shoulder through available ROM, avoiding lateral trunk flexion. Return limb to starting position. Performing passive movement provides an estimate of ROM and demonstrates to patient exact motion desired (see Fig. 3.21).
Goniometer alignment	Palpate the following bony landmarks (shown in Fig. 3.20) and align goniometer accordingly (Fig. 3.22).
Stationary arm	Parallel to sternum.
Axis	Anterior aspect of acromion process.

Fig. 3.21 End of shoulder adduction ROM, showing proper hand placement for stabilizing thorax and adducting shoulder. Bony landmarks for goniometer alignment (anterior aspect of acromion process, midline of sternum, medial humeral epicondyle) indicated by red line and dots.

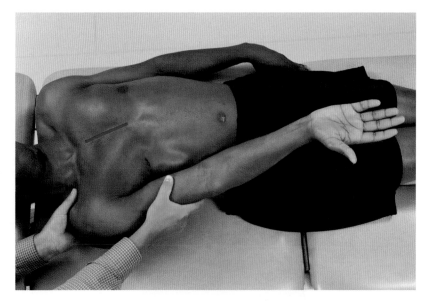

Fig. 3.22 Starting position for measurement of shoulder adduction, demonstrating proper initial alignment of goniometer.

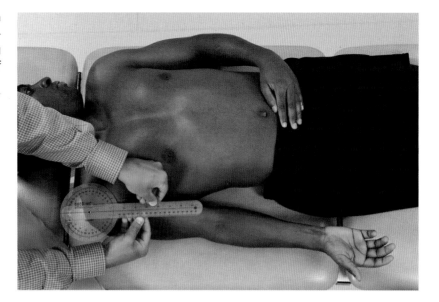

Moving arm	Anterior midline of humerus in line with medial humeral epicondyle.
	Read scale of goniometer.
Patient/Examiner action	Perform passive, or have patient perform active, shoulder adduction (Fig. 3.23).
Confirmation of alignment	Repalpate landmarks and confirm proper goniometric alignment at end of ROM, correcting alignment as necessary (see Note). Read scale of goniometer (see Fig. 3.23).
Documentation	Record patient's ROM.
Note	To prevent artificial inflation of ROM measurements, no lateral flexion of spine should be allowed during measurement of shoulder adduction.
Alternative patient position	Seated; goniometer alignment remains the same.

Fig. 3.23 End of shoulder adduction ROM, demonstrating proper alignment of goniometer at end of range.

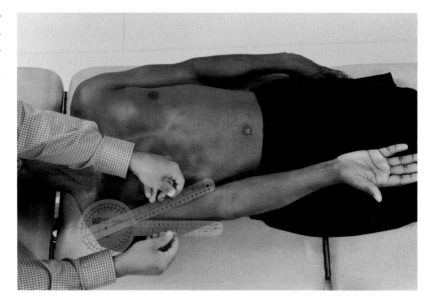

Shoulder Horizontal Abduction (Video 3.5)

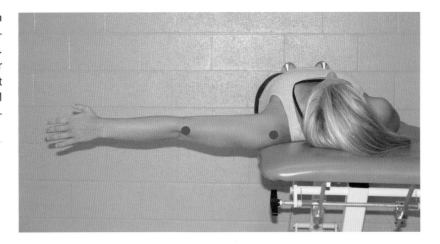

Fig. 3.24 Starting position for measurement of shoulder horizontal abduction. Landmarks for goniometer alignment (superior aspect of acromion process, lateral epicondyle of humerus) indicated by red dots.

Patient position	Supine with shoulder abducted to 90 degrees, glenohumeral joint at edge of table, elbow fully extended, and forearm in neutral rotation (Fig. 3.24).
Stabilization	Over superior aspect of ipsilateral shoulder, proximal to humeral head (Fig. 3.25).
Examiner action	After instructing patient in motion desired, horizontally abduct patient's shoulder through available ROM. Return limb to starting position. Performing passive movement provides an estimate of ROM and demonstrates to patient exact motion desired (see Fig. 3.25).
Goniometer alignment	Palpate the following bony landmarks (shown in Fig. 3.24), and align goniometer accordingly (Fig. 3.26).
Stationary arm	Parallel to floor.
Axis	Superior aspect of acromion process.

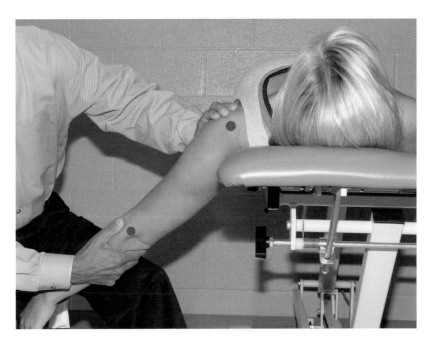

Fig. 3.25 End of shoulder horizontal abduction ROM, showing proper hand placement for stabilizing thorax and abducting shoulder in horizontal plane. Landmarks for goniometer alignment (superior aspect of acromion process, lateral epicondyle of humerus) indicated by red dots.

Fig. 3.26 Starting position for measurement of shoulder horizontal abduction, demonstrating proper initial alignment of goniometer.

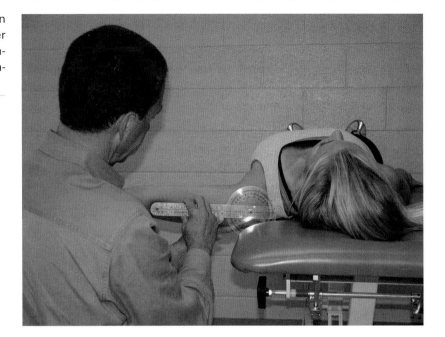

Moving arm	Midline of humerus toward lateral humeral epicondyle.
	Read scale of goniometer.
Patient/Examiner action	Perform passive, or have patient perform active, horizontal abduction of shoulder (Fig. 3.27).
Confirmation of alignment	Repalpate landmarks and confirm proper goniometer alignment at end of ROM, correcting alignment as necessary. Read scale of goniometer (see Fig. 3.27).
Documentation	Record patient's ROM.

Fig. 3.27 End of shoulder horizontal abduction ROM, demonstrating proper alignment of goniometer at end of range.

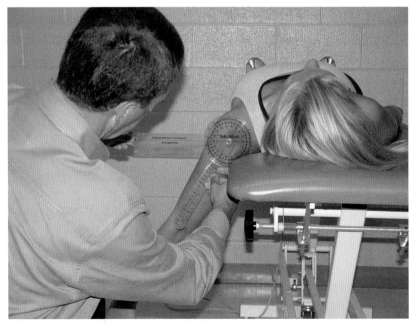

Shoulder Horizontal Adduction (Video 3.6)

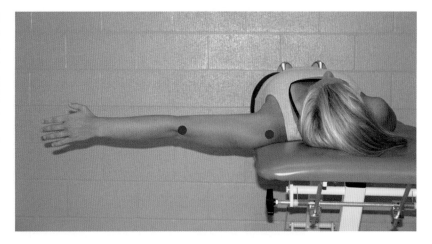

Fig. 3.28 Starting position for measurement of shoulder horizontal adduction. Landmarks for goniometer alignment (superior aspect of acromion process, lateral epicondyle of humerus) indicated by red dots.

Patient position	Supine with shoulder abducted to 90 degrees, glenohumeral joint at edge of table, elbow fully extended, and forearm in neutral rotation (Fig. 3.28).
Stabilization	Over ipsilateral shoulder and proximal humerus (Fig. 3.29).
Examiner action	After instructing patient in motion desired, horizontally adduct patient's shoulder through available ROM, making sure scapula does not lift off the table. Return limb to starting position. Performing passive movement provides an estimate of ROM and demonstrates to patient exact motion desired (see Fig. 3.29).
Goniometer alignment	Palpate the following bony landmarks (shown in Fig. 3.28) and align goniometer accordingly (Fig. 3.30).
Stationary arm	Parallel to floor.
Axis	Superior aspect of acromion process.

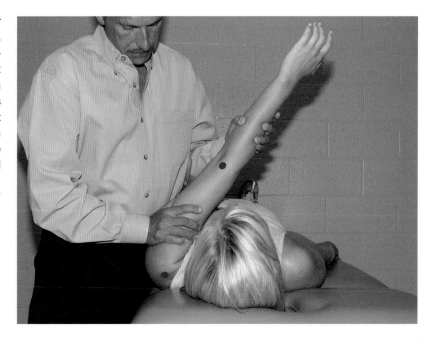

Fig. 3.29 End of shoulder horizontal adduction ROM, showing proper hand placement for stabilizing thorax and adducting shoulder in horizontal plane. Landmarks for goniometer alignment (superior aspect of acromion process, lateral epicondyle of humerus) indicated by red dots.

Fig. 3.30 Starting position for measurement of shoulder horizontal adduction, demonstrating proper initial alignment of goniometer.

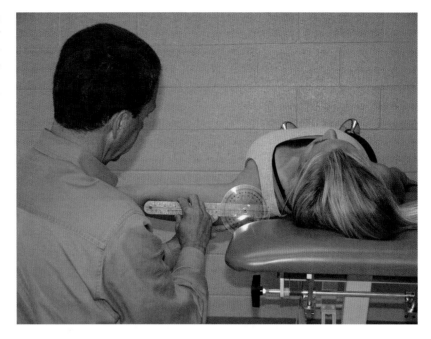

Moving arm	Midline of humerus toward lateral humeral epicondyle.
	Read scale of goniometer.
Patient/Examiner action	Perform passive, or have patient perform active, horizontal adduction of shoulder, stopping at point of elevation of scapula off the table (see Fig. 3.29).
Confirmation of alignment	Repalpate landmarks and confirm proper goniometer alignment at end of ROM, correcting alignment as necessary. Read scale of goniometer (Fig. 3.31).
Documentation	Record patient's ROM.

Fig. 3.31 End of shoulder horizontal adduction ROM, demonstrating proper alignment of goniometer at end of range.

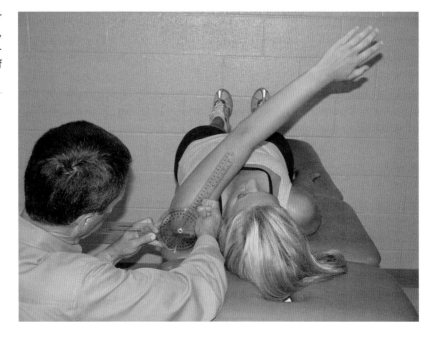

Shoulder Lateral Rotation: Goniometer (Video 3.7)

Fig. 3.32 Starting position for measurement of shoulder lateral rotation. Landmarks for goniometer alignment (olecranon and styloid processes of ulna) indicated by red dots.

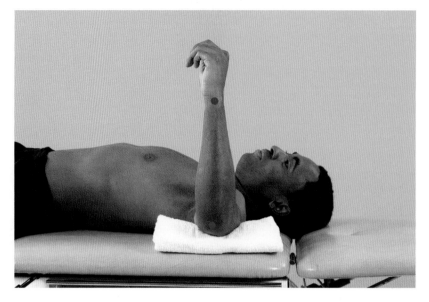

Normal ROM = 70–110 degrees.[49,52,53,58,63,65]

MDC for shoulder lateral rotation goniometry measured by a single examiner = 8–14 degrees in normal and 5–13 degrees in pathological shoulders.[45,51,58,61]

Patient position	Supine with shoulder abducted to 90 degrees, elbow flexed to 90 degrees, forearm pronated, and folded towel under humerus (Fig. 3.32).
Stabilization	Place heel of hand over superior aspect of ipsilateral shoulder, proximal to humeral head; fingers over ipsilateral scapula (Fig. 3.33).
Examiner action	After instructing patient in motion desired, laterally rotate patient's shoulder through available ROM, making sure the scapula does not lift off the table. Return limb to starting position. Performing passive movement provides an estimate of ROM and demonstrates to patient exact motion desired (see Fig. 3.33).
Goniometer alignment	Palpate the following bony landmarks (shown in Fig. 3.32) and align goniometer accordingly (Fig. 3.34).

Fig. 3.33 End of shoulder lateral rotation ROM, showing proper hand placement for stabilizing thorax and laterally rotating shoulder. Landmarks for goniometer alignment (olecranon and styloid processes of ulna) indicated by red dots.

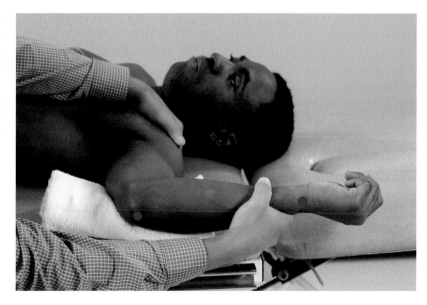

Fig. 3.34 Starting position for measurement of shoulder lateral rotation, demonstrating proper initial alignment of goniometer.

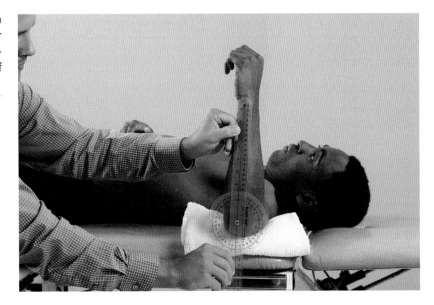

Stationary arm	Perpendicular to floor.
Axis	Olecranon process of ulna.
Moving arm	Ulnar border of forearm toward ulnar styloid process.
	Read scale of goniometer.
Patient/Examiner action	Perform passive, or have patient perform active, lateral rotation of the shoulder, stopping at the point of elevation of the scapula off the table (Fig. 3.35).
Confirmation of alignment	Repalpate landmarks and confirm proper goniometer alignment at end of ROM, correcting alignment as necessary. Read scale of goniometer (see Fig. 3.35).
Documentation	Record patient's ROM.
Alternative patient position	Prone; goniometer alignment remains same. Measurement also may be taken with shoulder positioned in less abduction. If such positioning is used, amount of abduction of shoulder must be documented.

Fig. 3.35 End of shoulder lateral rotation ROM, demonstrating proper alignment of goniometer at end of range.

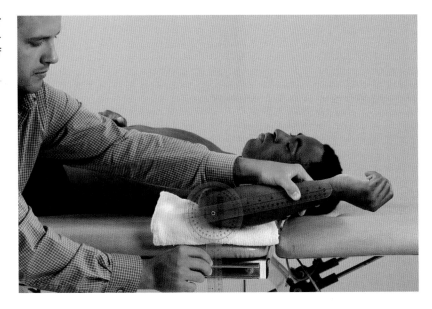

Shoulder Medial Rotation: Goniometer (Video 3.8)

Fig. 3.36 Starting position for measurement of shoulder medial rotation. Landmarks for goniometer alignment (olecranon and styloid processes of ulna) indicated by red dots.

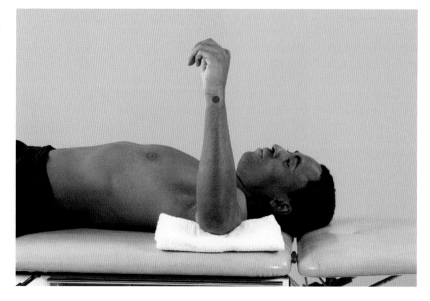

Normal ROM = 70–100 degrees.[49,52,53,58,63,65]

MDC for shoulder medial rotation goniometry measured by a single examiner = 5–11 degrees in normal and 14 degrees in pathological shoulders.[45,51,58,61]

Patient position

Supine with shoulder abducted to 90 degrees, elbow flexed to 90 degrees, forearm pronated, and folded towel under humerus (Fig. 3.36).

Stabilization

Place heel of hand over superior aspect of ipsilateral shoulder, proximal to humeral head, and fingers over ipsilateral scapula (Fig. 3.37).

Examiner action

After instructing patient in motion desired, medially rotate patient's shoulder through available ROM, making sure the scapula does not lift off the table. Return limb to starting position. Performing passive movement provides an estimate of ROM and demonstrates to patient exact motion desired (see Fig. 3.37).

Goniometer alignment

Palpate the following bony landmarks (shown in Fig. 3.36) and align goniometer accordingly (Fig. 3.38).

Fig. 3.37 End of shoulder medial rotation ROM, showing proper hand placement for stabilizing thorax and medially rotating shoulder. Landmarks for goniometer alignment (olecranon and styloid processes of ulna) indicated by red dots.

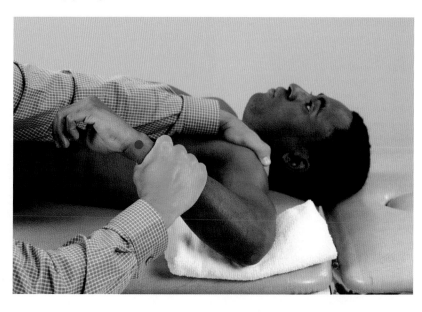

Fig. 3.38 Starting position for measurement of shoulder medial rotation, demonstrating proper initial alignment of goniometer.

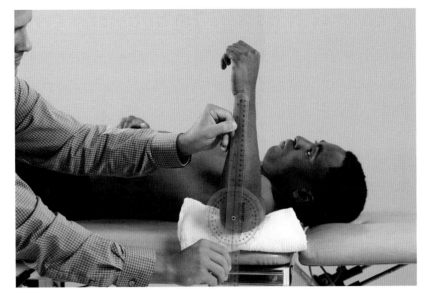

Stationary arm	Perpendicular to floor.
Axis	Olecranon process of ulna.
Moving arm	Ulnar border of forearm toward ulnar styloid process.
	Read scale of goniometer.
Patient/Examiner action	Perform passive, or have patient perform active, medial rotation of the shoulder, stopping at the point of elevation of the scapula off the table (Fig. 3.39).
Confirmation of alignment	Repalpate landmarks and confirm proper goniometer alignment at end of ROM, correcting alignment as necessary. Read scale of goniometer (see Fig. 3.39).
Documentation	Record patient's ROM.
Alternative patient position	Prone; goniometer alignment remains same. Measurement also may be taken with shoulder positioned in less abduction. If such positioning is used, amount of abduction of shoulder must be documented.

Fig. 3.39 End of shoulder medial rotation ROM, demonstrating proper alignment of goniometer at end of range.

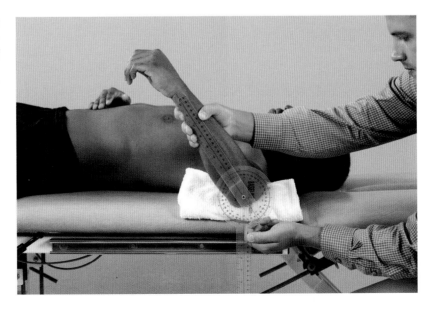

Shoulder Lateral Rotation: Inclinometer (Video 3.9)

Fig. 3.40 Starting position for measurement of shoulder lateral rotation.

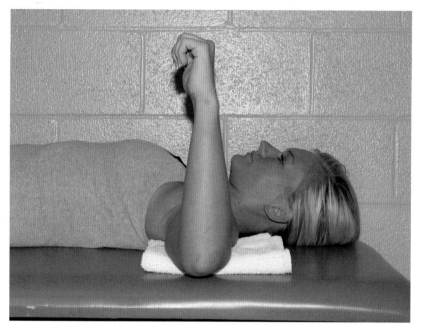

Normal ROM = 70–110 degrees.[52,53,58,63,65]

MDC for shoulder lateral rotation inclinometry measured by a single examiner = 5–16 degrees in normal and 13–29 degrees in pathological shoulders.[45,51,66–68]

Patient position

Supine with shoulder abducted to 90 degrees, elbow flexed to 90 degrees, forearm pronated, and folded towel under humerus (Fig. 3.40).

Stabilization

Place heel of hand over superior aspect of ipsilateral shoulder, proximal to humeral head; fingers over ipsilateral scapula (Fig. 3.41).

Examiner action

After instructing patient in motion desired, laterally rotate patient's shoulder through available ROM, making sure the scapula does not lift off the table. Return limb to starting position. Performing passive movement provides an estimate of ROM and demonstrates to patient exact motion desired (see Fig. 3.41).

Fig. 3.41 End of shoulder lateral rotation ROM, showing proper hand placement for stabilizing thorax and laterally rotating shoulder.

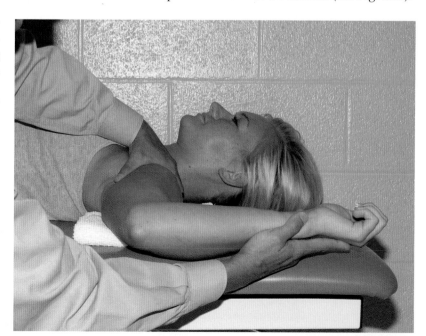

Fig. 3.42 Starting position for measurement of shoulder lateral rotation, demonstrating proper initial alignment of inclinometer.

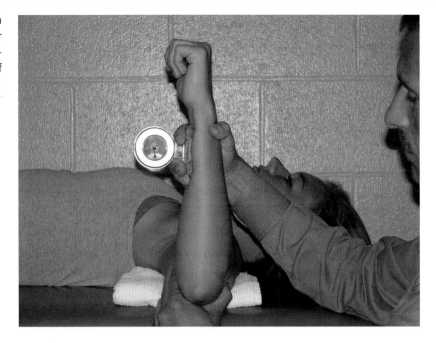

Inclinometer alignment

On ventral surface of ulna, proximal to wrist; legs of inclinometer parallel to forearm. Ensure that inclinometer is set to 0 degrees once it is positioned on patient (Fig. 3.42).

Patient/Examiner action

Perform passive, or have patient perform active, lateral rotation of the shoulder, stopping at the point of elevation of the scapula off the table (Fig. 3.43).

Inclinometer alignment

Ensure that inclinometer remains in firm contact with ventral surface of ulna. Read scale of inclinometer (see Fig. 3.43).

Alternative patient position

Prone; in this case, inclinometer should be positioned on dorsal surface of ulna (see inclinometer positioning for Shoulder Medial Rotation). Measurement also may be taken with shoulder positioned in less abduction. If such positioning is used, amount of abduction of shoulder must be documented.

Documentation

Record patient's ROM.

Fig. 3.43 End of shoulder lateral rotation ROM, demonstrating proper alignment of inclinometer at end of range.

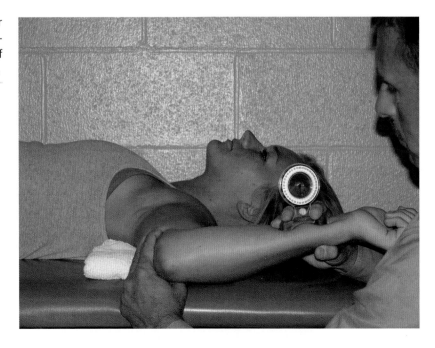

Shoulder Medial Rotation: Inclinometer (Video 3.10)

Fig. 3.44 Starting position for measurement of shoulder medial rotation.

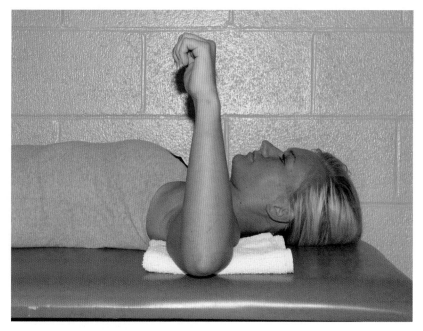

Normal ROM = 70–100 degrees.[49,52,53,58,63,65]

MDC for shoulder medial rotation inclinometry measured by a single examiner = 5–16 degrees in normal and 18 degrees in pathological shoulders.[45,51,61,66–68]

Patient position

Supine with shoulder abducted to 90 degrees, elbow flexed to 90 degrees, forearm pronated, and folded towel under humerus (Fig. 3.44).

Stabilization

Place heel of hand over superior aspect of ipsilateral shoulder, proximal to humeral head; fingers or thumb over ipsilateral scapula (Fig. 3.45).

Examiner action

After instructing patient in motion desired, medially rotate patient's shoulder through available ROM, making sure the scapula does not lift off the table. Return limb to starting position. Performing passive movement provides an estimate of ROM and demonstrates to patient exact motion desired (see Fig. 3.45).

Fig. 3.45 End of shoulder medial rotation ROM, showing proper hand placement for stabilizing thorax and medially rotating shoulder.

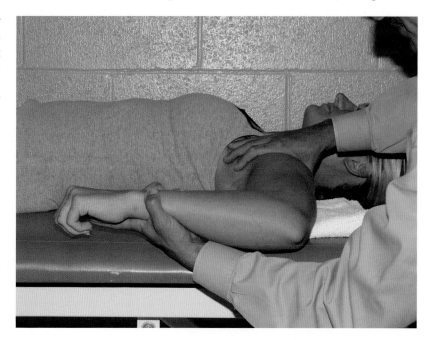

Fig. 3.46 Starting position for measurement of shoulder medial rotation, demonstrating proper initial alignment of inclinometer.

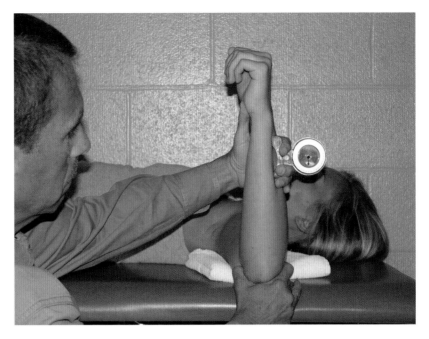

Inclinometer alignment

On dorsal surface of ulna, proximal to wrist; legs of inclinometer parallel to forearm. Ensure that inclinometer is set to 0 degrees once it is positioned on patient (Fig. 3.46).

Patient/Examiner action

Perform passive, or have patient perform active, medial rotation of the shoulder, stopping at the point of elevation of the scapula off the table (Fig. 3.47).

Inclinometer alignment

Ensure that inclinometer remains in firm contact with dorsal surface of ulna. Read scale of inclinometer (see Fig. 3.47).

Alternative patient position

Prone; in this case, inclinometer should be positioned on ventral surface of ulna (see inclinometer positioning for Shoulder Lateral Rotation). Measurement also may be taken with shoulder positioned in less abduction. If such positioning is used, amount of abduction of shoulder must be documented.

Documentation

Record patient's ROM.

Fig. 3.47 End of shoulder medial rotation ROM, demonstrating proper alignment of inclinometer at end of range.

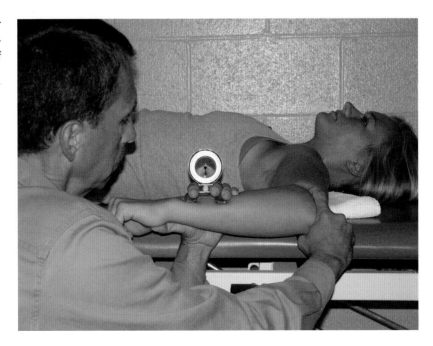

Shoulder Lateral Rotation: Smartphone Method

Fig. 3.48 Starting position for measurement of shoulder lateral rotation.

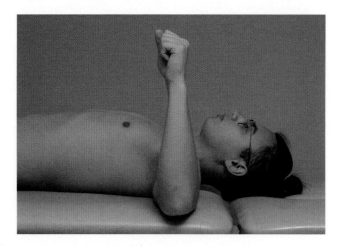

Patient position	Supine with shoulder abducted to 90 degrees, elbow flexed to 90 degrees, and forearm pronated. (Note—folded towel should be placed under humerus) (Fig. 3.48).
Stabilization	Place heel of hand over superior aspect of ipsilateral shoulder, proximal to humeral head; fingers over ipsilateral scapula (Fig. 3.49).
Examiner action	After instructing patient in motion desired, laterally rotate patient's shoulder through available ROM, making sure the scapula does not lift off the table. Return limb to starting position. Performing passive movement provides an estimate of ROM and demonstrates to patient exact motion desired (see Fig. 3.49).

Fig. 3.49 End of shoulder lateral rotation ROM, showing proper hand placement for stabilizing thorax and laterally rotating shoulder.

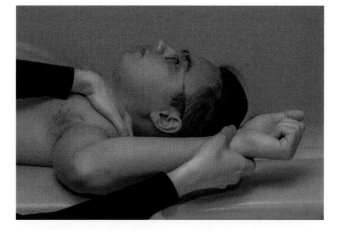

Fig. 3.50 Starting position for measurement of shoulder lateral rotation, demonstrating proper initial alignment of Smartphone.

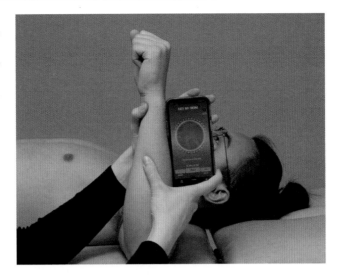

Smartphone alignment

Parallel with surface of ulna, proximal to wrist. Ensure that measurement app on Smartphone reads 0 degrees once it is positioned on patient (Fig. 3.50).

Patient/Examiner action

Perform passive, or have patient perform active, lateral rotation of the shoulder, stopping at the point of elevation of the scapula off the table (Fig. 3.51). Read angle on Smartphone at end of ROM.

Documentation

Record patient's ROM.

Fig. 3.51 End of shoulder lateral rotation ROM, demonstrating proper alignment of Smartphone at end of range.

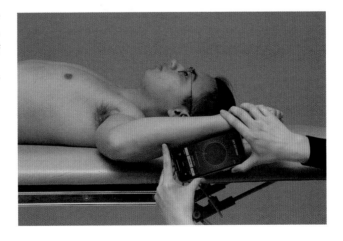

Shoulder Medial Rotation: Inclinometer

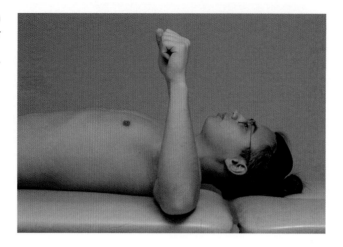

Fig. 3.52 Starting position for measurement of shoulder medial rotation.

Patient position

Supine with shoulder abducted to 90 degrees, elbow flexed to 90 degrees, forearm pronated. (Note—folded towel should be placed under humerus) (Fig. 3.52).

Stabilization

Place heel of hand over superior aspect of ipsilateral shoulder, proximal to humeral head; fingers or thumb over ipsilateral scapula (Fig. 3.53).

Examiner action

After instructing patient in motion desired, medially rotate patient's shoulder through available ROM, making sure the scapula does not lift off the table. Return limb to starting position. Performing passive movement provides an estimate of ROM and demonstrates to patient exact motion desired (see Fig. 3.53).

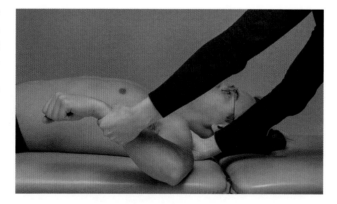

Fig. 3.53 End of shoulder medial rotation ROM, showing proper hand placement for stabilizing thorax and medially rotating shoulder.

Fig. 3.54 Starting position for measurement of shoulder medial rotation, demonstrating proper initial alignment of Smartphone.

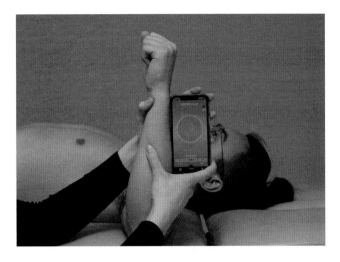

Smartphone alignment

Parallel with surface of ulna, proximal to wrist. Ensure that measurement app on Smartphone reads 0 degrees once it is positioned on patient (Fig. 3.54).

Patient/Examiner action

Perform passive, or have patient perform active, medial rotation of the shoulder, stopping at the point of elevation of the scapula off the table (Fig. 3.55). Read angle on Smartphone at end of ROM.

Documentation

Record patient's ROM.

Fig. 3.55 End of shoulder medial rotation ROM, demonstrating proper alignment of Smartphone at end of range.

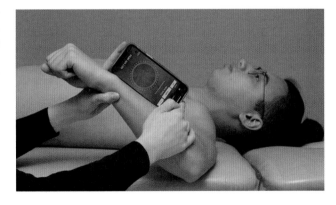

References

1. Kent BE. Functional anatomy of the shoulder complex. A review. *Phys Ther.* 1971;51(8):947.
2. Smith LE, Weiss L. *Lehmkuhl, Brunnstrom's Clinical Kinesiology.* 5th ed. Philadelphia: F.A. Davis; 1996.
3. Clemente C. *Gray's Anatomy of the Human Body.* 13th ed. Philadelphia: Lea & Febiger; 1985.
4. Massengill AD, Seeger LL, L Yao, et al. Labrocapsular ligamentous complex of the shoulder: Normal anatomy, anatomical variation, and pitfalls of MR imaging and MR arthrography. *Radiographics.* 1994;14(6):1211–1223.
5. Clark JM, Harryman DT. Tendons, ligaments, and capsule of the rotator cuff. Gross and microscopic anatomy. *J Bone Joint Surg Am.* 1992;74(5):713–725.
6. Culham E, Peat M. Functional anatomy of the shoulder complex. *J Orthop Sports Phys Ther.* 1993;18(1):342–350.
7. Pouliart N, Gagey OJ. The arthroscopic view of the glenohumeral ligaments compared with anatomy: fold or fact? *J Shoulder Elbow Surg.* 2005;14(3):324–328.
8. Turkel SJ, Panio MW, Marshall JL, et al. Stabilizing mechanisms preventing anterior dislocation of the glenohumeral joint. *J Bone Joint Surg Am.* 1981;63(8):1208–1217.
9. Ferrari DA. Capsular ligaments of the shoulder. Anatomical and functional study of the anterior superior capsule. *Am J Sports Med.* 1990;18(1):20–24.
10. Morrey B, An K. Biomechanics of the shoulder. In: *The Shoulder.* Philadelphia: WB Saunders; 1990.
11. Edelson JG, Taitz C, Grishkan A. The coracohumeral ligament. Anatomy of a substantial but neglected structure. *J Bone Joint Surg Br.* 1991;73(1):150–153.
12. O'Brien SJ, Neves MC, Arnoczky SP, et al. The anatomy and histology of the inferior glenohumeral ligament complex of the shoulder. *Am J Sports Med.* 1990;18(5):449–456.
13. Ovesen J, Nielsen S. Stability of the shoulder joint. Cadaver study of stabilizing structures. *Acta Orthop Scand.* 1985;56(2):149–151.
14. Neumann D. *Kinesiology of the Musculoskeletal System.* St Louis: Mosby; 2002.
15. Perry J. Normal upper extremity kinesiology. *Phys Ther.* 1978;58(3):265–278.
16. Soderberg G. *Kinesiology: Application to Pathological Motion.* 2nd ed. Baltimore: Williams & Wilkins; 1997.
17. Kapandji I. The physiology of joints. In: *Upper Limb.* vol. 1. 5th ed. New York: Churchill Livingstone; 1982.
18. Harris RI, Vu DH, Sonnabend DH, et al. Anatomical variance of the coracoclavicular ligaments. *J Shoulder Elbow Surg.* 2001;10(6):585–588.
19. Sellards R. Anatomy and biomechanics of the acromioclavicular joint. *Oper Tech Sports Med.* 2004;12:2–5.
20. Fukuda K, Craig EV, An KN, et al. Biomechanical study of the ligamentous system of the acromioclavicular joint. *J Bone Joint Surg Am.* 1986;68(3):434–440.
21. Inman VT, Saunders JB, Abbott LC. Observations of the function of the shoulder joint. *J Bone Joint Surg.* 1944;26:1–30.
22. Bagg SD, Forrest WJ. A biomechanical analysis of scapular rotation during arm abduction in the scapular plane. *Am J Phys Med Rehabil.* 1988;67(6):238–245.
23. Doody SG, Freedman L, Waterland JC. Shoulder movements during abduction in the scapular plane. *Arch Phys Med Rehabil.* 1970;51(10):595–604.
24. Freedman L, Munro RR. Abduction of the arm in the scapular plane: scapular and glenohumeral movements. A roentgenographic study. *J Bone Joint Surg Am.* 1966;48(8):1503–1510.
25. McClure PW, Michener LA, Sennett BJ, et al. Direct 3-dimensional measurement of scapular kinematics during dynamic movements in vivo. *J Shoulder Elbow Surg.* 2001;10(3):269–277.
26. Giphart JE, Brunkhorst JP, Horn NH, et al. Effect of plane of arm elevation on glenohumeral kinematics: a normative biplane fluoroscopy study. *J Bone Joint Surg Am.* 2013;95(3):238–245.
27. Poppen NK, Walker PS. Normal and abnormal motion of the shoulder. *J Bone Joint Surg Am.* 1976;58(2):195–201.
28. Cyriax JH, Coldham M. *Textbook of Orthopaedic Medicine.* London: Baillière Tindall; 1982.
29. Kaltenborn F. *Mobilization of the Extremity Joints.* 3rd ed. Oslo: Olaf Norlis Bokhandel; 1980.
30. Safaee-Rad R, Shwedyk E, Quanbury AO, et al. Normal functional range of motion of upper limb joints during performance of three feeding activities. *Arch Phys Med Rehabil.* 1990;71(7):505–509.
31. Cooper JE, Shwedyk E, Quanbury AO, et al. Elbow joint restriction: effect on functional upper limb motion during performance of three feeding activities. *Arch Phys Med Rehabil.* 1993;74(8):805–809.
32. Aizawa J, Masuda T, T Koyama, et al. Three-dimensional motion of the upper extremity joints during various activities of daily living. *J Biomech.* 2010;43(15):2915–2922.
33. Magermans DJ, Chadwick EK, Veeger HE, et al. Requirements for upper extremity motions during activities of daily living. *Clin Biomech (Bristol, Avon).* 2005;20(6):591–599.
34. Pearl ML, Harris SL, Lippitt SB, et al. A system for describing positions of the humerus relative to the thorax and its use in the presentation of several functionally important arm positions. *J Shoulder Elbow Surg.* 1992;1(2):13–18.
35. van Andel CJ, Wolterbeek N, Doorenbosch CA, et al. Complete 3D kinematics of upper extremity functional tasks. *Gait Posture.* 2008;27(1):120–127.
36. Henmi S, Yonenobu K, T Masatomi, et al. A biomechanical study of activities of daily living using neck and upper limbs with an optical three-dimensional motion analysis system. *Mod Rheumatol.* 2006;16(5):289–293.
37. O'Neill OR, Morrey BF, S Tanaka, et al. Compensatory motion in the upper extremity after elbow arthrodesis. *Clin Orthop Relat Res.* 1992;281:89–96.
38. Matsen FA, Sidles JA, Lippitt SB. *Practical Evaluation and Management of the Shoulder.* Philadelphia: WB Saunders; 1994.
39. Namdari S, Yagnik G, Ebaugh DD, et al. Defining functional shoulder range of motion for activities of daily living. *J Shoulder Elbow Surg.* 2012;21(9):1177–1183.
40. Petuskey K, Bagley A, E Abdala, et al. Upper extremity kinematics during functional activities: three-dimensional studies in a normal pediatric population. *Gait Posture.* 2007;25(4):573–579.
41. Mackey AH, Walt SE, Stott NS. Deficits in upper-limb task performance in children with hemiplegic cerebral palsy as defined by 3-dimensional kinematics. *Arch Phys Med Rehabil.* 2006;87(2):207–215.
42. Wu G, van der Helm FC, Veeger HE, et al. ISB recommendation on definitions of joint coordinate systems of various joints for the reporting of human joint motion—part II: shoulder, elbow, wrist and hand. *J Biomech.* 2005;38(5):981–992.
43. Oosterwijk AM, Nieuwenhuis MK, van der Schans CP, Mouton LJ. Shoulder and elbow range of motion for the performance of activities of daily living: a systematic review. *Physiother Theory Pract.* 2018;34(7):503–528.
44. Greene WB, Heckman JD. *The Clinical Measurement of Joint Motion.* Rosemont, IL: American Academy of Orthopaedic Surgeons; 1994.
45. Muir SW, Corea CL, Beaupre L. Evaluating change in clinical status: reliability and measures of agreement for the assessment of glenohumeral range of motion. *N Am J Sports Phys Ther.* 2010;5(3):98–110.
46. Southgate DF, Hill AM, S Alexander, et al. The range of axial rotation of the glenohumeral joint. *J Biomech.* 2009;42(9):1307–1312.
47. MacDermid JC, Chesworth BM, S Patterson, et al. Intratester and intertester reliability of goniometric measurement of passive lateral shoulder rotation. *J Hand Ther.* 1999;12(3):187–192.
48. Armstrong AD, MacDermid JC, S Chinchalkar, et al. Reliability of range-of-motion measurement in the elbow and forearm. *J Shoulder Elbow Surg.* 1998;7(6):573–580.
49. Boone DC, Azen SP. Normal range of motion of joints in male subjects. *J Bone Joint Surg Am.* 1979;61(5):756–759.
50. Shin SH, Ro du H, Lee OS, et al. Within-day reliability of shoulder range of motion measurement with a smartphone. *Man Ther.* 2012;17(4):298–304.
51. Cools AM, De Wilde L, Van Tongel A, et al. Measuring shoulder external and internal rotation strength and range of motion: comprehensive intra-rater and inter-rater reliability study of several testing protocols. *J Shoulder Elbow Surg.* 2014;23(10):1454–1461.
52. American Medical Association. *Guides to the Evaluation of Permanent Impairment.* 4th ed. Chicago: American Medical Association; 1993:339. xvii.
53. American Academy of Orthopaedic Surgeons. *Joint Motion: Method of Measuring and Recording.* Chicago: American Academy of Orthopaedic Surgeons; 1965.
54. Escalante A, Lichtenstein MJ, Hazuda HP. Determinants of shoulder and elbow flexion range: results from the San Antonio longitudinal study of aging. *Arthritis Care Res.* 1999;12(4):277–286.

55. Murray MP, Gore DR, Gardner GM, et al. Shoulder motion and muscle strength of normal men and women in two age groups. *Clin Orthop Relat Res.* 1985;192:268–273.

56. Sabari JS, Maltzev I, D Lubarsky, et al. Goniometric assessment of shoulder range of motion: comparison of testing in supine and sitting positions. *Arch Phys Med Rehabil.* 1998;79(6):647–651.

57. Soucie JM, Wang C, A Forsyth, et al. Range of motion measurements: reference values and a database for comparison studies. *Haemophilia.* 2011;17(3):500–507.

58. Macedo LG, Magee DJ. Effects of age on passive range of motion of selected peripheral joints in healthy adult females. *Physiother Theory Pract.* 2009;25(2):145–164.

59. de Jong LD, Dijkstra PU, Stewart RE, et al. Repeated measurements of arm joint passive range of motion after stroke: interobserver reliability and sources of variation. *Phys Ther.* 2012;92(8):1027–1035.

60. de Jong LD, Nieuwboer A, Aufdemkampe G. The hemiplegic arm: interrater reliability and concurrent validity of passive range of motion measurements. *Disabil Rehabil.* 2007;29(18):1442–1448.

61. Kolber MJ, Hanney WJ. The reliability and concurrent validity of shoulder mobility measurements using a digital inclinometer and goniometer: a technical report. *Int J Sports Phys Ther.* 2012;7(3):306–313.

62. Barnes CJ, Van Steyn SJ, Fischer RA. The effects of age, sex, and shoulder dominance on range of motion of the shoulder. *J Shoulder Elbow Surg.* 2001;10(3):242–246.

63. Gûnal I, Köse N, O Erdogan, et al. Normal range of motion of the joints of the upper extremity in male subjects, with special reference to side. *J Bone Joint Surg Am.* 1996;78(9):1401–1404.

64. Valentine RE, Lewis JS. Intraobserver reliability of 4 physiologic movements of the shoulder in subjects with and without symptoms. *Arch Phys Med Rehabil.* 2006;87(9):1242–1249.

65. Walker JM, Sue D, N Miles-Elkousy, et al. Active mobility of the extremities in older subjects. *Phys Ther.* 1984;64(6):919–923.

66. Kolber MJ, Vega F, K Widmayer, et al. The reliability and minimal detectable change of shoulder mobility measurements using a digital inclinometer. *Physiother Theory Pract.* 2011;27(2):176–184.

67. Tveitâ EK, Ekeberg OM, Juel NG, et al. Range of shoulder motion in patients with adhesive capsulitis; intra-tester reproducibility is acceptable for group comparisons. *BMC Musculoskelet Disord.* 2008;9:49.

68. Walker H, Pizzari T, Wajswelner H, et al. The reliability of shoulder range of motion measures in competitive swimmers. *Phys Ther Sport.* 2016;21:26–30.

69. Lizaur A, Marco L, Cebrian R. Acute dislocation of the acromioclavicular joint. Traumatic anatomy and the importance of deltoid and trapezius. *J Bone Joint Surg Br.* 1994;76(4):602–606.

4

MEASUREMENT of RANGE of MOTION of the ELBOW and FOREARM

Nancy Berryman Reese

ANATOMY

Within the elbow joint capsule are three articulations, two that make up the elbow joint complex and one that is part of the forearm complex. The humeroradial and humeroulnar joints form the joint complex known as the elbow (Figs. 4.1 and 4.2). The humeroradial joint consists of the articulation between the convex capitulum of the distal humerus and the slightly concave proximal surface of the radial head. The articulation between the somewhat hourglass-shaped trochlea of the humerus and the concave, semilunar-shaped trochlear notch of the ulna forms the humeroulnar joint. Both joints are located within a single joint capsule that also is shared by the proximal radioulnar joint.[1]

Ligamentous reinforcement of the elbow joint occurs primarily on the medial and lateral sides of the joint via the ulnar (Fig. 4.3) and radial (Fig. 4.4) collateral ligaments, respectively. These ligaments resist valgus and varus stresses to the joint throughout the full range of elbow motion.[2–4] Additional stability of the elbow joint is provided by the high degree of bony congruency among the articular surfaces that make up the joint.

OSTEOKINEMATICS

Although the elbow joint traditionally has been classified as a hinge joint, the hinge component occurs at the humeroulnar articulation, and the humeroradial joint is classified as a plane joint.[1] Motions at the elbow consist of flexion and extension, which occur in a plane oriented slightly oblique to the sagittal plane as a result of the angulation of the trochlea of the humerus.[5] The axis of rotation for flexion and extension of the elbow is centered on the trochlea, except at the extremes of flexion and extension, where the axis moves anteriorly and posteriorly, respectively.[6]

ARTHROKINEMATICS

During the movements of elbow flexion and extension, the concave surface of the trochlear notch of the ulna glides along the convex trochlea of the humerus. Simultaneously at the humeroradial joint, the concave head of the radius glides along the convex capitulum of the ulna. Both radial and ulnar articular surfaces glide anteriorly as the elbow flexes and posteriorly as it extends. At the extremes of flexion and extension, rolling motions of the ulna and radius replace the gliding motion.[6,7]

LIMITATIONS OF MOTION

Elbow flexion range of motion (ROM) is limited by soft-tissue approximation between the structures of the anterior arm and the forearm, particularly during active flexion of the joint when contact between contracting flexors of the arm and forearm stops the motion. The range of elbow flexion tends to be greater when the joint is moved passively because there is less interference by the contracting muscle bulk. Elbow extension ROM is limited by contact of the olecranon process of the ulna with the olecranon fossa of the humerus.[5] Information regarding normal ROM for the elbow is located in Appendix B.

END-FEEL

The normal end-feel for elbow flexion is soft because soft-tissue approximation normally limits motion. The normal end-feel for elbow extension is hard, because the olecranon process of the ulna becomes wedged in the olecranon fossa of the humerus.

CAPSULAR PATTERN

If elbow ROM is not full, the restrictions should be assessed for the presence of a capsular pattern. If elbow flexion is more restricted than elbow extension, then a capsular pattern is present, and involvement of the capsule should be suspected.[8,9]

ANATOMY

Gray's Anatomy[1] describes three articulations that interconnect the bones of the forearm: the proximal and distal

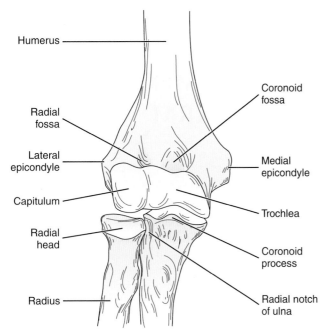

Fig. 4.1 Bony anatomy of the joints of the elbow—anterior view.

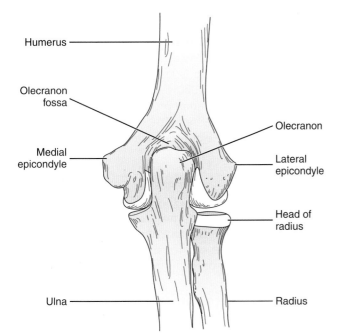

Fig. 4.2 Bony anatomy of the joints of the elbow—posterior view.

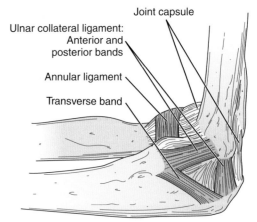

Fig. 4.3 Ligamentous reinforcement of the elbow and proximal radioulnar joint—medial view.

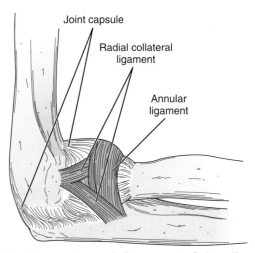

Fig. 4.4 Ligamentous reinforcement of the elbow and proximal radioulnar joint—lateral view.

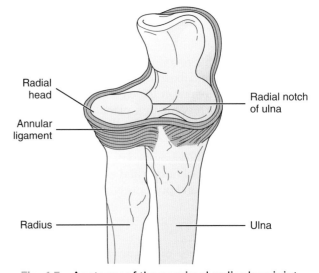

Fig. 4.5 Anatomy of the proximal radioulnar joint.

radioulnar joints and the middle radioulnar union. The proximal radioulnar joint is located anatomically within the capsule of the elbow joint and consists of the articulation between the rim of the radial head and the fibroosseous ring formed by the annular ligament and the radial notch of the ulna (Fig. 4.5). The distal radioulnar joint is located anatomically at the wrist, although inside a separate joint capsule. This joint is formed by the articulation between the concave ulnar notch of the radius and the

DISTAL RADIOULNAR JOINT

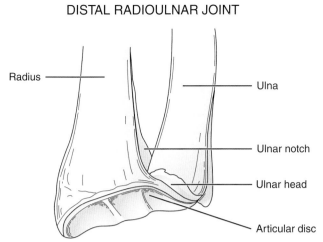

Fig. 4.6 Anatomy of the distal radioulnar joint.

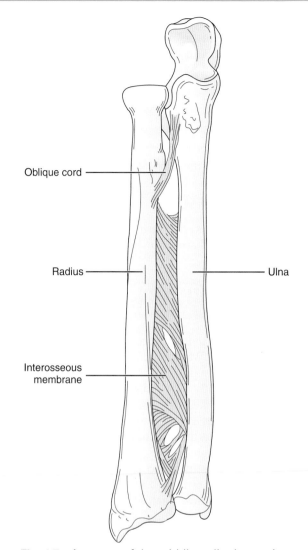

Fig. 4.7 Anatomy of the middle radioulnar union.

convex head of the ulna (Fig. 4.6).[10,11] A third articulation between the radius and ulna, the middle radioulnar union, has been classified as a syndesmosis, although this articulation is not classified as a joint at all by the Terminologia Anatomica.[12] The middle radioulnar union consists of the shafts of the radius and ulna held firmly together by the interosseous membrane and by the oblique cord, a small ligament that attaches from the ulnar tuberosity to just distal to the radial tuberosity (Fig. 4.7).[12] Ligamentous reinforcement of the proximal radioulnar joint occurs via two ligaments. The annular ligament is attached to the anterior and posterior margins of the radial notch of the ulna and encircles the radial head, holding it firmly against the radial notch (see Figs. 4.3–4.5).[12] A second ligament, the quadrate ligament, runs from the inferior aspect of the radial notch to the neck of the radius, reinforcing the joint capsule, and is considered to stabilize the proximal radioulnar joint during the extremes of pronation and supination.[13] The distal radioulnar joint is reinforced by a triangular articular disc that is positioned on the distal end of the ulna. This disc binds the distal ulna and radius together and is the primary reinforcement for the joint. The dorsal and palmar radioulnar ligaments assist in stabilization of the distal radioulnar joint.[14]

OSTEOKINEMATICS

Both proximal and distal radioulnar joints are classified as pivot joints, allowing rotation of the radius around the ulna in a transverse plane. When the forearm is fully supinated, the radius and the ulna lie parallel to each other. As the forearm pronates, the radius crosses anteriorly over the surface of the ulna. Very limited, if any, movement occurs at the middle radioulnar union.

ARTHROKINEMATICS

During pronation and supination of the forearm, motion occurs at the proximal and distal radioulnar joints simultaneously. At the proximal joint, the convex radial head spins within the ring formed by the radial notch of the ulna and the annular ligament. The radial head spins anteriorly during pronation and posteriorly during supination. Distally, the concave ulnar notch of the radius rolls and slides anteriorly on the ulnar head during pronation and posteriorly during supination.[3]

LIMITATIONS OF MOTION

Forearm Joints

Supination of the forearm is limited by tension in ligamentous structures (anterior radioulnar ligament and oblique cord).[15] Limitation of forearm pronation occurs as the result of contact between the bones of the forearm (radius crossing over ulna) and tension in the medial collateral ligament of the elbow and the dorsal radioulnar ligament of the distal radioulnar joint.[3,16] There is evidence that the range of supination increases and the range of pronation decreases as the angle of elbow flexion increases. The converse appears to be true for these respective motions as the angle of elbow flexion decreases.[17] Information regarding normal ranges of motion for forearm supination and pronation is located in Appendix B.

END-FEEL

The typical end-feel for forearm supination is firm as a result of ligamentous tension. Because bony contact limits pronation, the normal end-feel for that motion is hard.

CAPSULAR PATTERN

Capsular restrictions of forearm ROM result in relatively equal deficits of forearm pronation and supination.[8,9]

RANGE OF MOTION AND FUNCTIONAL ACTIVITY

Most functional activities require a fairly large amount of elbow flexion ROM (Figs. 4.8–4.10). A recent study by van Andel et al.[18] reported that all functional tasks examined in their study required a minimum of 85 degrees of elbow flexion. These results were similar to those reported by Vasen et al.[19] who used a motion-restricting brace to determine the functional ROM of the elbow. Of 50 subjects examined, 49 were able to perform all 12 functional activities included in the study, with elbow motion limited to a range of 75 to 120 degrees of flexion.

Numerous other investigators have attempted to quantify the amount of elbow and forearm motion required to perform various functional activities.[4,20–28] A summary of elbow and forearm ROM related to various functional activities is provided in Table 4.1. Most of the studies from which data were derived were performed in healthy adults, although some data were obtained from elderly and pediatric subjects. Characteristics of the study populations and the instrumentation used are included in

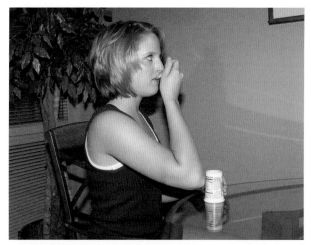

Fig. 4.9   Elbow and forearm motion required to eat with a spoon.

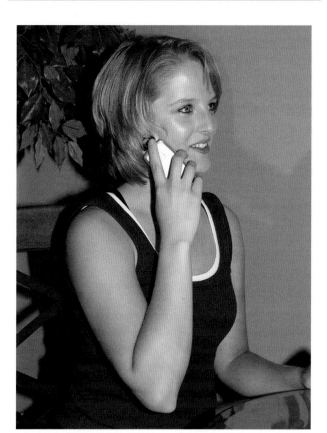

Fig. 4.10   Elbow and forearm motion required to use a telephone.

the table. Caution should be used in extrapolating these data to the general population because sample sizes for all studies were small. For more in-depth information on each study, the reader is referred to the reference list at the end of this chapter. Additional information on shoulder ROM required to perform functional tasks may be found in the review article by Oosterwijk and colleagues.[29] Figs. 4.8–4.10 demonstrate examples of elbow and forearm motion used during selected functional tasks.

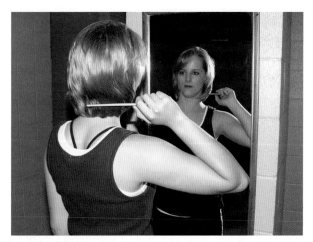

Fig. 4.8   Elbow and forearm motion required to comb one's hair.

	ELBOW FLEXION			FOREARM SUPINATION			FOREARM PRONATION			
FUNCTIONAL ACTIVITY	MIN.	MAX.	MEAN	MIN.	MAX.	MEAN	MIN.	MAX.	MEAN	COMMENTS
Combing Hair Magermans et al.[28]	112°	157°	136° ±15°				54°[oa]	143°[oa]	100° ±28°[oa]	Measured 24 healthy F, mean age 36.8 years, using Flock of Birds electromagnetic tracking device
Drink from Cup Morrey et al.[4]	45°	130°			13°			10°		Measured 33 healthy adults (18 F, 15 M) aged 21–57 years using triaxial electrogoniometer
Safaee-Rad[25]	72° ±6°	129° ±3°		3° ±7°	31° ±11°					Measured 10 M aged 20–29 years using 3-dimensional measurement system
Eat with Fork Morrey et al.[4]	85°	128°			52°			10°		Measured 33 healthy adults (18 F, 15 M) aged 21–57 years using triaxial electrogoniometer
Safaee-Rad[25]	94° ±6°	122° ±4°			59° ±8°		38° ±8°			Measured 10 M aged 20–29 years using 3-dimensional measurement system
Eat with Spoon Magermans et al.[28]	117°	143°	132° ±8°				33°[oa]	127°[oa]	72° ±31°[oa]	Measured 24 healthy F, mean age 36.8 years, using Flock of Birds electromagnetic tracking device
Eat with Spoon Packer et al.[26]	70°	115°								Measured 5 healthy adults aged 54–73 years (data in table) and compared with 5 adults with rheumatoid arthritis (data not shown) using uniaxial electrogoniometer
Safaee-Rad[25]	101° ±8°	132° ±5°			59° ±6°			23° ±15°		Measured 10 M aged 20–29 years using 3-dimensional measurement system
Lift Object from Floor Magermans et al.[28]	61°	130°	93° ±24°				38°[oa]	125°[oa]	76° ±28°[oa]	Measured 24 healthy F, mean age 36.8 years, using Flock of Birds electromagnetic tracking device
Cut with Knife Morrey et al.[4]	89°	107°					27°	42°		Measured 33 healthy adults (18 F, 15 M) aged 21–57 years using triaxial electrogoniometer
Perineal Care Magermans et al.[28]	35°	100°	61° ±20°				39°[oa]	155°[oa]	86° ±36°[oa]	Measured 24 healthy F, mean age 36.8 years, using Flock of Birds electromagnetic tracking device
Pour from Pitcher Morrey et al.[4]	36°	58°			22°			43°		Measured 33 healthy adults (18 F, 15 M) aged 21–57 years using triaxial electrogoniometer
Reach above Shoulder Level Magermans et al.[28]	20°	67°	39° ±18°				103°[oa]	147°[oa]	121° ±17°[oa]	Measured 24 healthy F, mean age 36.8 years, using Flock of Birds electromagnetic tracking device

Table 4.1   ELBOW/FOREARM ROM DURING FUNCTIONAL ACTIVITIES

Continued

Table 4.1   ELBOW/FOREARM ROM DURING FUNCTIONAL ACTIVITIES—cont'd

FUNCTIONAL ACTIVITY	ELBOW FLEXION			FOREARM SUPINATION			FOREARM PRONATION			COMMENTS
	MIN.	MAX.	MEAN	MIN.	MAX.	MEAN	MIN.	MAX.	MEAN	
Read Newspaper Morrey et al.[4]	78°	104°					7°	49°		Measured 33 healthy adults (18F, 15M) aged 21–57 years using triaxial electrogoniometer
Reach Forward to Receive Change Mackey et al.[22]	3°±7°	140°±27°			66°±27°			13°±34°		Measured 10 healthy children aged 6–12 years (data in table) and compared with 10 children with CP (data not shown) using 3-dimensional kinematic analysis
Hand to Mouth Mackey et al.[22]	53°±16°	153°±13°			79°±9°			5°±32°		Measured 10 healthy children aged 6–12 years (data in table) and compared with 10 children with CP (data not shown) using 3-dimensional kinematic analysis
Hand to Forehead Mackey et al.[22]	108°±22°	166°±8°			77°±22°			12°±30°		Measured 10 healthy children aged 6–12 years (data in table) and compared with 10 children with CP (data not shown) using 3-dimensional kinematic analysis
Rise from Chair Morrey et al.[4]	20°	95°					10°	34°		Measured 33 healthy adults (18F, 15M) aged 21–57 years using triaxial electrogoniometer
Packer et al.[26]	15°	100°								Measured 5 healthy adults aged 54–73 years (data in table) and compared with 5 adults with rheumatoid arthritis (data not shown) using uniaxial electrogoniometer
Use Telephone Morrey et al.[4]	43°	136°			23°			41°		Measured 33 healthy adults (18F, 15M) aged 21–57 years using triaxial electrogoniometer
Packer et al.[26]	75°	140°								Measured 5 healthy adults aged 54–73 years (data in table) and compared with 5 adults with rheumatoid arthritis (data not shown) using uniaxial electrogoniometer
Wash Axilla Magermans et al.[28]	104°	132°	118°±9°				42°*	124°*	77°±23°*	Measured 24 healthy F, mean age 36.8 years, using Flock of Birds electromagnetic tracking device

*Anatomical position of forearm defined as 0-degree pronation.

ELBOW FLEXION/EXTENSION

Elbow flexion and extension may be measured with the patient in the upright (standing or sitting), supine, or side-lying position. The supine position is preferred for measurement of ROM because it provides greater stability to the humerus. The American Academy of Orthopaedic Surgeons[30] recommends that the patient be in the upright position with the shoulder flexed to 90 degrees when measurements of elbow flexion and extension are taken. In patients in whom the long head of the triceps is tight, such positioning may limit flexion of the elbow. Therefore, motions of the elbow joint should be measured with the shoulder maintained in the anatomical position.

FOREARM PRONATION/SUPINATION

Forearm pronation and supination typically are measured with the elbow positioned in 90 degrees of flexion, with the shoulder fully adducted and the humerus held firmly against the lateral aspect of the thorax. In this position, the patient is prevented from substituting rotation of the shoulder for rotation of the forearm, and pronation and supination of the forearm can be visualized easily. Some authors recommend measuring forearm rotation with a rod or rod-like object held in the hand,[30] but errors of measurement have been shown to result from such methods.[31] Therefore, in this text, goniometric techniques involving measurement of forearm rotation will use the distal forearm rather than a hand-held object as the reference for the moving arm of the goniometer.

Elbow Flexion (Video 4.1)

Fig. 4.11 Starting position for measurement of elbow flexion. Bony landmarks for goniometer alignment (lateral aspect of acromion process, lateral humeral epicondyle, radial styloid process) indicated by red dots.

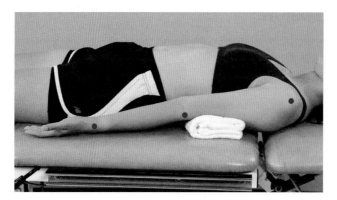

Normal ROM = 140 to 150 degrees.[27,32–39]

MDC for elbow flexion goniometry measured by a single examiner = 8 to 14 degrees in normal,[36,40] and 6 degrees in pathologic,[41] elbows.

Patient position

Supine with upper extremity in anatomical position (see Note), folded towel under humerus, proximal to humeral condyles (Fig. 4.11).

Stabilization

Over posterior aspect of proximal humerus (Fig. 4.12).

Examiner action

After instructing patient in motion desired, flex patient's elbow through available ROM. Return limb to starting position. Performing passive movement provides an estimate of ROM and demonstrates to patient exact motion desired (see Fig. 4.12).

Goniometer alignment

Palpate the following bony landmarks (shown in Fig. 4.11) and align goniometer accordingly (Fig. 4.13).

Fig. 4.12 End of elbow flexion ROM, showing proper hand placement for stabilizing humerus and flexing elbow. Bony landmarks for goniometer alignment (lateral aspect of acromion process, lateral humeral epicondyle, radial styloid process) indicated by red dots.

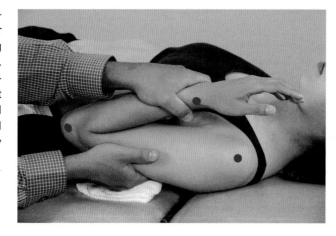

Fig. 4.13 Starting position for measurement of elbow flexion, demonstrating proper initial alignment of goniometer.

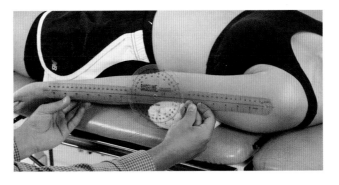

Stationary arm	Lateral midline of humerus toward acromion process.
Axis	Lateral epicondyle of humerus.
Moving arm	Lateral midline of radius toward radial styloid process (see Note).
	Read scale of goniometer.
Patient/Examiner action	Perform passive, or have patient perform active, elbow flexion (Fig. 4.14).
Confirmation of alignment	Repalpate landmarks and confirm proper goniometric alignment at end of ROM, correcting alignment as necessary. Read scale of goniometer (see Fig. 4.14).
Documentation	Record patient's ROM.
Note	Patient's forearm should be completely supinated at beginning of ROM or beginning reading of goniometer will be inaccurate and will make patient appear to lack full elbow extension.
Alternative patient position	Seated or side-lying; towel not needed; goniometer alignment remains the same. Stability of humerus is decreased in these positions; thus extra care must be taken to manually stabilize humerus.

Fig. 4.14 End of elbow flexion ROM, demonstrating proper alignment of goniometer at end of range.

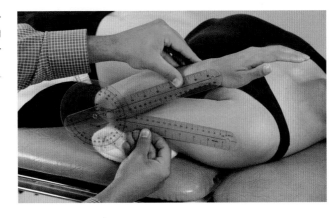

Elbow Extension (Video 4.2)

Fig. 4.15 Starting position for measurement of elbow extension. Bony landmarks for goniometer alignment (lateral aspect of acromion process, lateral humeral epicondyle, radial styloid process) indicated by red dots.

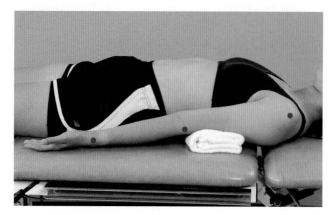

Normal ROM = 0 to 5 degrees.[27,32–39]

MDC for elbow extension goniometry measured by a single examiner = 6 degrees in normal[36] and 7 degrees in pathologic[41] elbows.

Patient position

Supine with upper extremity in anatomical position (see Note), elbow extended as far as possible, folded towel under distal humerus, proximal to humeral condyles (Fig. 4.15).

Stabilization

None needed.

Examiner action

Determine whether elbow is extended as far as possible by (1) asking patient to straighten elbow as far as possible (if measuring active ROM) or (2) providing pressure across the elbow in the direction of extension (if measuring passive ROM) (Fig. 4.16).

Fig. 4.16 End of elbow extension ROM, showing proper hand placement for stabilizing humerus and extending elbow. Bony landmarks for goniometer alignment (lateral aspect of acromion process, lateral humeral epicondyle, radial styloid process) indicated by red dots.

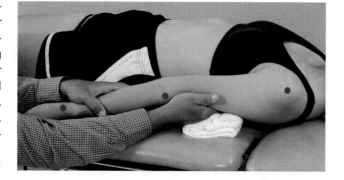

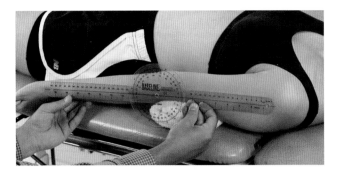

Fig. 4.17 Goniometer alignment for measurement of elbow extension.

Goniometer alignment	Palpate the following bony landmarks (shown in Fig. 4.15) and align goniometer accordingly (Fig. 4.17).
Stationary arm	Lateral midline of humerus toward acromion process.
Axis	Lateral epicondyle of humerus.
Moving arm	Lateral midline of radius toward radial styloid process (see Note).
	Read scale of goniometer (see Fig. 4.17).
Documentation	Record patient's amount of elbow extension.
Note	Patient's forearm should be completely supinated at beginning of ROM or initial goniometer reading will be inaccurate and will make patient appear to lack full elbow extension.
Alternative patient position	Seated or side-lying; towel not needed; goniometer alignment remains the same.

Forearm Supination: Goniometer (Video 4.3)

Fig. 4.18 Starting position for measurement of forearm supination. Bony landmarks for goniometer alignment (anterior midline of humerus and ulnar styloid process) indicated by red line and dot.

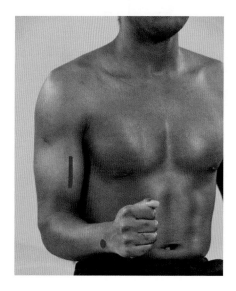

Normal ROM = 80 to 100 degrees.[32,33,36,37,39,42]

MDC for forearm supination goniometry measured by a single examiner = 7 to 14 degrees in normal[36,40] and 8 degrees in pathologic[41] forearms.

Patient position	Seated or standing with shoulder completely adducted, elbow flexed to 90 degrees, forearm in neutral rotation (Fig. 4.18).
Stabilization	Over lateral aspect of distal humerus, maintaining 0-degree shoulder adduction (Fig. 4.19).
Examiner action	After instructing patient in motion desired, supinate patient's forearm through available ROM, avoiding lateral rotation of shoulder or shoulder adduction past 0 degrees (see Note). Return limb to starting position. Performing passive movement provides an estimate of ROM and demonstrates to patient exact motion desired (see Fig. 4.19).
Goniometer alignment	Palpate the following bony landmarks (shown in Fig. 4.18) and align goniometer accordingly (Fig. 4.20).

Fig. 4.19 End of forearm supination ROM, showing proper hand placement for stabilizing humerus against thorax and supinating forearm. Bony landmark for goniometer alignment (anterior midline of humerus) indicated by red line.

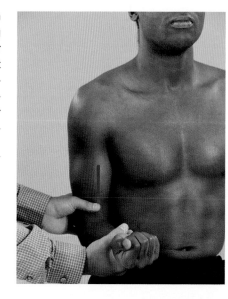

Fig. 4.20 Starting position for measurement of forearm supination, demonstrating proper initial alignment of goniometer.

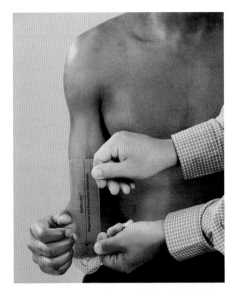

Stationary arm	Parallel with anterior midline of humerus.
Axis	On volar surface of wrist, in line with styloid process of ulna.*
Moving arm	Volar surface of wrist, at level of ulnar styloid process.
	Read scale of goniometer.
Patient/Examiner action	Perform passive supination or have patient perform active forearm supination (Fig. 4.21).
Confirmation of alignment	Repalpate landmarks and confirm proper goniometric alignment at end of ROM, correcting alignment as necessary (see Note). Read scale of goniometer (see Fig. 4.21).
Documentation	Record patient's ROM.
Note	To prevent artificial inflation of ROM measurements, no adduction or lateral rotation of shoulder should be allowed during measurement of forearm supination.

*Alignment of goniometer's axis opposite ulnar styloid process is possible at start of measuring forearm supination (see Fig. 4.20). By end of supination ROM, axis of goniometer will have moved to a position superior and medial to ulnar styloid (see Fig. 4.21). Alignment of arms and not axis of goniometer is the most critical element in this measurement.

Fig. 4.21 End of forearm supination ROM, demonstrating proper alignment of goniometer at end of range.

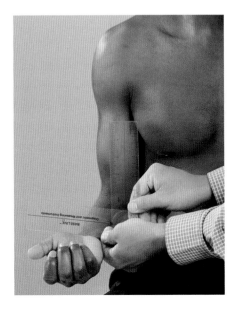

Forearm Pronation: Goniometer (Video 4.4)

Fig. 4.22 Starting position for measurement of forearm pronation. Bony landmarks for goniometer alignment (anterior midline of humerus and ulnar styloid process) indicated by red line and dot.

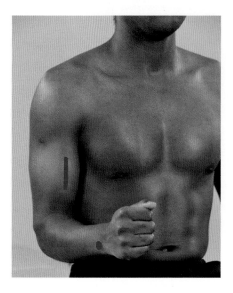

Normal ROM = 70 to 80 degrees.[32,33,37,39,42]

MDC for forearm pronation goniometry measured by a single examiner = 9 to 23 degrees in normal[36,40] and 8 degrees in pathologic[41] forearms.

Patient position   Seated or standing with shoulder completely adducted, elbow flexed to 90 degrees, forearm in neutral rotation (Fig. 4.22).

Stabilization   Over lateral aspect of distal humerus, maintaining shoulder adduction (Fig. 4.23).

Examiner action   After instructing patient in motion desired, pronate patient's forearm through available ROM, avoiding shoulder abduction and medial rotation (see Note). Return limb to starting position. Performing passive movement provides an estimate of ROM and demonstrates to patient exact motion desired (see Fig. 4.23).

Goniometer alignment   Palpate the following bony landmarks (shown in Fig. 4.22), and align goniometer accordingly (Fig. 4.24).

Stationary arm   Parallel with anterior midline of humerus.

Fig. 4.23 End of forearm pronation ROM, showing proper hand placement for stabilizing humerus against thorax and pronating forearm. Bony landmark for goniometer alignment (anterior midline of humerus) indicated by red line.

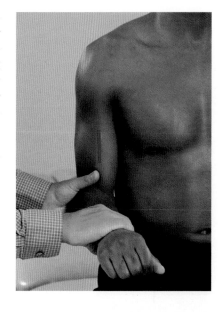

Fig. 4.24 Starting position for measurement of forearm pronation, demonstrating proper initial alignment of goniometer.

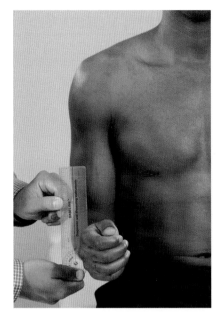

Axis	In line with, and just proximal to, styloid process of ulna.[*]
Moving arm	Dorsum of forearm, just proximal to ulnar styloid process.
	Read scale of goniometer.
Patient/Examiner action	Perform passive forearm pronation or have patient perform active forearm pronation (Fig. 4.25).
Confirmation of alignment	Repalpate landmarks and confirm proper goniometric alignment at end of ROM, correcting alignment as necessary (see Note). Read scale of goniometer (see Fig. 4.25).
Documentation	Record patient's ROM.
Note	To prevent artificial inflation of ROM measurements, no abduction or medial rotation of shoulder should be allowed during measurement of forearm pronation.

[*]Alignment of goniometer's axis with ulnar styloid process is possible at start of measuring forearm pronation (see Fig. 4.24). By end of pronation ROM, axis of goniometer will have moved to a position superior and lateral to ulnar styloid (see Fig. 4.25). Alignment of arms, and not axis, of goniometer is most critical element in this measurement.

Fig. 4.25 End of forearm pronation ROM, demonstrating proper alignment of goniometer at end of range.

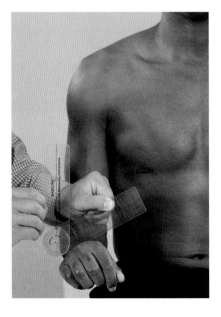

Forearm Supination: Inclinometer (Video 4.5)

Fig. 4.26 Starting position for measurement of forearm supination.

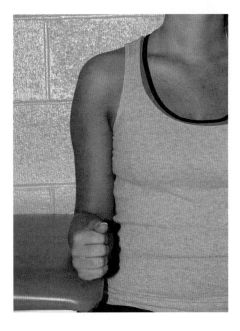

Patient position	Seated or standing with shoulder completely adducted, elbow flexed to 90 degrees, forearm in neutral rotation (Fig. 4.26).
Stabilization	Over lateral aspect of distal humerus, maintaining 0-degree shoulder adduction (Fig. 4.27).
Examiner action	After instructing patient in desired motion, supinate patient's forearm through available ROM, avoiding lateral rotation of shoulder or shoulder adduction (see Note). Return limb to starting position. Performing passive movement provides an estimate of ROM and demonstrates to patient exact motion desired (see Fig. 4.27).

Fig. 4.27 End of forearm supination ROM, showing proper hand placement for stabilizing humerus against thorax and supinating forearm.

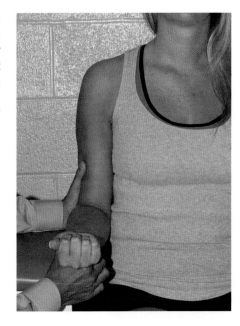

Fig. 4.28 Starting position for measurement of forearm supination, demonstrating proper initial alignment of inclinometer.

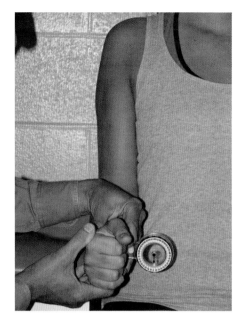

Inclinometer alignment	On ventral surface of forearm proximal to wrist. Ensure that the inclinometer is set to 0 degrees once it is positioned on patient (Fig. 4.28).
Patient/Examiner action	Perform passive, or have patient perform active, forearm supination.
Inclinometer alignment	Ensure that inclinometer remains in firm contact with ventral surface of forearm. Read scale of inclinometer (Fig. 4.29).
Documentation	Record patient's ROM.
Note	To prevent artificial inflation of ROM measurements, no adduction or lateral rotation of shoulder should be allowed during measurement of forearm supination.

Fig. 4.29 End of forearm supination ROM, demonstrating proper alignment of inclinometer at end range.

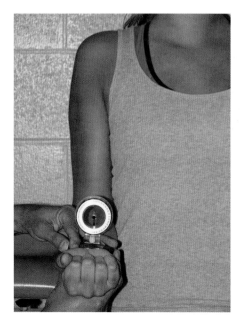

Forearm Pronation: Inclinometer (Video 4.6)

Fig. 4.30 Starting position for measurement of forearm pronation.

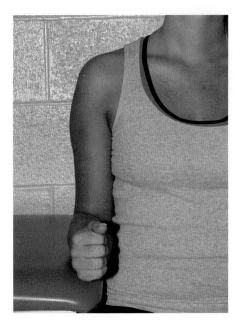

Patient position	Seated or standing with shoulder completely adducted, elbow flexed to 90 degrees, forearm in neutral rotation (Fig. 4.30).
Stabilization	Over lateral aspect of distal humerus, maintaining shoulder adduction (Fig. 4.31).
Examiner action	After instructing patient in motion desired, pronate patient's forearm through available ROM, avoiding shoulder abduction and medial rotation (see Note). Return limb to starting position. Performing passive movement provides an estimate of ROM and demonstrates to patient exact motion desired (see Fig. 4.31).

Fig. 4.31 End of forearm pronation ROM, showing proper hand placement for stabilizing humerus against thorax and pronating forearm.

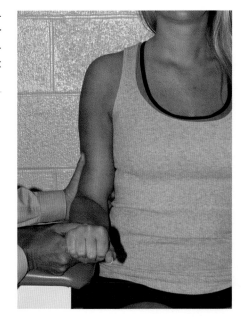

Fig. 4.32 Starting position for measurement of forearm pronation, demonstrating proper initial alignment of inclinometer.

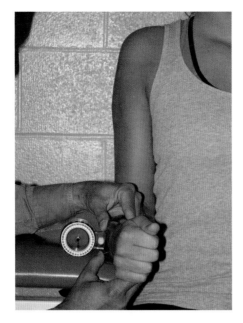

Inclinometer alignment	On dorsal surface of forearm proximal to wrist; across the forearm. Ensure that the inclinometer is set to 0 degrees once it is positioned on patient (Fig. 4.32).
Patient/Examiner action	Perform passive, or have patient perform active, forearm pronation.
Inclinometer alignment	Ensure that inclinometer remains in firm contact with dorsal surface of forearm. Read scale of inclinometer (Fig. 4.33).
Documentation	Record patient's ROM.
Note	To prevent artificial inflation of ROM measurement, no abduction or medial rotation of shoulder should be allowed during measurement of forearm pronation.

Fig. 4.33 End of forearm pronation ROM, demonstrating proper alignment of inclinometer at end of range.

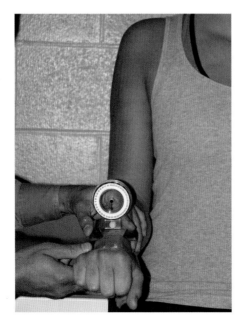

Forearm Supination: Smartphone Method

Fig. 4.34 Starting position for measurement of forearm supination.

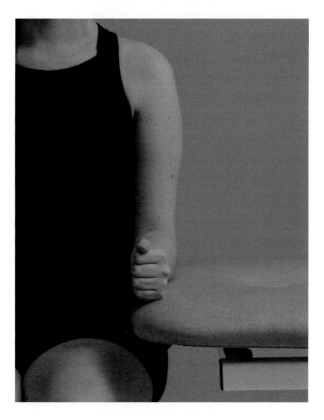

Patient position   Seated or standing with shoulder completely adducted, elbow flexed to 90 degrees, forearm in neutral rotation (Fig. 4.34).

Stabilization   Over lateral aspect of distal humerus, maintaining 0-degree shoulder adduction (Fig. 4.35).

Fig. 4.35 End of forearm supination ROM, showing proper hand placement for stabilizing humerus against thorax and supinating forearm.

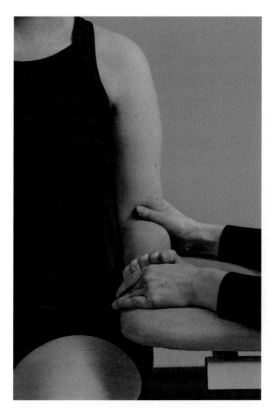

Fig. 4.36 Starting position for measurement of forearm supination, demonstrating proper initial alignment of Smartphone.

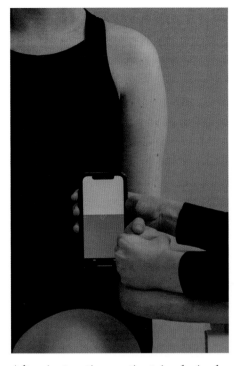

Examiner action

After instructing patient in desired motion, supinate patient's forearm through available ROM, avoiding lateral rotation of shoulder or shoulder adduction (see Note). Return limb to starting position. Performing passive movement provides an estimate of ROM and demonstrates to patient exact motion desired (see Fig. 4.35).

Smartphone alignment

Along surface of forearm proximal to wrist. Ensure that measurement app on Smartphone reads 0 degrees once it is positioned on patient (Fig. 4.36).

Patient/Examiner action

Perform passive, or have patient perform active, forearm supination. Read angle on Smartphone app at end of ROM (Fig. 4.37).

Documentation

Record patient's ROM.

Note

To prevent artificial inflation of ROM measurements, no adduction or lateral rotation of shoulder should be allowed during measurement of forearm supination.

Fig. 4.37 End of forearm supination ROM, demonstrating proper alignment of Smartphone at end range.

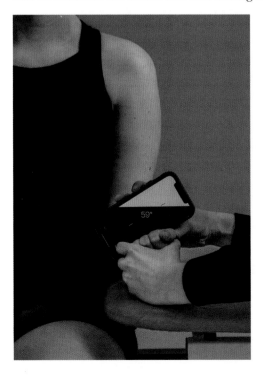

Forearm Pronation: Smartphone Method

Fig. 4.38 Starting position for measurement of forearm pronation.

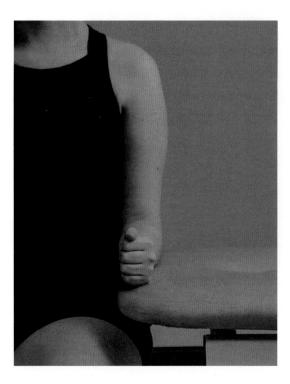

Patient position	Seated or standing with shoulder completely adducted, elbow flexed to 90 degrees, forearm in neutral rotation (Fig. 4.38).
Stabilization	Over lateral aspect of distal humerus, maintaining shoulder adduction (Fig. 4.39).
Examiner action	After instructing patient in motion desired, pronate patient's forearm through available ROM, avoiding shoulder abduction and medial rotation (see Note). Return limb to starting position. Performing passive movement provides an estimate of ROM and demonstrates to patient exact motion desired (see Fig. 4.39).

Fig. 4.39 End of forearm pronation ROM, showing proper hand placement for stabilizing humerus against thorax and pronating forearm.

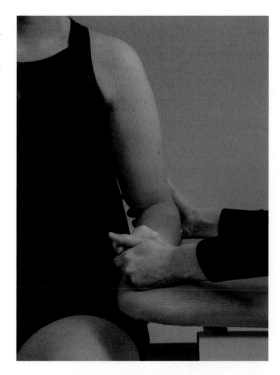

Fig. 4.40 Starting position for measurement of forearm pronation, demonstrating proper initial alignment of Smartphone.

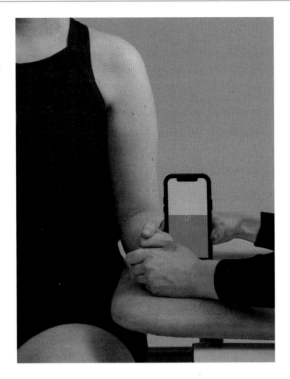

Smartphone alignment	Along surface of forearm proximal to wrist. Ensure that measurement app on Smartphone reads 0 degrees once it is positioned on patient (Fig. 4.40).
Patient/Examiner action	Perform passive, or have patient perform active, forearm pronation. Read angle on Smartphone app at end of ROM (Fig. 4.41).
Documentation	Record patient's ROM.
Note	To prevent artificial inflation of ROM measurement, no abduction or medial rotation of shoulder should be allowed during measurement of forearm pronation.

Fig. 4.41 End of forearm pronation ROM, demonstrating proper alignment of Smartphone at end of range.

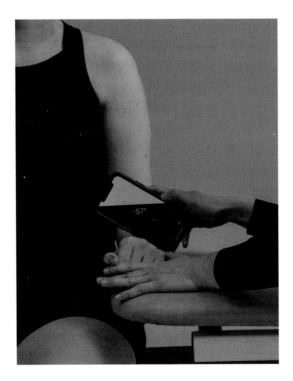

References

1. Clemente C. *Gray's Anatomy of the Human Body.* 13th ed. Philadelphia: Lea & Febiger; 1985.
2. Seki A, et al. Functional anatomy of the lateral collateral ligament complex of the elbow: configuration of Y and its role. *J Shoulder Elbow Surg.* 2002;11(1):53–59.
3. Neumann D. *Kinesiology of the Musculoskeletal System.* St Louis: Mosby; 2002.
4. Morrey BF, Askew LJ, Chao EY. A biomechanical study of normal functional elbow motion. *J Bone Joint Surg Am.* 1981;63(6):872–877.
5. Kapandji I. *The Physiology of Joints. Upper Limb.* Vol. 1. 5th ed. New York: Churchill Livingstone; 1982.
6. London JT. Kinematics of the elbow. *J Bone Joint Surg Am.* 1981;63(4):529–535.
7. Soderberg G. *Kinesiology: Application to Pathological Motion.* 2nd ed. Baltimore: Williams & Wilkins; 1997.
8. Cyriax JH, Coldham M. *Textbook of Orthopaedic Medicine.* London: Baillière Tindall; 1982.
9. Kaltenborn F. *Mobilization of the Extremity Joints.* 3rd ed. Oslo: Olaf Norlis Bokhandel; 1980.
10. Jaffe R, Chidgey LK, LaStayo PC. The distal radioulnar joint: anatomy and management of disorders. *J Hand Ther.* 1996;9(2):129–138.
11. Lees VC. Functional anatomy of the distal radioulnar joint in health and disease. *Ann R Coll Surg Engl.* 2013;95(3):163–170.
12. Martin BF. The annular ligament of the superior radio-ulnar joint. *J Anat.* 1958;92(3):473–482.
13. Spinner M, Kaplan EB. The quadrate ligament of the elbow—its relationship to the stability of the proximal radio-ulnar joint. *Acta Orthop Scand.* 1970;41(6):632–647.
14. LaStayo PC, Lee MJ. The forearm complex: anatomy, biomechanics and clinical considerations. *J Hand Ther.* 2006;19(2):137–144.
15. Schuind F, et al. The distal radioulnar ligaments: a biomechanical study. *J Hand Surg Am.* 1991;16(6):1106–1114.
16. Hotchkiss RN, Weiland AJ. Valgus stability of the elbow. *J Orthop Res.* 1987;5(3):372–377.
17. Shaaban H, et al. The effect of elbow position on the range of supination and pronation of the forearm. *J Hand Surg Eur.* 2008;33(1):3–8.
18. van Andel CJ, et al. Complete 3D kinematics of upper extremity functional tasks. *Gait Posture.* 2008;27(1):120–127.
19. Vasen AP, et al. Functional range of motion of the elbow. *J Hand Surg Am.* 1995;20(2):288–292.
20. Cooper JE, et al. Elbow joint restriction: effect on functional upper limb motion during performance of three feeding activities. *Arch Phys Med Rehabil.* 1993;74(8):805–809.
21. Henmi S, et al. A biomechanical study of activities of daily living using neck and upper limbs with an optical three-dimensional motion analysis system. *Mod Rheumatol.* 2006;16(5):289–293.
22. Mackey AH, Walt SE, Stott NS. Deficits in upper-limb task performance in children with hemiplegic cerebral palsy as defined by 3-dimensional kinematics. *Arch Phys Med Rehabil.* 2006;87(2):207–215.
23. Murray IA, Johnson GR. A study of the external forces and moments at the shoulder and elbow while performing everyday tasks. *Clin Biomech (Bristol, Avon).* 2004;19(6):586–594.
24. Petuskey K, et al. Upper extremity kinematics during functional activities: three-dimensional studies in a normal pediatric population. *Gait Posture.* 2007;25(4):573–579.
25. Safaee-Rad R, et al. Normal functional range of motion of upper limb joints during performance of three feeding activities. *Arch Phys Med Rehabil.* 1990;71(7):505–509.
26. Packer T, et al. Examining the elbow during functional activities. *OTJR.* 1990;10:323–333.
27. Smith J, Walker J. Knee and elbow range of motion in healthy older individuals. *Phys Occup Ther in Geriatr.* 1983;2:31–38.
28. Magermans DJ, et al. Requirements for upper extremity motions during activities of daily living. *Clin Biomech (Bristol, Avon).* 2005;20(6):591–599.
29. Oosterwijk AM, Nieuwenhuis MK, van der Schans CP, Mouton LJ. Shoulder and elbow range of motion for the performance of activities of daily living: a systematic review. *Physiother Theory Pract.* 2018;34(7):503–528.
30. Greene WB, Heckman JD. *The Clinical Measurement of Joint Motion.* Rosemont, IL: American Academy of Orthopaedic Surgeons; 1994.
31. Amis AA, Miller JH. The elbow. *Clin Rheum Dis.* 1982;8(3):571–593.
32. American Medical Association. *Guides to the Evaluation of Permanent Impairment.* 4th ed. Chicago: American Medical Association; 1993:xvii339.
33. Boone DC, Azen SP. Normal range of motion of joints in male subjects. *J Bone Joint Surg Am.* 1979;61(5):756–759.
34. Escalante A, Lichtenstein MJ, Hazuda HP. Determinants of shoulder and elbow flexion range: results from the San Antonio longitudinal study of aging. *Arthritis Care Res.* 1999;12(4):277–286.
35. Gûnal I, et al. Normal range of motion of the joints of the upper extremity in male subjects, with special reference to side. *J Bone Joint Surg Am.* 1996;78(9):1401–1404.
36. Macedo LG, Magee DJ. Effects of age on passive range of motion of selected peripheral joints in healthy adult females. *Physiother Theory Pract.* 2009;25(2):145–164.
37. Soucie JM, et al. Range of motion measurements: reference values and a database for comparison studies. *Haemophilia.* 2011;17(3):500–507.
38. Walker JM, et al. Active mobility of the extremities in older subjects. *Phys Ther.* 1984;64(6):919–923.
39. Surgeons AAOS. *Joint Motion: Method of Measuring and Recording.* Chicago: American Academy of Orthopaedic Surgeons; 1965.
40. Costa V, Ramirez O, Abraham O, Munoz-Garcia D, Uribarri S, Raya R. Validity and reliability of inertial sensors for elbow and wrist range of motion assessment. *PeerJ.* 2020;8:e9687. https://doi.org/10.7717/peerj.9687.
41. Armstrong AD, et al. Reliability of range-of-motion measurement in the elbow and forearm. *J Shoulder Elbow Surg.* 1998;7(6):573–580.
42. Gajdosik RL. Comparison and reliability of three goniometric methods for measuring forearm supination and pronation. *Percept Mot Skills.* 2001;93(2):353–355.

5

MEASUREMENT of RANGE of MOTION
of the WRIST and HAND

Nancy Berryman Reese

WRIST JOINT

ANATOMY: WRIST JOINT

Although *Gray's Anatomy* designates the radiocarpal joint as "the wrist joint proper,"[1] other authors describe a wrist joint complex that includes the more distal midcarpal joint as well as the radiocarpal joint.[2,3] The proximal articular surface of the radiocarpal joint is concave and is composed of the distal end of the radius and the triangular fibrocartilage of the radioulnar disk (Fig. 5.1). Distally, three of the carpal bones in the proximal row, specifically the scaphoid, lunate, and triquetrum, form the convex-shaped distal articular surface of the radiocarpal joint. The articulation between the proximal and distal rows of carpal bones makes up the midcarpal joint (see Fig. 5.1). Some sources have described the midcarpal joint as having medial and lateral joint compartments.[3,4] The medial compartment consists of the articulation of a concave proximal surface formed by the scaphoid, lunate, and triquetrum and a convex distal surface formed by the hamate and head of the capitate. Joint surfaces of the lateral compartment are fairly planar and consist of the articulation of the trapezium and trapezoid proximally with the scaphoid bone in the distal carpal row.

Several ligaments reinforce the wrist joint complex and guide the motions that occur at the radiocarpal and midcarpal joints. A number of intrinsic ligaments are present that interconnect the carpal bones, binding them together and providing stability to the wrist.[5] Limitation of wrist motion occurs primarily via ligaments arising external to the carpal bones. These so-called extrinsic ligaments of the wrist include the posteriorly located dorsal radiocarpal ligaments (Fig. 5.2), the anteriorly positioned palmar ulnocarpal and palmar radiocarpal ligaments (Fig. 5.3), and the radial and ulnar collateral ligaments, located on the radial and ulnar aspects of the wrist, respectively (see Figs. 5.2 and 5.3).[5-8]

OSTEOKINEMATICS: WRIST JOINT

Movement at both the radiocarpal and midcarpal joints is necessary to achieve the full range of motion (ROM) of the wrist, which has been classified as a condyloid joint with 2 degrees of freedom.[9] Motions present at the wrist include flexion, extension, abduction (radial deviation), and adduction (ulnar deviation). These movements occur around an axis passing through the head of the capitate.[10] The amounts of flexion and ulnar deviation exceed the amounts of extension and radial deviation available at the wrist.[11-13] Motions of the wrist are coupled such that wrist extension is accompanied by radial deviation, while ulnar deviation accompanies wrist flexion. Maximum range of motion in the sagittal plane (flexion/extension) occurs with the wrist in neutral abduction and vice versa.[14]

ARTHROKINEMATICS: WRIST JOINT

Motions of the bony surfaces making up the radiocarpal and midcarpal joints during motions of the wrist are fairly complex. Models have been proposed that, while not complete, account for much of the motion that occurs.[13,15,16] During flexion of the wrist, convex distal joint surfaces at the radiocarpal and midcarpal joints roll in a volar direction and slide dorsally on concave proximal joint surfaces. During extension, motion of the bony surfaces of these joints occurs in the opposite direction. Ulnar deviation is produced by ulnar roll and simultaneous radial slide of the convex distal joint surfaces of the radiocarpal and midcarpal joints on the concave proximal surfaces of these joints. Movement of the joint surfaces occurs in the opposite direction during radial deviation, with the majority of this motion being produced by the midcarpal joint.[3]

LIMITATIONS OF MOTION: WRIST JOINT

With the fingers free to move, limitation of wrist flexion and extension range of motion is produced by passive tension in the dorsal and palmar radiocarpal ligaments, respectively.[17] In addition, the palmar ulnocarpal ligament also restricts wrist extension. Limitation of ulnar deviation occurs secondary to tension in the radial collateral ligament. Radial deviation of the wrist is terminated by bony impingement of the trapezium upon the radial styloid process.[1,3,18,19] Information regarding normal ranges of motion for all movements of the wrist is found in Appendix B.

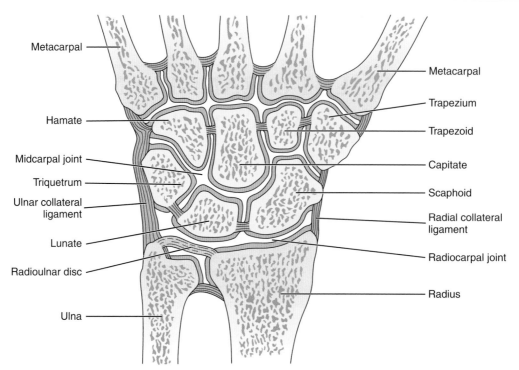

Fig. 5.1 Bony anatomy of the radiocarpal and midcarpal joints.

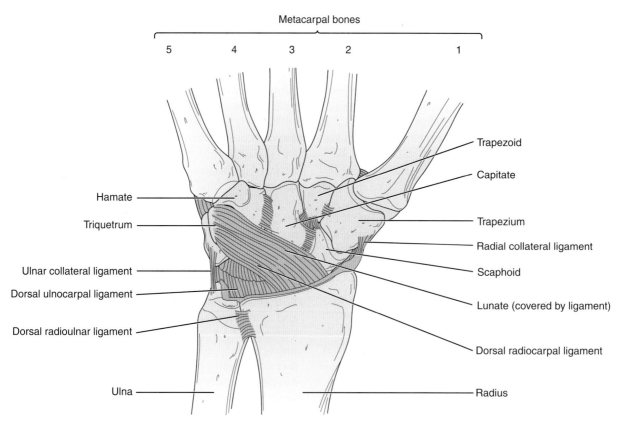

Fig. 5.2 Ligamentous reinforcement of the wrist–dorsal view.

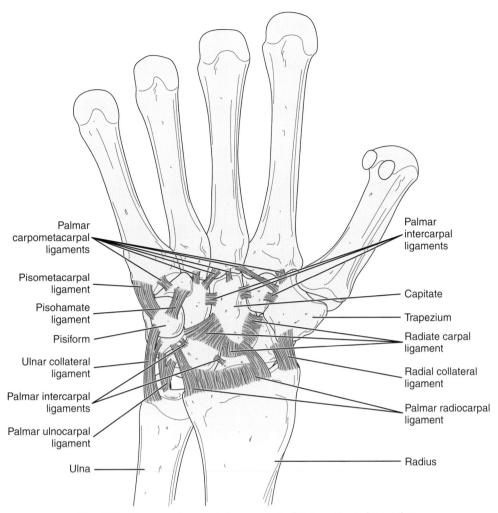

Fig. 5.3 Ligamentous reinforcement of the wrist–palmar view.

END-FEEL: WRIST JOINT

The end-feel for passive flexion and extension of the wrist is firm as a result of ligamentous limitation of the motion if the fingers are mobile. However, if the fingers are not free to move and are flexed, the position of the fingers will limit wrist flexion secondary to passive tension in the extrinsic finger extensors. Conversely, extension of the fingers will limit wrist extension owing to passive tension in the extrinsic finger flexors. Wrist adduction is also limited by ligamentous structures and thus possesses a firm end-feel. Wrist abduction is limited by bony contact between the radial styloid process and the trapezium, which produces a bony end-feel at the limit of motion.[1,18,19]

CAPSULAR PATTERN: WRIST JOINT

The capsular pattern for the wrist joint consists of equally limited flexion and extension. If this pattern of restriction is present, involvement of the capsule should be suspected.[20,21]

FIRST CARPOMETACARPAL (CMC) JOINT

ANATOMY: FIRST CMC JOINT

Unlike the carpometacarpal (CMC) joints of the fingers, the CMC joint of the thumb (first CMC joint) has a high degree of mobility. This joint is classified as a saddle joint and is formed by the articulation between the trapezium and the base of the first metacarpal bone (Fig. 5.4). The saddle classification of the joint defines the structure of the joint surfaces, which are each concave in one direction and convex in the other.[22] According to Neumann,[3] ligamentous reinforcement of the first CMC joint occurs via five ligaments: the anterior and posterior oblique, located, respectively, on the anterior and posterior aspects of the joint; the ulnar and radial collateral, located, respectively, on the ulnar and radial sides of the joint; and the first intermetacarpal ligament, connecting the bases of the first and second metacarpal bones.

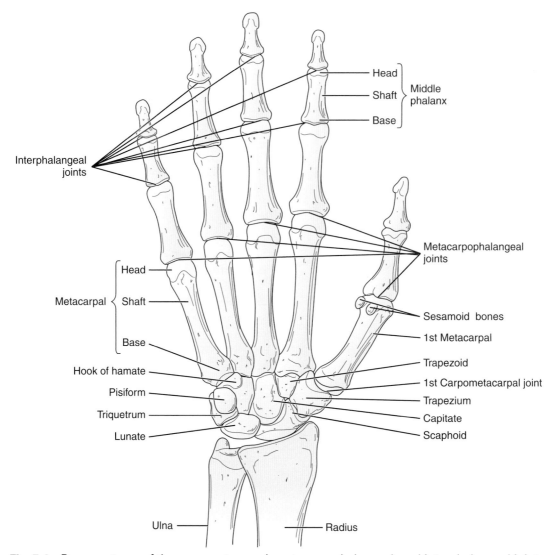

Fig. 5.4 Bony anatomy of the carpometacarpal, metacarpophalangeal, and interphalangeal joints.

OSTEOKINEMATICS: FIRST CMC JOINT

Motions occurring at the first CMC joint include flexion, extension, abduction, adduction, rotation, and opposition (Fig. 5.5). From the anatomical position, CMC flexion and extension occur in a plane parallel to the palm of the hand (frontal plane) (see Figs. 5.5, A and B), whereas abduction and adduction occur in a plane positioned perpendicular to the palm (sagittal plane) (see Figs. 5.5, C and D).[1,3] Rotation occurs as a result of rotation of the metacarpal around its longitudinal axis during flexion and extension of the first CMC joint and is normally not measured clinically. Opposition is a combination of flexion, medial rotation, and abduction of the first CMC joint (see Fig. 5.5, E).[1,3]

ARTHROKINEMATICS: FIRST CMC JOINT

During flexion and extension at the first CMC joint, the concave arch of the first metacarpal moves on the convex arch of the trapezium. Thus, according to the rules governing concave on convex movement, the first metacarpal rolls and slides in an ulnar direction during flexion and in a radial direction during extension at the first CMC joint. Conversely, since abduction and adduction at the first CMC joint involves movement of the convex arch of the first metacarpal on the concave arch of the trapezium, the first metacarpal rolls volarly and slides dorsally during abduction and moves in the reverse direction during adduction.[3,23]

LIMITATIONS OF MOTION: FIRST CMC JOINT

Motions of the first CMC joint are limited by a variety of structures, including soft tissues, ligaments, muscles, and joint capsule. Carpometacarpal joint flexion may be limited by contact between the thenar muscle mass and the soft tissue of the palm. When muscle mass of the thenar eminence is not well developed, limitation of CMC joint flexion is caused by tension in the extensor pollicis

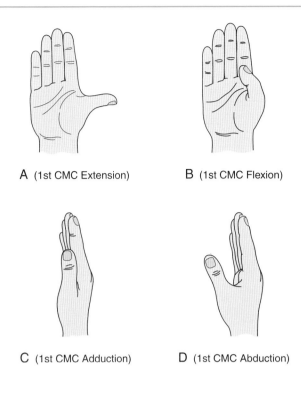

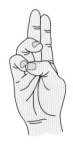

E (Opposition)

Fig. 5.5 Motions of the first carpometacarpal joint: (A) Extension, (B) Flexion, (C) Adduction, (D) Abduction, and (E) Opposition.

brevis and abductor pollicis brevis muscles, as well as by tension in the radial collateral ligament and the dorsal aspect of the CMC joint capsule. Extension of the first CMC joint is limited primarily by tension in muscles (adductor pollicis, flexor pollicis brevis, first dorsal interosseous, opponens pollicis), as well as by tension in the anterior oblique ligament. The limits of CMC abduction occur as a result of tension in the adductor pollicis and first dorsal interosseous muscles, all ligaments surrounding the first CMC joint, and secondary to stretching of the skin and connective tissue of the web space. Both opposition and adduction of the first CMC joint are limited by soft tissue approximation, the former between the pad of the thumb and the base of the fifth digit and the latter between the side of the thumb and the tissue overlying the second metacarpal.[3,18,22] Information regarding normal ranges of motion for all movements of the first CMC joint is found in Appendix B.

END-FEEL: FIRST CMC JOINT

A firm end-feel is present at the extremes of extension and abduction of the first CMC joint as a result of the limitation of motion by ligamentous and muscular structures. Flexion also may produce a firm end-feel if the muscle mass of the thenar eminence is poorly developed, but the end-feel for this motion is generally soft as long as sufficient thenar muscle mass is present. The end-feel for adduction and opposition of the first CMC joint is also soft secondary to soft tissue approximation.

CAPSULAR PATTERN: FIRST CMC JOINT

Decreased ROM at the first CMC joint may be caused by tightness of the joint capsule. If the capsule is involved, the patient will demonstrate full flexion, some limitation of extension, and an even greater limitation of abduction.[20,21]

METACARPOPHALANGEAL (MCP) AND INTERPHALANGEAL (IP) JOINTS

ANATOMY: MCP AND IP JOINTS

The metacarpophalangeal (MCP) joints of digits 1 through 5 are classified as condyloid joints and are formed by the articulation of the convex head of the metacarpal with the concave base of the proximal phalanx of the corresponding digit (see Fig. 5.4). Each MCP joint is reinforced along its sides by a pair of collateral ligaments and along its volar surface by a volar plate. The volar plates are fibrocartilaginous discs that reinforce the joint, resist hyperextension, and provide an expanded articular surface for the metacarpal heads.[3] The volar plates of the second through fifth MCP joints are interconnected via the deep transverse metacarpal ligaments[24] (Fig. 5.6).

Nine interphalangeal (IP) joints are present in the digits of the hand. Each finger possesses two IP joints: a proximal interphalangeal joint (PIP), which consists of the articulation of the convex head of the proximal phalanx with the concave base of the middle phalanx, and a distal interphalangeal joint (DIP), which consists of the articulation of the convex head of the middle phalanx with the concave base of the distal phalanx (see Fig. 5.4). The thumb possesses only a single IP joint, formed by the articulation of the convex head of the proximal phalanx with the concave base of the distal phalanx. Like the MCP joints, each IP joint is reinforced by a pair of collateral ligaments attached along the sides of the joint and by a volar plate on the volar surface (see Fig. 5.6). The function of these structures of the IP joints is analogous to their function at the MCP joints.[3,24,25]

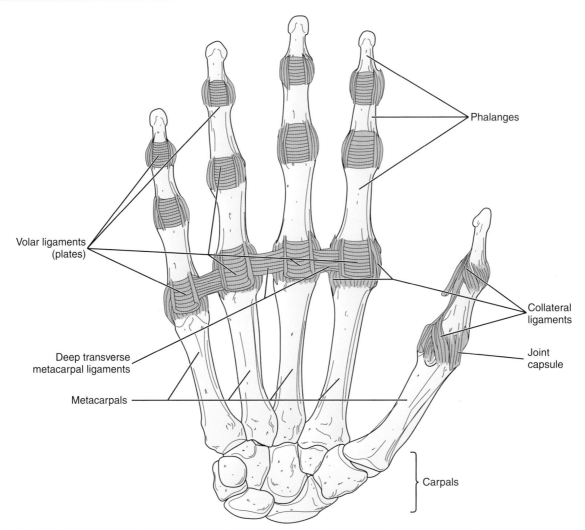

Fig. 5.6 Ligamentous reinforcement of the metacarpophalangeal and interphalangeal joints-palmar view.

OSTEOKINEMATICS: MCP AND IP JOINTS

Motions available at the MCP joints of digits two through five consist of flexion, extension, abduction, and adduction, while motion at the MCP joint of the thumb is essentially limited to flexion and extension.[26] The amount of MCP flexion generally increases from the first to the fifth digits, while MCP extension is greatest in the second and fifth digits.[27,28] The range of MCP joint abduction is most pronounced in the second and fifth digits, with less motion available in the third and fourth digits, and little to no motion available in the first MCP joint (in the thumb). Because of tightness of the collateral ligaments when the MCP joints are flexed, MCP abduction is least restricted when the MCP joints are extended and is severely limited to absent when the joints are flexed.

Each of the IP joints of the hand is classified as a hinge joint and is thus able to perform the motions of flexion and extension[1,18] There appears to be no significant difference in the amount of flexion and extension available at the PIP and DIP joints as one progresses across the hand.[27,28]

ARTHROKINEMATICS: MCP AND IP JOINTS

During movements at the MCP and IP joints, the concave distal joint surface (base of the phalanx) rolls and slides on the convex proximal joint surface in the same direction as the external motion. For example, during MCP extension, the base of the proximal phalanx rolls and slides dorsally, while during flexion, the roll and slide occur in a volar direction.[3]

LIMITATIONS OF MOTION: MCP AND IP JOINTS

Flexion of the MCP joints increases in range as one moves from the first digit (the thumb) toward the fifth digit, and is restricted by a variety of structures, including tension in the collateral ligaments and posterior joint capsule and bony contact between the anterior aspects of the metacarpal head and the base of the proximal phalanx. Limitation of MCP joint extension is produced by tension in the anterior joint capsule and volar plate. MCP joint abduction is limited by tension in the collateral ligaments and the skin of the interdigital web spaces. Adduction at these joints is restricted primarily by soft tissue contact with the adjacent digit.[2,3,18]

Limitation of IP joint flexion depends on the joint being moved. Flexion at the PIP joint usually is limited by contact of the soft tissue covering the anterior aspects of the proximal and middle phalanges of digits 2 through 5. Flexion at the IP (thumb) and DIP (fingers) joints (and occasionally flexion at the PIP joints of the fingers) is limited by tension in the posterior joint capsule and collateral ligaments. Extension of all IP joints is limited by tension in the anterior joint capsule and volar plate of the joint being moved.[2,3,18] Information regarding normal ranges of motion for all movements of the MCP and IP joints of the hand is found in Appendix B.

END-FEEL: MCP AND IP JOINTS

Depending on the particular individual, the end-feel for MCP joint flexion can be capsular or bony, while the end-feel for MCP extension is capsular. A capsular end-feel also is present at the extremes of MCP abduction, DIP flexion, flexion of the IP joint of the thumb, and extension of all interphalangeal joints. Adduction at the MCP joints and flexion at the PIP joints normally produce a soft end-feel due to soft tissue approximation.

CAPSULAR PATTERN: MCP AND IP JOINTS

The capsular pattern is the same for the metacarpophalangeal joints and the interphalangeal (PIP and DIP) joints. In each of these joints, the capsule should be suspected if flexion is more limited than extension.[18,20]

RANGE OF MOTION AND FUNCTIONAL ACTIVITY

Several authors have investigated the motion that occurs at the wrist during functional activities in healthy adults. In 1984, Brumfield and Champoux[29] used a uniaxial electrogoniometer to measure wrist flexion and extension in 19 healthy adults during seven hand placement motions and seven functional activities. The participants in the study consisted of 12 men and 7 women, aged 25 to 60 years of age. Based on the data gathered, the authors concluded that a range of 10 degrees of wrist flexion to 35 degrees of wrist extension was sufficient to perform the functional activities included in the study. A year later, Palmer et al.[30] used a triaxial goniometer to measure wrist flexion, extension, radial deviation, ulnar deviation, and rotation during 52 different tasks. The tasks included in the study were categorized according to activity including personal hygiene, culinary, other activities

of daily living (ADLs), carpentry, housekeeping, secretarial, mechanical, and surgical. Ten healthy subjects of unstated age were used to gather data for the tasks involved in personal hygiene, culinary, and other ADLs, and subgroups of five subjects were used for the other categories. Although specific ROM data were not provided by the authors, summary data for each category indicated that the ROM used to complete personal hygiene, culinary, and other ADL tasks consisted of a range of 33 degrees of wrist flexion to 59 degrees of wrist extension and 23 degrees of radial deviation to 22 degrees of ulnar deviation.

Other groups of investigators, including Safaee-Rad et al.[31] and Ryu et al.[12] have examined wrist motion during functional activities. The functions studied by Safaee-Rad et al.[31] were limited to feeding activities in a group of 10 healthy adult men, aged 20 to 29 years, using a three-dimensional motion analysis system. Ryu et al.[12] used a biaxial wrist electrogoniometer to measure motion in 40 subjects (20 men and 20 women of unstated age) during 7 hand placement and 24 functional activities. Table 5.1 contains a summary of selected data from the studies by Brumfield and Champoux,[29] Safaee-Rad et al.,[31] and Ryu et al.[12] Data from the study by Ryu et al. were translated from graphic data provided in the published report.

Fewer studies have investigated motion of the joints of the hand during functional activities. Hume et al.[32] used both standard and electrogoniometric methods to measure motion of the metacarpophalangeal and interphalangeal joints of the fingers and thumb during 11 functional activities in 35 adult males, aged 26 to 28 years. Based on data collected in this study, the authors concluded that only a small percentage of the total range of motion of the fingers was required for functional activities. They reported average flexion postures at each of the joints for all functional activities combined, as follows: metacarpophalangeal joint—61 degrees, proximal interphalangeal joint—60 degrees, distal interphalangeal joint—39 degrees, metacarpophalangeal joint of thumb—21 degrees, interphalangeal joint of thumb—18 degrees.

Some of the data reported by Hume et al.[32] were supported in a later study by Lee and Rim[33] who investigated the finger (but not thumb) joint angles and forces used by four different individuals when grasping five different-sized cylinders. In their results, Lee and Rim reported that flexion angles at the metacarpophalangeal joints and proximal interphalangeal joints increased as the size of the cylinder being grasped decreased. However, regardless of cylinder size, the position of the distal interphalangeal joint remained consistently at around 40 degrees of flexion (almost identical to the average 39 degrees of flexion reported for this joint by Hume et al.[32]). Figs. 5.7 to 5.9 illustrate motions of the wrist and hand used to perform selected functional activities.

Table 5.1 WRIST ROM DURING FUNCTIONAL ACTIVITIES				
FUNCTIONAL ACTIVITY	**FLEXION**	**EXTENSION**	**RADIAL DEVIATION**	**ULNAR DEVIATION**
Brush Teeth				
Ryu et al.[28]	30°	41°	9°	24°
Comb Hair				
Ryu et al.[28]	36°	31°	3°	39°
Cut with Knife				
Brumfield and Champoux[4]	4°	20°	−13°	28°
Ryu et al.[28]	31°	−6°		
Drink from Glass/Cup				
Brumfield and Champoux[4]	−11°	24°	−6°	19°
Ryu et al.[28]	−3°	22°	−8°	16°
Safaee-Rad[29]	8°	6°		
Eat with Fork				
Brumfield and Champoux[4]	−9°	37°	5°	3°
Safaee-Rad[29]	−3°	18°		
Eat with Spoon				
Safaee-Rad[29]	−8°	20°	4°	4°
Open/Close Jar Lid				
Ryu et al.[28]	35°	6°	12°	35°
Perineal Care				
Ryu et al.[28]	55°	−16°	4°	21°
Pour from Pitcher				
Brumfield and Champoux[4]	−9°	30°	−13°	31°
Ryu et al.[28]	20°	22°		
Pound with Hammer				
Ryu et al.[28]	−16°	44°	−8°	21°
Read Newspaper				
Brumfield and Champoux[4]	−2°	35°		
Rise from Chair				
Brumfield and Champoux[4]	−1°	63°	−3°	29°
Ryu et al.[28]	11°	61°		
Tie/Untie Shoe Laces				
Ryu et al.[28]	29°	36°	10°	33°
Tie/Untie Necktie/Scarf				
Ryu et al.[28]	51°	41°	13°	28°
Turn Doorknob				
Ryu et al.[28]	40°	45°	1°	32°
Turn Steering Wheel				
Ryu et al.[28]	17°	44°	17°	28°
Use Telephone				
Brumfield and Champoux[4]	0°	43°	10°	12°
Ryu et al.[28]	17°	42°		
Write				
Ryu et al.[28]	−16°	31°	−4°	17°

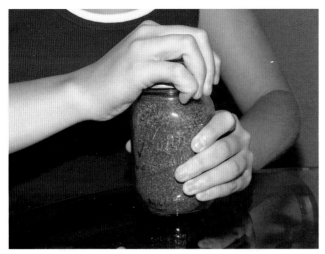

Fig. 5.7   Wrist motion used to open a jar.

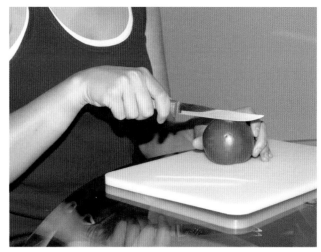

Fig. 5.9   Wrist motion used to cut with a knife.

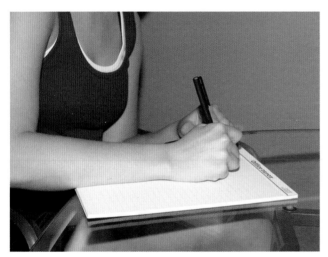

Fig. 5.8   Wrist motion used to write.

TECHNIQUES OF MEASUREMENT

WRIST JOINT

Recommended techniques for measuring flexion and extension of the wrist include positioning the goniometer along the radial, ulnar, and dorsal/volar surfaces of the wrist.[34–36] In a multicenter study of wrist flexion and extension goniometry, LaStayo and Wheeler[37] compared the reliability of all three positioning techniques and found that the dorsal-volar technique was consistently more reliable than the other two (see Chapter 7 for a full description of this study). In a cadaver study, Carter et al.[38] found no statistical difference in the intrarater reliability of the three measurement techniques but found the dorsal-volar technique to have the highest interrater reliability. Additionally, 73% of all therapists surveyed preferred the dorsal-volar technique to the other two placements when performing wrist ROM.[39] Therefore, in this text the dorsal-volar positioning technique is presented as the technique of choice, with radial positioning used as an alternative technique for measuring wrist flexion and extension. Wrist abduction and adduction are measured using the standard technique of positioning the goniometer over the dorsal surface of the joint.[35]

When measuring motion in one plane of movement at the wrist, a neutral position of the wrist with reference to the other plane should be maintained. For example, when measuring wrist flexion/extension, the subject's wrist should not be deviated in either a radial or ulnar direction. Conversely, when measuring radial and ulnar deviation, a neutral wrist position in terms of flexion and extension should be maintained. In a study of 54 subjects, Marshall et al.[40] found that wrist position in one plane could significantly affect wrist ROM in the perpendicular plane.

FIRST CARPOMETACARPAL JOINT

A variety of methods to measure motion of the first CMC joint have been presented in the literature.[34,35] Reported norms for ROM in this joint vary widely (see Appendix B), presumably because of differences in measurement techniques. Much of the variation in technique appears to be due, at least in part, to inconsistent terminology regarding motion of this joint. The majority of techniques used in this text are based on motions of the CMC joint as defined in *Gray's Anatomy.*[1]

Measurement of first CMC joint opposition involves the measurement of motions occurring at the first and fifth CMC joints, as well as motion occurring in at least one other joint of the first or fifth digit. To avoid measuring motion in any joint other than the first CMC joint, the technique described in this text for measuring first CMC opposition is one that was modified from two different techniques recommended by the American Academy of Orthopaedic Surgeons (AAOS)[41] and the American Medical Association (AMA).[34] The AAOS technique examines opposition by measuring the linear distance from the tip of the thumb to the base of the fifth metacarpal, stating that "opposition is usually considered complete when the tip of the thumb touches the base of the fifth finger."[41] Although the base (palmar digital crease) of the fifth digit provides a reproducible landmark against which first CMC joint opposition can be measured, included in this motion is measurement of metacarpophalangeal (MCP) and interphalangeal (IP) flexion of the thumb, which the AAOS considers part of opposition. The technique for examining opposition recommended by the AMA involves measuring the linear distance from the flexor crease of the thumb IP joint to the distal palmar crease over the third metacarpal, without allowing flexion at the MCP or IP joints of the thumb.[34] While the flexor crease of the thumb IP joint provides a more reproducible landmark than the tip of the thumb, the distal palmar crease runs obliquely across the third metacarpal, allowing a variety of points along which the distal end of the ruler may be placed during measurement (Fig. 5.10). Such a variety of possible placements could lend inconsistency to the results obtained when measuring opposition according to the AMA technique.

In an effort to use a technique that (1) measures only opposition occurring at the first CMC joint and (2) uses reproducible landmarks for both the proximal and the distal ends of the ruler, a technique that combines the best of the AAOS[41] and AMA[34] techniques is described in this text. The technique described herein examines first CMC joint opposition by measuring the linear distance between the flexor crease of the IP joint of the first digit (thumb) and the palmar digital crease of the fifth digit. Motion of the MCP and IP joints of the first and fifth digits is prevented during

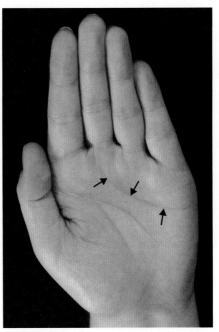

Fig. 5.10   Volar (palmar) surface of hand, demonstrating distal palmar crease (tip of arrows). Note oblique angle at which distal palmar crease crosses third metacarpal.

the measurement. Unfortunately, no standards for normal ROM are yet available for this technique of measuring opposition.

METACARPOPHALANGEAL AND INTERPHALANGEAL JOINTS

During goniometric measurement of MCP and IP joint motion, one must remain mindful of the fact that position of the proximal joints can greatly affect the ROM of the more distal joints of the hand.[27] Tension in the extrinsic finger extensors, when more proximal joints such as the wrist are flexed, can restrict the amount of flexion available in distal joints, such as the MCP joints.

Conversely, extension of the more proximal joints causes tension on the extrinsic finger flexors, which in turn restricts the amount of extension that can be obtained at more distal joints. Therefore, care should be taken to maintain the proximal joints of the wrist and hand in a neutral position during measurement of flexion and extension of the MCP and IP joints.

The standard technique for measuring MCP and IP joint flexion is with the goniometer positioned over the dorsal surface of the joint being examined.[34,41]

Extension of the MCP and IP joints may be measured with the goniometer positioned over either the dorsal or the volar surface of the joint. However, the soft tissue over the volar surface of the MCP joints may interfere with alignment of the goniometer during measurement of MCP extension using the volar positioning technique. Lateral positioning of the goniometer is a technique that is preferred by some examiners but one that has been reported to be slightly less reliable than dorsal placement.[39]

Wrist Flexion: Dorsal Alignment (Video 5.1)

Fig. 5.11 Starting position for measurement of wrist flexion using dorsal alignment technique. Bony landmarks for goniometer alignment (lateral epicondyle of humerus, lunate, dorsal midline of third metacarpal) indicated by red line and dots.

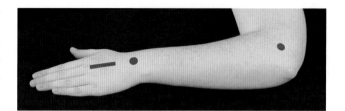

Normal ROM = 70 degrees to 95 degrees.[41–46]

MDC for wrist flexion goniometry measured by a single examiner = 8 degrees to 18 degrees.[37,47–49]

Patient position	Seated, with shoulder abducted 90 degrees; elbow flexed 90 degrees; forearm pronated; arm and forearm supported on table; hand off table with wrist in neutral position (Fig. 5.11).
Stabilization	Over dorsal surface of forearm (Fig. 5.12).
Examiner action	After instructing patient in motion desired, flex patient's wrist through available ROM (see Note). Return wrist to neutral position. Performing passive movement provides an estimate of ROM and demonstrates to patient exact motion desired (see Fig. 5.12).
Goniometer alignment	Palpate the following bony landmarks (shown in Fig. 5.11) and align goniometer accordingly (Fig. 5.13).
Stationary arm	Dorsal midline of forearm toward lateral epicondyle of humerus.

Fig. 5.12 End of wrist flexion ROM, showing proper hand placement for stabilizing forearm and flexing wrist. Bony landmarks for goniometer alignment (lateral epicondyle of humerus, lunate, dorsal midline of third metacarpal) indicated by red line and dots.

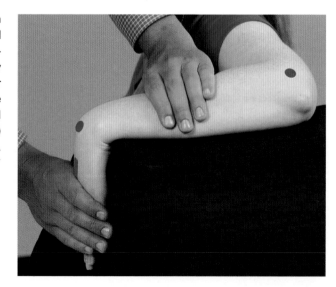

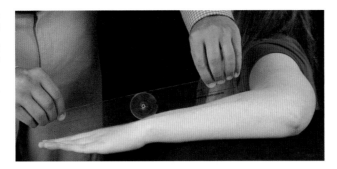

Fig. 5.13 Starting position for measurement of wrist flexion, demonstrating proper initial alignment of goniometer.

Axis	Lunate.
Moving arm	Dorsal midline of third metacarpal.
	Read scale of goniometer.
Patient/Examiner action	Perform passive, or have patient perform active, wrist flexion (Fig. 5.14).
Confirmation of alignment	Repalpate landmarks and confirm proper goniometric alignment at end of ROM, correcting alignment as necessary. Read scale of goniometer (see Fig. 5.14).
Documentation	Record patient's ROM.
Note	Flexion of fingers should be avoided during measurement of wrist flexion to prevent limitation of motion by tension in extrinsic finger extensors.
Alternative patient position	Patients unable to achieve 90 degrees of shoulder abduction may be positioned with shoulder adducted for this measurement. In such a case, stationary arm of goniometer should be aligned with dorsal midline of forearm toward bicipital tendon at elbow. Measurement may also be made with forearm in neutral rotation.

Fig. 5.14 End of wrist flexion ROM, demonstrating proper alignment of goniometer at end of range.

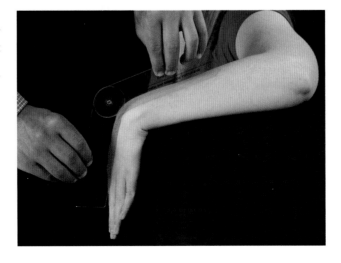

Wrist Flexion: Ulnar Alignment (Video 5.2)

Fig. 5.15 Starting position for measurement of wrist flexion using ulnar alignment technique. Bony landmarks for goniometer alignment (olecranon process of ulna, triquetrum, lateral midline of fifth metacarpal) indicated by red line and dots.

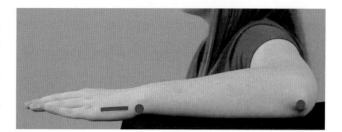

Normal ROM: See Wrist Flexion: Dorsal Alignment. One study demonstrated a significant difference in average ROM attained when using ulnar versus dorsal alignment of the goniometer during measurement of wrist flexion.[37]

MDC for wrist flexion goniometry measured by a single examiner = 8 degrees to 18 degrees.[37,47–49]

Patient position	Seated, with shoulder abducted 90 degrees; elbow flexed 90 degrees; forearm pronated; arm and forearm supported on table; hand off table with wrist in neutral position (Fig. 5.15).
Stabilization	Over dorsal surface of forearm (Fig. 5.16).
Examiner action	After instructing patient in motion desired, flex patient's wrist through available ROM (see Note). Return wrist to neutral position. Performing passive movement provides an estimate of ROM and demonstrates to patient exact motion desired (see Fig. 5.16).
Goniometer alignment	Palpate the following bony landmarks (shown in Fig. 5.15) and align goniometer accordingly (Fig. 5.17).
Stationary arm	Lateral midline of ulna toward olecranon process.
Axis	Triquetrum.

Fig. 5.16 End of wrist flexion ROM, showing proper hand placement for stabilizing forearm and flexing wrist. Bony landmarks for goniometer alignment (olecranon process of ulna, triquetrum, lateral midline of fifth metacarpal) indicated by red line and dots.

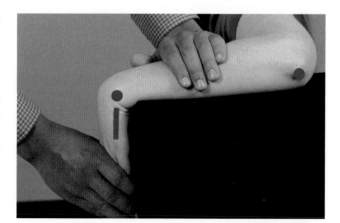

Fig. 5.17 Starting position for measurement of wrist flexion, demonstrating proper initial alignment of goniometer.

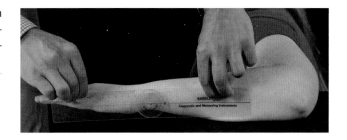

Moving arm   Lateral midline of fifth metacarpal.

Read scale of goniometer.

Patient/Examiner action   Perform passive, or have patient perform active, wrist flexion (Fig. 5.18).

Confirmation of alignment   Repalpate landmarks and confirm proper goniometric alignment at end of ROM, correcting alignment as necessary. Read scale of goniometer (see Fig. 5.18).

Documentation   Record patient's ROM.

Note   Flexion of fingers should be avoided during measurement of wrist flexion to prevent limitation of motion by tension in extrinsic finger extensors.

Alternative patient   Patients unable to achieve 90 degrees of shoulder abduction position may be positioned with shoulder adducted. In such a case, a dorsal alignment technique should be used, and the measurement also may be made with forearm in neutral rotation. Stationary arm of the goniometer should be aligned with the dorsal midline of the forearm toward the bicipital tendon at the elbow.

Fig. 5.18 End of wrist flexion ROM, demonstrating proper alignment of goniometer at end of range.

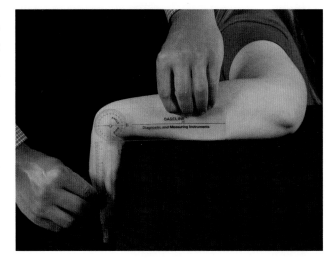

Wrist Extension: Volar Alignment (Video 5.3)

Fig. 5.19 Starting position for measurement of wrist extension using volar alignment technique. Bony landmarks for goniometer alignment (bicipital tendon at elbow, lunate, volar midline of third metacarpal) indicated by red line and dots.

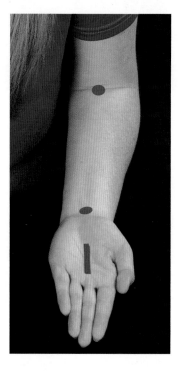

Normal ROM = 60 degrees to 85 degrees.[11,34,41–43,45,46,48]

MDC for wrist extension goniometry measured by a single examiner = 6 degrees to 18 degrees.[37,47–49]

Patient position

Seated, with shoulder adducted; elbow flexed 90 degrees; forearm supinated and supported on table; wrist and hand off table with wrist in neutral position (Fig. 5.19).

Stabilization

Over ventral surface of forearm (Fig. 5.20).

Fig. 5.20 End of wrist extension ROM, showing proper hand placement for stabilizing forearm and extending wrist. Bony landmarks for goniometer alignment (bicipital tendon at elbow, lunate, volar midline of third metacarpal) indicated by red line and dots.

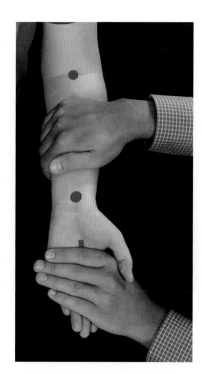

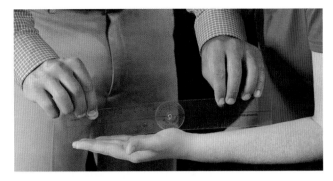

Examiner action	After instructing patient in motion desired, extend patient's wrist through available ROM (see Note). Return wrist to neutral position. Performing passive movement provides an estimate of ROM and demonstrates to patient exact motion desired (see Fig. 5.20).
Goniometer alignment	Palpate the following landmarks (shown in Fig. 5.19) and align goniometer accordingly (Fig. 5.21).
Stationary arm	Volar midline of forearm toward bicipital tendon at elbow.
Axis	Lunate.
Moving arm	Volar midline of third metacarpal.
	Read scale of goniometer.
Patient/examiner action	Perform passive, or have patient perform active, wrist extension (Fig. 5.22).
Confirmation of alignment	Repalpate landmarks and confirm proper goniometric alignment at end of ROM, correcting alignment as necessary.
	Read scale of goniometer (see Fig. 5.22).
Documentation	Record patient's ROM.
Note	Extension of fingers should be avoided during measurement of wrist extension to prevent limitation of motion by tension in extrinsic finger flexors.
Alternative patient position	Measurement also may be made with forearm in neutral rotation.

Fig. 5.22 End of wrist extension ROM, demonstrating proper alignment of goniometer at end of range.

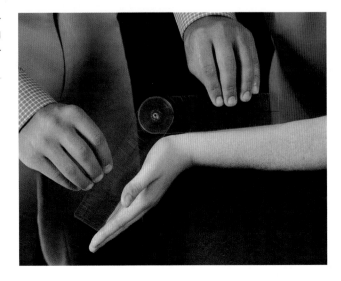

Wrist Extension: Ulnar Alignment (Video 5.4)

Fig. 5.23 Starting position for measurement of wrist extension using ulnar alignment technique. Bony landmarks for goniometer alignment (olecranon process of ulna, triquetrum, lateral midline of fifth metacarpal) indicated by red line and dots.

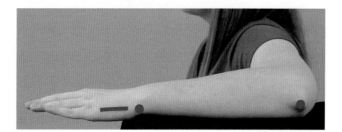

Normal ROM: See Wrist Extension: Dorsal Alignment. One study demonstrated a significant difference in average ROM attained when using ulnar versus dorsal alignment of the goniometer during measurement of wrist extension.[37]

MDC for wrist extension goniometry measured by a single examiner = 6 degrees to 18 degrees.[37,47-49]

Patient position   Seated, with shoulder abducted 90 degrees; elbow flexed 90 degrees; forearm pronated; arm and forearm supported on table; hand off table with wrist in neutral position (Fig. 5.23).

Stabilization   Over dorsal surface of forearm (Fig. 5.24).

Examiner action   After instructing patient in motion desired, extend patient's wrist through available ROM (see Note). Return wrist to neutral position. Performing passive movement provides an estimate of ROM and demonstrates to patient exact motion desired (see Fig. 5.24).

Goniometer alignment   Palpate the following bony landmarks (shown in Fig. 5.23) and align goniometer accordingly (Fig. 5.25).

Stationary arm   Lateral midline of ulna toward olecranon process.

Axis   Triquetrum.

Moving arm   Lateral midline of fifth metacarpal.

Fig. 5.24 End of wrist extension ROM, showing proper hand placement for stabilizing forearm and extending wrist. Bony landmarks for goniometer alignment (olecranon process of ulna, triquetrum, lateral midline of fifth metacarpal) indicated by red line and dots.

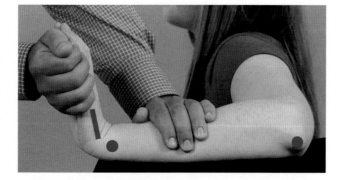

Fig. 5.25 Starting position for measurement of wrist extension, demonstrating proper initial alignment of goniometer.

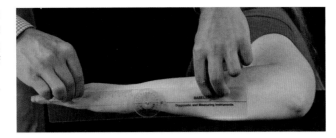

	Read scale of goniometer.
Patient/Examiner action	Perform passive, or have patient perform active, wrist extension (Fig. 5.26).
Confirmation of alignment	Repalpate landmarks and confirm proper goniometric alignment at end of ROM, correcting alignment as necessary. Read scale of goniometer (see Fig. 5.26).
Documentation	Record patient's ROM.
Note	Extension of fingers should be avoided during measurement of wrist extension to prevent limitation of motion by tension in extrinsic finger flexors.
Alternative patient position	Measurement also may be made with forearm in neutral rotation. In such a case, goniometer should be placed over volar surface of wrist with stationary arm aligned with midline of forearm toward bicipital tendon, axis over lunate, and moving arm aligned with volar midline of third metacarpal.

Fig. 5.26 End of wrist extension ROM, demonstrating proper alignment of goniometer at end of range.

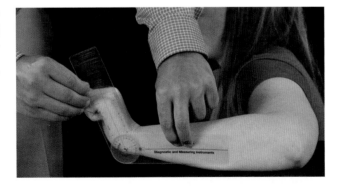

Wrist Adduction: Ulnar Deviation (Video 5.5)

Fig. 5.27 Starting position for measurement of wrist adduction. Bony landmarks for goniometer alignment (lateral epicondyle of humerus, capitate, dorsal midline of third metacarpal) indicated by red line and dots.

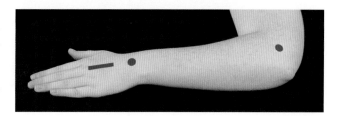

Normal ROM = 30 degrees to 40 degrees,[41–43,46,48] with values near 60 degrees if measured with the forearm in supination.[44,47]

MDC for wrist adduction goniometry measured by a single examiner = 8 degrees to 21 degrees.[47–49]

Patient position	Seated, with shoulder abducted 90 degrees; elbow flexed 90 degrees; forearm pronated; upper extremity (UE) supported on table; wrist and hand in neutral position (Fig. 5.27).
Stabilization	Over dorsal surface of distal forearm (Fig. 5.28).
Examiner action	After instructing patient in motion desired, adduct patient's wrist through available ROM. Return wrist to neutral position. Performing passive movement provides an estimate of ROM and demonstrates to patient exact motion desired (see Fig. 5.28).

Fig. 5.28 End of wrist adduction ROM, showing proper hand placement for stabilizing forearm and adducting wrist. Bony landmarks for goniometer alignment (lateral epicondyle of humerus, capitate, dorsal midline of third metacarpal) indicated by red line and dots.

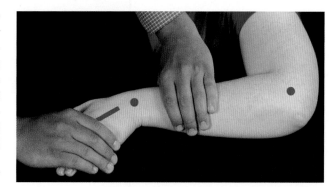

Fig. 5.29 Starting position for measurement of wrist adduction, demonstrating proper initial alignment of goniometer.

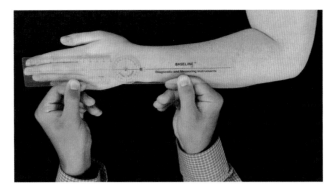

Goniometer alignment	Palpate the following bony landmarks (shown in Fig. 5.27) and align goniometer accordingly (Fig. 5.29).
Stationary arm	Dorsal midline of forearm toward lateral epicondyle of humerus.
Axis	Capitate.
Moving arm	Dorsal midline of third metacarpal.
	Read scale of goniometer.
Patient/examiner action	Perform passive, or have patient perform active, wrist adduction (Fig. 5.30).
Confirmation of alignment	Repalpate landmarks and confirm proper goniometric alignment at end of ROM, correcting alignment as necessary. Read scale of goniometer (see Fig. 5.30).
Documentation	Record patient's ROM.
Alternative patient position	Patients unable to achieve 90 degrees of shoulder adduction may be positioned with shoulder adducted for this measurement. In such a case, stationary arm of goniometer should be aligned with dorsal midline of forearm toward bicipital tendon at elbow.

Fig. 5.30 End of wrist adduction ROM, demonstrating proper alignment of goniometer at end of range.

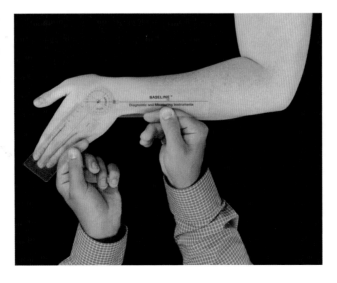

Wrist Abduction: Radial Deviation (Video 5.6)

Fig. 5.31 Starting position for measurement of wrist abduction. Landmarks for goniometer alignment (lateral epicondyle of humerus, capitate, dorsal midline of third metacarpal) indicated by red line and dots.

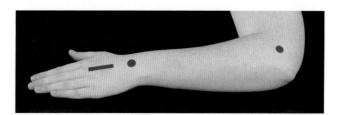

Normal ROM = 20 degrees to 25 degrees.[11,12,34,41,42,45,48,50]

MDC for wrist abduction goniometry measured by a single examiner = 7 degrees to 19 degrees.[47–49]

Patient position	Seated, with shoulder abducted 90 degrees; elbow flexed 90 degrees; forearm pronated; UE supported on table; wrist and hand in neutral position (Fig. 5.31).
Stabilization	Over dorsal surface of distal forearm (Fig. 5.32).
Examiner action	After instructing patient in motion desired, abduct patient's wrist through available ROM. Return wrist to neutral position. Performing passive movement provides an estimate of the ROM and demonstrates to patient exact motion desired (see Fig. 5.32).

Fig. 5.32 End of wrist abduction ROM, showing proper hand placement for stabilizing forearm and abducting wrist. Landmarks for goniometer alignment (lateral epicondyle of humerus, capitate, dorsal midline of third metacarpal) indicated by red line and dots.

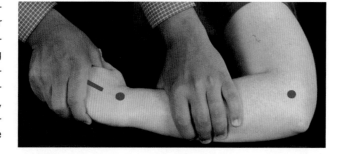

Fig. 5.33 Starting position for measurement of wrist abduction, demonstrating proper initial alignment of goniometer.

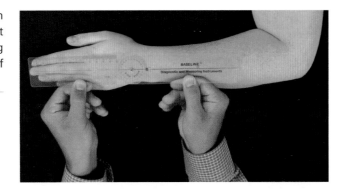

Goniometer alignment	Palpate the following bony landmarks (shown in Fig. 5.31) and align goniometer accordingly (Fig. 5.33).
Stationary arm	Dorsal midline of forearm toward lateral epicondyle of humerus.
Axis	Capitate.
Moving arm	Dorsal midline of third metacarpal.
	Read scale of goniometer.
Patient/Examiner action	Perform passive, or have patient perform active, wrist abduction (Fig. 5.34).
Confirmation of alignment	Repalpate landmarks and confirm proper goniometric alignment at end of ROM, correcting alignment as necessary. Read scale of goniometer (see Fig. 5.34).
Documentation	Record patient's ROM.
Alternative patient position	Patients unable to achieve 90 degrees of shoulder abduction may be positioned with shoulder adducted for this measurement. In such a case, stationary arm of goniometer should be aligned with dorsal midline of forearm toward bicipital tendon at elbow.

Fig. 5.34 End of wrist abduction ROM, demonstrating proper alignment of goniometer at end of range.

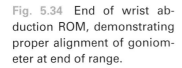

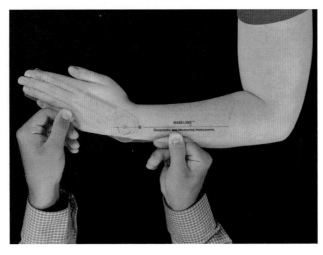

Metacarpophalangeal (MCP) Abduction (Video 5.7)

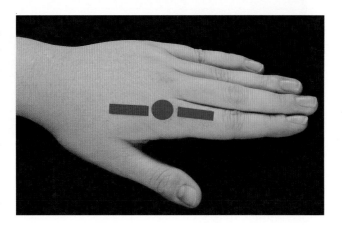

Fig. 5.35 Starting position for measurement of MCP abduction. Landmarks for goniometer alignment (dorsal midline of metacarpal, dorsum of MCP joint, dorsal midline of proximal phalanx) indicated by red lines and dot.

Normal ROM: Variable, depending on specific finger being measured.[51]

No values for MDC for goniometry of this joint were found in the literature.

Patient position

Seated, with forearm pronated; UE supported on table; wrist and hand in neutral position (Fig. 5.35).

Stabilization

Over metacarpals (Fig. 5.36).

Examiner action

After instructing patient in motion desired, abduct MCP joint to be examined through available ROM. Return finger to neutral position. Performing passive movement provides an estimate of ROM and demonstrates to patient exact motion desired (see Fig. 5.36).

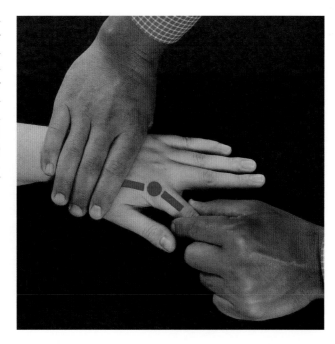

Fig. 5.36 End of MCP abduction ROM, showing proper hand placement for stabilizing metacarpals and abducting MCP joint. Landmarks for goniometer alignment (dorsal midline of metacarpal, dorsum of MCP joint, dorsal midline of proximal phalanx) indicated by red lines and dot.

Fig. 5.37 Starting position for measurement of MCP abduction, demonstrating proper initial alignment of goniometer.

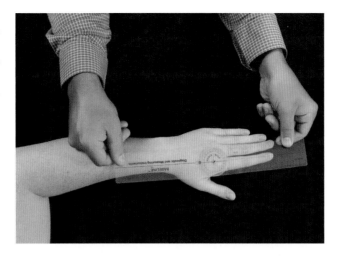

Goniometer alignment	Palpate the following bony landmarks (shown in Fig. 5.35) and align goniometer accordingly (Fig. 5.37).
Stationary arm	Dorsal midline of metacarpal.
Axis	Dorsum of MCP joint.
Moving arm	Dorsal midline of proximal phalanx.
	Read scale of goniometer.
Patient/examiner action	Perform passive, or have patient perform active, MCP abduction (Fig. 5.38).
Confirmation of alignment	Repalpate landmarks and confirm proper goniometric alignment at end of ROM, correcting alignment as necessary.
	Read scale of goniometer (see Fig. 5.38).
Documentation	Record patient's ROM.

Fig. 5.38 End of MCP abduction ROM, demonstrating proper alignment of goniometer at end of range.

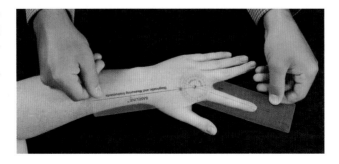

Metacarpophalangeal (MCP) or interphalangeal (PIP or DIP) Flexion (Video 5.8)

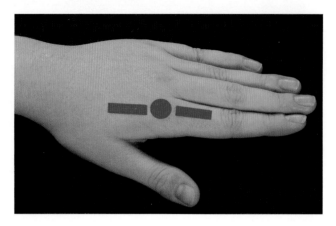

Fig. 5.39 Starting position for measurement of MCP flexion. Landmarks for goniometer alignment (dorsal midline of metacarpal, dorsum of MCP joint, dorsal midline of proximal phalanx) indicated by red lines and dot.

Normal ROM: MCP = 85 degrees to 100 degrees.[27,34,41,51,52]

MDC for finger flexion goniometry measured by a single examiner = 18 to 24 degrees for the MCP joint, 12 to 15 degrees for the PIP joint, and 14 to 18 degrees for the DIP joint.[49]

(Measurement of Second MCP Joint Shown.)

Patient position	Seated, with UE supported on table; wrist and hand in neutral position* (Fig. 5.39).
Stabilization	Over more proximal bone of joint (in this case, stabilization of metacarpals is shown) (Fig. 5.40).
Examiner action	After instructing patient in motion desired, flex joint to be examined through available ROM. Return finger to neutral position. Performing passive movement provides an estimate of ROM and demonstrates to patient exact motion desired (see Fig. 5.40).

*Proximal joints should remain in neutral position during measurement to prevent obstruction of full ROM by tension in extrinsic and intrinsic finger extensor muscles.

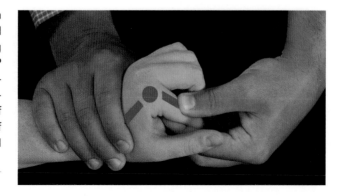

Fig. 5.40 End of MCP flexion ROM, showing proper hand placement for stabilizing metacarpals and flexing MCP joint. Landmarks for goniometer alignment (dorsal midline of metacarpal, dorsum of MCP joint, dorsal midline of proximal phalanx) indicated by red lines and dot.

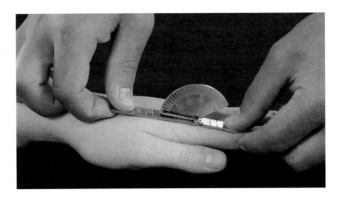

Fig. 5.41 Starting position for measurement of MCP flexion, demonstrating proper initial alignment of goniometer.

Goniometer alignment	Palpate the following bony landmarks (shown in Fig. 5.39) and align goniometer accordingly (Fig. 5.41).
Stationary arm	Dorsal midline of more proximal bone of joint (in this case, a metacarpal).
Axis	Dorsum of joint being examined (in this case, MCP joint).
Moving arm	Dorsal midline of more distal bone joint (in this case, a proximal phalanx).
	Read scale of goniometer.
Patient/examiner action	Perform passive, or have patient perform active, flexion of the joint (Fig. 5.42).
Confirmation of alignment	Repalpate landmarks and confirm proper goniometric alignment at end of ROM, correcting alignment as necessary.
	Read scale of goniometer (see Fig. 5.42).
Documentation	Record patient's ROM.
Note	This technique may be used to measure flexion of the MCP, PIP, or DIP joints of the fingers. The figures shown here depict the measurement of MCP flexion of the second digit (index finger).

Fig. 5.42 End of MCP flexion ROM, demonstrating proper alignment of goniometer at end of range.

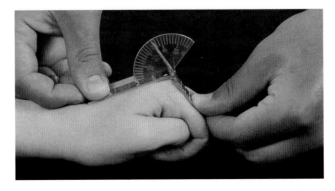

Metacarpophalangeal (MCP) or Interphalangeal (PIP or DIP) Extension (Video 5.9)

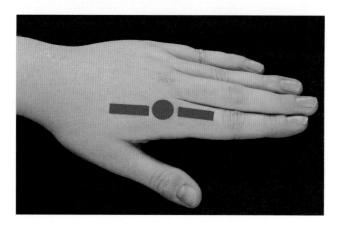

Fig. 5.43 Starting position for measurement of MCP extension. Landmarks for goniometer alignment (dorsal midline of metacarpal, dorsum of MCP joint, dorsal midline of proximal phalanx) indicated by red lines and dot.

Normal ROM: MCP = 20 degrees to 25 degrees.[27,51]

No values for MDC for goniometry of this joint were found in the literature.

(Measurement of Second MCP Joint Shown.)

Patient position	Seated, with UE supported on table; wrist and hand in neutral position* (Fig. 5.43).
Stabilization	Over more proximal bone of joint being examined (in this case, stabilization of metacarpals is shown) (Fig. 5.44).
Examiner action	After instructing patient in motion desired, extend MCP joint to be examined through available ROM. Return finger to neutral position. Performing passive movement provides an estimate of ROM and demonstrates to patient exact motion desired (see Fig. 5.44).

*Proximal joints should remain in neutral position during measurement to prevent obstruction of full ROM by tension in extrinsic or intrinsic finger flexor muscles.

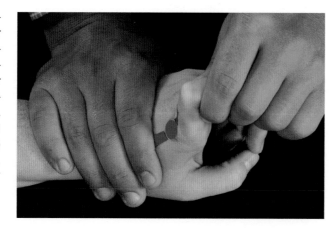

Fig. 5.44 End of MCP extension ROM, showing proper hand placement for stabilizing metacarpals and extending MCP joint. Landmarks for goniometer alignment (dorsal midline of metacarpal, dorsum of MCP joint, dorsal midline of proximal phalanx) indicated by red lines and dot.

Fig. 5.45 Starting position for measurement of MCP extension, demonstrating proper initial alignment of goniometer.

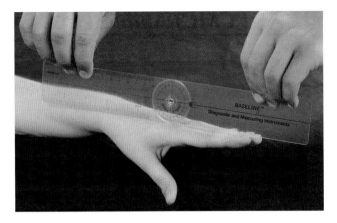

Goniometer alignment	Palpate the following bony landmarks (shown in Fig. 5.43) and align goniometer accordingly (Fig. 5.45).
Stationary arm	Dorsal midline of more proximal bone of joint (in this case, a metacarpal).
Axis	Dorsum of joint being examined (in this case, MCP joint).
Moving arm	Dorsal midline of more distal bone of joint (in this case, a proximal phalanx).
	Read scale of goniometer.
Patient/Examiner Action	Perform passive, or have patient perform active, extension of the joint (Fig. 5.46).
Confirmation of alignment	Repalpate landmarks and confirm proper goniometric alignment at end of ROM, correcting alignment as necessary. Read scale of goniometer (see Fig. 5.46).
Documentation	Record patient's ROM.
Note	This technique may be used to measure extension of the MCP, PIP, or DIP joints of the fingers. The figures shown here depict the measurement of MCP extension of the second digit (index finger).

Fig. 5.46 End of MCP extension ROM, demonstrating proper alignment of goniometer at end of range.

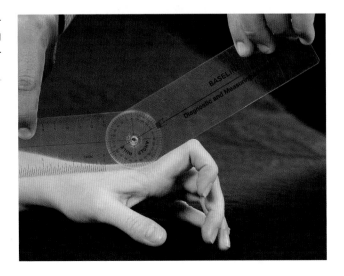

Carpometacarpal (First CMC) Abduction (Video 5.10)

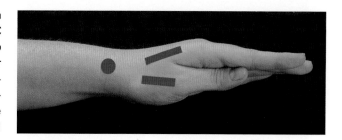

Fig. 5.47 Starting position for measurement of first CMC abduction. Note that thumb is positioned alongside volar surface of second metacarpal. Landmarks for goniometer alignment (lateral midline of second metacarpal, radial styloid process, dorsal midline of first metacarpal) indicated by red lines and dot.

Normal ROM = 45 degrees to 70 degrees.[53,54]

MDC for CMC abduction goniometry measured by a single examiner = 8 degrees to 12 degrees.[53,55]

Patient position	Seated, with forearm neutral; UE supported on table; wrist and hand in neutral position; thumb positioned along volar surface of second metacarpal (Fig. 5.47).
Stabilization	Over second metacarpal (Fig. 5.48).
Examiner action	After instructing patient in motion desired, abduct first CMC joint by grasping first metacarpal and moving thumb perpendicularly away from palm. Return thumb to starting position. Performing passive movement provides an estimate of ROM and demonstrates to patient exact motion desired (see Fig. 5.48).
Goniometer alignment	Palpate the following bony landmarks (shown in Fig. 5.47) and align goniometer accordingly (Fig. 5.49).
Stationary arm	Lateral midline of second metacarpal.

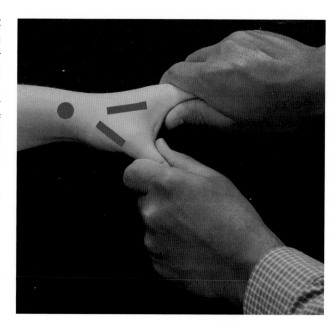

Fig. 5.48 End of first CMC abduction ROM, showing proper hand placement for stabilizing second metacarpal and abducting first CMC joint. Landmarks for goniometer alignment (lateral midline of second metacarpal, radial styloid process, dorsal midline of first metacarpal) indicated by red lines and dot.

Fig. 5.49 Starting position for measurement of first CMC abduction, demonstrating proper initial alignment of goniometer.

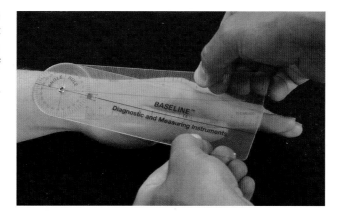

Axis	Radial styloid process.
Moving arm	Dorsal midline of first metacarpal.
	Read scale of goniometer (see Note).
Patient/Examiner Action	Perform passive, or have patient perform active, abduction of first CMC joint (Fig. 5.50).
Confirmation of Alignment	Repalpate landmarks and confirm proper goniometric alignment at end of ROM, correcting alignment as necessary (see Fig. 5.50). Read scale of goniometer (see Note).
Documentation	Calculate and record patient's ROM (see Note).
Note	Goniometer will not read 0 degrees at the beginning of first CMC abduction. However, this initial reading should be translated as 0 degrees starting position. Number of degrees of abduction through which a joint moves is calculated by subtracting the *initial* goniometer reading from the *final* reading. Motion is then recorded as 0 degrees to X degrees first CMC abduction. For example, if goniometer reads 25 degrees at beginning of first CMC abduction and 52 degrees at end of ROM, then first CMC abduction = 52 degrees – 25 degrees, or 0 degrees to 27 degrees first CMC abduction.

Fig. 5.50 End of first CMC abduction ROM, demonstrating proper alignment of goniometer at end of range.

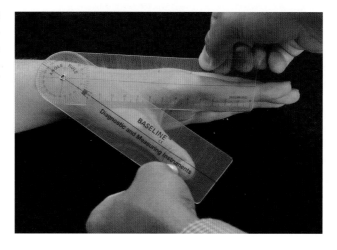

Carpometacarpal (First CMC) Flexion (Video 5.11)

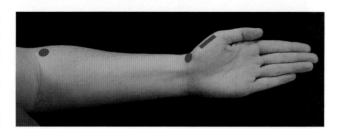

Fig. 5.51 Starting position for measurement of first CMC flexion. Note that thumb is positioned alongside lateral surface of second metacarpal. Landmarks for goniometer alignment (radial head, ventral surface of first CMC joint, ventral midline of first metacarpal) indicated by red line and dots.

Patient position	Seated, with forearm supinated; UE supported on table; wrist and hand in neutral position; thumb positioned along lateral side of second metacarpal (Fig. 5.51).
Stabilization	Over ventral surface of wrist (Fig. 5.52).
Examiner action	After instructing patient in motion desired, flex first CMC joint by grasping first metacarpal and moving thumb across palm. Return thumb to starting position. Performing passive movement provides an estimate of ROM and demonstrates to patient exact motion desired (see Fig. 5.52).
Goniometer alignment	Palpate the following bony landmarks (shown in Fig. 5.51) and align goniometer accordingly (Fig. 5.53).
Stationary arm	Ventral midline of radius toward radial head.
Axis	Ventral surface of first CMC joint.
Moving arm	Ventral midline of first metacarpal.

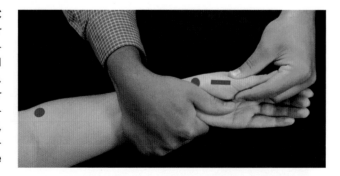

Fig. 5.52 End of first CMC flexion ROM, showing proper hand placement for stabilizing second metacarpal and flexing first CMC joint. Landmarks for goniometer alignment (radial head, ventral surface of first CMC joint, ventral midline of first metacarpal) indicated by red line and dots.

Fig. 5.53 Starting position for measurement of first CMC flexion, demonstrating proper initial alignment of goniometer.

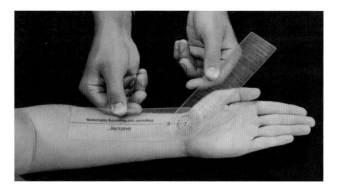

Read scale of goniometer (see Note).

Patient/examiner action

Perform passive, or have patient perform active, flexion of first CMC joint (Fig. 5.54).

Confirmation of alignment

Repalpate landmarks and confirm proper goniometric alignment at end of ROM, correcting alignment as necessary (see Fig. 5.54).

Read scale of goniometer (see Note).

Documentation

Calculate and record patient's ROM (see Note).

Note

Goniometer will not read 0 degrees at beginning of first CMC flexion. However, this initial reading should be translated as 0 degrees starting position. Number of degrees of flexion through which joint moves is calculated by subtracting the *final* goniometer reading from the *initial* reading. Motion is then recorded as 0 degrees to X degrees first CMC flexion. For example, if goniometer reads 36 degrees at beginning of first CMC flexion, and 4 degrees at end of ROM, then first CMC flexion = 36 degrees – 4 degrees, or 0 degrees to 32 degrees first CMC flexion.

Fig. 5.54 End of first CMC flexion ROM, demonstrating proper alignment of goniometer at end of range.

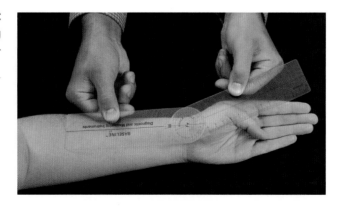

Carpometacarpal (First CMC) Extension (Video 5.12)

Fig. 5.55 Starting position for measurement of first CMC extension. Note that thumb is positioned alongside lateral surface of second metacarpal. Landmarks for goniometer alignment (radial head, ventral surface of first CMC joint, ventral midline of first metacarpal) indicated by red line and dots.

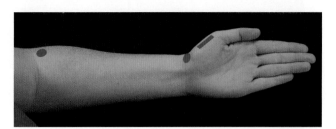

Patient position	Seated, with forearm supinated; UE supported on table; wrist and hand in neutral position, thumb positioned along lateral side of second metacarpal (Fig. 5.55).
Stabilization	Over ventral surface of wrist (Fig. 5.56).
Examiner action	After instructing patient in motion desired, extend first CMC joint by grasping first metacarpal and moving thumb away from, but parallel to, palm. Return thumb to starting position. Performing passive movement provides an estimate of ROM and demonstrates to patient exact motion desired (see Fig. 5.56).
Goniometer alignment	Palpate the following bony landmarks (shown in Fig. 5.55) and align goniometer accordingly (Fig. 5.57).
Stationary arm	Ventral midline of radius toward radial head.
Axis	Ventral surface of first CMC joint.
Moving arm	Ventral midline of first metacarpal.
	Read scale of goniometer (see Note).

Fig. 5.56 End of first CMC extension ROM, showing proper hand placement for stabilizing second metacarpal and extending first CMC joint. Landmarks for goniometer alignment (radial head, ventral surface of first CMC joint, ventral midline of first metacarpal) indicated by red line and dots.

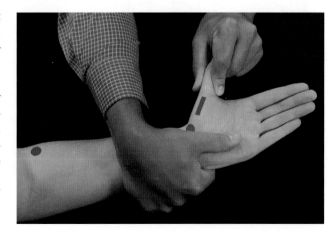

Fig. 5.57 Starting position for measurement of first CMC extension, demonstrating proper initial alignment of goniometer.

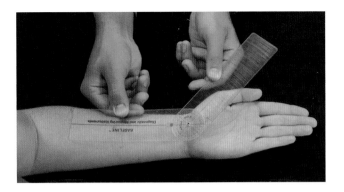

Patient/Examiner Action

Perform passive, or have patient perform active, extension of first CMC joint (Fig. 5.58).

Confirmation of Alignment

Repalpate landmarks and confirm proper goniometric alignment at end of ROM, correcting alignment as necessary (see Fig. 5.58). Read scale of goniometer (see Note).

Documentation

Calculate and record patient's ROM (see Note).

Note

Goniometer will not read 0 degrees at beginning of first CMC extension. However, this initial reading should be translated as 0-degree starting position. Number of degrees of extension through which joint moves is calculated by subtracting *initial* goniometer reading from *final* reading. Motion is then recorded as 0 degrees to X degrees first CMC extension. For example, if goniometer reads 36 degrees at beginning of first CMC extension and 65 degrees at end of ROM, then first CMC extension = 65 degrees – 36 degrees, or 0 degrees to 29 degrees first CMC extension.

Fig. 5.58 End of first CMC extension ROM, demonstrating proper alignment of goniometer at end of range.

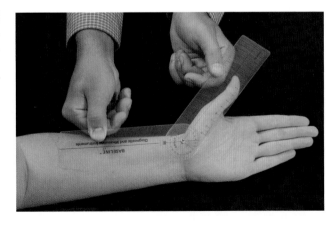

Carpometacarpal (First CMC) Opposition (Video 5.13)

Fig. 5.59 Starting position for measurement of first CMC opposition. Note that thumb is positioned alongside lateral surface of second metacarpal. Measurement is made with a ruler, rather than with a goniometer. Landmarks for alignment of ruler (palmar digital crease of fifth digit, flexor crease of IP joint of thumb) indicated by red lines.

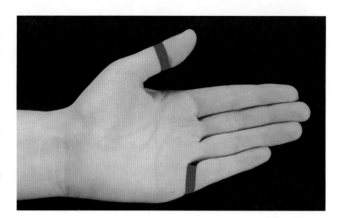

Patient position

Seated, with forearm supinated; UE supported on table, wrist and hand in neutral position, thumb positioned along lateral side of second metacarpal (Fig. 5.59).

Stabilization

Over ventral surface of fifth metacarpal with one hand, and over MCP and IP joints of thumb with other hand, preventing flexion of MCP and IP joints of thumb (Fig. 5.60).

Examiner action

After instructing patient in motion desired, move first CMC joint into opposition by bringing flexor crease of IP joint of patient's thumb toward palmar digital crease of fifth digit. No flexion of MCP or IP joints of thumb should be allowed. Return thumb to starting position. Performing passive movement provides an estimate of ROM and demonstrates to patient exact motion desired (see Fig. 5.60).

Fig. 5.60 End of first CMC opposition ROM, showing proper hand placement for stabilizing digits 2 through 5 and moving thumb into opposition toward fifth digit. Landmarks for alignment of ruler (palmar digital crease of fifth digit, flexor crease of IP joint of thumb) indicated by red lines.

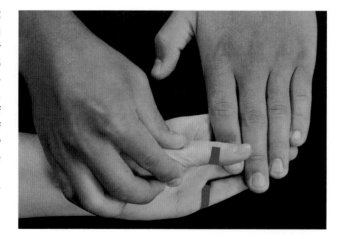

Fig. 5.61 End of list CMC opposition ROM, demonstrating proper alignment of ruler. Measurement is made of distance between flexor crease of IP joint of thumb and palmar digital crease of fifth digit.

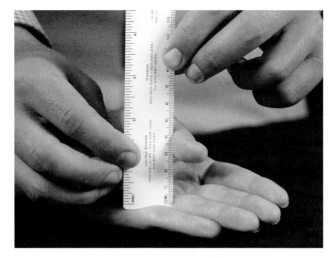

Instrument Alignment	Place end of ruler at palmar digital crease of fifth digit (Fig. 5.61).
Patient/Examiner Action	Perform passive, or have patient perform active, opposition of first CMC joint without flexing MCP or IP joints of thumb (see Fig. 5.61).
Measurement of Motion	Measure distance between flexor crease of IP joint of patient's thumb and palmar digital crease of fifth digit, keeping end of ruler in contact with palmar digital crease (see Fig. 5.61).
Documentation	Record distance as measured.

Metacarpophalangeal (MCP) or Interphalangeal (IP) Flexion of Thumb (Video 5.14)

Fig. 5.62 Starting position for measurement of first MCP flexion (thumb). Note that CMC joint of thumb is positioned in slight abduction. Landmarks for goniometer alignment (dorsal midline of first metacarpal, dorsum of first MCP joint, dorsal midline of proximal phalanx) indicated by red lines and dot.

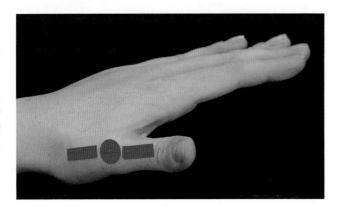

Normal ROM: MCP = 50 degrees – 60 degrees.[26,56,57]

MDC for 1st MCP and IP flexion goniometry measured by a single examiner = 19 to 30 degrees, respectively.[49]

(Measurement of First MCP Joint Shown.)

Patient position	Seated, with forearm neutral; UE supported on table; wrist in neutral position*; first CMC joint in slight abduction (Fig. 5.62).
Stabilization	First metacarpal (MCP) or proximal phalanx of thumb (IP). In this case, stabilization of first MCP is shown (Fig. 5.63).
Examiner action	After instructing patient in motion desired, flex joint through available ROM. Return thumb to neutral position. Performing passive movement provides an estimate of ROM and demonstrates to patient exact motion desired (see Fig. 5.63).

*Proximal joints should remain in neutral position (not flexed or extended) during testing to prevent obstruction of full ROM by tension in thumb extensor muscles.

Fig. 5.63 End of first MCP flexion ROM, showing proper hand placement for stabilizing metacarpal and flexing first MCP joint. Landmarks for goniometer alignment (dorsal midline of first metacarpal, dorsum of first MCP joint, dorsal midline of proximal phalanx) indicated by red lines and dot.

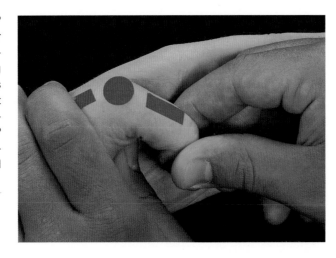

Fig. 5.64 Starting position for measurement of first MCP flexion, demonstrating proper initial alignment of goniometer.

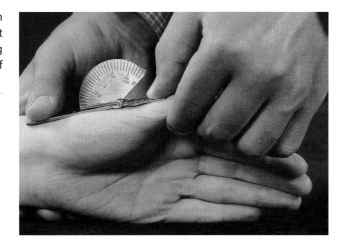

Goniometer alignment	Palpate the following bony landmarks (shown in Fig. 5.62) and align goniometer accordingly (Fig. 5.64).
Stationary arm	Dorsal midline of first metacarpal (MCP) or of proximal phalanx of thumb (IP).
Axis	Dorsum of first MCP or IP joint.
Moving arm	Dorsal midline of proximal phalanx of thumb (MCP) or distal phalanx of thumb (IP).
	Read scale of goniometer.
Patient/Examiner action	Perform passive, or have patient perform active, flexion of joint to be measured (Fig. 5.65).
Confirmation of alignment	Repalpate landmarks and confirm proper goniometric alignment at end of ROM, correcting alignment as necessary. Read scale of goniometer (see Fig. 5.65).
Documentation	Record patient's ROM.
Note	This technique may be used to measure flexion of the MCP or IP joints of the thumb. The figures shown here depict the measurement of MCP flexion of the thumb.

Fig. 5.65 End of first MCP flexion ROM, demonstrating proper alignment of goniometer at end of range.

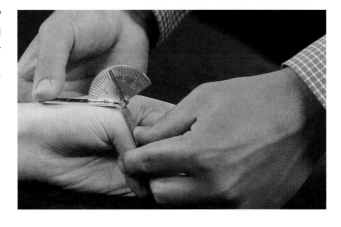

Metacarpophalangeal (MCP) or Interphalangeal (IP) Extension of Thumb (Video 5.15)

Fig. 5.66 Starting position for measurement of IP extension (thumb). Note that CMC joint of thumb is positioned in slight abduction. Landmarks for goniometer alignment (dorsal midline of proximal phalanx, dorsum of IP joint, dorsal midline of distal phalanx) indicated by red lines and dot.

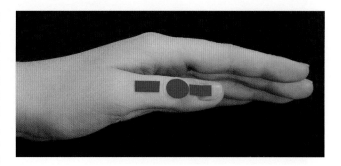

(Measurement of IP Joint Shown.)

Patient position	Seated, with forearm neutral; UE supported on table; wrist in neutral position*; first CMC joint in slight abduction (Fig. 5.66).
Stabilization	Over first metacarpal (MCP) or proximal phalanx of thumb (IP). In this case, stabilization of proximal phalanx is shown (Fig. 5.67).
Examiner action	After instructing patient in motion desired, extend joint through available ROM. Return finger to neutral position. Performing passive movement provides an estimate of ROM and demonstrates to patient exact motion desired (see Fig. 5.67).

*Proximal joints should remain in neutral position during testing to prevent obstruction of full ROM by tension in flexor pollicis longus muscle.

Fig. 5.67 End of IP extension ROM, showing proper hand placement for stabilizing proximal phalanx and extending IP joint. Landmarks for goniometer alignment (dorsal midline of proximal phalanx, dorsum of IP joint, dorsal midline of distal phalanx) indicated by red lines and dot.

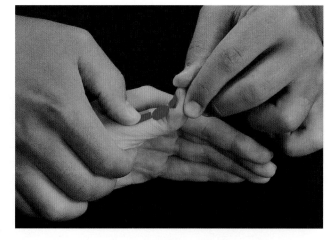

Fig. 5.68 Starting position for measurement of IP extension, demonstrating proper initial alignment of goniometer.

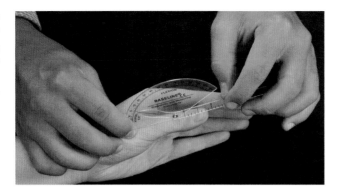

Goniometer alignment	Palpate the following bony landmarks (shown in Fig. 5.66) and align goniometer accordingly (Fig. 5.68).
Stationary arm	Dorsal midline of first metacarpal (MCP) or of proximal phalanx of thumb (IP).
Axis	Dorsum of first MCP or IP joint.
Moving arm	Dorsal midline of proximal phalanx of thumb (MCP) or distal phalanx of thumb (IP).
	Read scale of goniometer.
Patient/Examiner action	Perform passive, or have patient perform active, extension of joint to be measured (Fig. 5.69).
Confirmation of alignment	Repalpate landmarks and confirm proper goniometric alignment at end of ROM, correcting alignment as necessary. Read scale of goniometer (see Fig. 5.69).
Documentation	Record patient's ROM.
Note	This technique may be used to measure extension of the MCP or IP joints of the thumb. The figures shown here depict the measurement of IP flexion of the thumb.

Fig. 5.69 End of IP extension ROM, demonstrating proper alignment of goniometer at end of range.

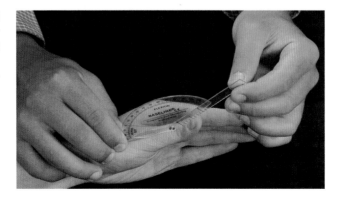

References

1. Clemente C. *Gray's Anatomy of the Human Body.* 13th ed. Philadelphia: Lea & Febiger; 1985.
2. Levangie PK, Norkin CC. *Joint Structure and Function: A Comprehensive Analysis.* 3rd ed. Philadelphia: Davis; 2001. 495. Xv.
3. Neumann D. *Kinesiology of the Musculoskeletal System.* St. Louis: Mosby; 2002.
4. Werner SL, Plancher KD. Biomechanics of wrist injuries in sports. *Clin Sports Med.* 1998;17(3):407–420.
5. Berger RA. The ligaments of the wrist. A current overview of anatomy with considerations of their potential functions. *Hand Clin.* 1997;13(1):63–82.
6. Mayfield JK, Johnson RP, Kilcoyne RF. The ligaments of the human wrist and their functional significance. *Anat Rec.* 1976;186(3):417–428.
7. Mizuseki T, Ikuta Y. The dorsal carpal ligaments: their anatomy and function. *J Hand Surg Br.* 1989;14(1):91–98.
8. Viegas SF. The dorsal ligaments of the wrist. *Hand Clin.* 2001;17(1):65–75. vi.
9. Bird HA, Stowe J. The wrist. *Clin Rheum Dis.* 1982;8(3):559–569.
10. Youm Y, et al. Kinematics of the wrist. I. an experimental study of radial-ulnar deviation and flexion-extension. *J Bone Joint Surg Am.* 1978;60(4):423–431.
11. Gûnal I, et al. Normal range of motion of the joints of the upper extremity in male subjects, with special reference to side. *J Bone Joint Surg Am.* 1996;78(9):1401–1404.
12. Ryu JY, et al. Functional ranges of motion of the wrist joint. *J Hand Surg Am.* 1991;16(3):409–419.
13. Sarrafian SK, Melamed JL, Goshgarian GM. Study of wrist motion in flexion and extension. *Clin Orthop Relat Res.* 1977;126:153–159.
14. Li ZM, et al. Coupling between wrist flexion-extension and radial-ulnar deviation. *Clin Biomech (Bristol, Avon).* 2005;20(2):177–183.
15. Kauer JM. The mechanism of the carpal joint. *Clin Orthop Relat Res.* 1986;202:16–26.
16. Ruby LK, et al. Relative motion of selected carpal bones: a kinematic analysis of the normal wrist. *J Hand Surg Am.* 1988;13(1):1–10.
17. Savelberg HH, et al. Strains and forces in selected carpal ligaments during in vitro flexion and deviation movements of the hand. *J Orthop Res.* 1992;10(6):901–910.
18. Kapandji I. Upper Limb. In: *The Physiology of Joints.* Vol. 1. 5th ed. New York: Churchill Livingstone; 1982.
19. Smith L, Weiss E, Lehmkuhl L. *Brunnstrom's Clinical Kinesiology.* 5th ed. Phiadelphia: FA: Davis; 1996.
20. Cyriax JH, Coldham M. *Textbook of Orthopaedic Medicine.* London: Baillière Tindall; 1982.
21. Kaltenborn F. *Mobilization of the Extremity Joints.* 3rd ed. Oslo: Olaf Norlis Bokhandel; 1980.
22. Zancolli EA, Ziadenberg C, Zancolli E. Biomechanics of the trapeziometacarpal joint. *Clin Orthop Relat Res.* 1987;220:14–26.
23. Imaeda T, et al. Kinematics of the normal trapeziometacarpal joint. *J Orthop Res.* 1994;12(2):197–204.
24. Moore M. Clinical assessment of joint motion. In: *Therapeutic Exercise.* Baltimore: Williams & Wilkins; 1978.
25. Leibovic SJ, Bowers WH. Anatomy of the proximal interphalangeal joint. *Hand Clin.* 1994;10(2):169–178.
26. Shaw SJ, Morris MA. The range of motion of the metacarpophalangeal joint of the thumb and its relationship to injury. *J Hand Surg Br.* 1992;17(2):164–166.
27. Mallon WJ, Brown HR, Nunley JA. Digital ranges of motion: normal values in young adults. *J Hand Surg Am.* 1991;16(5):882–887.
28. Skvarilová B, Plevková A. Ranges of joint motion of the adult hand. *Acta Chir Plast.* 1996;38(2):67–71.
29. Brumfield RH, Champoux JA. A biomechanical study of normal functional wrist motion. *Clin Orthop Relat Res.* 1984;187:23–25.
30. Palmer AK, et al. Functional wrist motion: a biomechanical study. *J Hand Surg Am.* 1985;10(1):39–46.
31. Safaee-Rad R, et al. Normal functional range of motion of upper limb joints during performance of three feeding activities. *Arch Phys Med Rehabil.* 1990;71(7):505–509.
32. Hume MC, et al. Functional range of motion of the joints of the hand. *J Hand Surg Am.* 1990;15(2):240–243.
33. Lee JW, Rim K. Measurement of finger joint angles and maximum finger forces during cylinder grip activity. *J Biomed Eng.* 1991;13(2):152–162.
34. American Medical Association. *Guides to the Evaluation of Permanent Impairment.* 4th ed. Chicago: American Medical Association; 1993:339.
35. Greene WB, Heckman JD. *The Clinical Measurement of Joint Motion.* Rosemont, IL: American Academy of Orthopaedic Surgeons; 1994.
36. Moore KL, Dalley AF, Agur AMR. *Clinically Oriented Anatomy.* 5th ed. Philadelphia: Lippincott Williams & Wilkins; 2006:1209.
37. LaStayo PC, Wheeler DL. Reliability of passive wrist flexion and extension goniometric measurements: a multicenter study. *Phys Ther.* 1994;74(2):162–176.
38. Carter TI, et al. Accuracy and reliability of three different techniques for manual goniometry for wrist motion: a cadaveric study. *J Hand Surg Am.* 2009;34(8):1422–1428.
39. Groth GN, et al. Goniometry of the proximal and distal interphalangeal joints, part II: placement prefereces, interrater reliability, and concurrent validity. *J Hand Ther.* 2001;14(1):23–29.
40. Marshall MM, Mozrall JR, Shealy JE. The effects of complex wrist and forearm posture on wrist range of motion. *Hum Factors.* 1999;41(2):205–213.
41. AAoO Surgeons. *Joint Motion: Method of Measuring and Recording.* Chicago: American Academy of Orthopaedic Surgeons; 1965.
42. Boone DC, Azen SP. Normal range of motion of joints in male subjects. *J Bone Joint Surg Am.* 1979;61(5):756–759.
43. Cobe HM. The range of active motion at the wrist of white adults. *J Bone Joint Surg Am.* 1928;10(4):763–774.
44. Macedo LG, Magee DJ. Differences in range of motion between dominant and nondominant sides of upper and lower extremities. *J Manipulative Physiol Ther.* 2008;31(8):577–582.
45. Stubbs NBF, Jeffrey EG, William M. Normative data on joint ranges of motion of 25- to 54-year old males. *Int J Ind Ergonomics.* 1993;12:265–272.
46. Hewitt D. The range of active motion at the wrist of women. *J Bone Joint Surg.* 1928;10:775–787.
47. Horger MM. The reliability of goniometric measurements of active and passive wrist motions. *Am J Occup Ther.* 1990;44(4):342–348.
48. Macedo LG, Magee DJ. Effects of age on passive range of motion of selected peripheral joints in healthy adult females. *Physiother Theory Pract.* 2009;25(2):145–164.
49. Reissner L, Fischer G, List R, Taylor WR, Giovanoli P, Calcagni M. Minimal detectable difference of the finger and wrist range of motion: comparison of goniometry and 3D motion analysis. *J Orthop Surg Res.* 2019;14:173. https://doi.org/10.1186/s13018-019-1177-y.
50. Walker JM, et al. Active mobility of the extremities in older subjects. *Phys Ther.* 1984;64(6):919–923.
51. Smahel Z, Klímová A. The influence of age and exercise on the mobility of hand joints: 1: metacarpophalangeal joints of the three-phalangeal fingers. *Acta Chir Plast.* 2004;46(3):81–88.
52. Lewis E, Fors L, Tharion WJ. Interrater and intrarater reliability of finger goniometric measurements. *Am J Occup Ther.* 2010;64(4):555–561.
53. de Kraker M, et al. Palmar abduction: reliability of 6 measurement methods in healthy adults. *J Hand Surg Am.* 2009;34(3):523–530.
54. Goubier JN, et al. Normal range-of-motion of trapeziometacarpal joint. *Chir Main.* 2009;28(5):297–300.
55. Holzbauer M, Hopfner M, Haslhofer D, Kwasny O, Duscher D, Froschauer SM. Radial and palmar active range of motion measurement: reliability of six methods in healthy adults. *J Plast Surg Hand Surg.* 2020. https://doi.org/10.1080/2000656X.2020.1828899.
56. Jenkins M, et al. Thumb joint flexion. What is normal? *J Hand Surg Br.* 1998;23(6):796–797.
57. De Smet L, et al. Metacarpophalangeal and interphalangeal flexion of the thumb: influence of sex and age, relation to ligamentous injury. *Acta Orthop Belg.* 1993;59(4):357–359.

6

MUSCLE LENGTH TESTING
of the UPPER EXTREMITY

William D. Bandy

In contrast to those for the lower extremity, there are only a few tests for examining the length of muscles in the upper extremity. Moreover, very little research has been conducted on the reliability of tests described in the literature. The purpose of this section is to describe some early tests suggested in the literature for measurement of muscle length of the upper extremity and the rationale for not including these tests in this chapter on upper extremity muscle length measurement techniques. Additionally, 12 tests for the examination of upper extremity muscle length are presented.

APLEY'S SCRATCH TEST

In 1959, a physical education text published by Scott and French[1] introduced a test for upper extremity flexibility, called the "opposite arm across the back" test. Hoppenfeld[2] later referred to this test as "Apley's scratch test." In 1960, Myers[3] described these tests to measure the muscle length of the shoulder and elbow, referring to this combination of tests as the "'y' position of the arms." The test (herein referred to as Apley's scratch test) consists of two parts that, depending on the author, could be performed on one extremity at a time or on two extremities simultaneously. One part involves asking the individual who is being tested to place the palm of the hand on the back by reaching behind the head and down between the shoulder blades as far as possible (Fig. 6.1). Hoppenfeld[2] suggested that this maneuver yielded a measurement of shoulder lateral rotation and abduction, and Sullivan and Hawkins[4] suggested that the test was a measurement for shoulder lateral rotation.

The second part of Apley's scratch test consists of asking the subject to place the dorsum of the hand against the back and to reach behind the back and up the spine as far as possible (see Fig. 6.1). Hoppenfeld[2] suggested that this maneuver measured shoulder medial rotation and adduction; Sullivan and Hawkins[4] suggested that the test examined shoulder medial rotation; and Mallon

et al.[5] suggested that the test measured shoulder medial rotation and extension, elbow flexion, and scapular movement.

Techniques for documentation of the measurement have varied. Scott and French[1] suggested measuring the distance between the tips of the fingers of both hands when the two parts of the test are performed simultaneously. Goldstein[6] suggested performing the test one upper extremity at a time and recording the distance between the spinous process of C7 and the tips of the fingers. Finally, an alternative measurement presented by Magee[7] consists of performing the test one extremity at a time and recording the levels of the vertebrae that the fingers most closely approximate.

As is suggested by the variety of interpretations of Apley's scratch test, the movement that takes place during testing is poorly defined, and the actual muscles being examined for flexibility are not known. Therefore, the "opposite arm across the back test," Apley's scratch test, is not included among the flexibility tests for the upper extremity presented in this chapter.

SHOULDER AND WRIST ELEVATION TEST

In a text on flexibility written in 1977, Johnson[8] described the shoulder and wrist elevation test used to measure shoulder flexibility. This test requires the individual to lift a stick or broom handle until the upper extremities are fully elevated overhead while the individual is lying in a prone position with the chin on a stable surface (Fig. 6.2). The individual raises the stick upward as high as possible by flexion at the shoulders.

Two methods have been described for documenting the amount of shoulder elevation achieved in this test. The first is simply to measure the distance from the stable surface to the stick.[9] In the second, which takes into consideration the length of the individual's upper extremity, the length of the upper extremity is measured,

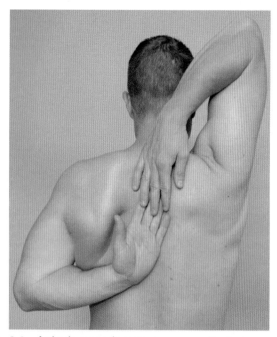

Fig. 6.1 Apley's scratch test, a composite test measuring multiple motions and muscles, is not included in this chapter. (From Magee DJ. *Orthopedic Physical Therapy Assessment*. 6th ed. St. Louis: Saunders; 2014.)

and the test score is determined by subtracting the height to which the stick is raised from the length of the arm.[8] A score of 0 is considered perfect.

As the techniques to be included in this chapter were selected, an effort was made to present techniques that can be performed easily and have the option of being performed passively or actively. The shoulder and wrist elevation test was not included because of the need for a minimal strength level in the shoulder and trunk musculature of the subject for the test to be performed, the difficulty in controlling back extension by the individual during testing, and the inability of the test to be performed passively.

TECHNIQUES FOR TESTING MUSCLE

Length: Upper Extremity

Figs. 6.3–6.41 illustrate the techniques for flexibility testing of the upper extremity that are included in this chapter. These measurement techniques were chosen because they can be performed passively by the clinician or actively by the patient, the tests do not require patient strength, and the examination can be performed easily.

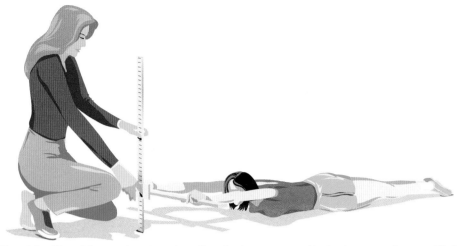

Fig. 6.2 Shoulder and wrist elevation test, a composite test measuring multiple motions and muscles, is not included in this chapter.

Latissimus Dorsi Muscle Length

Fig. 6.3 End ROM for latissimus dorsi muscle length. Bony landmarks for goniometer alignment (lateral midline of trunk; shoulder, lateral to acromion; lateral epicondyle of humerus) indicated by red line and dots.

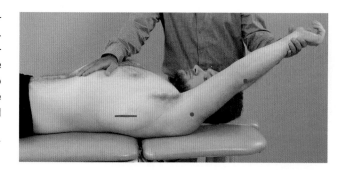

Patient position	Supine, upper extremities at sides with elbows extended; lumbar spine flat against support surface.
Examiner action	After instructing patient in motion desired, examiner flexes shoulder through available range of motion (ROM) while maintaining elbow in full extension and keeping arms close to head; lumbar spine should remain flat against support surface. (*Note:* Examiner ordinarily would perform this task while standing on same side as extremity being flexed. Examiner is standing on opposite side in photo so landmarks can be seen.) This passive movement allows an estimate of available ROM and demonstrates to patient exact motion required (Fig. 6.3).
Patient/Examiner action	Patient flexes shoulder through full available ROM, keeping arm close to head. Examiner must ensure that elbow remains extended and lumbar spine remains flat against support surface (see Fig. 6.3).
Goniometer method (Video 6.1)	Palpate bony landmarks shown in Fig. 6.3 and align goniometer accordingly (Fig. 6.4).

Fig. 6.4 Patient position for measurement of latissimus dorsi muscle length using goniometer.

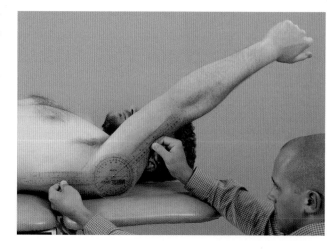

Fig. 6.5 Patient position for measurement of latissimus dorsi muscle length using tape measure.

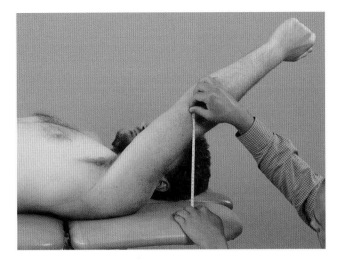

Stationary arm	Aligned with lateral midline of trunk.
Axis	Shoulder, lateral to acromion.
Moving arm	Lateral epicondyle of humerus.
	Maintaining proper goniometric alignment, note amount of shoulder flexion (see Fig. 6.4).
Tape measure method (Video 6.2)	Using tape measure or ruler, measure distance (inches or centimeters) between lateral epicondyle of humerus and support surface (Fig. 6.5).
Documentation	Record patient's amount of shoulder flexion or distance from lateral epicondyle of humerus to support surface.

Pectoralis Major Muscle Length: General (Video 6.3)

Fig. 6.6 Starting position for measurement of pectoralis major muscle length.

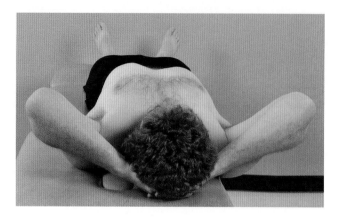

Patient position

Supine, with hands clasped together behind head; cervical spine should not flex any more than necessary to place clasped hands behind head (Fig. 6.6).

Patient/Examiner action

Examiner ensures that patient maintains clasped hands and does not flex cervical spine. Patient relaxes shoulder muscles, allowing elbows to move toward support surface; lumbar spine should remain flat against support surface (see Fig. 6.6).

Fig. 6.7 Patient position for measurement of pectoralis major muscle length using tape measure.

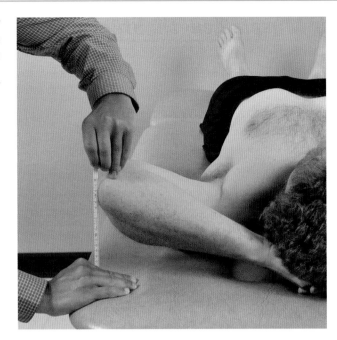

Tape measure

Using tape measure or ruler, measure distance (inches or centimeters) between olecranon process of humerus and support surface (Fig. 6.7).

Documentation

Record distance from support surface to olecranon process.

Pectoralis Major Muscle Length: Sternal (Lower) Portion

Fig. 6.8 Starting position for measurement of lower portion of pectoralis major muscle length.

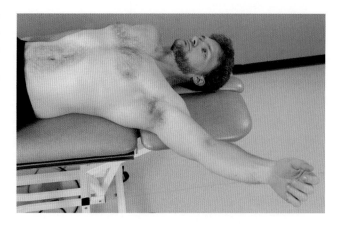

Patient position	Supine, with shoulder laterally rotated and abducted to 135 degrees; elbow fully extended, and forearm supinated; lumbar spine flat against support surface (Fig. 6.8).
Patient/Examiner action	While ensuring that patient maintains shoulder in lateral rotation at 135 degrees of abduction, as well as full extension of elbow and supination of forearm, examiner asks patient to relax all shoulder muscles, allowing shoulder to move into maximal horizontal abduction. Examiner must ensure that patient maintains lumbar spine flat against support surface and does not allow trunk rotation (especially to side of extremity being measured) (see Fig. 6.8).
Goniometer method (Video 6.4)	Palpate bony landmarks and align goniometer accordingly (Fig. 6.9).
Stationary arm	Parallel to support surface.
Axis	Lateral tip of acromion.

Fig. 6.9 Patient position for measurement of lower portion of pectoralis major muscle length using goniometer. Goniometer aligned with bony landmarks (parallel to support surface, lateral tip of acromion, midline of humerus toward lateral epicondyle).

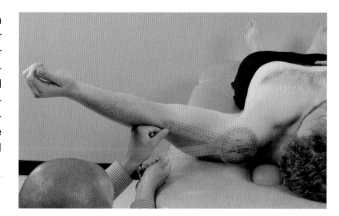

Fig. 6.10 Patient position for measurement of lower portion of pectoralis major muscle length using tape measure.

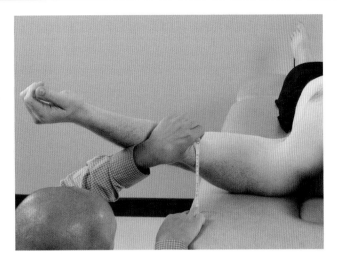

Moving arm

Along midline of humerus toward lateral epicondyle.

Maintaining proper goniometric alignment, note amount of shoulder horizontal abduction (see Fig. 6.9).

Tape measure method (Video 6.5)

Using tape measure or ruler, measure distance (inches or centimeters) between lateral epicondyle of humerus and support surface (Fig. 6.10).

Documentation

Record patient's ROM or distance from support surface and lateral epicondyle of humerus.

Note

Fig. 6.11 illustrates patient with excessive length in lower portion of pectoralis major muscle, which is not uncommon.

Fig. 6.11 Example of excessive length in lower portion of pectoralis major muscle.

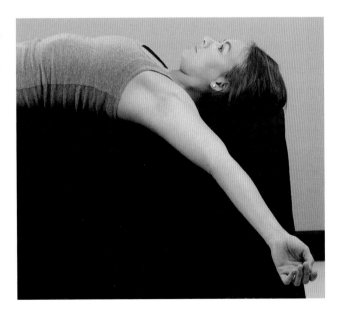

Pectoralis Major Muscle Length: Clavicular (Upper) Portion

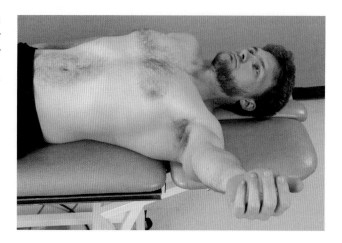

Fig. 6.12 Starting position for measurement of upper portion of pectoralis major muscle length.

Patient position	Supine, with shoulder laterally rotated and abducted to 90 degrees; elbow fully extended; forearm supinated; lumbar spine flat against support surface (Fig. 6.12).
Patient/Examiner action	Ensuring that patient maintains shoulder in lateral rotation and 90 degrees of abduction, as well as full extension of elbow and supination of forearm, examiner asks patient to relax all shoulder muscles, allowing shoulder to move into maximal horizontal abduction. Examiner must ensure that patient maintains lumbar spine flat against support surface and does not allow trunk rotation (especially to side of extremity being measured) (see Fig. 6.12).
Goniometer method (Video 6.6)	Palpate bony landmarks and align goniometer accordingly (Fig. 6.13).
Stationary arm	Parallel to support surface.
Axis	Lateral tip of acromion.

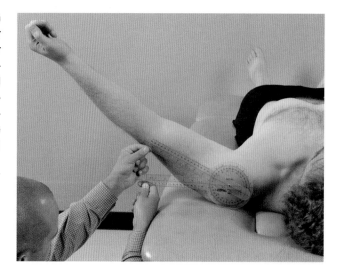

Fig. 6.13 Patient position for measurement of upper portion of pectoralis major muscle length using goniometer. Goniometer aligned with bony landmarks (parallel to support surface, lateral tip of acromion, midline of humerus toward lateral epicondyle).

Fig. 6.14 Patient position for measurement of upper portion of pectoralis major muscle length using tape measure.

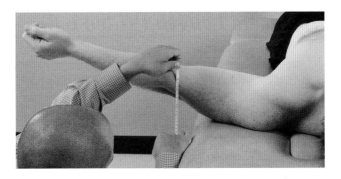

Moving arm	Along midline of humerus toward lateral epicondyle.
	Maintaining proper goniometric alignment, note amount of shoulder horizontal abduction (see Fig. 6.13).
Tape measure method (Video 6.7)	Using tape measure, measure distance (inches or centimeters) between lateral epicondyle of humerus and support surface (Fig. 6.14).
Documentation	Record patient's ROM or distance from support surface and lateral epicondyle of humerus.
Note	Fig. 6.15 illustrates patient with excessive length in upper portion of pectoralis major muscle, which is not uncommon.

Fig. 6.15 Example of excessive length in upper portion of pectoralis major muscle.

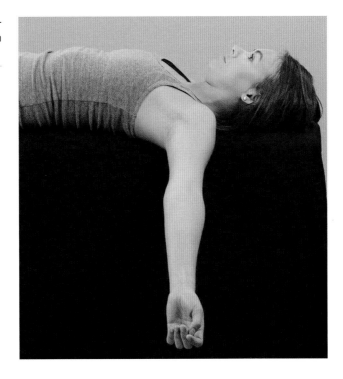

Pectoralis Minor Muscle Length (Video 6.8)

Fig. 6.16 Starting position for measurement of pectoralis minor muscle length. Bony landmark for goniometer alignment (posterior acromial border) for tape measure alignment indicated by red dot.

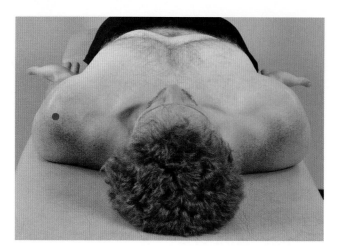

Patient position	Supine, with arms at side; shoulders laterally rotated; forearm supinated (palms up); lumbar spine should be flat against support surface (Fig. 6.16).
Patient/Examiner action	Examiner ensures that patient maintains arms at sides with palms up and lumbar spine flat against the support surface. Patient relaxes shoulder muscles, allowing the posterior border of the acromion process to move toward support surface (see Fig. 6.16).

Fig. 6.17 Patient position for measurement of pectoralis minor muscle length using tape measure. Bony landmark (posterior acromial border) indicated by red dot.

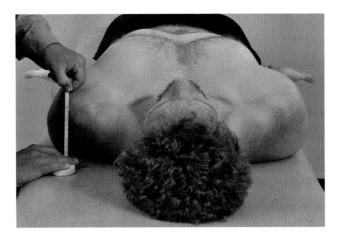

Tape measure alignment   Palpate posterior acromial border (see Fig. 6.16). Using tape measure or ruler, measure distance (inches or centimeters) between posterior border of acromion process and support surface (Fig. 6.17).

Documentation   Record distance from posterior border of acromion process and support surface.

Triceps Muscle Length (Video 6.9)

Fig. 6.18 Starting position for measurement of triceps muscle length. Bony landmarks for goniometer alignment (humeral head, lateral epicondyle of humerus, radial styloid process) indicated by red dots.

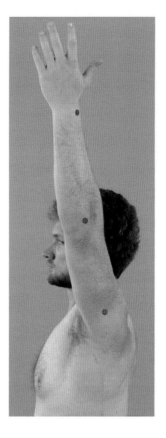

Patient position   Sitting, with shoulder in full flexion; elbow extended; forearm supinated (Fig. 6.18).

Examiner action   After instructing patient in motion desired, examiner flexes elbow through available ROM while maintaining full flexion of shoulder. This passive movement allows an estimate of available ROM and demonstrates to patient exact motion required (Fig. 6.19).

Fig. 6.19 End ROM of triceps muscle length. Bony landmarks for goniometer alignment (humeral head, lateral epicondyle of humerus, radial styloid process) indicated by red dots.

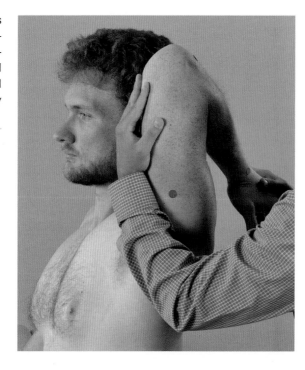

Fig. 6.20 Patient position and goniometer alignment at end of triceps muscle length.

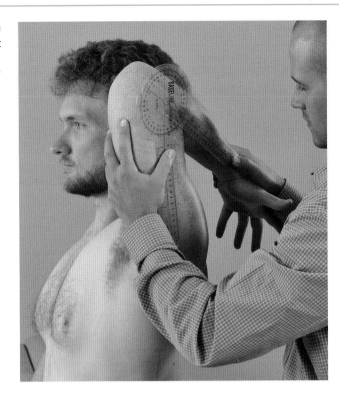

Patient/Examiner action	Maintaining full shoulder flexion, perform passive, or have patient perform active, flexion of the elbow (see Fig. 6.19).
Goniometer alignment	Palpate landmarks shown in Fig. 6.18 and align goniometer accordingly (Fig. 6.20).
Stationary arm	Lateral midline of humerus toward humeral head.
Axis	Lateral epicondyle of humerus.
Moving arm	Lateral midline of radius toward radial styloid.
	Maintaining proper goniometric alignment, read scale of goniometer (see Fig. 6.20).
Documentation	Record patient's maximum amount of elbow flexion.

Biceps Muscle Length (Video 6.10)

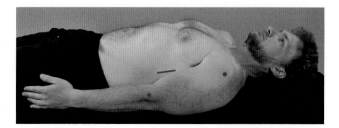

Fig. 6.21 Starting position for measurement of biceps muscle length. Bony landmarks for goniometer alignment (lateral midline of thorax, lateral aspect of acromion process, lateral epicondyle of humerus) indicated by red line and dots. (Note: as indicated in the text, the forearm should be pronated.)

Patient position	Supine, with shoulder at edge of plinth; elbow extended; forearm pronated (Fig. 6.21).
Examiner action	After instructing patient in motion desired, examiner extends shoulder through available ROM while maintaining elbow in full extension. This passive movement allows an estimate of available ROM and demonstrates to patient exact motion required (Fig. 6.22).
Patient/Examiner action	Maintaining full elbow extension, perform passive, or have patient perform active, extension of the shoulder (see Fig. 6.22).

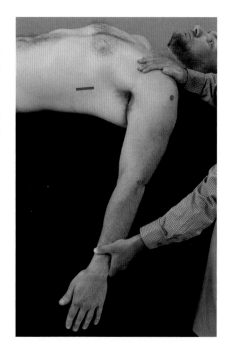

Fig. 6.22 End ROM of biceps muscle length. Bony landmarks for goniometer alignment (lateral midline of thorax, lateral aspect of acromion process, lateral epicondyle of humerus) indicated by red line and dots. (Note: forearm should be pronated.)

Fig. 6.23 Patient position and goniometer alignment at end of biceps muscle length. (Note: forearm should be pronated.)

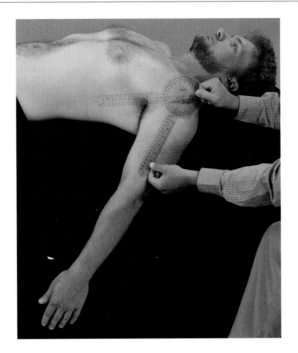

Goniometer alignment	Palpate landmarks shown in Fig. 6.21 and align goniometer accordingly (Fig. 6.23).
Stationary arm	Lateral midline of thorax.
Axis	Lateral midline of humerus toward lateral aspect of acromion process.
Moving arm	Lateral epicondyle of humerus.
	Maintaining proper goniometric alignment, read scale of goniometer (see Fig. 6.23).
Documentation	Record patient's maximum amount of shoulder extension.

Sternocleidomastoid (SCM) Muscle Length: Inclinometer

Fig. 6.24 Starting position for measurement of SCM muscle length. Bony land-mark (base of head) indicated by red dot.

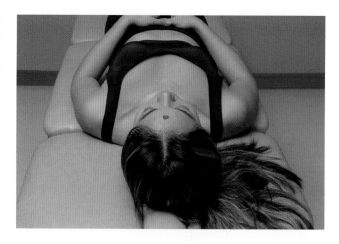

Patient position

Supine with top of patient's head at the edge of the table, nose pointed toward ceiling (Fig.6.24).

Patient action

After being instructed in motion desired, the patient actively moves their head as far as possible into first lateral flexion away and, second, rotation toward the muscle to be measured. Patient then returns to starting position. This movement provides an estimate of ROM and demonstrated to patient exact motion desired (Fig. 6.25).

Fig. 6.25 End ROM of SCM muscle length. (*Note*—the picture shown in this figure is not accurate. The subject should be taken to the end of the muscle length and held without the inclinometer held on the forehead.)

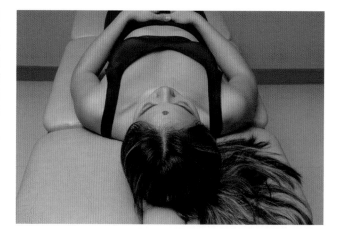

Fig. 6.26 Initial inclinometer alignment for measurement of left SCM muscle.

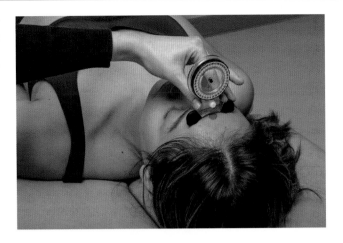

Inclinometer alignment	Palpate base of forehead (Fig. 6.24) and align inclinometer accordingly (Fig. 6.26).
Patient/Examiner action	Examiner, first, passively side bends cervical spine away to end range; then, second, rotate toward to end range the muscle being tested (Fig. 6.27).
Documentation	Record patient's ROM

Fig. 6.27 Inclinometer at end of left SCM length.

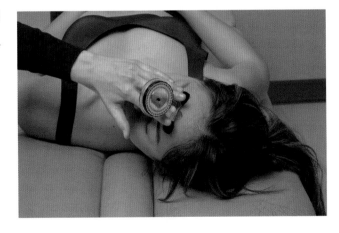

Sternocleidomastoid (SCM) Muscle Length: Smartphone Method

Fig. 6.28 Starting position for measurement of SCM muscle length. Bony landmark (base of head) indicated by red dot.

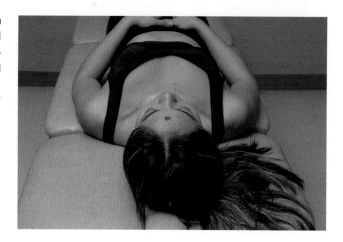

Patient position	Supine with top of patient's head at the edge of the table, nose pointed toward ceiling (Fig.6.28).
Patient action	After being instructed in motion desired, the patient actively moves their head as far as possible into first lateral flexion away and, second, rotation toward the muscle to be measured. Patient then returns to starting position. This movement provides an estimate of ROM and demonstrates to patient exact motion desired (Fig. 6.29).

Fig. 6.29 End ROM of SCM muscle length. (*Note*—the picture shown in this figure is not accurate. The subject should be taken to the end of the muscle length and held without the inclinometer held on the forehead.)

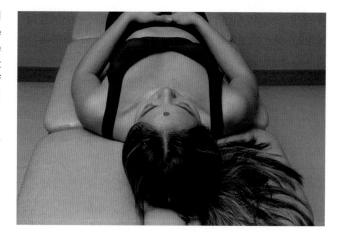

Fig. 6.30 Initial Smartphone alignment for measurement of left SCM.

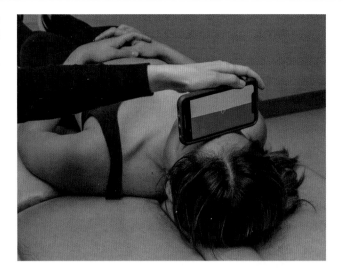

Smartphone alignment	Palpate base of forehead and align border of Smartphone accordingly (Fig. 6.30) with Smartphone screen facing toward therapist. Ensure the Smartphone application starts at 0 degrees before initiating motion, and cue the patient to adjust neck as needed.
Patient/Examiner action	Holding the Smartphone in place, examiner, first, passively side bends cervical spine away to end range; then, second, rotates toward to end range the muscle being tested (Fig. 6.31). Read scale of Smartphone.
Documentation	Record patient's ROM

Fig. 6.31 Smartphone alignment at end range of left SCM.

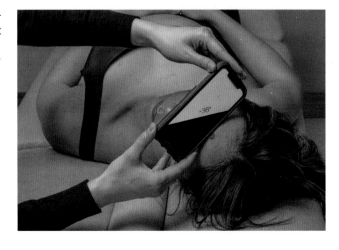

Flexor Digitorum Superficialis, Flexor Digitorum Profundus, and Flexor Digiti Minimi Muscle Length (Video 6.11)

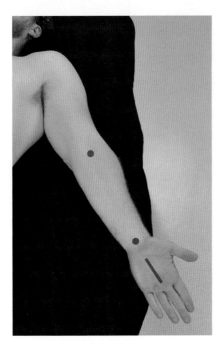

Fig. 6.32 Starting position for measurement of length of forearm flexor muscles. Landmarks for goniometer alignment (insertion of biceps muscle, lunate, volar midline of third metacarpal) indicated by red line and dots.

Patient position	Supine, with shoulder abducted 70–90 degrees; elbow extended; forearm supinated; fingers extended (Fig. 6.32).
Examiner action	After instructing patient in motion desired, examiner extends patient's wrist through available ROM while maintaining elbow and fingers in extension (Fig. 6.33). This passive movement allows an estimate of available ROM and demonstrates to patient exact motion required.

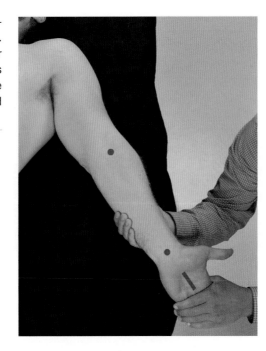

Fig. 6.33 End ROM of forearm flexor muscle length. Landmarks for goniometer alignment (insertion of biceps muscle, lunate, volar midline of third metacarpal) indicated by red line and dots.

Fig. 6.34 Patient position and goniometer alignment at end of forearm flexor muscle length.

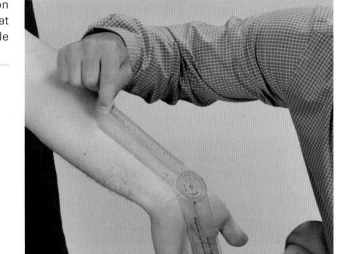

Patient/Examiner action	Maintaining elbow and fingers in full extension, perform passive, or have patient perform active, extension of the wrist (see Fig. 6.32).
Goniometer alignment	Palpate landmarks shown in Fig. 6.33 and align goniometer accordingly (Fig. 6.34).
Stationary arm	Insertion of biceps muscle.
Axis	Lunate.
Moving arm	Volar midline of third metacarpal.
	Maintaining proper goniometric alignment, read scale of goniometer (see Fig. 6.34). Note: Elbow must be maintained in full extension.
Documentation	Record patient's maximum amount of wrist extension.

Extensor Digitorum, Extensor Indicis, and Extensor Digiti Minimi Muscle Length (Video 6.12)

Fig. 6.35 Starting position for measurement of length of forearm extensor muscles. Bony landmarks (lateral epicondyle of humerus, lunate, dorsal midline of third metacarpal) indicated by red line and dots.

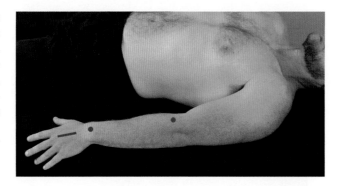

Patient position	Supine, with shoulder abducted 70–90 degrees; elbow extended; forearm pronated; fingers flexed (Fig. 6.35).
Examiner action	After instructing patient in motion desired, examiner flexes patient's wrist through available ROM while maintaining elbow in extension and fingers in flexion (Fig. 6.36). This passive movement allows an estimate of available ROM and demonstrates to patient exact motion required.
Patient/Examiner action	Maintaining elbow in extension and fingers in flexion, perform passive, or have patient perform active, flexion of the wrist (see Fig. 6.36).
Goniometer alignment	Palpate landmarks shown in Fig. 6.35 and align goniometer accordingly (Fig. 6.37).
Stationary arm	Lateral epicondyle of humerus.

Fig. 6.36 End ROM of forearm extensor muscle length. Bony landmarks for goniometer alignment (lateral epicondyle of humerus, lunate, dorsal midline of third metacarpal) indicated by red line and dots.

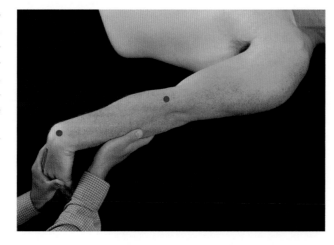

Fig. 6.37 Patient position and goniometer alignment at end of forearm extensor muscle length.

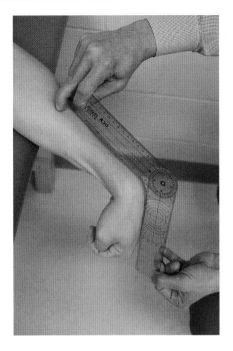

Axis	Lunate.
Moving arm	Dorsal midline of third metacarpal.
	Maintaining proper goniometric alignment, read scale of goniometer (see Fig. 6.37). Note: Elbow must be maintained in full extension.
Documentation	Record patient's maximum amount of wrist flexion.

Lumbricals: Palmer and Dorsal Interossei Muscle Length (Video 6.13)

Fig. 6.38 Starting position for measurement of length of lumbricals and palmar and dorsal interossei. Bony landmarks for goniometer alignment (dorsal midline of the metacarpal, dorsal aspect of MCP joint, dorsal midline of proximal phalanx) indicated by red lines and dot.

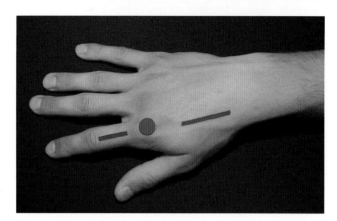

Patient position	Seated, with forearm supported on table; wrist and hand in neutral position (Fig. 6.38).
Examiner action	After instructing patient in motion desired, examiner extends metacarpophalangeal joint (MCP) into full available ROM while keeping proximal interphalangeal joint (PIP) and distal interphalangeal joint (DIP) in full flexion (Fig. 6.39). This passive movement allows an estimate of available ROM and demonstrates to patient exact motion required.
Patient/Examiner action	Keeping the PIP and DIP in full flexion, examiner extends MCP through available ROM (see Fig. 6.39).
Goniometer alignment	Palpate landmarks shown in Fig. 6.38 and align goniometer accordingly (first finger, Fig. 6.40; second finger, Fig. 6.41).

Fig. 6.39 End ROM of lumbricals and palmar and dorsal interossei muscle length of the first finger. Bony landmarks for goniometer alignment (dorsal midline of the metacarpal, dorsal aspect of MCP joint, dorsal midline of proximal phalanx) indicated by red lines and dot.

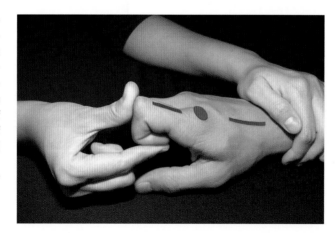

Fig. 6.40 Patient position and goniometer alignment at end of lumbricals and palmar and dorsal interossei muscle length of the first finger.

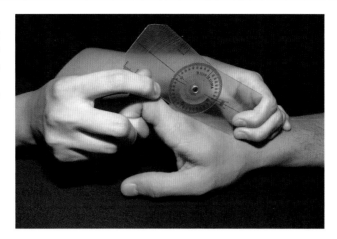

Stationary arm	Dorsal midline of the metacarpal.
Axis	Dorsal aspect of MCP joint.
Moving arm	Dorsal midline of proximal phalanx.
	While maintaining proper goniometric alignment, read scale of goniometer.
Documentation	Record patient's maximum amount of MCP extension.

Fig. 6.41 Patient position and goniometer alignment at end of lumbricals and palmar and dorsal interossei muscle length of the second finger.

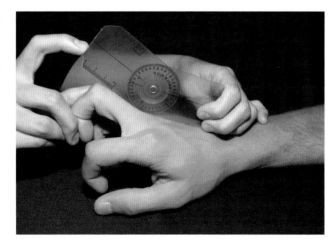

References

1. Scott MG, French E. Flexibility. In: *Measurement and Evaluation in Physical Education.* Dubuque, IA: Wm. C. Brown; 1959.
2. Hoppenfeld S. Physical Examination of the Spine and Extremities. Norwalk: CT: Appleton & Lange; 1976.
3. Myers H. Range of motion and flexibility. *Phys Ther Rev.* 1960;41:177–182.
4. Sullivan JF, Hawkins RJ. Clinical examination of the shoulder complex. In: Andrews JR, Wilk KE, eds. *The Athlete's Shoulder.* 2nd ed. New York: Churchill Livingstone; 2008.
5. Mallon WJ, Herring CL, Sallay PI, et al. Use of vertebral levels to measure presumed internal rotation of the shoulder: A radiographic analysis. *J Shoulder Elbow Surg.* 1996;5:299–306.
6. Goldstein TS. Functional Rehabilitation in Orthopedics. Gaithersburg, MD: Aspen Publications; 1995.
7. Magee DJ. Orthopedic Physical Assessment. 5th ed. Philadelphia: WB Saunders; 2007.
8. Johnson BL. Practical Flexibility Measurement With the Flexomeasure. Portland, TX: Brown and Littleman; 1977.
9. Corbin CB. Flexibility. *Clin Sports Med.* 1984;3:101–117.

RELIABILITY and VALIDITY of MEASUREMENTS of RANGE of MOTION and MUSCLE LENGTH TESTING of the UPPER EXTREMITY

Nancy Berryman Reese and William D. Bandy

Chapters 3 through 6 described techniques for measuring joint range of motion (ROM) and muscle length of the upper extremity. Research regarding reliability and validity of ROM techniques, including goniometer and inclinometer measurements, is presented in this chapter (no studies examining reliability of upper extremity muscle length testing were found). Only those studies providing information about both relative and absolute reliability or validity are included. More detailed information regarding appropriate analysis of reliability and validity is presented in Chapter 2.

RELIABILITY AND VALIDITY OF UPPER EXTREMITY GONIOMETRY AND INCLINOMETRY

Shoulder Complex and Glenohumeral Flexion/Extension

A moderate amount of research has focused on the reliability of goniometric and inclinometric measurements of the shoulder complex and glenohumeral flexion and extension. In the following sections on the shoulder complex and glenohumeral joint, the term *shoulder* is used to refer to measurements of shoulder complex motion where no attempt was made to prevent scapular rotation during the movement. *Glenohumeral* is used to refer to motions in which the examiners attempted to prevent scapular rotation and measure only glenohumeral motion.

Passive

The reliability of passive shoulder flexion and extension goniometry was studied by Riddle et al.[1] This group of investigators examined both intrarater and interrater reliability of passive shoulder flexion and extension ROM in a group of 100 adult patients aged 19–77 years. The investigators did not use standardized goniometric technique or patient positioning in this study. To determine whether the size of the goniometer used made a difference in the reliability of results, two different sizes of universal goniometers were used in the study. Intraclass correlation coefficients (ICCs) were calculated both within and between raters for each type of goniometer used. Intrarater reliability did not vary, and interrater reliability varied only slightly with the type of goniometer used to measure both shoulder flexion and extension. However, although intrarater reliabilities for shoulder flexion and extension were good (0.98 for flexion and 0.94 for extension) (Table 7.1), interrater reliability for shoulder flexion was not as high (0.87 and 0.89, respectively), and interrater reliability for shoulder extension was poor (0.26 and 0.27, respectively) (Table 7.2).

Passive shoulder flexion was measured via goniometry in 695 subjects as part of the San Antonio Longitudinal Study of Aging.[19] Before initiating the study, the four examiners who measured ROM participated in a preliminary investigation to determine interrater reliability. Passive shoulder flexion in 24 adults aged 65–80 years was measured by each of the four examiners. Measurements were taken with the subjects' supine using a standardized measurement technique. Interrater reliability was analyzed using an ICC. Results indicated only fair reliability for the measurement of shoulder flexion (ICC = 0.42; see Table 7.2).

Macedo and Magee[6] examined intrarater reliability of goniometric measurements of shoulder and glenohumeral flexion and extension ROM (in addition to the reliability of several other joint ROM measurements) as part of a larger study of changes in ROM with age in healthy adult females.[6] Reliability was tested in 12 subjects before initiation of the larger study. A single examiner measured passive shoulder and glenohumeral flexion and extension ROM along with 26 additional movements twice within a 6-h period using standardized measurement techniques. Shoulder and glenohumeral flexion were measured with the subjects supine, while extension was measured with the subjects prone. ICCs were 0.98 for both shoulder and glenohumeral flexion, 0.94 for shoulder extension, and 0.78 for glenohumeral extension (see Table 7.1).

Table 7.1   INTRARATER RELIABILITY: SHOULDER FLEXION/EXTENSION ROM

SHOULDER FLEXION—GONIOMETRY

STUDY	TECHNIQUE	n	SAMPLE	r*	ICC†
Correll et al.[2]	AROM; supine; standardized technique; 2 examiners (third year DPT students); goniometer (G) vs HALO (laser-guided digital inclinometer) (H)	42 (75 shoulders)	Healthy adults (30 F, 11 M) (18–70 years) ($\bar{x}=32.3\pm2.12$)		0.83–0.84 (G)
Greene and Wolf[3]	AROM; technique not described	20	Healthy adults (18–55 years)		0.96
Hayes et al.[4]	AROM; sitting; standardized technique	9	Adults with shoulder pathology (29–74 years)		0.53
Kolber and Hanney[5]	AROM; seated with back support; standardized technique; flexion performed with palm down; examiners were third-year DPT students	30	Healthy adults; (21 F, 9 M) ($\bar{x}=26\pm4.2$ years)		0.89–0.98
Macedo and Magee[6]	PROM; supine; shoulder in 0° abduction, and rotation; elbow extended; forearm neutral	12	Healthy Caucasian females (18–59 years) ($\bar{x}=37.2$ years)		0.98
Mullaney et al.[7]	AROM, supine; standardized technique; affected (A) and nonaffected (NA) extremity tested; 2 examiners (PTs)	20	Adults with shoulder pathology (11 F, 9 M) (19–79 years)		0.96–0.97 (A) 0.91–0.97 (NA)
Muir et al.[8]	AROM; standing (ST) and supine (SU); 2 examiners; each measured shoulder ROM twice using goniometer; standardized technique	17 (34 shoulders)	Adults with and without shoulder pathology (23 normal shoulders, NS, 11 shoulders with pathology, PS) (14 F, 3 M) ($\bar{x}=45.1$ years)		0.86 AROM (ST, NS) 0.92 AROM (SU, NS) 0.85 PROM (SU, NS) 0.63 AROM (ST, PS) 0.90 AROM (SU, PS) 0.92 PROM (SU, PS)
Riddle et al.[1]	PROM; small goniometer; nonstandardized technique	100	Adults with shoulder pathology (19–77 years)		0.98
	PROM; large goniometer; nonstandardized technique	100	Adults with shoulder pathology (19–77 years)		0.98
Sabari et al.[9]	AROM; sitting; standardized technique	30	Healthy adults (17–92 years)		0.97
	AROM; supine; standardized technique	30			0.95
	PROM; sitting; standardized technique	30			0.95
	PROM; supine; standardized technique	30			0.94
Shin et al.[10]	AROM and PROM; standing; standardized technique; affected extremity tested; 3 examiners (MDs); goniometer (G) vs smartphone inclinometer application (SI)	41	Adults with shoulder pathology (21 F, 20 M) (19–79 years)		0.80–0.96 AROM (G) 0.95–0.99 PROM (G)
Walker et al.[11]	AROM; AAOS technique and shoulder complex motion	4	Healthy adults; no ages provided	>0.81	

GLENOHUMERAL FLEXION—GONIOMETRY

STUDY	TECHNIQUE	n	SAMPLE	r*	ICC†
Macedo and Magee[6]	PROM; supine; shoulder in 0° abduction and adduction; elbow extended; forearm neutral; examiner stabilized over lateral border of scapula to prevent posterior tilting and upward rotation of scapula	12	Healthy Caucasian females (18–59 years) ($\bar{x}=37.2$ years)		0.98

SHOULDER FLEXION—INCLINOMETRY

STUDY	TECHNIQUE	n	SAMPLE	r*	ICC†
Correll et al.[2]	AROM; supine; standardized technique; 2 examiners (third year DPT students); goniometer (G) vs HALO (laser-guided digital inclinometer) (H)	42 (75 shoulders)	Healthy adults (30 F, 11 M) (18–70 years) ($\bar{x}=32.3\pm2.12$)		0.86–0.88 (H)
Dougherty et al.[12]	PROM; seated; standardized technique; digital inclinometer; measured total shoulder flexion	90 (168 shoulders)	Healthy adults (54 F, 36 M) ($\bar{x}=23.5\pm8.9$ years)		0.74–0.88

Table 7.1	INTRARATER RELIABILITY: SHOULDER FLEXION/EXTENSION ROM—cont'd				
STUDY	**TECHNIQUE**	**n**	**SAMPLE**	**r***	**ICC†**
SHOULDER FLEXION—INCLINOMETRY—cont'd					
Geertzen et al.[13]	AROM; standing with heels and back against wall; standardized technique; affected (A) and nonaffected (NA) extremities tested using digital inclinometer; 2 experienced examiners	29	Adults with reflex sympathetic dystrophy (19 F, 10 M) (x̄ = 49.1 ± 13.3 years)		0.91–0.95 (A) 0.95–0.97 (NA)
Green et al.[14]	AROM; seated, palms facing medially; motion stopped at point of first pain; affected extremity tested by six "manipulative physiotherapists" using a gravity inclinometer	6	Adults with shoulder pain (2 F, 4 M) (x̄ = 57.3 years)		0.49–0.80
Hoving et al.[15]	AROM; gravity inclinometer; 2 sets of raters; 6 rheumatologists, 6 physiotherapists	6	Adults with shoulder pain and stiffness (4 F, 2 M) (54–82 years) (x̄ = 72)		0.83
Kolber et al.[16]	AROM; seated with back support; standardized; flexion performed with palm down; 2 examiners (PTs) measured nondominant arm with digital inclinometer using digital inclinometer; 2 experienced examiners	30	Healthy adults (18 F, 12 M) (x̄ = 25.93 ± 3.10 years)		0.83
Kolber and Hanney[5]	AROM; seated with back support; standardized technique; flexion performed with palm down; examiners were third-year DPT students	30	Healthy adults; (21 F, 9 M) (x̄ = 26 ± 4.2 years)		0.90–0.98 (DI)
Shin et al.[10]	AROM and PROM; standing standardized technique; affected extremity tested; 3 examiners (MDs); goniometer (G) vs smartphone inclinometer application (SI)	41	Adults with shoulder pathology (21 F, 20 M) (19–79 years)		0.97–0.99 AROM (SI) 0.96–0.99 PROM (SI)
Tveitå et al.[17]	AROM; standing, palms facing medially; standardized technique; affected (A) and nonaffected (NA) extremity tested by single examiner using digital inclinometer	32	Adults with adhesive capsulitis of the shoulder (19 F, 13 M) (x̄ = 50 ± 6 years)		0.83 (A) 0.75 (NA)
Valentine and Lewis[18]	AROM; standing; affected (A) and nonaffected (NA) extremities tested in subjects with shoulder pain; right (R) and left (L) extremity tested in subjects without shoulder pain; 1 examiner (PT) using a gravity inclinometer measurements made with 12-in. goniometer (G) and digital inclinometer (DI)	90	45 adults with shoulder pain; 45 adults without shoulder pain (>18 years)		0.82 (A) 0.89 (NA) 0.91 (L) 0.94 (R)
GLENOHUMERAL FLEXION—INCLINOMETRY					
Dougherty et al.[12]	PROM; seated; scapula stabilized; standardized technique; digital inclinometer	90 (168 shoulders)	Healthy adults (54 F, 36 M) (x̄ = 23.5 ± 8.9 years)		0.63–0.83
Green et al.[14]	AROM; seated; palms facing medially; scapula stabilized by downward pressure on acromion; motion stopped at first pain; affected extremity tested by six "manipulative physiotherapists" using a gravity inclinometer	6	Adults with shoulder pain (2 F, 4 M) (x̄ = 57.3 years)		0.47–0.65
Hoving et al.[15]	AROM; gravity inclinometer; 2 sets of raters; 6 rheumatologists, 6 physiotherapists	6	Adults with shoulder pain and stiffness (4 F, 2 M) (54–82 years) (x̄ = 72)		0.62

Continued

STUDY	TECHNIQUE	n	SAMPLE	r*	ICC[†]
Table 7.1　INTRARATER RELIABILITY: SHOULDER FLEXION/EXTENSION ROM—cont'd					
GLENOHUMERAL FLEXION—INCLINOMETRY—cont'd					
Tveitå et al.[17]	PROM; standing, palms facing medially; motion stopped upon initiation of scapular rotation; standardized technique; affected (A) and nonaffected (NA) extremity tested by single examiner using digital inclinometer	32	Adults with adhesive capsulitis of the shoulder (19 F, 13 M) ($\bar{x}=50\pm6$ years)		0.76 (A) 0.61 (NA)
SHOULDER EXTENSION—GONIOMETRY					
Greene and Wolf[3]	AROM; technique not described	20	Healthy adults (aged 18–55 years)		0.98
Macedo and Magee[6]	PROM; prone; shoulder 0° abduction and rotation; elbow slightly flexed; forearm neutral	12	Healthy Caucasian Females (18–59 years) ($\bar{x}=37.2$ years)		0.94
Muir et al.[8]	AROM; standing (ST) and supine (SU); 2 examiners; each measured shoulder ROM twice using goniometer; standardized technique	17 (34 shoulders)	Adults with and without shoulder pathology (23 normal shoulders, NS, 11 shoulders with pathology, PS) (14 F, 3 M) ($\bar{x}=45.1$ years)		0.86 AROM (ST, NS) 0.92 AROM (SU, NS) 0.85 PROM (SU, NS) 0.63 AROM (ST, PS) 0.90 AROM (SU, PS) 0.92 PROM (SU, PS)
Riddle et al.[1]	PROM; small goniometer; nonstandardized technique	100	Adults with shoulder pathology (19–77 years)		0.94
	PROM; large goniometer; nonstandardized technique	100	Adults with shoulder pathology (19–77 years)		0.94
Walker et al.[11]	AROM; AAOS technique	4	Healthy adults; no ages provided	>0.81	
GLENOHUMERAL EXTENSION—GONIOMETRY					
Macedo and Magee[6]	PROM; prone; shoulder 0° abduction, adduction, and rotation; elbow slightly flexed; forearm neutral; examiner stabilized over inferior angle of scapula to prevent elevation or anterior tilting of scapula	12	Healthy Caucasian females (18–59 years) ($\bar{x}=37.2$ years)		0.78

AAOS, American Academy of Orthopaedic Surgeons; *AROM*, active ROM; *PROM*, passive ROM.

*Pearson's r.

[†]Intraclass correlation coefficient.

In a report published in 1998, a group of investigators performed a study designed to determine whether intrarater reliability of goniometric measurements of active and passive shoulder flexion and abduction changed when the subjects were placed in a seated compared with a supine position.[9] Two measurements were taken of each motion in each position in 30 adult subjects, aged 17–92 years. Data were analyzed using ICCs, which ranged from 0.94 to 0.97 for intrarater reliability of shoulder flexion, regardless of the type of motion measured (active or passive) or of the patient's position during the measurement (supine or sitting) (see Table 7.1). However, paired *t*-tests between goniometric readings taken in trial 1 compared with trial 2 revealed a significant difference ($P<0.05$) in the measurement of passive shoulder flexion taken in a supine position.

Muir et al.[8] assessed both intrarater and interrater reliability of numerous goniometric measurements of the shoulder (including passive shoulder flexion and active shoulder flexion and extension) in adults with and without shoulder pathology. Movement in a total of 17 subjects (34 shoulders; 23 without pathology, 11 with pathology) with an average age of 45.1 years was measured by two physical therapist examiners using standardized techniques. Passive shoulder flexion was measured with the subjects' supine, while active shoulder flexion was measured with subjects positioned in supine and in standing positions. The patients were also standing for the measurement of active shoulder extension; passive shoulder extension was not measured. In addition to ICCs, the authors reported the standard error of the measurement (SEM) and minimum clinical difference (MCD) for each measurement. The highest intrarater reliability was reported for active shoulder flexion measured in supine (ICC = 0.92, SEM = 4 degrees, MCD = 11 degrees), followed by active shoulder flexion measured in standing (ICC = 0.86, SEM = 5 degrees, MCD = 12 degrees), passive shoulder flexion measured in supine (ICC = 0.85, SEM = 3 degrees, MCD = 7 degrees), and

Table 7.2   INTERRATER RELIABILITY: SHOULDER FLEXION/EXTENSION ROM

SHOULDER FLEXION—GONIOMETRY

STUDY	TECHNIQUE	n	SAMPLE	ICC*
Correll et al.[2]	AROM; supine; standardized technique; 2 examiners (third year DPT students); goniometer (G) vs HALO (laser-guided digital inclinometer) (H)	42 (75 shoulders)	Healthy adults (30 F, 11 M) (18–70 years) ($\bar{x}=32.3\pm2.12$)	0.90 (G)
Escalante et al.[19]	PROM; supine; standardized technique	24	Ambulatory Adults (65–80 years)	0.42
Hayes et al.[4]	AROM; sitting; standardized technique	8	Adults with shoulder pathology	0.69
Mullaney et al.[7]	AROM, supine; standardized technique; affected (A) and nonaffected (NA) extremity tested; 2 examiners (PTs)	20	Adults with shoulder pathology (11 F, 9 M) (19–79 years)	0.88–0.93 (A) 0.74–0.79 (NA)
Muir et al.[8]	AROM; standing (ST) and supine (SU); 2 examiners; each measured shoulder ROM twice using standardized technique	17 (34 shoulders)	Adults with and without shoulder pathology (23 normal shoulders, NS, 11 shoulders with pathology, PS) (14 F, 3 M) ($\bar{x}=45.1$ years)	0.76 AROM (ST, NS) 0.74 AROM (SU, NS) 0.78 PROM (SU, NS) 0.55 AROM (ST, PS) 0.89 AROM (SU, PS) 0.88 PROM (SU, PS)
Riddle et al.[1]	PROM; small goniometer; nonstandardized technique	100	Adults with shoulder pathology (19–77 years)	0.87
	PROM; large goniometer; nonstandardized technique	100	Adults with shoulder pathology (19–77 years)	0.89
Shin et al.[10]	AROM and PROM; standing standardized technique; affected extremity tested; 3 examiners (MDs); goniometer (G) vs smartphone inclinometer application (SI)	41	Adults with shoulder pathology (21 F, 20 M) (19–79 years)	0.77–0.86 AROM (G) 0.84–0.89 PROM (G)

SHOULDER FLEXION—INCLINOMETRY

STUDY	TECHNIQUE	n	SAMPLE	ICC*
Correll et al.[2]	AROM; supine; standardized technique; 2 examiners (third year DPT students); goniometer (G) vs HALO (laser-guided digital inclinometer) (H)	42 (75 shoulders)	Healthy adults (30 F, 11 M) (18–70 years) ($\bar{x}=32.3\pm2.12$)	0.89 (H)
de Jong et al.[20]	PROM; supine; standardized techniques; affected extremity tested using "hydrogoniometer" (gravity inclinometer); 2 examiners (PTs); subjects tested at baseline and at 5 and 10 weeks	19	Adults after CVA of middle cerebral artery (9 F, 10 M) ($\bar{x}=54\pm10$ years)	0.98–0.99
de Jong et al.[21]	PROM; supine standardized technique; affected extremity tested using "hydrogoniometer" (gravity inclinometer); 2 examiners (PTs); subjects tested at baseline and at 4, 8, and 20 weeks	38–43	Adults after CVA (20 F, 28 M) ($\bar{x}=57.8\pm11.9$ years)	0.93–0.97
Geertzen et al.[13]	AROM; standing with heels and back against wall; standardized technique; affected (A) and nonaffected (NA) extremities tested using digital inclinometer; 2 experienced examiners	29	Adults with reflex sympathetic dystrophy (19 F, 10 M) ($\bar{x}=49.1\pm13.3$ years)	0.92–0.99 (A) 0.88–0.90 (NA)
Green et al.[14]	AROM; seated, palms facing medially; motion stopped at point of first pain; affected extremity tested by six "manipulative physiotherapists" using a gravity inclinometer	6	Adults with shoulder pain (2 F, 4 M) ($\bar{x}=57.3$ years)	0.58–0.82
Hoving et al.[15]	AROM; gravity inclinometer; 2 sets of raters; 6 rheumatologists, 6 physiotherapists	6	Adults with shoulder pain and stiffness (4 F, 2 M) (54–82 years) ($\bar{x}=72$)	0.72

Continued

STUDY	TECHNIQUE	n	SAMPLE	ICC*
Table 7.2 INTERRATER RELIABILITY: SHOULDER FLEXION/EXTENSION ROM—cont'd				
SHOULDER FLEXION—INCLINOMETRY—cont'd				
Kolber et al.[16]	AROM; seated with back support; standardized technique; flexion performed with palm down; 2 examiners (PTs) measured nondominant arm with digital inclinometer	30	Healthy adults (18 F, 12 M) ($\bar{x} = 25.93 \pm 3.10$ years)	0.58
Shin et al.[10]	AROM and PROM; standing; standardized technique; affected extremity tested; 3 examiners (MDs); goniometer (G) vs smartphone inclinometer application (SI)	41	Adults with shoulder pathology (21 F, 20 M) (19–79 years)	0.83–0.84 AROM (SI) 0.73–0.74 PROM (SI)
GLENOHUMERAL FLEXION—INCLINOMETRY				
Green et al.[14]	AROM; seated, palms facing medially; motion stopped at point of first pain; affected extremity tested by six "manipulative physiotherapists" using a gravity inclinometer	6	Adults with shoulder pain (2 F, 4 M) ($\bar{x} = 57.3$ years)	0.45–0.73
Hoving et al.[15]	AROM; gravity inclinometer; 2 sets of raters; 6 rheumatologists, 6 physiotherapists	6	Adults with shoulder pain and stiffness (4 F, 2 M) (54–82 years) ($\bar{x} = 72$)	0.65
SHOULDER EXTENSION-GONIOMETRY				
Muir et al.[8]	AROM; standing (ST) and supine (SU); 2 examiners; each measured shoulder ROM twice using goniometer; standardized technique	17 (34 shoulders)	Adults with and without shoulder pathology (23 normal shoulders, NS, 11 shoulders with pathology, PS) (14 F, 3 M) ($\bar{x} = 45.1$ years)	0.77 AROM (ST, NS) 0.47 AROM (ST, PS)
Riddle et al.[1]	PROM; small goniometer; nonstandardized technique	100	Adults with shoulder pathology (19–77 years)	0.26
	PROM; large goniometer; nonstandardized technique	100	Adults with shoulder pathology (19–77 years)	0.27

AROM, Active ROM; *CVA*, cerebrovascular accident; *PROM*, passive ROM.
*Intraclass correlation coefficient.

finally active shoulder extension measured in standing (ICC = 0.76, SEM = 4 degrees, MCD = 11 degrees) (see Table 7.1). Interrater reliability was lower in almost all cases, ranging from a high of 0.78 for passive shoulder flexion measured supine (ICC = 0.78, SEM = 3 degrees, MCD = 9 degrees), to a low of 0.74 for active shoulder flexion measured supine (ICC = 0.74, SEM = 4 degrees, MCD = 12 degrees).[8]

In two separate studies, de Jong et al.[20,21] examined interrater reliability of passive shoulder flexion as well as several other upper extremity movements in subjects at various time points following a cerebrovascular accident (CVA). Their 2007 study included 19 subjects (12 of whom completed the study) whose ROM was measured by each of two physical therapist examiners at an average of 39 days after the patients had a middle cerebral artery stroke, with follow-up measurements occurring 5 and 10 weeks later.[20] Their 2012 study included 48 subjects (38 of whom completed the study) whose ROM was measured by each of two physical

therapist examiners at an undefined "baseline" point and then at 4, 8, and 20 weeks following initial measurements.[21] In each of the studies, a "hydrogoniometer" (gravity-based inclinometer) was used to measure ROM, standardized measurement techniques were used, and the examiners were trained in the measurement procedures before testing. The authors reported interrater reliability for each study using ICCs, SEMs, and smallest detectable differences (SDD, equivalent in this case to MDC). For the 2007 study, ICCs ranged from 0.98 to 0.99, with SEM ranging from 3.00 degrees to 4.56 degrees and SDD (or MDC) ranging from 8.31 degrees to 12.64 degrees.[20] Authors in the 2012 study reported "overall" reliability, which they defined as reliability of the examiners over all measurement sessions, and data for observers, which they defined as differences between examiners in a single measurement session.[21] The overall ICC for shoulder flexion was 0.96, with overall SEM of 6.6 degrees and SDD (MDC) of 18.3 degrees. The SEM and SDD for a single measurement session were reported as 1.9 degrees and 5.2 degrees, respectively.

A recently published study examined the reliability of measurements of shoulder and glenohumeral ROM using a digital inclinometer.[12] Dougherty et al. measured passive shoulder and glenohumeral flexion and five additional motions in a group of 90 healthy adults. Both shoulders were measured in the majority of the subjects, yielding data from 168 asymptomatic shoulders. Standardized measurement techniques were used, and a single examiner performed all of the measurements. Passive flexion ROM was measured with the subject seated and the back against the chair to stabilize the trunk. For glenohumeral motions, the spine of the scapula was stabilized to prevent scapular movement. The authors reported intrarater reliability (ICC) of 0.82 with a SEM of 12.3 degrees for shoulder flexion and an ICC of 0.75 with a SEM of 9.4 degrees for glenohumeral flexion.[12]

Another group of investigators compared the reliability of measurements of shoulder flexion (as well as four other motions of the shoulder) when using visual estimation, a goniometer, and a smartphone "clinometer" (inclinometer).[22] Bilateral shoulder ROM measurements were taken in 24 healthy college students and in 15 subjects 6–12 weeks after total shoulder replacement surgery. Five examiners (three physicians with varying experience, one physician's assistant, and one medical student) performed the visual estimations and ROM measurements in college students. The postsurgical subjects were measured only by the physicians. Measurements of shoulder flexion and abduction were taken with the subjects in a standing position, and the remaining motions (lateral rotation with the shoulder in 0-degree and 90-degree abduction and medial rotation with the shoulder in 90-degree abduction) were performed with the subject supine. ROM was visually estimated before measuring motion with either the goniometer or the smartphone inclinometer. No additional details were provided about the procedures used during ROM measurements with either device. The authors reported ICCs and SEM values for interrater reliability for all measurements across all three methods of assessing ROM. The interrater reliability of shoulder flexion in healthy subjects using all five raters was highest with the smartphone inclinometer (ICC = 0.75, SEM = 1 degree), followed by the goniometer (ICC = 0.57, SEM = 2 degrees), and then visual estimation (ICC = 0.43, SEM = 6 degrees). Reliability between raters was higher in postsurgical subjects, where only two experienced examiners performed the measurements. As with the healthy subjects, interrater reliability was highest in postsurgical subjects with the smartphone inclinometer (ICC = 0.97, SEM = 3 degrees), followed by the goniometer (ICC = 0.90, SEM = 8 degrees), and then visual estimation (ICC = 0.63, SEM = 12 degrees).[22]

Active

A greater number of investigators have examined active shoulder flexion and extension measurement than have examined passive flexion and extension goniometry. In a study designed to compare reliability of the Ortho Ranger (an electronic, computerized goniometer) and the universal goniometer, Greene and Wolf[3] examined intrarater reliability of active shoulder flexion and extension goniometry in addition to 12 other motions of the upper extremity in 20 healthy adults. Measurements of shoulder flexion and extension were each taken three times per session across three testing sessions by the same examiner. Intrarater reliability for the measurements was analyzed using an ICC. Results revealed high reliability for the universal goniometer (0.96 for flexion, 0.98 for extension) for both active shoulder flexion and extension (see Table 7.1). The 95% confidence interval (CI) for the universal goniometer was 3.9 degrees for shoulder flexion and 2.4 degrees for shoulder extension.

Walker et al.[11] also examined intrarater reliability of active shoulder flexion and extension goniometry. In a study designed to determine the normal active ROM of 26 movements of the upper and lower extremities in older adults, measurements were taken in 60 persons aged 60–84 years. Techniques recommended by the American Academy of Orthopaedic Surgeons (AAOS) were used for all measurements. Before data collection, intrarater reliability was determined using four subjects. Although the exact number of motions measured to determine reliability was unclear from the authors' description of their methods, they reported Pearson product moment correlation coefficients (Pearson's *r*) for intrarater reliability "above 0.81" for active shoulder flexion and extension measurements (see Table 7.1) and a mean error between repeated measures of 5 degrees.

In a study that examined a variety of methods of assessing shoulder ROM, Hayes et al.[4] used two separate groups of subjects with shoulder pathology to determine intrarater and interrater reliability of active shoulder flexion, abduction, and external rotation measurements taken with a goniometer. Ten shoulders were measured in nine subjects (aged 29–74 years) for the intrarater reliability trial, and eight subjects (aged 57–72 years) were used to investigate interrater reliability. Measurements of shoulder flexion were taken with subjects seated on the edge of a treatment table and the stationary arm of the goniometer aligned with "a vertical line in the coronal plane."[4] Subjects were asked to flex the shoulder and stop at the point of pain. A single examiner (an orthopedic surgeon) performed measurements for the intrarater reliability study. Four examiners (an orthopedic surgeon, a sports medicine resident, and two physical therapists) participated in the interrater reliability study, with each examiner measuring each subject using five different

ROM measurement methods. ICCs and SEMs were calculated for both intrarater and interrater reliability trials. Intrarater reliability for shoulder flexion was fair to good (0.53; Table 7.1), while interrater reliability was higher at 0.69 (see Table 7.2). Standard errors ranged from 17 degrees for a single rater to 25 degrees between raters (see Table 7.2). Although the authors of this study did not address specific reasons for the lower reliability found in this study compared with others,[3,9,11] several possibilities are apparent, including the lack of trunk stabilization during ROM measurements and the possibility that pain patterns changed in subjects during the course of multiple measurements.

Mullaney et al.[7] reported higher reliability coefficients for intrarater and interrater reliability of shoulder flexion goniometry when they measured active assistive shoulder flexion ROM in subjects with unilateral shoulder pathology in a supine position. Two physical therapists measured shoulder flexion ROM in the affected (A) and nonaffected (NA) extremity of 20 adults with unilateral should pathology, aged 18–79 years. Each subject was measured by each of the examiners using a standard goniometer and a digital construction level. A standardized technique was used to take each measurement. Analysis of the goniometric measurements revealed high intrarater reliability with ICCs ranging from 0.91 to 0.97 for the nonaffected shoulder and from 0.96 to 0.97 for the affected shoulder (see Table 7.1). Interrater reliability was somewhat lower, ranging from 0.88 to 0.93 for the affected shoulder and 0.74 to 0.79 for the nonaffected shoulder (see Table 7.2).

Numerous researchers have investigated the reliability of measurements of active shoulder and glenohumeral flexion using an inclinometer. No studies examining the reliability of shoulder or glenohumeral extension using an inclinometer were located. Four studies examined active shoulder flexion ROM using an inclinometer in healthy adults, and all reported good to excellent intrarater reliability, with lower interrater reliability.[2,5,10,16] Kolber et al.[16] measured shoulder flexion ROM in the nondominant arm of 30 healthy adults, with an average age of 25.9 years, using a digital inclinometer. Subjects were seated with the back supported during measurements. Shoulder flexion was performed with the palm facing downward, and standardized measurement techniques were used by the two physical therapist examiners. The researchers found a higher level of intrarater reliability (ICC = 0.83; Table 7.1) than interrater reliability (ICC = 0.58; see Table 7.2) in this group of subjects.

Two studies[2,5] compared reliability of measurements of active shoulder ROM using a digital inclinometer and a universal goniometer. In both studies, measurements were made by third-year doctor of physical therapy (DPT) students using standardized measuring techniques. One of these studies measured only active shoulder flexion and reported nearly identical intrarater reliability for the two instruments, with ICCs for the goniometer ranging from 0.89 to 0.98 and from 0.90 to 0.98

for the inclinometer.[5] The other study[2] examined active shoulder flexion, abduction, medial rotation, and lateral rotation and reported both relative and absolute reliability. Values for relative reliability ranged from ICCs of 0.82 to 0.91 for the digital inclinometer (HALO device) and from 0.83 to 0.95 for the universal goniometer, while absolute reliability ranged from minimal detectable change (MDC) values of 6.9–21.1 for the digital inclinometer and values of 6.8–15.1 for the universal goniometer.

Shin et al.[10] compared reliability of measurements of active and passive shoulder flexion ROM but used a goniometer and a smartphone inclinometer application. Measurements were taken in the affected limb of 41 adults with shoulder pathology by three physicians (two orthopedic residents and one orthopedic surgeon) using each instrument. ICCs, SEMs, and minimal detectable change at the 90% confidence level (MDC_{90}) were calculated for both intrarater and interrater reliability trials. The highest intrarater reliability was reported for active shoulder flexion measured with the smartphone app (ICC = 0.97–0.99; SEM = 2.69 degrees; MDC_{90} = 12 degrees), followed by passive shoulder flexion measured with the smartphone app (ICC = 0.96–0.99; SEM = 2.30 degrees; MDC_{90} = 2 degrees); passive shoulder flexion measured with the goniometer (ICC = 0.95–0.99; SEM = 5.36 degrees; MDC_{90} = 4 degrees); and active shoulder flexion measured with the goniometer (ICC = 0.80–0.96; SEM = 6.28 degrees; MDC_{90} = 27 degrees). The highest interrater reliability was reported for passive shoulder flexion measured with the goniometer (ICC = 0.84–0.89; SEM = 6.30–7.53 degrees; MDC_{90} = 15–18 degrees), followed by active shoulder flexion measured with the smartphone app (ICC = 0.83–0.84; SEM = 9.56–9.99 degrees; MDC_{90} = 22–23 degrees), active shoulder flexion measured with the goniometer (ICC = 0.77–0.86; SEM = 8.80–12.03 degrees; MDC_{90} = 21–28 degrees), and passive shoulder flexion measured with the smartphone app (ICC = 0.73–0.74; SEM = 10.09–10.32 degrees; MDC_{90} = 24 degrees).

Valentine and Lewis[18] examined the intrarater reliability of shoulder flexion and abduction ROM measurements using a gravity inclinometer as part of a study that also included tape measure and visual estimation methods. A single investigator measured active shoulder flexion and abduction in two groups of subjects during two separate testing sessions using standardized methods. One of the groups consisted of 45 individuals (23 F, 22 M) aged 19–84 years with shoulder pathology, while the second group contained 45 individuals (24 F, 21 M) aged 23–56 years who were free of shoulder symptoms. Shoulder flexion was performed in the sagittal plane, and shoulder abduction was performed in a plane 45 degrees off the sagittal and frontal planes. The inclinometer was aligned parallel to the humerus, just distal to the insertion of the deltoid muscle. Each motion was measured three times in each subject during each testing session, and the average of the three measurements was used for data analysis. Intrarater reliability was determined through the calculation of ICCs (model 3.1) along with 95% CIs and calculation of standard errors of the measurement (SEMs). For the asymptomatic group, intrarater reliability ranged from 0.91 for flexion and abduction measurements of the left shoulder to 0.94 for flexion measurements of the right shoulder (see Table 7.1). SEM in this group fell between approximately 2 degrees and 3 degrees for each motion. Intrarater reliability for the group with shoulder pathology was slightly lower and, with the exception of flexion in the painful shoulder, ranged from 0.88 to 0.98 with SEMs between approximately 4 degrees and 5 degrees (see Table 7.1). Measurements of shoulder flexion in patients with painful shoulders had a reliability of 0.82 with a standard error of 14 degrees, unless outliers were eliminated from the data. With the elimination of outliers, the ICC improved to 0.97 and the SEM declined to approximately 5 degrees.

At least four studies[13–15,17] in addition to the study by Valentine and Lewis[18] have examined the reliability of measurements of active shoulder or glenohumeral flexion ROM using an inclinometer in patients with shoulder pathology. Geertzen et al.[13] used an inclinometer to measure active shoulder flexion and external rotation as well as forearm supination and wrist flexion, extension, radial deviation, and ulnar deviation. Two examiners measured each motion once per session for two sessions in 29 patients with upper extremity reflex sympathetic dystrophy. Measurements were taken from both the affected and the unaffected extremities. A standardized protocol for performing measurements was followed, and the examiners trained in executing the measurements for 10 h before data collection. Although not defined in the article, the authors appear to have used the Pearson's correlation coefficient to calculate reliability. Intrarater reliability for active shoulder flexion ranged from 0.91 to 0.95 for the affected side and from 0.95 to 0.97 for the nonaffected side (see Table 7.1). Interrater reliability ranged from 0.92 to 0.96 for the affected side and from 0.88 to 0.90 for the nonaffected side (see Table 7.2). In addition to correlation coefficients, the authors calculated the smallest detectable difference (SDD, or MDC) for each motion. These values were reported as 17.0 degrees for the affected side and 11.3 degrees for the nonaffected side.

In a study designed to develop and test a standardized protocol for the use of a gravity inclinometer to measure shoulder ROM, Green et al.[14] examined intrarater and interrater reliability of the inclinometer. Six "manipulative physiotherapists"[14] participated in the study in which active shoulder flexion, abduction, external rotation (in two different positions), and internal rotation as well as glenohumeral flexion and abduction and hand behind back were measured using standardized procedures with a gravity inclinometer. All six examiners underwent a 1-h training and supervised practice session before data collection. Subjects for the study consisted of six patients (4 M, 2 F; aged 45–66 years) with varying amounts of shoulder pain and stiffness. Measurements were performed in two separate sessions with a 1-h break

between sessions. During both sessions, each of the six examiners measured all motions in each patient once, following a randomized order of the patients and motions measured. Intrarater and interrater reliability were determined by comparing the combined measurements of all six examiners for each patient for sessions one and two and then calculating ICCs. Based on these calculations, intrarater reliability ranged from 0.49 to 0.80 for shoulder flexion and from 0.47 to 0.65 for glenohumeral flexion (see Table 7.1). Interrater reliability ranged from 0.58 to 0.82 for shoulder flexion and from 0.45 to 0.73 for glenohumeral flexion (see Table 7.2).

This same group of investigators conducted a similar study in which reliability of a gravity inclinometer in measuring the same set of shoulder motions was examined but with a group of rheumatologists rather than physical therapists.[15] Identical research protocols were used for the two studies. Intrarater reliability for shoulder flexion was 0.83 and for glenohumeral flexion was 0.62 (see Table 7.1). Interrater reliability was 0.72 for shoulder flexion and 0.65 for glenohumeral flexion (see Table 7.2).

Tveitå et al.[17] measured active shoulder flexion and passive glenohumeral flexion ROM (along with six other shoulder motions) in 32 adult subjects with adhesive capsulitis of the shoulder (19 F, 13 M; average age 50 ± 6 years) using a digital inclinometer. All measurements were taken twice in both the affected and nonaffected extremity by the same examiner within a 1-week period using standardized measurement techniques. Intrarater reliability (ICC) and SDDs were reported for each measurement. Results revealed higher reliability for measurements of shoulder flexion (ICCs = 0.83 for affected shoulder and 0.75 for nonaffected shoulder) than for glenohumeral flexion (ICC = 0.76 for affected shoulder and 0.61 for nonaffected shoulder). However, SDD was lowest (14 degrees) for measurements of active shoulder flexion on the nonaffected side and highest for measurements of active shoulder flexion on the affected side (28 degrees).

The previous three studies comparing shoulder to glenohumeral flexion revealed higher intrarater and interrater reliability for shoulder flexion than for glenohumeral flexion when measured with an inclinometer. However, only one of the studies reported minimal detectable change (SDD), and these data did not provide clear evidence that the reliability of one measurement was superior to that of the other.

Shoulder Complex and Glenohumeral Abduction

Passive

Four groups of researchers[1,6,8,9] have investigated the reliability of passive shoulder abduction goniometry in healthy adult subjects. These studies, which have been described elsewhere (see Section "Shoulder Flexion/ Extension"), yielded ICCs for intrarater reliability of

Table 7.3   INTRARATER RELIABILITY: SHOULDER ABDUCTION ROM

SHOULDER ABDUCTION—GONIOMETRY

STUDY	TECHNIQUE	n	SAMPLE	r*	ICC†
Correll et al.[2]	AROM; supine; standardized technique; 2 examiners (third year DPT students); goniometer (G) vs HALO (laser-guided digital inclinometer) (H)	42 (75 shoulders)	Healthy adults (30 F, 11 M) (18–70 years) ($\bar{x}=32.3\pm2.12$)		0.94–0.95 (G)
Greene and Wolf[3]	AROM; technique not described	20	Healthy adults (18–55 years)		0.96
Hayes et al.[4]	AROM; sitting; standardized technique	9	Adults with shoulder pathology (29–74 years)		0.58
Kolber and Hanney[5]	AROM; seated with back support; standardized technique; flexion performed with palm down; examiners were third-year DPT students; measurements made with 12-in. goniometer (G) and digital inclinometer (DI)	30	Healthy adults; (21 F, 9 M) ($\bar{x}=26\pm4.2$ years)		0.94–0.99 (G)
Macedo and Magee[6]	PROM; supine; shoulder in lateral rotation; 0° adduction and flexion; palm facing anteriorly; elbow extended	12	Healthy Caucasian females (18–59 years) ($\bar{x}=37.2$ years)		0.95
Muir et al.[8]	AROM; standing (ST) and supine (SU); 2 examiners; each measured shoulder ROM twice using goniometer; standardized technique	17 (34 shoulders)	Adults with and without shoulder pathology (23 normal shoulders, NS, 11 shoulders with pathology, PS) (14 F, 3 M) ($\bar{x}=45.1$ years)		0.91 AROM (ST, NS) 0.87 AROM (SU, NS) 0.91 PROM (SU, NS) 0.93 AROM (ST, PS) 0.95 AROM (SU, PS) 0.94 PROM (SU, PS)
Pandya et al.[23]	PROM; supine; AAOS technique	150	Patients with Duchenne muscular dystrophy (<1–20 years)		0.84
Riddle et al.[1]	PROM; small goniometer; nonstandardized technique	100	Adults with shoulder pathology (19–77 years)		0.98
	PROM; large goniometer; nonstandardized technique	100	Adults with shoulder pathology (19–77 years)		0.98
Sabari et al.[9]	AROM; sitting; standardized technique	30	Healthy adults (17–92 years)		0.97
	AROM; supine; standardized technique	30			0.99
	PROM; sitting; standardized technique	30			0.95
	PROM; supine; standardized technique	30			0.98
Shin et al.[10]	AROM and PROM; standing; standardized technique; affected extremity tested; 3 examiners (MDs); goniometer (G) vs smartphone inclinometer application (SI)	41	Adults with shoulder pathology (21 F, 20 M) (19–79 years)		0.94–0.99 AROM (G) 0.95–0.99 PROM (G)
Walker et al.[11]	AROM; AAOS technique	4	Healthy adults; no ages provided	>0.81	

GLENOHUMERAL ABDUCTION—GONIOMETRY

STUDY	TECHNIQUE	n	SAMPLE	r*	ICC†
Macedo and Magee[6]	PROM; supine; shoulder in lateral rotation; 0° adduction; palm facing anteriorly; elbow extended; examiner stabilized over lateral border of scapula to prevent upward rotation and elevation of scapula	12	Healthy Caucasian females (18–59 years) ($\bar{x}=37.2$ years)		0.84

SHOULDER ABDUCTION—INCLINOMETRY

STUDY	TECHNIQUE	n	SAMPLE	r*	ICC†
Correll et al.[2]	AROM; supine; standardized technique; 2 examiners (third year DPT students); goniometer (G) vs HALO (laser-guided digital inclinometer) (H)	42 (75 shoulders)	Healthy adults (30 F, 11 M) (18–70 years) ($\bar{x}=32.3\pm2.12$)		0.86–0.91 (H)
Dougherty et al.[12]	PROM; seated; standardized technique; digital inclinometer; measured total shoulder abduction	90 (168 shoulders)	Healthy adults (54 F, 36 M) ($\bar{x}=23.5\pm8.9$ years)		0.61–0.82
Green et al.[14]	AROM; seated, thumb pointed upward; motion stopped at point of first pain; affected extremity tested by 6 "manipulative physiotherapists" using a gravity inclinometer	6	Adults with shoulder pain (2F, 4 M) ($\bar{x}=57.3$ years)		0.38–0.75

	Table 7.3	INTRARATER RELIABILITY: SHOULDER ABDUCTION ROM—cont'd				
STUDY	**TECHNIQUE**		**n**	**SAMPLE**	**r***	**ICC†**
		SHOULDER ABDUCTION—INCLINOMETRY—cont'd				
Hoving et al.[15]	AROM; gravity inclinometer; 2 sets of raters; 6 rheumatologists, 6 physiotherapists		6	Adults with shoulder pain and stiffness (4 F, 2 M) (54–82 years) ($\bar{x}$=72)		0.56
Kolber et al.[16]	AROM; seated with back support; standardized technique; abduction performed with thumb pointing upward; 2 examiners (PTs) measured nondominant arm with digital inclinometer		30	Healthy adults (18 F, 12 M) ($\bar{x}$=25.93±3.10 years)		0.91
Kolber and Hanney[5]	AROM; seated with back support; standardized technique; flexion performed with palm down; examiners were third-year DPT students; measurements made with 12-in. goniometer (G) and digital inclinometer (DI)		30	Healthy adults; (21 F, 9 M) ($\bar{x}$=26±4.2 years)		0.94–0.98 (DI)
Shin et al.[10]	AROM and PROM; standing; standardized technique; affected extremity tested; 3 examiners (MDs); goniometer (G) vs smartphone inclinometer application (SI)		41	Adults with shoulder pathology (21 F, 20 M) (19–79 years)		0.96–0.99 AROM (SI) 0.97–0.99 PROM (SI)
Tveitå et al.[17]	AROM; standing, elbow flexed to 90°; standardized technique; affected (A) and nonaffected (NA) extremity tested by single examiner using digital inclinometer		32	Adults with adhesive capsulitis of the shoulder (19 F, 13 M) ($\bar{x}$=50±6 years)		0.93(A) 0.61 (NA)
Valentine and Lewis[18]	AROM; standing; affected (A) and nonaffected (NA) extremities tested in subjects with shoulder pain; right (R) and left (L) extremity tested in subjects without shoulder pain; 1 examiner (PT) using a gravity inclinometer		90	Adults with (45) and without (45) shoulder pain (>18 years)		0.98 (A) 0.88 (NA) 0.91 (L) 0.93 (R)
		GLENOHUMERAL ABDUCTION—INCLINOMETRY				
Dougherty et al.[12]	PROM; seated; scapula stabilized; standardized technique; digital inclinometer		90 (168 shoulders)	Healthy adults (54 F, 36 M) ($\bar{x}$=23.5±8.9 years)		0.64–0.84
Green et al.[14]	AROM; seated, thumb pointed upward; motion stopped at point of first pain; affected extremity tested by six "manipulative physiotherapists" using a gravity inclinometer		6	Adults with shoulder pain (2 F, 4 M) ($\bar{x}$=57.3 years)		0.43–0.62
Hoving et al.[15]	AROM; gravity inclinometer; 2 sets of raters; 6 rheumatologists, 6 physiotherapists		6	Adults with shoulder pain and stiffness (4 F, 2 M) (54–82 years) ($\bar{x}$=72)		0.35
Tveitå et al.[17]	AROM; standing, elbow flexed to 90°; standardized technique; motion stopped upon initiation of scapular rotation; affected (A) and nonaffected (NA) extremity tested by single examiner using digital inclinometer		32	Adults with adhesive capsulitis of the shoulder (19 F, 13 M) ($\bar{x}$=50±6 years)		0.72 (A) 0.89 (NA)

AAOS, American Academy of Orthopaedic Surgeons; *AROM,* active ROM; *PROM,* passive ROM.
*Pearson's *r*.
†Intraclass correlation coefficient.

passive shoulder abduction measurements ranging from 0.91 to 0.98 (Table 7.3). All four groups of investigators[1,6,8,9] measured passive shoulder abduction with the subjects in the supine position, and Sabari et al.[9] also measured shoulder abduction in the sitting position in their subjects. Two groups of investigators[6,8]

calculated SEM and MDC at the 95% confidence level as a follow-up to ICC calculations. These authors reported SEMs ranging from 3.4 degrees to 4 degrees and MDCs ranging from 9.5 degrees to 12 degrees when measuring passive shoulder abduction in supine. When Sabari et al.[9] followed up their ICC calculations with paired *t*-tests between goniometric readings taken in trial 1 compared with trial 2, they found a significant difference ($P < 0.05$) in the measurement of passive shoulder abduction taken with the subject in a sitting but not in a supine position. Two groups of investigators[1,8] also analyzed interrater reliability of passive shoulder abduction in healthy adult subjects and reported slightly lower reliability, with ICCs ranging from 0.84 to 0.88[1,8] (Table 7.4) and SEM and MDC reported as 5 degrees and 14 degrees, respectively.[8]

Table 7.4   INTERRATER RELIABILITY: SHOULDER ABDUCTION ROM

SHOULDER ABDUCTION—GONIOMETRY

STUDY	TECHNIQUE	n	SAMPLE	ICC*
Correll et al.[2]	AROM; supine; standardized technique; 2 examiners (third year DPT students); goniometer (G) vs HALO (laser-guided digital inclinometer) (H)	42 (75 shoulders)	Healthy adults (30 F, 11 M) (18–70 years) ($\bar{x} = 32.3 \pm 2.12$)	0.97 (G)
Hayes et al.[4]	AROM; sitting; standardized technique	8	Adults with shoulder pathology (57–72 years)	0.69
Muir et al.[8]	AROM; standing (ST) and supine (SU); (23 normal shoulders, NS, 11 shoulders with pathology, PS); 2 examiners; each measured shoulder ROM twice using goniometer; standardized technique	17 (34 shoulders)	Adults with and without shoulder pathology (14 F, 3 M) ($\bar{x} = 45.1$ years)	0.80 AROM (SU, NS) 0.67 AROM (ST, NS) 0.88 PROM (SU, NS) 0.57 AROM (ST, PS) 0.91 AROM (SU, PS) 0.92 PROM (SU, PS)
Pandya et al.[23]	PROM; supine; AAOS technique	21	Patients with Duchenne muscular dystrophy (<1–20 years)	0.67
Riddle et al.[1]	PROM; small goniometer; nonstandardized technique	100	Adults with shoulder pathology (19–77 years)	0.84
	PROM; large goniometer; nonstandardized technique	100	Adults with shoulder pathology (19–77 years)	0.87
Shin et al.[10]	AROM and PROM; standing; standardized technique; affected extremity tested; 3 examiners (MDs); goniometer (G) vs smartphone inclinometer application (SI)	41	Adults with shoulder pathology (21 F, 20 M) (19–79 years)	0.85–0.89 AROM (G) 0.78–0.83 PROM (G)

SHOULDER ABDUCTION—INCLINOMETRY

STUDY	TECHNIQUE	n	SAMPLE	ICC*
Correll et al.[2]	AROM; supine; standardized technique; 2 examiners (third year DPT students); goniometer (G) vs HALO (laser-guided digital inclinometer) (H)	42 (75 shoulders)	Healthy adults (30 F, 11 M) (18–70 years) ($\bar{x} = 32.3 \pm 2.12$)	0.93 (H) 0.97 (G)
de Jong et al.[20]	PROM; seated with back supported; standardized techniques; affected extremity tested using "hydrogoniometer" (gravity inclinometer); 2 examiners (PTs); subjects tested at baseline and at 5 and 10 weeks	19	Adults after cerebrovascular accident of middle cerebral artery (9 F, 10 M) ($\bar{x} = 54 \pm 10$ years)	0.84–0.87
de Jong et al.[21]	PROM; seated with back supported: standardized techniques; affected extremity tested using "hydrogoniometer" (gravity inclinometer); 2 examiners (PTs); subjects tested at baseline and at 4, 8, and 20 weeks	38–43	Adults post-CVA (20 F, 28 M) ($\bar{x} = 57.8 \pm 11.9$ years)	0.95–0.98
Green et al.[14]	AROM; seated, thumb pointed upward; motion stopped at point of first pain; affected extremity tested by 6 "manipulative physiotherapists" using a gravity inclinometer	6	Adults with shoulder pain (2 F, 4 M) ($\bar{x} = 57.3$ years)	0.62–0.88
Hoving et al.[15]	AROM; gravity inclinometer; 2 sets of raters; 6 rheumatologists, 6 physiotherapists	6	Adults with shoulder pain and stiffness (4 F, 2 M) (54–82 years) ($\bar{x} = 72$)	0.49
Kolber et al.[16]	AROM; seated with back support; standardized technique; abduction performed with thumb pointing upward; 2 examiners (PTs) measured nondominant arm with digital inclinometer	30	Healthy adults (18 F, 12 M) ($\bar{x} = 25.93 \pm 3.10$ years)	0.95
Shin et al.[10]	AROM and PROM; standing; standardized technique; affected extremity tested; 3 examiners (MDs); goniometer (G) vs smartphone inclinometer application (SI)	41	Adults with shoulder pathology (21 F, 20 M) (19–79 years)	0.78–0.79 AROM (SI) 0.70–0.72 PROM (SI)

STUDY	TECHNIQUE	n	SAMPLE	ICC*
	Table 7.4 INTERRATER RELIABILITY: SHOULDER ABDUCTION ROM—cont'd			
	GLENOHUMERAL ABDUCTION—INCLINOMETRY			
de Winter et al.[24]	PROM; seated with shoulder in neutral rotation; standardized technique; motion stopped upon initiating scapular rotation; affected (A) and nonaffected (NA) extremity tested using digital inclinometer; 2 examiners (PTs)	155	Adults with shoulder pathology (101 F, 54 M) ($\bar{x} = 47 \pm 12.6$ years)	0.83 (A) 0.28 (NA)
Green et al.[14]	AROM; seated, thumb pointed upward; motion stopped at point of first pain; affected extremity tested by 6 "manipulative physiotherapists" using a gravity inclinometer	6	Adults with shoulder pain (2 F, 4 M) ($\bar{x} = 57.3$ years)	0.46–0.69
Hoving et al.[15]	AROM; gravity inclinometer; 2 sets of raters: 6 rheumatologists, 6 physiotherapists	6	Adults with shoulder pain and stiffness (4 F, 2 M) (54–82 years) ($\bar{x} = 72$)	0.51
Sharma et al.[25]	PROM; standing; gravity inclinometer; standardized technique; scapula was stabilized; measured affected (A) and nonaffected (NA) shoulders; 2 examiners with experience measuring ROM	50 (100 shoulders)	Adults with adhesive shoulder capsulitis (28 F, 22 M) (38–75 years) ($\bar{x} = 52 + 9.3$ years)	0.64–0.91 (NA) 0.83–0.90 (A)

AAOS, American Academy of Orthopaedic Surgeons; *AROM*, active ROM; *CVA*, cerebrovascular accident; *PROM*, passive ROM.
*Intraclass correlation coefficient.

Both intrarater and interrater reliabilities have been reported for passive shoulder abduction measurements using a goniometer in children. Pandya et al.[23] examined intrarater reliability of passive shoulder abduction ROM in 150 children with Duchenne muscular dystrophy.[23] ICCs were used to analyze the data, and reliability was reported as 0.84 (see Table 7.3). Interrater reliability of passive shoulder abduction in a subgroup of 21 children with Duchenne muscular dystrophy also was examined, and reliability of 0.67 was reported (see Table 7.4).

The reliability of passive shoulder or glenohumeral abduction ROM measurements made with an inclinometer has been studied by at least seven groups of investigators.[10,12,17,20,21,24,25] Three of these studies, which have been described previously, measured intrarater reliability of passive shoulder abduction,[10,12,17] and the other four studies focused exclusively on examination of interrater reliability.[20,21,24,25] All but one of the seven studies examined subjects with shoulder pain or pathology. Intrarater reliability reported in the study by Shin et al.[10] was high, with ICCs ranging from 0.97 to 0.99 for measures of passive shoulder abduction using a smartphone inclinometer application. The reliability reported by Tveitå et al.[17] was lower, with ICCs ranging from 0.72 in the affected extremity to 0.89 in the nonaffected side for measures of glenohumeral abduction using a digital inclinometer. Dougherty et al.[12] also reported lower intrarater reliability for both shoulder and glenohumeral abduction using a digital inclinometer, with an ICC of 0.73 and SEM of 15.8 degrees for shoulder abduction, and an ICC of 0.75 and SEM of 7.3 degrees for glenohumeral abduction.[12]

In two studies published in 2007 and 2012 that have been described previously (see Section "Passive Shoulder Complex and Glenohumeral Flexion and Extension"), de Jong et al. examined the interrater reliability of inclinometric measurements of passive shoulder abduction ROM in patients after stroke.[20,21] For both studies, the authors reported the ICC, SEM, and SDD for each motion measured. For the 2007 study, ICCs ranged from 0.84 to 0.87, with the SEM ranging from 4.32 degrees to 6.54 degrees and SDD (or MDC) ranging from 11.97 degrees to 18.13 degrees.[20] Authors in the 2012 study reported "overall" reliability, which they defined as reliability of the examiners' overall measurement sessions, and data for observers, which they defined as differences between examiners in a single measurement session. The overall ICC for shoulder abduction was 0.97, with an overall SEM of 7.6 degrees and SDD (MDC) of 21.2 degrees. The SEM and SDD for a single measurement session was reported as 1.9 degrees and 5.2 degrees, respectively.[20,21]

Two studies not previously described examined the interrater reliability of measurements of passive glenohumeral abduction using an inclinometer.[24,25] Both studies involved the examination of subjects with shoulder pain or pathology. The pool of subjects used by de Winter et al.[24] consisted of 155 adults with shoulder pain (101 F, 54 M; average age 47 ± 12.6 years). Measurements of glenohumeral abduction were taken using a digital inclinometer by two physical therapist examiners with the patient in a seated position. Measuring techniques were standardized, and motion was stopped upon initiation of scapular rotation or when pain limited further motion. ROM data from both the affected and nonaffected extremity were taken and included in the data analysis. Interrater reliability was assessed using ICCs, and 95% limits of agreement also were reported. Reliability (ICC) for measurements of the affected side was 0.83 with a limit of agreement of 0.8 ± 19.6 degrees. For the nonaffected side, reliability was 0.28 and limit of agreement was 0.9 ± 18.8 degrees.[24]

Sharma et al.[25] examined the interrater reliability of measurements of ROM in passive glenohumeral abduction as well as rotation. Both shoulders of 50 adult subjects with a diagnosis of adhesive shoulder capsulitis were measured by two examiners using a gravity inclinometer. Measurements were taken on three separate visits (baseline, 4, and 8 weeks) with the subject standing and the inferior angle of the scapula stabilized between the thumb and forefinger of the examiner's hand. Interrater reliability (ICC) ranged from 0.64 to 0.91 for measurements of the nonaffected extremity and from 0.83 to 0.90 for measurements of the affected extremity.

In a study described previously, Werner et al.[22] compared the interrater reliability of measurements of shoulder abduction (and four additional motions) in healthy adults and in postsurgical subjects using a goniometer, a smartphone inclinometer, and visual estimation. Interrater reliability in healthy subjects was highest using the smartphone inclinometer or visual estimation (ICC = 0.72, SEM = 3 degrees for both methods) and lowest when using the goniometer (ICC = 0.63, SEM = 7 degrees). In subjects following total shoulder replacement, reliability was highest when using the goniometer (ICC = 0.93, SEM = 0.2 degrees), followed by the smartphone inclinometer (ICC = 0.91, SEM = 0.3 degrees), and then visual estimation (ICC = 0.90, SEM = 0.1 degrees).

Active

Intrarater reliability of active shoulder abduction measured with a goniometer has been examined by several groups of investigators whose studies have been described previously.[2–5,8–11] Six of the studies used standardized measurement techniques, [2–5,8,10] while the remaining two studies were not specific regarding the measuring techniques employed.[9,11] Five of the studies were performed in healthy adult subjects,[2,3,5,9,11] one study compared subjects with and without shoulder pathology,[8] and two studies used only subjects with shoulder pathology.[4,10] Multiple of these groups of investigators analyzed their data using ICCs and performed follow-up measures of concordance on the data.[2–5,8–11] Sabari et al.[9] reported correlations ranging from 0.97 to 0.99 for active shoulder abduction goniometry, depending on the patient position used (see Table 7.3). Paired t-tests revealed no significant difference ($P > 0.05$) between measures of active shoulder abduction ROM taken in the two trials, regardless of

patient position. Greene and Wolf[3] analyzed their data using the ICC and reported intrarater reliability of 0.96 (see Table 7.3) and a 95% confidence level of 6.4 degrees. Kolber and Hanney[5] reported similarly high intrarater reliability (ICC = 0.97) with a SEM of 2 degrees.

Several studies[2,8,10] examining the intrarater reliability of shoulder abduction ROM using a goniometer reported ICCs, SEMs, and MDCs. Intrarater reliability for the studies ranged from ICCs of 0.86–0.99 while SEM calculations ranged from 4 to 14.7 degrees and MDC values ranged from 3.5 to 16 degrees (see Table 7.3). Hayes et al.[4] reported a lower intrarater reliability of 0.54 for measurements of active shoulder abduction with a 95% confidence level of 46 degrees in their population of patients with shoulder pathology. Walker et al.[11] used Pearson's r for data analysis and reported a correlation of greater than 0.81 (see Table 7.3) and a mean error of 5 degrees (± 1 degree).

In the same studies described previously, Hayes et al.,[4] Muir et al.,[8] and Shin et al.[10] also examined interrater reliability of active shoulder abduction. Data analysis revealed ICCs ranging from 0.57 to 0.91 (see Table 7.4), with follow-up concordance data including a 95% CI of 42 degrees in the study by Hayes et al.[4]; SEM of 9 degrees and 10 degrees, and MDC of 24 degrees and 28 degrees for measurements in supine and standing, respectively, in the study by Muir et al.[8]; and SEMs ranging from 10.01 degrees to 11.85 degrees and MDC[90] of 23 degrees to 28 degrees in the study by Shin et al.[10]

Seven groups of investigators, whose studies have been described previously, have examined the intrarater reliability of active shoulder or glenohumeral abduction ROM measured using an inclinometer.[5,10,14–18] Standardized measuring techniques were used in all studies. All studies examined reliability of active shoulder abduction, and three of the studies also examined the reliability measurements of active glenohumeral abduction ROM. Two studies included only healthy adults,[5,16] one study included subjects with and without shoulder pain,[18] and the remaining four studies focused on subjects with shoulder pathology.[10,14,15,17] Intrarater reliability (ICCs) of measurements of active shoulder abduction using the inclinometer ranged from 0.91 to 0.98 for subjects without shoulder pain or known pathology,[5,16,18] and from 0.38 to 0.99 for subjects with shoulder pain or pathology.[10,14,15,17,18] For those reporting such data, SEMs ranged from 2.0 degrees to 2.7 degrees for subjects without shoulder pain or known pathology,[5,16,18] and from 4.8 degrees to 6.3 degrees for the affected side in subjects with shoulder pain or pathology.[10,17,18]

Although none of the studies measuring healthy adults examined glenohumeral motion, two of the studies of subjects with shoulder pain or pathology did examine the reliability of measurements of active glenohumeral abduction using an inclinometer.[14,15] Intrarater reliability (ICCs) of glenohumeral ROM measurements in these studies ranged from 0.35 to 0.62 for the affected side; SEMs were not reported in these two studies. One reason for the low intrarater reliability may have been the low number of subjects ($n = 6$) measured in each study.

Four groups of investigators, whose studies have been described previously, have examined the inter-rater reliability of active shoulder or glenohumeral abduction ROM measured using an inclinometer.[10,14–16] Standardized measuring techniques were used in all studies. Two of the studies examined only active shoulder abduction,[10,16] while the other two examined both active shoulder and active glenohumeral abduction.[14,15] Only the study by Kolber et al.[16] examined healthy adults. The remaining studies examined the reliability of measurements in subjects with shoulder pain or pathology.[10,14,15] Intrarater reliability (ICCs) of measurements of active shoulder abduction using the inclinometer were 0.95 for subjects without shoulder pain or known pathology[16] and ranged from 0.49 to 0.88 for subjects with shoulder pain or pathology.[10,14,15] The interrater reliability of measurements of active glenohumeral abduction were lower than for shoulder abduction and ranged from 0.46 to 0.69 for subjects with shoulder pain or pathology.[10,14,15] No studies were found that examined interrater reliability of active glenohumeral abduction measurements using an inclinometer in healthy adults. Standard errors of measurement and MDC_{90} were reported for the two studies focusing exclusively on the measurement of active shoulder abduction with an inclinometer. For healthy adult subjects, the authors reported a SEM of 1.63 degrees and an MDC_{90} of 4 degrees.[16] For subjects with shoulder pain or pathology, the authors reported SEMs ranging from 13.21 degrees to 13.84 degrees and MDC_{90} ranging from 31 degrees to 32 degrees.[10]

Shoulder Complex and Glenohumeral Medial/Lateral Rotation

Passive

Reliability of passive shoulder and glenohumeral rotation goniometry has been studied by at least 10 groups of investigators. Seven of these groups either focused on[6,26–29] or included[8,22] healthy adults in the study. Boon and Smith[26] examined the intrarater and interrater reliability of medial and lateral rotation of the shoulder with the subject's scapula "stabilized" (glenohumeral rotation) or "nonstabilized" (shoulder rotation). Subjects consisted of 50 high school athletes (32 F, 18 M; aged 12–18 years), each of whom had their passive shoulder rotation ROM measured by two groups of two experienced physical therapist examiners. Measurements were taken with the subjects supine and the upper extremity in 90 degrees of shoulder ab-

duction and 90 degrees of elbow flexion. Each group of examiners measured both medial and lateral rotation on every subject, once with the scapula stabilized and once without scapular stabilization. Stabilization of the scapula was accomplished via posteriorly directed pressure over the subject's coracoid process and clavicle by the heel of the examiner's hand. Both of the subjects' extremities were measured, and the entire process was repeated 5 days following the initial measurement session. The authors calculated ICCs and SEMs within and between examiners for measurements of each motion in both the stabilized and nonstabilized situation. Intrarater reliability of medial rotation measurements was higher with the scapula stabilized (ICC = 0.60, SEM = 8.03 degrees) than nonstabilized (ICC = 0.23, SEM = 20.18 degrees), and interrater reliability showed a similar trend (ICC = 0.38, SEM = 9.99 degrees with the scapula stabilized; ICC = 0.13, SEM = 21.45 degrees with scapula nonstabilized). In measurements of lateral rotation, both intrarater and interrater reliability were higher with the scapula nonstabilized. Intrarater reliability calculations yielded ICCs and SEMs of 0.58 and 9.14 degrees, respectively, with the scapula stabilized and 0.79 and 5.63 degrees in the nonstabilized situation. Interrater reliability showed a similar pattern with ICCs and SEMs at 0.78 and 6.61 degrees, respectively, with the scapula stabilized vs 0.84 and 4.92 degrees without stabilization.

Macedo and Magee[6] also examined the reliability of goniometric measurements of both shoulder and glenohumeral rotation ROM. These investigators reported intrarater reliability in the form of ICCs, SEMs, and MDCs for both measurements in a group of 12 healthy adults (see study details in Section "Shoulder Complex and Glenohumeral Flexion/Extension"). As in the study by Boon and Smith,[26] all measurements were taken with the subjects positioned in supine with the shoulder in 90-degree abduction and the elbow flexed to 90 degrees. During measurements of glenohumeral rotation, stabilization was provided "over the superior trapezius positioning the thumb over the clavicle to prevent posterior tilting or retraction of the scapula."[6] Unlike the findings in the study by Boon and Smith,[26] Macedo and Magee[6] reported identical intrarater ICCs for shoulder and glenohumeral medial rotation measurements (ICC = 0.97) and slightly lower SEM and MDC for shoulder medial rotation (SEM = 2.5 degrees, MDC = 6.8 degrees) than for glenohumeral medial rotation (SEM = 2.8 degrees, MDC = 7.6 degrees). Additionally, measurements of shoulder lateral rotation demonstrated higher reliability (ICC = 0.96, SEM = 2.8 degrees, MDC = 7.8 degrees) than did measurements of glenohumeral lateral rotation (ICC = 0.84, SEM = 5.5 degrees, MDC = 15.3 degrees).[6]

Lunden et al.[27] studied reliability of goniometric measurements of passive glenohumeral but not shoulder medial rotation ROM in 51 healthy adults (21 F, 30 M;

average age 29.5±7.6 years) and in 19 subjects with shoulder pathology (9F, 10M; average age 52.9±14.6 years). Each subject was measured by two different physical therapist examiners using standardized testing procedures. Two testing positions were used in the study, supine and side-lying. Each examiner measured each subject in both testing positions. When supine, the subject's upper extremity was positioned in 90 degrees of shoulder abduction and 90 degrees of elbow flexion. The scapula was stabilized during ROM measurements via posteriorly applied pressure over the subject's acromion and coracoid processes by the examiner. For side-lying measurements, the subject was positioned on the side to be measured with the shoulder and elbow in 90 degrees of flexion and the shoulder in 0 degrees of rotation. No manual stabilization was applied to the scapula, but the examiner ensured visually that the acromion process maintained a perpendicular position in relation to the surface of the examining table. The authors reported ICCs for intrarater and interrater reliability that were consistently higher for measurements taken in the side-lying position compared with the supine position, regardless of group (healthy or with shoulder pathology) being measured (Tables 7.5 and 7.6). However, MDC levels were higher in the groups measured in the side-lying position (2.3–4.1 degrees in the supine position vs 3.0–6.1 degrees in the side-lying position).[27]

In an effort to compare the reliability and resultant ROM of various methods of measuring glenohumeral medial rotation ROM, Wilk et al.[28] examined this motion in asymptomatic subjects using three different scapular stabilization methods. The subjects were 20 adult males with an average age of 27±6 years who were free of shoulder pathology. All measurements were performed with the subjects' supine with the shoulder in 90-degree abduction and 10-degree horizontal adduction (which the authors refer to as the "scapular plane") and the elbow flexed to 90 degrees. Three teams of two examiners measured passive medial rotation using a standard goniometer with a bubble level and three different techniques for stabilizing the scapula. For the first technique, the examiner stabilized the scapula by applying posterior pressure with the heel of the hand over the clavicle, coracoid process, and humeral head of the subject's tested shoulder. Scapular stabilization was provided in the second technique by the examiner's grasping the subject's coracoid process and scapular spine. In the third technique, the scapula was not manually stabilized, but visual inspection was used to detect the point at which the scapula elevated from the table, indicating the end of medial rotation ROM. Intrarater and interrater reliability of the three methods was assessed using ICCs. Intrarater reliability ranged from 0.62 for the second technique (stabilization of coracoid process and scapular spine) to 0.48 for the third technique (no stabilization). Interrater reliability was actually highest for the technique using no stabilization (ICC=0.47), followed

by the first technique (stabilization of the clavicle, coracoid process, and humeral head; ICC=0.45), and finally the second technique (stabilization of the coracoid process and scapular spine; ICC=0.43).[28]

In a study that also focused on the reliability of measurements of glenohumeral rotation under a variety of conditions, Cools et al.[29] measured passive medial and lateral rotation using 14 different procedures. Measurements of shoulder rotation were recorded from 30 young, healthy adults by two examiners using both a goniometer and a digital inclinometer. Lateral rotation was measured with the goniometer while the subject was in both the seated and supine positions and with the shoulder in 0-degree and 90-degree abduction. The same measurements of lateral rotation were taken with the inclinometer, with the exception of lateral rotation with the subject seated and the shoulder in 0-degree abduction. Medial rotation was measured using both the goniometer and the inclinometer with the subject supine and in a seated position and the shoulder in 90-degree abduction. Additional measurements of medial rotation were made using the goniometer with the subject in seated and supine positions and the shoulder in 90 degrees of flexion. Finally, medial rotation was measured with the inclinometer with the subject seated and the shoulder in 90 degrees of flexion. Thus a total of seven different procedures were used to measure lateral rotation, with another seven procedures used to measure medial rotation. The authors reported intrarater and interrater reliability for measurements made using the inclinometer and only intrarater reliability for goniometric measurements. Reliability was acceptable for all measurement techniques (intrarater ICCs=0.85–0.99, interrater ICCs=0.96–0.98), and the highest levels of reliability were found when using the inclinometer (see Tables 7.5 and 7.6). The highest reliability for measurements of lateral rotation were found using the inclinometer with the subject supine and the shoulder in 0-degree abduction (Intrarater: ICC=0.98, SEM=2 degrees, MDC=4 degrees; Interrater: ICC=0.98, SEM=2 degrees, MDC=5 degrees). Although ICC levels were slightly lower, the lowest SEM and MDC values were reported for measurements of medial rotation using the inclinometer with the subject in the seated position and the shoulder in 90 degrees of flexion (Intrarater: ICC=0.89, SEM=1–2 degrees, MDC=3–4 degrees; Interrater: ICC=0.96, SEM=1 degrees, MDC=3 degrees). The lowest reliability levels were reported for measurements made using the goniometer (see Table 7.5). These authors found the least reliable method of measuring lateral rotation was with the subject supine and the shoulder in 90-degree abduction using the goniometer (Intrarater: ICC=0.94, SEM=3 degrees, MDC=8 degrees). The least reliable method of measuring medial rotation appeared to be with the subject seated and the shoulder in 90-degree abduction using the goniometer (Intrarater: ICC=0.98, SEM=3 degrees, MDC=6 degrees).[29]

Table 7.5	INTRARATER RELIABILITY: SHOULDER MEDIAL/LATERAL ROTATION ROM

SHOULDER MEDIAL ROTATION—GONIOMETRY

STUDY	TECHNIQUE	n	SAMPLE	r*	ICC†
Boon and Smith[26]	PROM; supine; standardized techniques; 2 groups of 2 examiners (PTs) measured glenohumeral and shoulder complex motion	50	High school athletes (32 F, 18 M) (12–18 years)		°0.23
Correll et al.[2]	AROM; supine; standardized technique; 2 examiners (third year DPT students); goniometer (G) vs HALO (laser-guided digital inclinometer) (H)	42 (75 shoulders)	Healthy adults (30 F, 11 M) (18–70 years) ($\bar{x}=32.3\pm2.12$)		0.83–0.87 (G)
Fieseler et al.[30]	AROM; supine; shoulder in 90° abduction, elbow in 90° flexion, neutral wrist, shoulder stabilized; compared throwing arm (TA) and non-throwing arm (NTA)	47	Female handball athletes (HB) ($\bar{x}=21.0\pm3.7$ years) Healthy adults (HA) (13 F, 12 M) ($\bar{x}=21.9\pm1.2$ years)		0.96 (TA, HA) 0.98 (NTA, HA) 0.97 (TA, HB) 0.97 (NTA, HB)
Greene and Wolf[3]	AROM; technique not described	20	Healthy adults (18–55 years)		0.93
Kolber and Hanney[5]	AROM; seated with back support; standardized technique; flexion performed with palm down; examiners were third-year DPT students; measurements made with 12-in. goniometer (G) and digital inclinometer (DI)	30	Healthy adults; (21 F, 9 M) ($\bar{x}=26\pm4.2$ years)		0.89–0.98 (G)
Lunden et al.[27]	PROM; supine (SU) vs side-lying (SL); affected (A) shoulder tested in subjects with pathology; dominant (D) shoulder tested in subjects without pathology; 2 examiners (PTs)	70	Adults with (19) and without (51) shoulder pathology (30 F, 40 M) (average 36.8 years)		0.86–0.88 (SU, D) 0.94–0.95 (SL, D) 0.70–0.93 (SU, A) 0.96–0.98 (SL, A)
Macedo and Magee[6]	PROM; supine; shoulder in 90° abduction; elbow in 90° flexion; forearm neutral	12	Healthy Caucasian females (18–59 years) ($\bar{x}=37.2$ years)		0.97
Mullaney et al.[7]	AROM, supine; standardized technique; affected (A) and nonaffected (NA) extremity tested; 2 examiners (PTs)	20	Adults with shoulder pathology (11 F, 9 M) (19–79 years)		0.94–0.95 (A) 0.91–0.96 (NA)
Muir et al.[8]	AROM; standing (ST) and supine (SU); 2 examiners; each measured shoulder ROM twice using goniometer; standardized technique	17 (34 shoulders)	Adults with and without shoulder pathology (23 normal shoulders, NS, 11 shoulders with pathology, PS) (14 F, 3 M) ($\bar{x}=45.1$ years)		0.87 (NS) 0.69 (PS)
Riddle et al.[1]	PROM; small goniometer; nonstandardized technique	100	Adults with shoulder pathology (19–77 years)		0.93
	PROM; large goniometer; nonstandardized technique	100	Adults with shoulder pathology (19–77 years)		0.94
Shin et al.[10]	AROM and PROM; standing; standardized technique; affected extremity tested; 3 examiners (MDs); goniometer (G) vs smartphone inclinometer application (SI)	41	Adults with shoulder pathology (21 F, 20 M) (19–79 years)		0.94–0.98 AROM (G) 0.89–0.97 PROM (G)
Walker et al.[11]	AROM; AAOS technique and shoulder complex motion	4	Healthy adults; no ages provided	>0.81	

GLENOHUMERAL MEDIAL ROTATION—GONIOMETRY

STUDY	TECHNIQUE	n	SAMPLE	r*	ICC†
Boon and Smith[26]	PROM; supine; standardized techniques; 2 groups of 2 examiners (PTs) measured glenohumeral and shoulder complex motion	50	High school athletes (32 F, 18 M) (12–18 years)		0.60

Continued

Table 7.5	INTRARATER RELIABILITY: SHOULDER MEDIAL/LATERAL ROTATION ROM—cont'd				
STUDY	**TECHNIQUE**	**n**	**SAMPLE**	**r***	**ICC†**
GLENOHUMERAL MEDIAL ROTATION—GONIOMETRY—cont'd					
Macedo and Magee[6]	PROM; supine; shoulder in 90° abduction; elbow in 90° flexion; forearm neutral examiner stabilized over superior trapezius positioning the thumb over clavicle to prevent anterior tilting and protraction of scapula	12	Healthy Caucasian females (18–59 years) ($\bar{x}=37.2$ years)	0.97	
Wilk et al.[28]	PROM; supine with shoulder at 90° abduction and 10° horizontal adduction, 90° elbow flexion. 3 methods measuring IR: (1) stabilization of clavicle, coracoid process and humeral head; (2) stabilization of coracoid process and scapular spine; and (3) no stabilization provided	20	Asymptomatic overhead athletes (20 M) ($\bar{x}=27\pm6$ years)	0.51 (1) 0.62 (2) 0.48 (3)	
SHOULDER MEDIAL ROTATION—INCLINOMETRY					
Correll et al.[2]	AROM; supine; standardized technique; 2 examiners (third year DPT students); goniometer (G) vs HALO (laser-guided digital inclinometer) (H)	42 (75 shoulders)	Healthy adults (30 F, 11 M) (18–70 years) ($\bar{x}=32.3\pm2.12$)		0.82–0.85 (H)
Dougherty et al.[12]	PROM; seated; shoulder abducted to 90°; elbow flexed to 90°; forearm in neutral rotation; standardized technique; digital inclinometer	90 (168 shoulders)	Healthy adults (54 F, 36 M) ($\bar{x}=23.5\pm8.9$ years)		0.48–0.75
Furness et al.[31]	AROM; standard technique; tested in prone (P) and supine (S); single examiner (new graduate PT); used gravity-dependent inclinometer (I) and HALO device (H); compared within and between sessions	15 (30 shoulders)	Healthy adults (7 F, 8 M) ($\bar{x}=26.8\pm6.5$ years)		0.99 (P, I) (within session) 0.99 (P, H) (within session) 0.98 (S, I) (within session) 0.98 (S, H) (within session) 0.96 (P, I) (between sessions) 0.96 (P, H) (between sessions) 0.96 (S, I) (between sessions) 0.84 (S, H) (between sessions)
Green et al.[14]	AROM; supine with shoulder abducted to 45°, elbow flexed to 90°; forearm fully pronated; motion stopped at point of first pain; affected extremity tested by six "manipulative physiotherapists" using a gravity inclinometer	6	Adults with shoulder pain (2 F, 4 M) ($\bar{x}=57.3$ years)		0.79–0.82
Kolber et al.[16]	AROM; prone with shoulder in 90° abduction; standardized technique; abduction performed with thumb pointing upward; 2 examiners (PTs) measured nondominant arm with digital inclinometer	30	Healthy adults (18 F, 12 M) ($\bar{x}=25.93\pm3.10$ years)		0.87
Kolber and Hanney[5]	AROM; seated with back support; standardized technique; flexion performed with palm down; examiners were third-year DPT students; measurements made with 12-in. goniometer (G) and digital inclinometer (DI)	30	Healthy adults (21 F, 9 M) ($\bar{x}=26\pm4.2$ years)		0.93–0.98 (DI)

STUDY	TECHNIQUE	n	SAMPLE	r*	ICC†
Table 7.5 INTRARATER RELIABILITY: SHOULDER MEDIAL/LATERAL ROTATION ROM—cont'd					
SHOULDER MEDIAL ROTATION—INCLINOMETRY—cont'd					
Shin et al.[10]	AROM and PROM; standing; standardized technique; affected extremity tested; 3 examiners (MDs); goniometer (G) vs smartphone inclinometer application (SI)	41	Adults with shoulder pathology (21 F, 20 M) (19–79 years)		0.79–0.99 AROM (SI) 0.90–0.97 PROM (SI)
Tveitå et al.[17]	AROM; supine with shoulder in 45° abduction, elbow flexed to 90°; standardized technique; affected (A) and nonaffected (NA) extremity tested by single examiner using digital inclinometer	32	Adults with adhesive capsulitis of the shoulder (19 F, 13 M) ($\bar{x}=50\pm6$ years)		0.77 (A) 0.69 (NA)
Valentine and Lewis[18]	AROM; standing; affected (A) and nonaffected (NA) extremities tested in subjects with shoulder pain; right (R) and left (L) extremity tested in subjects without shoulder pain; 1 examiner (PT) using a gravity inclinometer	90	Adults with (45) and without (45) shoulder pain (>18 years)		0.82 (A) 0.89 (NA) 0.91 (L) 0.94 (R)
Walker et al.[32]	AROM; supine; shoulder in 90° abduction, elbow in 90° flexion, wrist and forearm in neutral, scapula stabilized with caudal and posterior force; 2 examiners (PTs)	16	Competitive swimmers (8 F, 8 M) ($\bar{x}=17\pm3$ years)		0.85–0.96
GLENOHUMERAL MEDIAL ROTATION—INCLINOMETRY					
Kevern et al.[33]	PROM; 3 measuring methods: (1) supine, shoulder in 90° abduction, elbow flexed to 90°; examiner determine end of ROM by palpation of capsular end feel (2) supine, shoulder in 90° abduction, elbow flexed to 90°; gravity determined end of ROM (3) sidelying with non-dominant UE uppermost; shoulder in 90° flexion, elbow flexed to 90°, scapula retracted	38	NCAA Division I baseball and softball players over 18 years (30 baseball, 8 softball players)		0.94–0.98 (Method 1) 0.97–0.98 (Method 2) 0.98–0.99 (Method 3)
Tveitå et al.[17]	AROM; supine with shoulder in 45° abduction, elbow flexed to 90°; standardized technique; affected (A) and nonaffected (NA) extremity tested by single examiner using digital inclinometer	32	Adults with adhesive capsulitis of the shoulder (19 F, 13 M) ($\bar{x}=50\pm6$ years)		0.81 (A) 0.88 (NA)
SHOULDER LATERAL ROTATION—GONIOMETRY					
Boone et al.[34]	AROM; AAOS technique	12	Adult males (26–54 years)		0.96
Correll et al.[2]	AROM; supine; standardized technique; 2 examiners (third year DPT students); goniometer (G) vs HALO (laser-guided digital inclinometer) (H)	42 (75 shoulders)	Healthy adults (30 F, 11 M) (18–70 years) ($\bar{x}=32.3\pm2.12$)		0.88–0.90 (G)

Continued

Table 7.5   INTRARATER RELIABILITY: SHOULDER MEDIAL/LATERAL ROTATION ROM—cont'd

STUDY	TECHNIQUE	n	SAMPLE	r*	ICC[†]
			SHOULDER LATERAL ROTATION—GONIOMETRY—cont'd		
Fieseler et al.[30]	AROM; supine; shoulder in 90° abduction, elbow in 90° flexion, neutral wrist, shoulder stabilized; compared throwing arm (TA) and non-throwing arm (NTA)	47	Female handball athletes (HB) (x̄ = 21.0 ± 3.7 years) Healthy adults (HA) (13 F, 12 M) (x̄ = 21.9 ± 1.2 years)		0.98 (TA, HA) 0.98 (NTA, HA) 0.95 (TA, HB) 0.96 (NTA, HB)
Greene and Wolf[3]	AROM; technique not described	20	Healthy adults (18–55 years)		0.91
Hayes et al.[4]	AROM; sitting; standardized technique	9	Patients with shoulder pathology (29–74 years)		0.65
Kolber and Hanney[5]	AROM; supine with shoulder in 90° abduction; standardized technique; examiners were third-year DPT students measurements made with 12-in. goniometer (G) and digital inclinometer (DI)	30	Healthy adults (21 F, 9 M) (x̄ = 26 ± 4.2 years)		0.87–0.97 (G)
MacDermid et al.[35]	PROM; supine; shoulder abducted 20°–30°	34	Patients with shoulder pathology (>55 years)		0.89/0.94[‡]
Macedo and Magee[6]	PROM; supine; shoulder in 90° abduction; elbow in 90° flexion; forearm neutral	12	Healthy Caucasian females (18–59 years) (x̄ = 37.2 years)		0.97
Mitchell et al.[36]	AROM; supine with shoulder abducted to 90°; folded towel under arm; compared smartphone goniometer apps, GetMyROM (GMR) and Dr. Goniometer (DG), to standard goniometry (SG); 4 examiners (2 novice DPT students; 2 experienced PTs with >15 years of experience); intratester reliability included only novice examiners	94	Recruited DPT students from Texas Woman's University in Houston (57 F, 37 M) (x̄ = 26.4 ± 7.6 years)		0.70–0.86 (GMR) 0.72–0.87 (DG) 0.74–0.88 (SG)
Mullaney et al.[7]	AROM; supine; standardized technique; affected (A) and nonaffected (NA) extremity tested; 2 examiners (PTs)	20	Adults with shoulder pathology (11 F, 9 M) (19–79 years)		0.99 (A) 0.97–0.98 (NA)
Muir et al.[8]	AROM and PROM; shoulder in 0° adduction (AD) or 90° abduction (AB); 2 examiners; each measured shoulder ROM twice using goniometer; standardized technique	17 (34 shoulders)	Adults with and without shoulder pathology (23 normal shoulders, NS, 11 shoulders with pathology, PS) (14 F, 3 M) (x̄ = 45.1 years)		0.91 (AROM, AD, NS) 0.94 (PROM, AD, NS) 0.86 (PROM, AB, NS) 0.89 (AROM, AD, PS) 0.93 (AROM, AB, PS) 0.94 (AROM, AD, PS) 0.95 (AROM, AB, PS)
Riddle et al.[1]	PROM; small goniometer; nonstandardized technique	100	Adults with shoulder pathology (19–77 years)		0.98
	PROM; large goniometer; nonstandardized technique	100	Adults with shoulder pathology (19–77 years)		0.99
Shin et al.[10]	AROM and PROM; supine with shoulder in 0° adduction (AD) or 90° abduction (AB); involved extremity tested; 3 examiners (MDs); goniometer (G) vs smartphone inclinometer application (SI)	41	Adults with shoulder pathology (21 F, 20 M) (19–79 years)		0.96–0.98 AROM (AD, G) 0.96–0.99 AROM (AB, G) 0.93–0.99 PROM (AD, G) 0.97–0.97 PROM (AB, G)
Walker et al.[11]	AROM; AAOS technique	4	Healthy adults, no ages provided	0.78	

Table 7.5	INTRARATER RELIABILITY: SHOULDER MEDIAL/LATERAL ROTATION ROM—cont'd				
STUDY	**TECHNIQUE**	**n**	**SAMPLE**	**r***	**ICC†**
GLENOHUMERAL LATERAL ROTATION—GONIOMETRY

STUDY	TECHNIQUE	n	SAMPLE	r*	ICC†
Macedo and Magee[6]	PROM; supine; shoulder in 90° abduction; elbow in 90° flexion; forearm neutral; examiner stabilized over superior trapezius positioning the thumb over clavicle to prevent posterior tilting or retraction of scapula	12	Healthy Caucasian females (18–59 years) ($\bar{x}=37.2$ years)	0.84	

SHOULDER LATERAL ROTATION—INCLINOMETRY

STUDY	TECHNIQUE	n	SAMPLE	r*	ICC†
Correll et al.[2]	AROM; supine; standardized technique; 2 examiners (third year DPT students); goniometer (G) vs HALO (laser-guided digital inclinometer) (H)	42 (75 shoulders)	Healthy adults (30 F, 11 M) (18–70 years) ($\bar{x}=32.3\pm2.12$)		0.89–0.90 (H)
Dougherty et al.[12]	PROM; seated; elbow flexed to 90°; forearm in neutral rotation; lateral rotation was measured with the shoulder in neutral abduction (N) and with the shoulder abducted to 90° (ABD); standardized technique; digital inclinometer	90 (168 shoulders)	Healthy adults (54 F, 36 M) ($\bar{x}=23.5\pm8.9$ years)		0.06–0.47 (N) 0.52–0.77 (ABD)
Furness et al.[31]	AROM; standard technique; tested in prone (P) and supine (S); single examiner (new graduate PT); used gravity-dependent inclinometer (I) and HALO device (H); compared within and between sessions	15 (30 shoulders)	Healthy adults (7 F, 8 M) ($\bar{x}=26.8\pm6.5$ years)		0.98 (P, I) (within session) 0.97 (P, H) (within session) 0.93 (S, I) (within session) 0.97 (S, H) (within session) 0.82 (P, I) (between sessions) 0.85 (P, H) (between sessions) 0.88 (S, I) (between sessions) 0.93 (S, H) (between sessions)
Geertzen et al.[13]	AROM; supine with shoulder at 0°, elbow flexed to 90°; standardized technique; affected (A) and nonaffected (NA) extremities tested using digital inclinometer (DI); 2 experienced examiners	29	Adults with reflex sympathetic dystrophy (19 F, 10 M) ($\bar{x}=49.1\pm13.3$ years)		0.85–0.89 (A) 0.77–0.91 (N)
Green et al.[14]	AROM; supine with elbow flexed to 90°; shoulder in 0° abduction (N) or 90° abduction (ABD); forearm fully pronated; motion stopped at point of first pain; affected extremity tested by six "manipulative physiotherapists" using a gravity inclinometer	6	Adults with shoulder pain (2 F, 4 M) ($\bar{x}=57.3$ years)		0.85–0.93 (AD) 0.75–0.82 (AB)
Kolber et al.[16]	AROM; supine with shoulder in 90° abduction; standardized technique; 2 examiners (PTs) measured nondominant arm with digital inclinometer	30	Healthy adults (18 F, 12 M) ($\bar{x}=25.93\pm3.10$ years)		0.94
Kolber and Hanney[5]	AROM; supine with shoulder in 90° abduction; standardized technique; examiners were third-year DPT students; measurements made with 12-in. goniometer (G) and digital inclinometer (DI)	30	Healthy adults; (21 F, 9 M) ($\bar{x}=26\pm4.2$ years)		0.96–0.99 (DI)

Continued

Table 7.5 INTRARATER RELIABILITY: SHOULDER MEDIAL/LATERAL ROTATION ROM—cont'd					
STUDY	**TECHNIQUE**	**n**	**SAMPLE**	**r***	**ICC[†]**
SHOULDER LATERAL ROTATION—INCLINOMETRY—cont'd					
Shin et al.[10]	AROM and PROM; supine with shoulder in 0°adduction (AD) or 90° abduction (AB); involved extremity tested; 3 examiners (MDs); goniometer (G) vs smartphone inclinometer application (SI)	41	Adults with shoulder pathology (21 F, 20 M) (19–79 years)		0.95–0.97 AROM (AD, SI) 0.96–0.98 AROM (AB, SI) 0.97–0.98 PROM (AD, SI) 0.98–0.98 PROM (AB, SI)
Tveitå et al.[17]	AROM; supine with shoulder in 45° abduction, elbow flexed to 90°; standardized technique; affected (A) and nonaffected (NA) extremity tested by single examiner using digital inclinometer	32	Adults with adhesive capsulitis of the shoulder (19 F, 13 M) ($\bar{x} = 50 \pm 6$ years)		0.91 (A) 0.85 (NA)
Valentine and Lewis[18]	AROM; standing; affected (A) and nonaffected (NA) extremities tested in subjects with shoulder pain; right (R) and left (L) extremity tested in subjects without shoulder pain; 1 examiner (PT) using a gravity inclinometer	90	Adults with (45) and without (45) shoulder pain (>18 years)		0.82 (A) 0.89 (NA) 0.91 (L) 0.94 (R)
Walker et al.[32]	AROM; supine; shoulder in 90° abduction, elbow in 90° flexion, wrist and forearm in neutral, scapula stabilized with caudal and posterior force; 2 experienced examiners (PTs)	16 (32 shoulders)	Competitive swimmers (8 F, 8 M) (12–24 years) ($\bar{x} = 17 \pm 3$ years)		0.90–0.95
GLENOHUMERAL LATERAL ROTATION—INCLINOMETRY					
Kevern et al.[33]	PROM; 3 measuring methods: (1) supine, shoulder in 90° abduction, elbow flexed to 90°; examiner determine end of ROM by palpation of capsular end feel (2) supine, shoulder in 90° abduction, elbow flexed to 90°; gravity determined end of ROM (3) sidelying with non-dominant UE uppermost; shoulder in 90° flexion, elbow flexed to 90°, scapula retracted	38	NCAA Division I baseball and softball players over 18 years (30 baseball, 8 softball players)		0.98–0.99 (Method 1) 0.99 (Method 2) 0.99 (Method 3)
Tveitå et al.[17]	AROM; supine with shoulder in 45° abduction, elbow flexed to 90°; standardized technique; affected (A) and nonaffected (NA) extremity tested by single examiner using digital inclinometer	32	Adults with adhesive capsulitis of the shoulder (19 F, 13 M) ($\bar{x} = 50 \pm 6$ years)		0.91 (A) 0.86 (NA)

AAOS, American Academy of Orthopaedic Surgeons; *AROM*, active ROM; *PROM*, passive ROM.

*Pearson's *r*.

[†]Intraclass correlation coefficient.

[‡]Two separate examiners.

Table 7.6 INTERRATER RELIABILITY: SHOULDER MEDIAL/LATERAL ROTATION ROM

SHOULDER MEDIAL ROTATION—GONIOMETRY

STUDY	TECHNIQUE	n	SAMPLE	ICC*
Boon and Smith[26]	PROM; supine; standardized techniques; 2 groups of 2 examiners (PTs) measured glenohumeral and shoulder complex motion	50	High school athletes (32 F, 18 M) (12–18 years)	0.13
Correll et al.[2]	AROM; supine; standardized technique; 2 examiners (third year DPT students); goniometer (G) vs HALO (laser-guided digital inclinometer) (H)	42 (75 shoulders)	Healthy adults (30 F, 11 M) (18–70 years) ($\bar{x}=32.3\pm2.12$)	0.96 (G)
Lunden et al.[27]	PROM; supine (SU) vs side-lying (SL); affected (A) shoulder tested in subjects with pathology; dominant (D) shoulder tested in subjects without pathology; 2 examiners (PTs)	70	Adults with (19) and without (51) shoulder pathology (30 F, 40 M) (average 36.8 years)	0.81 (SU, D) 0.88 (SL, D) 0.74 (SU, A) 0.96 (SL, A)
Mullaney et al.[7]	AROM, supine; standardized technique; affected (A) and nonaffected (NA) extremity tested; 2 examiners (PTs)	20	Adults with shoulder pathology (11 F, 9 M) (19–79 years)	0.82–0.87 (A) 0.62–0.63 (NA)
Muir et al.[8]	AROM; supine; 2 examiners; each measured shoulder ROM twice using goniometer; standardized technique	17 (34 shoulders)	Adults with and without shoulder pathology (23 normal shoulders, NS, 11 shoulders with pathology, PS) (14 F, 3 M) ($\bar{x}=45.1$ years)	0.62 (NS) 0.39 (PS)
Riddle et al.[1]	PROM; small goniometer; nonstandardized technique	100	Adults with shoulder pathology (19–77 years)	0.43
	PROM; large goniometer; nonstandardized technique	100	Adults with shoulder pathology (19–77 years)	0.55
Shin et al.[10]	AROM & PROM; supine with shoulder in 0° adduction (AD) or 90° abduction (AB); involved extremity tested, 3 examiners (MDs) goniometer (G) vs smartphone inclinometer application (SI)	41	Adults with shoulder pathology (21 F, 20 M) (19–79 years)	
Wilk et al.[28]	PROM; supine with shoulder at 90° abduction and 10° horizontal adduction, 90° elbow flexion. 3 methods measuring IR: (1) stabilization of clavicle, coracoid process and humeral head; (2) stabilization of coracoid process and scapular spine; and (3) no stabilization provided	20	Asymptomatic overhead athletes (20 M) ($\bar{x}=27\pm6$ years)	0.45 (1) 0.43 (2) 0.47 (3)

GLENOHUMERAL MEDIAL ROTATION—GONIOMETRY

STUDY	TECHNIQUE	n	SAMPLE	ICC*
Boon and Smith[26]	PROM; supine; standardized techniques; 2 groups of 2 examiners (PTs) measured glenohumeral and shoulder complex motion	50	High school athletes (32 F, 18 M) (12–18 years)	0.38

SHOULDER MEDIAL ROTATION—INCLINOMETRY

STUDY	TECHNIQUE	n	SAMPLE	ICC*
Correll et al.[2]	AROM; supine; standardized technique; 2 examiners (third year DPT students); goniometer (G) vs HALO (laser-guided digital inclinometer) (H)	42 (75 shoulders)	Healthy adults (30 F, 11 M) (18–70 years) ($\bar{x}=32.3\pm2.12$)	0.96 (H)
Green et al.[14]	AROM; supine with shoulder abducted to 45°, elbow flexed to 90°; forearm fully pronated; motion stopped at point of first pain; affected extremity tested by six "manipulative physiotherapists" using a gravity inclinometer	6	Adults with shoulder pain (2 F, 4 M) ($\bar{x}=57.3$ years)	0.41–0.48

Continued

Table 7.6	INTERRATER RELIABILITY: SHOULDER MEDIAL/LATERAL ROTATION ROM—cont'd			
STUDY	TECHNIQUE	n	SAMPLE	ICC*
	SHOULDER MEDIAL ROTATION—INCLINOMETRY—cont'd			
Kevern et al.[33]	PROM; 3 measuring methods: (1) supine, shoulder in 90° abduction, elbow flexed to 90°; examiner determine end of ROM by palpation of capsular end feel (2) supine, shoulder in 90° abduction, elbow flexed to 90°; gravity determined end of ROM (3) sidelying with non-dominant UE uppermost; shoulder in 90° flexion, elbow flexed to 90°, scapula retracted	38	NCAA Division I baseball and softball players over 18 years (30 baseball, 8 softball players)	0.54 (Method 1) 0.63 (Method 2) 0.68 (Method 3)
Kolber et al.[16]	AROM; prone with shoulder in 90° abduction; standardized technique; 2 examiners (PTs) measured nondominant arm with digital inclinometer	30	Healthy adults (18 F, 12 M) ($\bar{x}=25.93\pm3.10$ years)	0.93
Sharma et al.[25]	PROM; supine; gravity inclinometer; standardized technique; scapula not stabilized; measured affected (A) and nonaffected (NA) shoulders; 2 examiners with experience measuring ROM	50 (100 shoulders)	Adults with adhesive shoulder capsulitis (28 F, 22 M) (38–75 years) ($\bar{x}=52\pm9.3$ years)	0.63–0.78 (NA) 0.85–0.89 (A)
Shin et al.[10]	AROM & PROM; supine with shoulder in 0° adduction (AD) or 90° abduction (AB); involved extremity tested, 3 examiners (MDs) goniometer (G) vs smartphone inclinometer application (SI)	41	Adults with shoulder pathology (21 F, 20 M) (19–79 years)	0.66–0.67 AROM (SI) 0.63–0.68 PROM (SI)
	SHOULDER LATERAL ROTATION—GONIOMETRY			
Boone et al.[34]	AROM; AAOS technique	12	Adult males (26–54 years)	0.97
Boon and Smith[26]	PROM; supine; standardized techniques; 2 groups of 2 examiners (PTs) measured glenohumeral and shoulder complex motion	50	High school athletes (32 F, 18 M) (12–18 years)	0.84
Correll et al.[2]	AROM; supine; standardized technique; 2 examiners (third year DPT students); goniometer (G) vs HALO (laser-guided digital inclinometer) (H)	42 (75 shoulders)	Healthy adults (30 F, 11 M) (18–70 years) ($\bar{x}=32.3\pm2.12$)	0.98 (G)
Hayes et al.[4]	AROM; sitting; standardized technique	8	Adults with shoulder pathology (57–72 years)	0.64
Kevern et al.[33]	PROM; 3 measuring methods: (1) supine, shoulder in 90° abduction, elbow flexed to 90°; examiner determine end of ROM by palpation of capsular end feel (2) supine, shoulder in 90° abduction, elbow flexed to 90°; gravity determined end of ROM (3) sidelying with non-dominant UE uppermost; shoulder in 90° flexion, elbow flexed to 90°, scapula retracted	38	NCAA Division I baseball and softball players over 18 years (30 baseball, 8 softball players)	0.57 (Method 1) 0.77 (Method 2) 0.68 (Method 3)
MacDermid et al.[35]	PROM; supine; shoulder abducted 20°–30°	34	Patients with shoulder pathology (over age 55 years)	0.85/0.96[†]
Mitchell et al.[36]	AROM; supine with shoulder abducted to 90°; folded towel under arm; compared smartphone goniometer apps, GetMyROM (GMR) and Dr. Goniometer (DG), to standard goniometry (SG); 4 examiners (2 novice DPT students; 2 experienced PTs with >15 years experience)	94	Recruited DPT students from Texas Woman's University in Houston (57 F, 37 M) ($\bar{x}=26.4\pm7.6$ years)	0.87–0.98 (GMR) 0.85–0.96 (DG) 0.64–0.97 (SG)

Table 7.6 INTERRATER RELIABILITY: SHOULDER MEDIAL/LATERAL ROTATION ROM—cont'd				
STUDY	**TECHNIQUE**	**n**	**SAMPLE**	**ICC***
		SHOULDER LATERAL ROTATION—GONIOMETRY—cont'd		
Mullaney et al.[7]	AROM, supine with shoulder in 90° abduction; standardized technique; affected (A) and nonaffected (NA) extremity tested; 2 examiners (PTs)	20	Adults with shoulder pathology (11 F, 9 M) (19–79 years)	0.99 (A) 0.97–0.98 (NA)
Muir et al.[8]	AROM and PROM; supine with shoulder in 0° adduction (AD) or 90° abduction (AB); 2 examiners; each measured shoulder ROM twice using goniometer; standardized technique	17 (34 shoulders)	Adults with and without shoulder pathology (23 normal shoulders, NS, 11 shoulders with pathology, PS) (14 F, 3 M) ($\bar{X}$ = 45.1 years)	0.91 (AROM, AD, NS) 0.72 (AROM, AB, NS) 0.85 (PROM, AD, NS) 0.49 (PROM, AB, NS) 0.76 (AROM, AD, PS) 0.89 (AROM, AB, PS) 0.86 (AROM, AD, PS) 0.89 (AROM, AB, PS)
Riddle et al.[1]	PROM; small goniometer; nonstandardized technique	100	Adults with shoulder pathology (19–77 years)	0.90
	PROM; large goniometer; nonstandardized technique	100	Adults with shoulder pathology (19–77 years)	0.88
Shin et al.[10]	AROM and PROM; supine with shoulder in 0° adduction (AD) or 90° abduction (AB); involved extremity tested, 3 examiners (MDs) goniometer (G) vs smartphone inclinometer application (SI)	41	Adults with shoulder pathology (21 F, 20 M) (19–79 years)	0.67–0.67 AROM (G) 0.64–0.68 PROM (G)
		GLENOHUMERAL LATERAL ROTATION—GONIOMETRY		
Boon and Smith[26]	PROM; supine; standardized techniques; 2 groups of 2 examiners (PTs) measured glenohumeral and shoulder complex motion	50	High school athletes (12–18 years) (32 F, 18 M)	0.78
		SHOULDER LATERAL ROTATION—INCLINOMETRY		
Correll et al.[2]	AROM; supine; standardized technique; 2 examiners (third year DPT students); goniometer (G) vs HALO (laser-guided digital inclinometer) (H)	42 (75 shoulders)	Healthy adults (30 F, 11 M) (18–70 years) ($\bar{x}$ = 32.3 ± 2.12)	0.98 (H)
de Jong et al.[20]	PROM; supine; standardized technique; affected extremity tested using "hydrogoniometer" (gravity inclinometer); 2 examiners (PTs); subjects tested at baseline and at 5 and 10 weeks	19	Adults after CVA of middle cerebral artery (9 F, 10 M) ($\bar{x}$ = 54 ± 10 years)	0.94–0.99
de Jong et al.[21]	PROM; supine; standardized technique; affected extremity tested using "hydrogoniometer" (gravity inclinometer); 2 examiners (PTs); subjects tested at baseline and at 4, 8, and 20 weeks	38–43	Adults after CVA (20 F, 28 M) ($\bar{x}$ = 57.8 ± 11.9 years)	0.91–0.96
de Winter et al.[24]	PROM; supine with shoulder in 0° abduction and rotation; elbow flexed to 90°; standardized technique; affected (A) and nonaffected (NA) extremity tested using digital inclinometer; 2 examiners (PTs)	155	Adults with shoulder pathology (101 F, 54 M) ($\bar{x}$ = 47 ± 12.6 years)	0.90 (A) 0.56 (NA)
Geertzen et al.[13]	AROM; supine with shoulder in 0°, elbow flexed to 90°; standardized technique; affected (A) and nonaffected (NA) extremities tested using digital inclinometer (DI); 2 experienced examiners	29	Adults with reflex sympathetic dystrophy (19 F, 10 M) ($\bar{x}$ = 49.1 ± 13.3 years)	0.76–0.83 (A) 0.74–0.90 (N)

Continued

	Table 7.6 INTERRATER RELIABILITY: SHOULDER MEDIAL/LATERAL ROTATION ROM—cont'd			
STUDY	**TECHNIQUE**	**n**	**SAMPLE**	**ICC***
	SHOULDER LATERAL ROTATION—INCLINOMETRY—cont'd			
Green et al.[14]	AROM; supine with elbow flexed to 90°; shoulder in 0° abduction (N) or 90° abduction (ABD); forearm fully pronated; motion stopped at point of first pain; affected extremity tested by six "manipulative physiotherapists" using a gravity inclinometer	6	Adults with shoulder pain (2 F, 4 M) ($\bar{x}$ = 57.3 years)	0.85–0.95 (AD) 0.64–0.73 (AB)
Kolber et al.[16]	AROM; supine with shoulder in 90° abduction; standardized technique; 2 examiners (PTs) measured nondominant arm with digital inclinometer	30	Healthy adults (18 F, 12 M) ($\bar{x}$ = 25.93 ± 3.10 years)	0.88
Sharma et al.[25]	PROM; supine; gravity inclinometer; standardized technique; scapula not stabilized; measured affected (A) and nonaffected (NA) shoulders; 2 examiners with experience measuring ROM	50 (100 shoulders)	Adults with adhesive shoulder capsulitis (28 F, 22 M) (38–75 years) ($\bar{x}$ = 52 ± 9.3 years)	0.69–0.83 (NA) 0.89–0.91 (A)
Shin et al.[10]	AROM and PROM; supine with shoulder in 0° adduction (AD) or 90° abduction (AB); involved extremity tested; 3 examiners (MDs); goniometer (G) vs smartphone inclinometer application (SI)	41	Adults with shoulder pathology (21 F, 20 M) (19–79 years)	0.80–0.81 AROM (AD, SI) 0.87–0.91 (AB, SI) 0.79–0.80 (AD, SI) 0.87–0.91 (AB, SI)

AAOS, American Academy of Orthopaedic Surgeons; *AROM,* active ROM; *CVA,* cerebrovascular accident; *PROM,* passive ROM.
*Intraclass correlation coefficient.
†See text for further explanation.

Muir et al.[8] examined intrarater and interrater reliability of goniometric measurements of passive and active shoulder but not glenohumeral rotation ROM in 17 adult subjects with and without shoulder pathology. Only lateral rotation was measured passively, with subjects supine and the shoulder in 0-degree and in 90-degree abduction. Both medial and lateral rotation were measured actively. Subjects were supine, and lateral rotation was measured with the shoulder in 0-degree and in 90-degree abduction. Medial rotation was measured with the shoulder in 90-degree abduction. Other details of the study have been described previously (see study details in Section "Shoulder Complex and Glenohumeral Flexion/Extension.") In addition to ICCs, the authors reported the SEM and MDC for each measurement. The highest intrarater reliability was reported for passive shoulder lateral rotation measured with the shoulder in 0-degree abduction (ICC = 0.94, SEM = 4 degrees, MDC = 11 degrees), followed by active shoulder lateral rotation measured with the shoulder in 0-degree abduction (ICC = 0.91, SEM = 5 degrees, MDC = 13 degrees), active shoulder medial rotation (ICC = 0.87, SEM = 4 degrees, MDC = 11 degrees), passive shoulder lateral rotation measured with the shoulder in 90-degree abduction (ICC = 0.86, SEM = 5 degrees, MDC = 13 degrees), and finally, active

shoulder lateral rotation measured with the shoulder in 90-degree abduction (ICC = 0.81, SEM = 5 degrees, MDC = 14 degrees) (see Table 7.5). Interrater reliability was lower in almost all cases, ranging from a high of 0.91 for active shoulder lateral rotation measured with the shoulder in 0-degrees abduction (ICC = 0.91, SEM = 5 degrees, MDC = 14 degrees) to a low of 0.49 for passive shoulder lateral rotation with the shoulder in 90-degree abduction (ICC = 0.49, SEM = 9 degrees, MDC = 24 degrees).

Riddle et al.[1] examined both intrarater and interrater reliability of measurements of passive shoulder ROM, including shoulder medial and lateral rotation, using two different sizes of universal goniometers. ROM was measured in 100 patients aged 19–77 years with shoulder pathology without the use of standardized measuring or positioning techniques. Intrarater reliability (ICC) for passive shoulder rotation ranged from 0.93 for medial rotation using a small goniometer to 0.99 for lateral rotation using a large goniometer (see Table 7.5). Reliability between raters for lateral rotation remained high and was reported as 0.90 and 0.88 for a small and a large goniometer, respectively. However, interrater reliability for passive shoulder medial rotation was fairly low, equaling 0.43 with a small goniometer and 0.55 with a large goniometer (see Table 7.6).

MacDermid et al.[35] also examined reliability of passive shoulder rotation goniometry but focused exclusively on passive lateral rotation measurements. In a study of 34 patients older than 55 years with shoulder pathology, they measured passive lateral rotation of the shoulder while the patient was supine with the shoulder abducted 20–30 degrees. Both intrarater and interrater reliabilities were calculated using ICCs. Intrarater reliability was reported as 0.89 and 0.94 (see Table 7.5), and the SEM was 7.0 degrees and 4.9 degrees, depending on the examiner performing the measurement. Interrater reliability was 0.85 and 0.86 (see Table 7.6) with the SEM reported as 7.5 degrees and 8.0 degrees, depending on whether the first or second measurement was used in the calculation.

In a study described previously, Shin et al.[10] measured passive as well as active shoulder medial and lateral rotation ROM in a group of subjects with shoulder pain. All measurements were taken with the subjects positioned in supine using both a standard goniometer and a smartphone inclinometer application. Measurements of internal rotation were taken with the subject's shoulder in 90-degree abduction and the elbow in 90 degrees of flexion. Lateral rotation was measured in two different positions: with the subject's shoulder in 0-degree abduction and the elbow in 90 degrees of flexion, and with the subject's shoulder in 90-degree abduction and the elbow in 90 degrees of flexion. Intrarater and interrater reliability for all measurements was calculated using ICCs, with SEMs and MDC_{90} also reported. Intrarater reliability for all measurements in all positions, regardless of the instrument used, was above 0.91, with the exception of the measurement of passive medial rotation by one examiner using the smartphone inclinometer application (ICC = 0.79) and the measurement of passive medial rotation by one examiner using the goniometer (ICC = 0.89). SEMs ranged from 1.86 degrees for measurement of active medial rotation with the smartphone inclinometer application, to 7.61 degrees for the measurement of active lateral rotation with the shoulder in 0-degree abduction using the goniometer. The highest interrater reliabilities were reported for active shoulder lateral rotation measured with the goniometer with the shoulder in 90-degree abduction (ICC = 0.87–0.91; SEM = 6.33–7.49 degrees; MDC_{90} = 15–17 degrees), followed by passive shoulder lateral rotation measured with the goniometer with the shoulder in 90-degree abduction (ICC = 0.88–0.90; SEM = 6.83–7.71 degrees; MDC_{90} = 16–18 degrees), passive shoulder lateral rotation measured with the smartphone inclinometer application with the shoulder in 90-degree abduction (ICC = 0.89–0.90; SEM = 7.15–7.34 degrees; MDC_{90} = 17 degrees), and active shoulder lateral rotation measured with the smartphone inclinometer application with the shoulder in 90-degree abduction (ICC = 0.87; SEM = 7.76–7.80 degrees; MDC_{90} = 18 degrees). The lowest interrater reliabilities

were reported for measurements of active and passive medial rotation measured with either instrument. Intraclass correlation coefficients for these measurements ranged from 0.63 to 0.68, with SEMs ranging from 10.29 to 11.70 degrees and MDC_{90} ranging from 24 to 27 degrees.

Werner et al.[22] also compared the reliability of measurements of medial and lateral rotation using a goniometer, a smartphone inclinometer, and visual estimation. Bilateral measurements of medial and lateral rotation were taken in 24 healthy college students and in 15 subjects 6–12 weeks after they had total shoulder replacement surgery. Additional details of the study have been described previously. Measurements of lateral rotation were taken with the subject supine and the shoulder in 0-degree and 90-degree abduction, while medial rotation was measured only with the shoulder in 90-degree abduction (subject supine). ROM was visually estimated before measuring motion with either the goniometer or the smartphone inclinometer. No additional details were provided about the procedures used during ROM measurements with either device. The authors reported ICCs and SEM values for interrater reliability for all measurements across all three methods of assessing ROM. The interrater reliability of lateral rotation in healthy subjects using all five raters was highest with the smartphone inclinometer, regardless of the testing position (ICC = 0.86, SEM = 4 degrees), followed by the goniometer (0-degree abduction: ICC = 0.78, SEM = 13 degrees; 90-degree abduction: ICC = 0.83, SEM = 4 degrees), and then visual estimation (0-degree abduction: ICC = 0.74, SEM = 12 degrees; 90-degree abduction: ICC = 0.57, SEM = 19 degrees). Reliability between raters was higher in postsurgical subjects, where only two experienced examiners performed the measurements. As with the healthy subjects, interrater reliability was highest in postsurgical subjects with the smartphone inclinometer (0-degree abduction: ICC = 0.85, SEM = 9 degrees; 90-degree abduction: ICC = 0.88, SEM = 0.1 degrees), although reliability using the goniometer (0-degree abduction: ICC = 0.73, SEM = 10 degrees; 90-degree abduction: ICC = 0.84, SEM = 1 degree) and visual estimation were similar (0-degree abduction: ICC = 0.79, SEM = 3 degrees; 90-degree abduction: ICC = 0.81, SEM = 6 degrees).

Six additional groups of investigators examined the reliability of measurements of passive shoulder or glenohumeral rotation ROM using an inclinometer.[12,20,21,24,25,33] The details of most of these studies have been presented previously (see previous sections on the shoulder). In the study by de Winter et al.,[24] the subjects were positioned supine with the shoulder in 0-degree abduction and the elbow in 90 degrees of flexion for measurements of lateral rotation. Interrater reliability was assessed using ICCs, and 95% limits of agreement also were reported. Reliability (ICC) for measurement of lateral rotation on the affected side was 0.90 with a limit of agreement of 4.6 ± 18.8 degrees. For the nonaffected side, reliability was 0.56 and limit of agreement was 6.6 ± 18.62 degrees.[24]

Dougherty et al.[12] investigated the reliability of measurements of passive lateral rotation in healthy adults using two testing positions (supine with the shoulder in 0-degree abduction and in 90-degree abduction). They also measured medial rotation with the shoulder in 90-degree abduction. Measurements were made with a digital inclinometer, and ICCs and SEMs for intrarater reliability were reported. Intrarater reliability for measurement of lateral rotation in 0-degree abduction was lower (ICC=0.28, SEM=8.4 degrees) than for measurements taken in 90-degree abduction (ICC=0.66, SEM=12.1 degrees). Intrarater reliability for measurements of medial rotation (ICC=0.64, SEM=10.6 degrees) were similar to that for lateral rotation in 90-degree abduction.

The reliability of glenohumeral rotation measurements with the subjects in different testing positions also was examined by Kevern et al.[33] These investigators measured passive medial and lateral rotation with the subjects in either a supine or side-lying position. Measurements made with the subjects supine were done with or without the application of passive overpressure at the end of the motion. All measurements were taken in National Collegiate Athletic Association Division I baseball and softball players by two examiners who were physical therapists. Each examiner was trained on the measurement techniques before data collection. Scapular motion was monitored via palpation of the coracoid process, and the inclinometer was positioned on the dorsum of the forearm just proximal to the ulnar styloid process. The authors reported intrarater and interrater reliability for the measurements (see Tables 7.5 and 7.6). Intrarater reliability was high, regardless of the position used for the measurements (ICCs=0.94–0.99). Interrater reliability was lower, with ICCs ranging from 0.54 for measurements of medial rotation with passive overpressure to 0.77 for measurements of lateral rotation without passive overpressure.

Sharma et al.[25] measured passive shoulder medial and lateral rotation in subjects with adhesive shoulder capsulitis with the subjects supine and in 45 degrees shoulder abduction using a gravity inclinometer. They reported only interrater reliability, with values ranging from 0.69 to 0.83 in the non affected extremity and 0.89–0.91 in the affected extremity for lateral rotation. Values for medial rotation ranged from 0.63 to 0.78 for the non affected extremity and from 0.85 to 0.89 for the affected extremity.[25]

Positioning of the subjects' shoulders was not described in the two studies by de Jong et al.[20,21] In both of these the authors reported the ICC, SEM, and SDD for motions measured at three separate time points. For the 2007 study, ICCs ranged from 0.94 to 0.99, with the SEM ranging from 2.42 to 3.53 degrees and SDD (or MDC) ranging from 6.71 to 9.78 degrees. In the 2012 study, the investigators reported overall reliability, which

they defined as reliability of the examiners over all measurement sessions, and data for observers, which they defined as differences between examiners in a single measurement session. The overall ICC for shoulder lateral rotation was 0.94, with an overall SEM of 5.9 degrees and SDD (MDC) of 16.3 degrees. The SEM and SDD for a single measurement session was reported as 2.0 degrees and 5.4 degrees, respectively.

Active

Several groups have examined the intrarater reliability of goniometric measurements of active shoulder and glenohumeral rotation.[3,11,30]. The study by Walker et al.[11] included four healthy adults, Greene and Wolf[3] examined 20 healthy adults, and Fieseler et al.[30] measured shoulder rotation in 22 female handball players and 25 male and female volunteers. Relative reliability for all studies was good to high, while absolute reliability, reported as SEM by the Fieseler et al. study[30], ranged from 1.07 to 1.14 degrees for medial rotation and from 2.08–2.16 for lateral rotation (see Table 7.5).

The reliability of goniometric measurements of active shoulder lateral rotation only was examined by Boone et al.[34] in a group of 12 adult males aged 26–54 years. Four different examiners with varied experience in goniometry performed the measurements using AAOS measurement techniques. Measurements were taken once per week for 4 weeks by each of the four examiners. Average intrarater reliability was 0.96 (see Table 7.5), and repeated measures analysis of variance (ANOVA) revealed no significant intratester variation for measurements of shoulder lateral rotation. However, although average interrater reliability was 0.97 (see Table 7.6), repeated measures ANOVA demonstrated significant differences between two of the four examiners for measurements of shoulder lateral rotation.

In a study described previously (see Section "Active Shoulder Flexion/Extension"), Hayes et al.[4] examined both intrarater and interrater reliability of active shoulder lateral rotation goniometry. Measurements were taken in two separate groups of patients with symptomatic shoulder pathology. Lateral rotation measurements were taken with the shoulder positioned in 0 degrees abduction. Investigators reported an ICC of 0.67 for intrarater reliability (see Table 7.5) and 0.64 for interrater reliability (see Table 7.6). In both instances 95% CIs were 28 degrees.

Three groups of investigators compared the reliability of measurements of either active or active assistive shoulder rotation using a goniometer compared with another device. Each of these studies[2,5,7] has been described previously, and investigators reported reliability of active[2,5] or active assistive[7] shoulder medial and lateral rotation range of motion measurements. Mullaney et al.[7] compared measurements taken with a universal goniometer and a digital construction level, Kolber and Hanney[5] compared measurements taken with a 12-in. goniometer and a digital inclinometer, and Correll and colleagues[2] compared measurements taken with a universal goniometer and an inclinometer (HALO). All reported relative reliability using the ICC (see Tables 7.5 and 7.6), and two of the studies[2,5] reported absolute reliability. Kolber and Hanney[5] reported SEMs ranging from 0.98 and 2 degrees, respectively for measurements of lateral rotation taken with the inclinometer, to 0.94 and 3 degrees for measurements of lateral rotation taken with the goniometer. Correll and colleagues[2] reported SEMs for medial rotation of 5.7 degrees for the Halo inclinometer and 5.2–5.5 degrees for the goniometer. For lateral rotation, SEMs were 4.2–4.3 degrees for the Halo inclinometer and 4.0–4.2 degrees for the goniometer. This group also reported MDC values (cited in the article as "smallest real difference") ranging from a low of 11.1 degrees when measuring lateral rotation with a goniometer to a high of 15.9 degrees when measuring medial rotation with the Halo inclinometer.

In a recently published study, Mitchell et al.[36] compared the reliability of measurements of active shoulder lateral rotation using a universal goniometer with measurements obtained using two smartphone applications: GetMyROM, which is an inclinometer-based application, and DrGoniometer, a photo-based method of measuring ROM. The study was conducted in 94 healthy young adults using four examiners: two DPT students (novice examiners) and two examiners with at least 15 years of experience (expert examiners). For all three devices, intrarater reliability was determined for the novice examiners and interrater reliability was determined between novice and expert examiners. In addition, concurrent validity between each of the two smartphone applications and the universal goniometer was calculated using the measurements of the novice examiners. Intrarater reliability was similar for all three devices (GetMyROM, 0.79; DrGoniometer, 0.81; goniometer, 0.82), as was interrater reliability (GetMyROM, 0.94; DrGoniometer, 0.92; goniometer, 0.91). Both smartphone applications showed high concurrent validity with the universal goniometer, with ICCs of 0.4 and 0.93 for the GetMyROM and DrGoniometer, respectively.

Several groups of investigators, have examined active shoulder rotation ROM using an inclinometer.[13,14,16–18,31,32] Four of these studies included the examination of reliability of shoulder rotation measurements in healthy adults.[16,18,31,32] Only healthy subjects were included in all studies in this group except Valentine and Lewis[18] who examined subjects with and without shoulder pathology. Measurement techniques differed among the studies. Kolber et al.[16] measured shoulder lateral rotation with subjects supine and shoulder medial rotation with subjects prone, while Furness et al.[31] measured both motions in prone and in supine, and Walker et al.[32] measured both motions only in supine. In all three of these studies, the shoulders were abducted to 90 degrees and the elbow flexed to 90 degrees.[16,31,32] Alternatively, Valentine and Lewis measured both medial and lateral rotation with the subject in a standing position with the shoulder in 0 degrees abduction and the elbow flexed to 90 degrees.[18] All of these studies reported intrarater reliability using ICCs and SEMs, and two of the studies also reported MDC values.[31,32] Kolber et al.[16] and Walker et al.[32] also reported data for interrater reliability. Intrarater reliability was high and similar across all studies (see Tables 7.5 and 7.6).

The remaining studies examining reliability of measurements of active shoulder rotation using an inclinometer all focused exclusively on subjects with shoulder pathology.[13,14,17] Each of these studies has been described previously. Both Green et al.[14] and Tveitå et al.[17] measured shoulder rotation with the subjects supine. Tveitå[17] positioned the subject's shoulder in 45 degrees abduction with the elbow flexed to 90 degrees and measured both active shoulder and passive glenohumeral rotation. Green[14] positioned the patient's shoulder in either 0-degree or 90-degree abduction with the elbow flexed to 90 degrees for measurements of lateral rotation. Medial rotation was measured with the shoulder in 45 degrees abduction with the elbow flexed to 90 degrees. Similar intrarater reliability for measurements of the affected shoulder was reported by both groups. Tveitå et al.[17] reported ICCs of 0.77 for shoulder medial rotation, 0.81 for glenohumeral medial rotation, 0.91 for shoulder lateral rotation, and 0.91 for glenohumeral lateral rotation. Green et al.[14] reported ICCs of 0.79–0.82 for shoulder medial rotation, 0.85–0.93 for lateral rotation with the shoulder in 0 degrees abduction, and 0.75–0.82 for lateral rotation with the shoulder in 90 degrees abduction. Interrater reliability was also reported by Green et al.[14] and was highest for measurements of lateral rotation with the shoulder in 0 degrees adduction (ICC = 0.85–0.95), and lowest for measurements of medial rotation (ICC = 0.41–0.48).

Geertzen et al.[13] examined only measurements of lateral shoulder ROM using a goniometer and reported both intrarater and interrater reliability. Reliability of measurements of the affected shoulder in subjects with reflex sympathetic dystrophy ranged from 0.85 to 0.89 for intrarater reliability and from 0.76 to 0.83 for interrater reliability.

Elbow Flexion/Extension

Active

Several groups of researchers have investigated the reliability of elbow flexion and extension goniometry. The majority of studies on the reliability of measuring elbow flexion ROM involve measurements of active elbow flexion. In contrast, reports of reliability of elbow extension goniometry include about equal numbers of measurements of active and passive joint motion.

Armstrong et al.[37] examined intrarater and interrater reliability of active elbow and forearm goniometric measurements in a group of 38 patients aged 14–72 years. Each of the subjects had undergone a surgical procedure for an injury to the elbow, the forearm, or the wrist a minimum of 6 months before measurement. Standardized measuring techniques and patient positioning were used during the testing, in which three different instruments were employed to assess ROM. The instruments used for the study included a universal goniometer, a computerized goniometer, and "a mechanical rotation measuring device."[37] Only the universal goniometer and the computerized goniometer were used to measure elbow flexion and extension, because the rotation measuring device was capable only of measuring forearm rotation. Active elbow flexion and extension ROM were measured twice for each instrument on all subjects. Five different examiners who had varying amounts of experience in performing goniometry measured the amount of elbow flexion and extension in each subject. Both intrarater and interrater reliability were analyzed using ICCs. Intrarater reliability for active elbow flexion using the universal goniometer ranged from 0.55 to 0.98, depending on which examiner performed the measurements (Table 7.7). Similar intrarater reliability levels were obtained for active elbow extension, ranging from 0.45 to 0.98 (see Table 7.7). Of interest is the fact that the lowest reliability levels were produced by an experienced hand therapist, while less experienced examiners demonstrated higher reliability. Within raters, 95% CIs averaged 6 degrees for elbow flexion and 7 degrees for elbow extension. Interrater reliability for elbow flexion using the universal goniometer was reported as 0.58 and 0.62, depending on which set of measurements was used for the analysis. Elbow extension interrater reliability using the universal goniometer was reported as 0.58 and 0.87 (Table 7.8), again depending on which set of measurements was used for the analysis. Between raters, 95% CIs averaged 10 degrees for both elbow flexion and extension.

Individuals with established elbow contractures were used to examine the interrater reliability and validity of visual estimation of elbow ROM compared with goniometric measurements.[43] The motion in 50 elbows in 43 adults with established elbow contractures was evaluated by four examiners (elbow surgeon, physician assistant, clinical fellow, and study coordinator). Visual estimates of ROM were made before measurements with the goniometer. All measurements were performed with the subject standing and the shoulder in 90 degrees flexion. Goniometer alignment techniques were left to the individual examiners. Interrater reliability of all measurements was reported using ICCs. Validity was reported using Bland–Altman analysis. Reliability of goniometric measurements was high between all

examiners (ICCs = 0.94–0.98), with the exception of comparisons between an experienced examiner and the study coordinator (ICCs = 0.76–0.86). Reliability of visual estimates was somewhat lower among experienced examiners (ICCs = 0.87–0.96), and much lower when comparisons were made between experienced examiners and the study coordinator (ICCs = 0.38–0.53). Agreement between visual estimates and goniometric measurements was highest for the elbow surgeon, with ICC scores of 0.97 for flexion and extension and 95% limits of agreement of −7 to 9 degrees for extension and −6 to 7 degrees for flexion. The authors concluded that the human eye is capable of accurately estimating ROM and that this ability is dependent on the experience of the examiner.[43]

Goodwin et al.[41] also used a variety of examiners and instruments in their study of the reliability of measurements of active elbow flexion ROM. These investigators compared the reliability of the universal goniometer, of a fluid goniometer, and of an electrogoniometer using three experienced examiners measuring a group of 24 healthy females, aged 18–31 years. Active elbow flexion was measured in each subject on two separate occasions by all three examiners using each of the three instruments. Standardized measurement techniques and patient positioning were employed by all three examiners in all subjects. Test–retest reliability for each examiner using each type of measuring device was calculated using both Pearson's r and the ICC. Reliabilities for the universal goniometer ranged from 0.61 to 0.92 using Pearson's r and from 0.56 to 0.91 using ICCs, depending on which of the three examiners performed the measurements (see Table 7.7).

As part of a study investigating the validity and reliability of inertial sensors in measuring active elbow, forearm, and wrist range of motion, Costa and colleagues[39] compared ROM measurements obtained from 29 asymptomatic adults using inertial sensors to those obtained using a universal goniometer. Elbow flexion was measured with subjects standing in the anatomical position. Intrarater and interrater reliability of both methods of measurement were investigated as part of the study. Relative reliability was reported using ICCs, and absolute reliability was reported via the MDC_{90}. Intrarater reliability of goniometric measurement of elbow flexion ranged from 0.75 to 0.86 with MDC values of 8–14 degrees (see Table 7.7). Interrater reliability ranged from 0.86 to 0.92 with MDC values from 8 to 9 degrees (see Table 7.8).

Chapleau et al.[38] compared goniometric measurements to radiographic measurements of joint ROM of the elbow in 51 healthy adults to assess the validity of the goniometric measurements. In addition, they calculated the reliability of both methods using ICCs and 95% CIs. Measurements of ROM and radiographs of elbow motion were taken with subjects in the same position. Subjects were seated with the shoulder flexed (degrees not indicated) and the forearm in

Table 7.7 INTRARATER RELIABILITY: ELBOW FLEXION/EXTENSION ROM

ELBOW FLEXION

STUDY	TECHNIQUE	n	SAMPLE	r*	ICC[†]
Armstrong et al.[37]	AROM; standardized technique	38	Patients (14–72 years)		0.55–0.98[§]
Boone et al.[34]	AROM; AAOS technique	12	Healthy adult males (26–54 years)		0.94
Chapleau et al.[38]	AROM; seated with shoulder in anterior flexion; standardized technique; distal landmark midline of wrist; 1 examiner (MD); 3 trials per elbow	51 (102 elbows)	Healthy adults (31 F, 20 M) (19–50 years; $\bar{x}=31.7\pm9.3$ years)		0.945
Costa et al.[39]	AROM; standing in anatomical position; compared goniometer (G) to inertial sensors (IS); 2 examiners (PTs)	29	Healthy adults (9 F, 20 M) (F $\bar{x}==21.33\pm1.50$, M $\bar{x}=24.10\pm3.86$)		0.75–0.86 (G) 0.79–0.83 (IS)
Fieseler et al.[30]	AROM; supine; humerus stabilized against body; compared throwing arm (TA) and non-throwing arm (NTA)	47	Female handball athletes (HB) ($\bar{x}=21.0\pm3.7$ years) Healthy adults (HA) (13 F, 12 M) ($\bar{x}=21.9\pm1.2$ years)		0.96 (TA, HA) 0.95 (NTA, HA) 0.82 (TA, HB) 0.79 (NTA, HB)
Geertzen et al.[13]	AROM; standing with forearm in neutral rotation; distal landmark midline of wrist; standardized technique; affected (A) and nonaffected (NA) extremities tested using goniometer; 2 experienced examiners	29	Adults with reflex sympathetic dystrophy (19 F, 10 M) ($\bar{x}=49.1\pm13.3$ years)		0.84 (A) 0.66–0.84 (NA)
Golden et al.[40]	AROM; seated or standing with shoulder adducted and in approximately 45° flexion; elbow, wrist, and IP joints extended; 1 examiner; 3 measurements per elbow; first measurement compared with average of the three	35 (70 elbows)	Healthy children (2–18 years)		0.94
Goodwin et al.[41]	AROM; standardized technique	23	Healthy females (18–31 years)	0.61–0.92[‡]	0.56–0.91[‡]
Greene and Wolf[3]	AROM; technique not described	20	Healthy adults (18–55 years)		0.94
Macedo and Magee[6]	PROM; supine; upper extremity in anatomical position	12	Healthy Caucasian females (18–59 years) ($\bar{x}=37.2$ years)		0.90
Rothstein et al.[42]	PROM; nonstandardized technique	12	Patients; no ages provided	0.95–0.99[‖]	0.86–0.96[‖]
Walker et al.[11]	AROM; AAOS technique	4	Healthy adults; no ages provided	>0.81	

ELBOW EXTENSION

STUDY	TECHNIQUE	n	SAMPLE	r*	ICC[†]
Armstrong et al.[37]	AROM; standardized technique	38	Patients (14–72 years)		0.45–0.98[§]
Chapleau et al.[38]	AROM; seated with shoulder in anterior flexion; standardized technique; distal landmark midline of wrist; 1 examiner (MD); 3 trials per elbow	51 (102 elbows)	Healthy adults (31 F, 20 M) (19–50 years) ($\bar{x}=31.7\pm9.3$ years)		0.973
Fieseler et al.[30]	AROM; supine; humerus stabilized against body; compared throwing arm (TA) and non-throwing arm (NTA)	47	Female handball athletes (HB) ($\bar{x}=21.0\pm3.7$ years) Healthy adults (HA) (13 F, 12 M) ($\bar{x}=21.9\pm1.2$ years)		0.87 (TA, HA) 0.95 (NTA, HA) 0.82 (TA, HB) 0.80 (NTA, HB)
Geertzen et al.[13]	AROM; standing with forearm in neutral rotation; distal landmark midline of wrist; standardized technique; affected (A) and nonaffected (NA) extremities tested using goniometer; 2 experienced examiners	29	Adults with reflex sympathetic dystrophy (19 F, 10 M) ($\bar{x}=49.1\pm13.3$ years)		0.90–0.92 (A) 0.88 (NA)
Golden et al.[40]	AROM; seated or standing; with shoulder adducted and in approximately 45° flexion; elbow, wrist, and IP joints extended; 1 examiner; 3 measurements per elbow; first measurement compared with average of the three	35 (70 elbows)	Healthy children (2–18 years)		0.96
Greene and Wolf[3]	AROM; technique not described	20	Healthy adults (18–55 years)		0.95
Macedo and Magee[6]	PROM; supine; upper extremity in anatomical position	12	Healthy Caucasian females (18–59 years) ($\bar{x}=37.2$ years)		0.88
Pandya et al.[23]	PROM; AAOS technique	150	Patients with Duchenne muscular dystrophy (<1–20 years)		0.87
Rothstein et al.[42]	PROM; nonstandardized technique	12	Patients; no ages provided	0.95–0.99″	0.94–0.96″
Walker et al.[11]	AROM; AAOS technique	4	Healthy adults; no ages provided	>0.81	

AAOS, American Academy of Orthopaedic Surgeons; *AROM*, active ROM; *PROM*, passive ROM.
*Pearson's r.
[†]Intraclass correlation coefficient.
[‡]Three separate examiners.
[§]Five separate examiners.
[‖]Correlation depended on type of goniometer used.

Table 7.8   INTERRATER RELIABILITY: ELBOW FLEXION/EXTENSION ROM

STUDY	TECHNIQUE	n	SAMPLE	r*	ICC[†]
ELBOW FLEXION					
Armstrong et al.[37]	AROM; standardized technique	38	Patients (14–72 years)		0.58/0.62[‡]
Boone et al.[34]	AROM; AAOS technique	12	Healthy adult males (26–54 years)		0.88
Blonna et al.[43]	AROM; standing with shoulder flexed to 90°, forearm fully supinated; compared goniometry (G) to visual estimation (VE); 4 examiners; 3 "experts" (EE), 1 novice (NE)	43 (50 elbows)	Adults with established elbow contractures (18–85 years; $\bar{x}=51$ years)		0.96–0.98 (G; EE) 0.81–0.86 (G; NE) 0.87–0.93 (VE; EE) 0.38–0.53 (VE; NE)
Costa et al.[39]	AROM; standing in anatomical position; compared goniometer (G) to inertial sensors (IS); 2 examiners (PTs)	29	Healthy adults (9 F, 20 M) (F $\bar{x}=21.33\pm1.50$, M $\bar{x}=24.10\pm3.86$)		0.86–0.92 (G) 0.95–0.97 (IS)
Escalante et al.[19]	PROM; supine; standardized technique	24	Ambulatory adults (65–80 years)		0.84
Geertzen et al.[13]	AROM; standing with forearm in neutral rotation; distal landmark midline of wrist; standardized technique; affected (A) and nonaffected (NA) extremities tested using goniometer; 2 experienced examiners	29	Adults with reflex sympathetic dystrophy (19 F, 10 M) ($\bar{x}=49.1\pm13.3$ years)		0.57–0.72 (A) 0.64–0.75 (NA)
Petherick et al.[44]	AROM; standardized technique	30	Healthy adults (mean age 24 years)		0.53
Rothstein et al.[42]	PROM; nonstandardized technique	12	Patients; no ages provided	0.95–0.99″	0.94–0.96″
ELBOW EXTENSION					
Armstrong et al.[37]	AROM; standardized technique	38	Patients (14–72 years)		0.58/0.87[†]
Blonna et al.[43]	AROM; standing with shoulder flexed to 90°, forearm fully supinated; compared goniometry (G) to visual estimation (VE); 4 examiners; 3 "experts" (EE), 1 novice (NE)	43 (50 elbows)	Adults with established elbow contractures (18–85 years; $\bar{x}=51$ years)		0.94–0.98 (G; EE) 0.76–0.78 (G; NE) 0.91–0.96 (VE; EE) 0.51–0.52 (VE; NE)
de Jong et al.[20]	PROM; supine; standardized technique; affected extremity tested using "hydrogoniometer" (gravity inclinometer); 2 examiners (PTs); subjects tested at baseline and at 5 and 10 weeks	19	Adults after CVA of middle cerebral artery (9 F, 10 M) ($\bar{x}=54\pm10$ years)		0.78–0.97 (GI)
de Jong et al.[21]	PROM; supine; standardized technique; affected extremity tested using "hydrogoniometer" (gravity inclinometer); 2 examiners (PTs); subjects tested at baseline and at 4, 8, and 20 weeks	38–43	Adults after CVA (20 F, 28 M) ($\bar{x}=57.8\pm11.9$ years)		0.89–0.95 (GI)
Geertzen et al.[13]	AROM; standing with forearm in neutral rotation; distal landmark midline of wrist; standardized technique; affected (A) and nonaffected (NA) extremities tested using goniometer; 2 experienced examiners	29	Adults with reflex sympathetic dystrophy (19 F, 10 M) ($\bar{x}=49.1\pm13.3$ years)		0.68–0.73 (A) 0.70–0.78 (NA)
Pandya et al.[23]	PROM; AAOS technique	150	Patients with Duchenne muscular dystrophy (<1–20 years)		0.91
Rothstein et al.[42]	PROM; nonstandardized technique	12	Patients; no ages provided		0.92–0.96[†]

AAOS, American Academy of Orthopedic Surgeons; *AROM,* active ROM; *CVA,* cerebrovascular accident; *PROM,* passive ROM.

*Pearson's (r).

[†]Intraclass correlation coefficient.

[‡]See text for further explanation.

neutral. Measurements of ROM using the goniometer were found to be slightly lower using radiographic measurement than with the goniometer for both elbow flexion (150.9 degrees ±4.5 for radiography vs 153.5 degrees ±3.5 for goniometry) and extension (11.9 degrees ±6.7 for radiography vs 13.0 degrees ±6.5 for goniometry). For extension, 95% of goniometric measurements were within 10.3 degrees of radiographic measures. For flexion, 95% of goniometric measurements were within 7.0 degrees of radiographic measures. Intrarater reliability for ROM measurements using the goniometer was 0.945 with a 95% CI of 0.905–0.985 for elbow flexion, and 0.973 with a 95% CI of 0.958–0.990 for elbow extension.

Golden et al.[40] examined the intrarater reliability of elbow flexion and extension ROM using a goniometer as part of a larger study in which they compared elbow ROM to body mass index (BMI) in a group of 113 healthy children. The first 35 of the children who enrolled served as the pool of subjects for the reliability study. Measurements were made with the subjects either seated or standing with the shoulder adducted and flexed (degrees not indicated). Intrarater reliability was calculated using the Pearson correlation coefficient and was reported as 0.94 for elbow flexion and 0.96 for elbow extension.[40]

Several other groups of researchers, whose studies have been described previously, have investigated the reliability of measurements of active elbow flexion and extension.[3,11,13] Fieseler et al.,[30] Greene and Wolf,[3] Geertzen et al.,[13] and Walker et al.[11] all examined the intrarater reliability of active elbow flexion and extension goniometry in healthy adults. Reliability was analyzed using either Pearson's r[11] or the ICC.[3] Fieseler et al.[30] found ICCs ranging from 0.80 to 0.96 and SEM values ranging from 0.98 to 1.59 in their study of handball players and healthy controls (see Table 7.7). Geertzen et al.[13] and Walker et al.[11] reported reliability as greater than 0.81 (see Table 7.7), with a mean error of 5 degrees. Greene and Wolf[3] reported reliability of 0.94 for elbow flexion and 0.95 for elbow extension (see Table 7.7), with 95% CIs of 3.0 degrees for elbow flexion and 1.9 degrees for elbow extension. Geertzen et al.[13] reported ICCs and SDDs for intrarater and interrater reliability of measures of active elbow flexion and extension using a goniometer in patients with reflex sympathetic dystrophy. The authors reported ICCs of 0.66–0.84 for elbow flexion and higher reliability (0.88–0.92) for elbow extension, depending on whether the affected or unaffected extremity was tested (see Table 7.7). ICCs for interrater reliability were 0.57–0.75 for elbow flexion and 0.68–0.78 for elbow extension, again depending on whether the affected or unaffected extremity was measured (see Table 7.8).[13] Smallest detectable differences for elbow flexion were 7.1 degrees for elbow flexion of the non-affected side and 9.6 degrees for the affected side. For elbow extension, the SDD was 12.1 degrees, regardless of the side being measured.

The reliability (intrarater and interrater) of goniometric measurements of active elbow flexion ROM was examined by Boone et al.[34] in a group of 12 healthy males aged 26–54 years. Measuring techniques advocated by the AAOS were used in the study. Average intrarater reliability was 0.94 (see Table 7.7), and repeated measures of ANOVA revealed no significant intratester variation for measurements of elbow flexion. Although average interrater reliability was 0.88 (see Table 7.8), repeated measures of ANOVA demonstrated significant differences among all four of the examiners for measurements of elbow flexion.

One other group of researchers examined the reliability of active elbow flexion goniometry, but this group confined their investigation to interrater reliability of this motion. Petherick et al.[44] compared the interrater reliability of active elbow flexion measurements taken with the universal goniometer with those taken with a "fluid-based goniometer" (inclinometer) in a group of 30 healthy subjects, with a mean age of 24 years. Two examiners measured active elbow flexion in each subject three times with both instruments. Standardized measuring techniques and patient positioning were used during the testing procedure. The mean of the three measurements was used to calculate the ICC for each instrument. Intrarater reliability was not reported for either of the two examiners. Interrater reliability using the universal goniometer to measure active elbow flexion was reported as 0.53 (see Table 7.8), whereas reliability using the inclinometer was 0.92. The reliability level using the universal goniometer was similar to that reported by Armstrong et al.[37] but lower than that reported by Boone et al[36] (see Table 7.8).

Passive

Although the majority of the studies examining the reliability of measurements of passive elbow motion have focused on passive elbow extension, fewer researchers have investigated the reliability of goniometric measurements of passive elbow flexion ROM.[19,23,42] Rothstein et al.[42] measured passive elbow flexion and extension in 12 patients of unstated age using three different commonly used goniometers. Twelve different examiners performed the measurements, although measurements in any one patient were done by only two different examiners. Data were analyzed using both Pearson's r and the ICC. Intrarater reliability ranged from 0.86 to 0.99 for elbow flexion and from 0.94 to 0.98 for elbow extension (see Table 7.7). Interrater reliability ranged from 0.85 to 0.97 for elbow flexion and from 0.92 to 0.96 for elbow extension (see Table 7.8). In the case of both intrarater and interrater reliability levels, values obtained were dependent on the type of goniometer used and the type of statistical analysis performed. Additionally, interrater reliability levels were dependent on which measurement was used for comparison purposes (first measurement, second measurement, or mean).

As part of the San Antonio Longitudinal Study of Aging, 695 subjects underwent evaluation of passive elbow flexion ROM.[19] Before collecting the data, the four examiners who took ROM measurements participated in a preliminary investigation to determine interrater reliability of elbow flexion goniometry. A group of 24 adults aged 65–80 years had passive elbow flexion ROM measured by four examiners using a universal goniometer. All measurements were taken with the subjects positioned supine, and a standardized measurement protocol was followed. ICC was calculated and reported as 0.84 for elbow flexion.

Reliability of passive elbow extension but not of flexion was investigated in a pediatric population by Pandya et al.[23] AAOS techniques were used to measure passive elbow extension with the universal goniometer. Intrarater reliability of passive elbow extension measurements was analyzed on 150 subjects with Duchenne muscular dystrophy, and interrater reliability was analyzed in a subgroup of 21 of those subjects. In this group of children with muscular dystrophy, intrarater reliability was 0.87 (see Table 7.7) and interrater reliability was 0.91 (see Table 7.8).

In two separate studies, de Jong et al.[20,21] examined the reliability of measurements of passive elbow extension ROM in patients at various points following stroke, using a gravity-based inclinometer. Details of these two studies have been described previously (see Section "Shoulder Complex and Glenohumeral Flexion/Extension"). The authors reported interrater reliability for each study using ICCs, SEMs, and smallest detectable differences (SDD, equivalent in this case to MDC). For the 2007 study, ICCs ranged from 0.78 to 0.97, with SEM ranging from 2.32 to 4.86 degrees and SDD (or MDC) ranging from 6.43 to 13.47 degrees.[20] Authors in the 2012 study reported "overall" reliability, which they defined as reliability of the examiners over all measurement sessions, and data for observers, which they defined as differences between examiners in a single measurement session. The overall ICC for elbow extension was 0.92, with overall SEM at 2.4 degrees and SDD (MDC) at 6.8 degrees. The SEM and SDD for a single measurement session was reported as 1.0 degree and 2.7 degrees, respectively.[21]

Macedo and Magee[6] also examined intrarater reliability of elbow flexion and extension ROM (in additional to the reliability of several other joint ROM measurements) as part of a larger study of changes in ROM with age in healthy adult females. Reliability was tested in 12 subjects before initiation of the larger study. A single examiner measured passive elbow flexion and extension ROM along with 28 additional movements twice within a 6-h period using standardized measurement techniques. Measurements were conducted with the subjects in a supine position with the shoulder in 0 degrees flexion and a pad positioned under the humerus so that it was level with the acromion process. ICCs were 0.98 for elbow flexion and 0.88 for elbow extension (see Table 7.7).

Forearm Pronation/Supination

Some investigators who examined the reliability of goniometric measurements of elbow flexion and extension also examined the reliability of goniometric measurements of forearm pronation and supination. Three studies were found that investigated the reliability of passive forearm ROM.[6,20,21] In two separate studies, de Jong et al.[20,21] examined the reliability of measurements of passive forearm supination ROM using a gravity-based inclinometer in patients at various points after a stroke. Details of these two studies have been described previously (see Section "Shoulder Complex and Glenohumeral Flexion/Extension"). The authors reported interrater reliability for each study using ICCs, SEMs, and smallest detectable differences (SDD, equivalent in this case to MDC). For the 2007 study, ICCs ranged from 0.94 to 0.98, with SEM ranging from 3.02 to 4.42 degrees and SDD (or MDC) ranging from 8.37 to 12.25 degrees. Authors in the 2012 study reported "overall" reliability, which they defined as reliability of the examiners over all measurement sessions, and data for observers, which they defined as differences between examiners in a single measurement session. The overall ICC for forearm supination was 0.89, with overall SEM at 4.9 degrees and SDD (MDC) at 13.8 degrees. The SEM and SDD for a single measurement session was reported as 2.2 degrees and 6.2 degrees, respectively.

As part of an investigation of the effects of age on passive ROM in women, Macedo and Magee[6] calculated ICCs for intrarater reliability of passive forearm pronation and supination ROM. Details of this study have been described previously (see Section "Shoulder Complex and Glenohumeral Flexion/Extension"). Intrarater reliability for measurements of forearm supination were higher (ICC = 0.95, SEM = 3 degrees, MDC = 7 degrees) than for measures of forearm pronation (ICC = 0.84, SEM = 3, MDC = 9 degrees) (Table 7.9).[6]

Both Greene and Wolf[3] and Walker et al.[11] examined the intrarater reliability of active forearm pronation and supination in healthy adults. In their study comparing the reliability of the universal goniometer and the Ortho Ranger (see the more complete description of the study in Section "Shoulder Flexion/Extension"), Greene and Wolf[3] measured active forearm pronation and supination in 20 healthy subjects aged 18–55 years. Data were analyzed using the ICC, and intrarater reliability was 0.90 for forearm pronation and 0.98 for forearm supination (see Table 7.9). For forearm pronation and supination, 95% CIs were 9.1 degrees and 8.2 degrees, respectively. Walker et al[11] measured active forearm pronation and supination in a group of four healthy adults and obtained intrarater reliability levels of greater than 0.81 and a mean error of 5 degrees for both measurements using Pearson's r (see Table 7.9).

Both intrarater and interrater reliability of active forearm pronation and supination were investigated by Armstrong et al.[37] in a group of 38 subjects aged 14–72 years. Each subject had undergone a surgical procedure to the upper extremity a minimum of 6 months before measurement. Three separate instruments and five examiners were used in the study (see the full description in Section "Elbow Flexion/Extension").

Table 7.9	INTRARATER RELIABILITY: FOREARM PRONATION/SUPINATION ROM				
STUDY	**TECHNIQUE**	**n**	**SAMPLE**	**r***	**ICC†**
Armstrong et al.[37]	AROM; standardized technique	38	Patients (14–72 years)		0.96–0.99‡
Colaris et al.[45]	AROM; elbow positioned against chest to prevent shoulder and elbow motions; elbow flexed to 90°; forearm and wrist in neutral; 3 measurements repeated twice by 1 observer; goniometer; standardized technique	47	Children within 2 years after forearm fracture (13 F, 34 M) (6–16 years) ($\bar{x}$ = 11.1 ± 3.1 years)		0.73–0.96
Costa et al.[39]	AROM; seated with elbow flexed at 90° on support surface, hand protruding off support surface in neutral; compared goniometer (G) to inertial sensors (IS); 2 examiners (PTs)	29	Healthy adults (9 F, 20 M) (F $\bar{x}$ = 21.33 ± 1.50, M $\bar{x}$ = 24.10 ± 3.86)		0.62–0.74 (G) 0.86–0.89 (IS)
Flowers et al.[46]	PROM; compared traditional goniometry (TM) to newly designed plumbline goniometer (NM) for forearm pronation and supination; 3 examiners (therapists experienced in hand therapy)	30 (31 wrists)	Adults with orthopedic conditions of the hand, wrist, or forearm (15 F, 15 M) (21–79 years)		0.87 (NM) 0.79 (TM)
Gajdosik[47]	AROM; 3 standardized testing methods; seated, R arm adducted to trunk, elbow flexed to 90°, forearm neutral	31	Nondisabled adults (19–40 years)		0.81–0.97 (within session) 0.86–0.96 (between sessions)
Greene and Wolf[3]	AROM; technique not described	20	Healthy adults (18–55 years)		0.90
Karagiannopoulos et al.[48]	AROM; hand-held pencil method; seated with knees and hips flexed to 90°, feet flat on the floor; ipsilateral arm fully adducted, elbow flexed to 90°; forearm unsupported and neutral	40	Adults: 20 injured (ages 31–80 years) 20 noninjured (20–74 years)		0.95/0.97§ 0.86/0.98§
	AROM; plumbline goniometer method; patient position not described	40	Adults: 20 injured (ages 31–80 years) 20 noninjured (20–74 years)		0.96/0.98§ 0.95/0.97§
Macedo and Magee[6]	PROM; supine; shoulder in 0° flexion; extension, and abduction; flexion; extension, elbow in 90° flexion	12	Healthy Caucasian females (18–59 y) ($\bar{x}$ = 37.2 years)		0.84
Walker et al.[11]	AROM; AAOS technique	4	Healthy adults; no ages provided	>0.81	
	FOREARM SUPINATION				
Armstrong et al.[37]	AROM; standardized technique	38	Patients (14–72 years)		0.96–0.99‡
Colaris et al.[45]	AROM; elbow positioned against chest to prevent shoulder and elbow motions; elbow flexed to 90°; forearm and wrist in neutral; 3 measurements repeated twice by 1 observer; goniometer; standardized technique	47	Children within 2 years after forearm fracture (13 F, 34 M) (6–16 years) ($\bar{x}$ = 11.1 ± 3.1 years)		0.80–0.97
Costa et al.[39]	AROM; seated with elbow flexed at 90° on support surface, hand protruding off support surface in neutral; compared goniometer (G) to inertial sensors (IS); 2 examiners (PTs)	29	Healthy adults (9 F, 20 M) (F $\bar{x}$ = 21.33 ± 1.50, M $\bar{x}$ = 24.10 ± 3.86)		0.91–0.96 (G) 0.92–0.96 (IS)

Continued

	Table 7.9	INTRARATER RELIABILITY: FOREARM PRONATION/SUPINATION ROM—cont'd				
STUDY	**TECHNIQUE**	**n**	**SAMPLE**	**r***	**ICC[†]**	
		FOREARM SUPINATION—cont'd				
Flowers et al.[46]	PROM; compared traditional goniometry (TM) to newly designed plumbline goniometer (NM) for forearm pronation and supination; 3 examiners (therapists experienced in hand therapy)	30 (31 wrists)	Adults with orthopedic conditions of the hand, wrist, or forearm (15 F, 15 M) (21–79 years)		0.95 (NM) 0.95 (TM)	
Gajdosik[47]	AROM; 3 standardized testing methods; seated, R arm adducted to trunk, elbow flexed to 90°, forearm neutral	31	Nondisabled adults (19–40 years)		0.81–0.97 (within session) 0.86–0.96 (between sessions)	
Geertzen et al.[13]	AROM; standing with forearm in neutral rotation; distal landmark midline of wrist; standardized technique; affected (A) and nonaffected (NA) extremities tested using goniometer; 2 experienced examiners	29	Adults with reflex sympathetic dystrophy (19 F, 10 M) ($\bar{x}$ = 49.1 ± 13.3 years)		0.57–0.72 (A) 0.64–0.75 (NA)	
Geertzen et al.[13]	AROM; standing with heels and back against the wall; standardized technique; affected (A) and nonaffected (NA) extremities tested using digital inclinometer (DI); 2 experienced examiners	29	Adults with reflex sympathetic dystrophy (19 F, 10 M) ($\bar{x}$ = 49.1 ± 13.3 years)		0.92–0.93 (A, DI) 0.92–0.94 (NA, DI)	
Greene and Wolf[3]	AROM; technique not described	20	Healthy adults (18–55 years)		0.98	
Karagiannopoulos et al.[48]	AROM; hand-held pencil method; Patient seated with knees and hips flexed to 90°, feet flat on the floor; ipsilateral arm fully adducted, elbow flexed to 90°; forearm unsupported and neutral	40	Adults: 20 injured (ages 31–80 years) 20 noninjured (20–74 years)		0.98/0.98[d] 0.96/0.96[d]	
	AROM; plumbline goniometer method; patient position not described	40	Adults: 20 injured (ages 31–80 years) 20 noninjured (20–74 years)		0.98/0.98[d] 0.94/0.98[d]	
Macedo and Magee[6]	PROM; supine; shoulder in 0° flexion; extension, and abduction; flexion; extension, elbow in 90° flexion	12	Healthy Caucasian Females (18–59 years) ($\bar{x}$ = 37.2 years)		0.95	
Walker et al.[11]	AROM; AAOS technique	4	Healthy adults; no ages provided	>0.81		

AAOS, American Academy of Orthopaedic Surgeons; *AROM,* active ROM.
*Pearson's r.
[†]Intraclass correlation coefficient.
[‡]Five separate examiners.
[§]Two separate examiners.

Intrarater reliability for the universal goniometer ranged from 0.96 to 0.99 for both active forearm pronation and supination motions, depending on the examiner performing the measurement (see Table 7.9). Interrater reliability was slightly lower for the two measurements, with reliability coefficients reported as 0.83 and 0.86 for forearm pronation and 0.90 and 0.93 for forearm supination, depending on which set of measurements was used for the analysis (Table 7.10). Within raters, 95% CIs averaged 8 degrees for both forearm pronation and supination, whereas CIs between raters averaged 10 degrees for pronation and 11 degrees for supination.

Costa et al.,[39] whose study has been described previously, compared the intrarater and interrater reliability of measurements of active forearm pronation and supination using a universal goniometer and wearable inertial sensors. Intrarater reliability of forearm pronation measurements using the goniometer ranged from ICCs of 0.62–0.74 with MDC$_{90}$ values ranging from 19 to 23 degrees. Values for forearm supination ranged from ICCs of 0.91 to 0.96 with MDC$_{90}$ values from 10 to 14 degrees (see Table 7.9). Interrater reliability was higher with ICC ranging from 0.83 to 0.93 for forearm pronation and from 0.91 to 0.95 for supination. MDC$_{90}$ values

Table 7.10 INTERRATER RELIABILITY: FOREARM PRONATION/SUPINATION ROM

FOREARM PRONATION

STUDY	TECHNIQUE	n	SAMPLE	ICC*
Armstrong et al.[37]	AROM; standardized technique	38	Patients (14–72 years)	0.83/0.86[†]
Cimatti et al.[49]	AROM; 2 experienced examiners; standardized goniometric methods with (w HHP) and without (w/o HHP) a hand-held pencil; seated, arm adducted to trunk, elbow flexed to 90°, forearm neutral	33	Healthy subjects: HS ($n = 20$) and subjects with previous elbow trauma: IS ($n = 13$)	0.76 (HS; w HHP) 0.92 (HS; w/o HHP) 0.93 (IS; w HHP) 0.94 (IS; w/o HHP)
Colaris et al.[45]	AROM; elbow positioned against chest to prevent shoulder and elbow motions; elbow flexed to 90°; forearm and wrist in neutral; 3 measurements repeated twice by 1 observer; used a goniometer (G) standardized technique and visual estimation (VE)	47	Children within 2 years after forearm fracture (13 F, 34 M) (6–16 years) ($\bar{x} = 11.1 \pm 3.1$ years)	0.65–0.92 (G) 0.77–0.87 (VE)
Costa et al.[39]	AROM; seated with elbow flexed at 90° on support surface, hand protruding off support surface in neutral; compared goniometer (G) to inertial sensors (IS); 2 examiners (PTs)	29	Healthy adults (9 F, 20 M) (F $\bar{x} = 21.33 \pm 1.50$, M $\bar{x} = 24.10 \pm 3.86$)	0.83–0.93 (G) 0.94–0.95 (IS)
Karagiannopoulos et al.[48]	AROM; hand-held pencil method; seated with knees and hips flexed to 90°, feet flat on the floor; ipsilateral arm fully adducted, elbow flexed to 90°; forearm unsupported and neutral	40	Adults: 20 injured (ages 31–80 years) 20 noninjured (20–74 years)	0.95 0.92
	AROM; plumbline goniometer method; patient position not described	40	Adults: 20 injured (31–80 years) 20 noninjured aged (20–74 years)	0.92 0.91

FOREARM SUPINATION

STUDY	TECHNIQUE	n	SAMPLE	ICC*
Armstrong et al.[37]	AROM; standardized technique	38	Patients (14–72 years)	0.90/0.93[†]
Cimatti et al.[49]	AROM; 2 experienced examiners; standardized goniometric methods with (w HHP) and without (w/o HHP) a hand-held pencil; seated, arm adducted to trunk, elbow flexed to 90°, forearm neutral	33	Healthy subjects: HS ($n = 20$) and subjects with previous elbow trauma: IS ($n = 13$)	0.92 (HS; w HHP) 0.95 (HS; w/o HHP) 0.97 (IS; w HHP) 0.97 (IS; w/o HHP)
Colaris et al.[45]	AROM; elbow positioned against chest to prevent shoulder and elbow motions; elbow flexed to 90°; forearm and wrist in neutral; 3 measurements repeated twice by 1 observer; used a goniometer (G) standardized technique and visual estimation (VE)	47	Children within 2 years after forearm fracture (13 F, 34 M) (6–16 years) ($\bar{x} = 11.1 \pm 3.1$ years)	0.63–0.96 (G) 0.70–0.89 (VE)
Costa et al.[39]	AROM; seated with elbow flexed at 90° on support surface, hand protruding off support surface in neutral; compared goniometer (G) to inertial sensors (IS); 2 examiners (PTs)	29	Healthy adults (9 F, 20 M) (F $\bar{x} = 21.33 \pm 1.50$, M $\bar{x} = 24.10 \pm 3.86$)	0.91–0.95 (G) 0.96–0.97 (IS)
de Jong et al.[20]	PROM; supine; standardized techniques; affected extremity tested using "hydrogoniometer" (gravity inclinometer); 2 examiners (PTs); subjects tested at baseline and at 5 and 10 weeks	19	Adults after CVA of middle cerebral artery (9 F, 10 M) ($\bar{x} = 54 \pm 10$ years)	0.94–0.98 (GI)
de Jong et al.[21]	PROM; supine standardized techniques; affected extremity tested using "hydrogoniometer" (gravity inclinometer); 2 examiners (PTs); subjects tested at baseline and at 4,8, and 20 weeks	38–43	Adults after CVA (20 F, 28 M) ($\bar{x} = 57.8 \pm 11.9$ years)	0.84–0.93 (GI)
Geertzen et al.[13]	AROM; standing with heels and back against the wall; standardized technique; affected and nonaffected (NA) extremities tested using digital inclinometer (DI); 2 experienced examiners	29	Adults with reflex sympathetic dystrophy (19 F, 10 M) ($\bar{x} = 49.1 \pm 13.3$ years)	0.92–0.93 (A, DI) 0.85–0.91 (NA, DI)
Karagiannopoulos et al.[48]	AROM; hand-held pencil method; seated with knees and hips flexed to 90°, feet flat on the floor; ipsilateral arm fully adducted, elbow flexed to 90°; forearm unsupported and neutral	40	Adults: 20 injured (31–80 years) 20 noninjured (20–74 years)	0.96 0.94
	AROM; plumbline goniometer method; patient position not described	40	Adults: 20 injured (31–80 years) 20 noninjured (20–74 years)	0.96 0.96

AROM, Active ROM; *CVA,* cerebrovascular accident.
*Intraclass correlation coefficient.
[†]See text for further information.

ranged from 11 to 14 degrees for pronation and from 10 to 14 degrees for supination (see Table 7.10).

Colaris et al.[45] compared the reliability of measurements of active forearm pronation and supination using conventional goniometry and visual estimation. Subjects consisted of 47 children aged 6–16 years who had a forearm fracture within the previous 2 years. Two examiners (graduate students who had been trained in pediatric goniometry by the primary investigator) visually estimated pronation and supination ROM in each subject and also measured each motion six times (two sessions of three measurements each) using a universal goniometer. Results of the three measurements for each session were averaged and the averages used to calculate ICCs for intrarater and interrater reliability. The authors also reported smallest detectable difference (SDD). Intrarater reliability, calculated only for the goniometric method, was high (pronation: ICC = 0.94, SDD = 7 degrees; supination: ICC = 0.93, SDD = 6 degrees). Interrater reliability was calculated for both methods and was generally higher for the goniometric method, for which SDDs also were lower. Results for pronation included an ICC of 0.89 with an SDD of 10 degrees when using a goniometer, while visual estimation for this motion yielded an ICC of 0.82 and an SDD of 26 degrees (see Table 7.9). Similarly, measurement of supination using a goniometer produced an interrater reliability of 0.84 with an SDD of 10 degrees, while visual estimation of this motion resulted in interrater reliability of 0.75 and an SDD of 16 degrees (see Table 7.10).

Geertzen et al.,[13] whose study has been described previously, examined intrarater and interrater reliability of forearm supination using a digital inclinometer in a group of adults with reflex sympathetic dystrophy. Both the affected and nonaffected arms of these subjects were measured by two separate examiners. The authors reported ICCs of 0.92–0.93 for both intrarater and interrater reliability for the affected extremity. Levels of intrarater reliability for the nonaffected extremity ranged from 0.92 to 0.94 while interrater reliability was slightly lower, ranging from 0.85 to 0.91. In addition to ICCs, these investigators reported SDDs of 19.3 degrees for the affected side and 16.5 degrees for the nonaffected side.[13]

All previously described studies involving forearm ROM measured pronation and supination by positioning the goniometer along the distal forearm as described in this text (see Chapter 4). However, other sources recommend measuring forearm rotation by aligning the goniometer with a pencil or other rod-like object held in the subject's hand.[46] Several groups of investigators have investigated the reliability of this measurement method.[46–49] Flowers et al.[46] examined the intrarater reliability of measurements of passive pronation and supination ROM using a newly developed "plumb line" goniometer (PLG). Measurements were taken by three examiners experienced in hand

therapy in subjects with orthopedic conditions of the hand, wrist, or forearm. In addition to measurements taken using the PLG, measurements also were taken using a standard goniometer, and the reliability of the two methods was compared. Results demonstrated higher reliability using the PLG when measuring pronation (ICC = 0.87, SEM = 6 degrees) than when using the standard goniometer (ICC = 0.79, SEM = 7 degrees). Reliability for measurements of supination was higher and basically identical for the two instruments (PLG: ICC = 0.95. SEM = 4 degrees; standard goniometer: ICC = 0.95, SEM = 4 degrees).[46]

Karagiannopoulos et al.[48] compared the intrarater and interrater reliability of two different methods of measuring active forearm rotation: the hand-held pencil (HHP) method and the PLG method. The HHP method involved having the subject hold a pencil in the closed fist with the pencil extending from the radial aspect of the subject's fist. The arms of the goniometer were aligned parallel to the pencil and perpendicular to the floor, with the axis positioned over the head of the third metacarpal. The PLG method involved the use of a single-arm goniometer modified to include a handle attached perpendicular to the arm and a plumb line attached to the center of the scale. Active forearm pronation and supination were measured using both devices in two groups of 20 subjects each, one group with elbow, forearm, or hand trauma and the other group free of pathology. Two examiners measured forearm pronation and supination three times with each testing method on each subject during a single testing session. Each examiner was a novice regarding the two testing methods but received formal training and practice in each of the methods before the study. Both ICCs and SEMs were calculated on the data. Intrarater reliability was based on the second and third trials of each motion for each tester, while the mean of the three trials was used to calculate interrater reliability. Intrarater reliability for the HHD method ranged from 0.86 to 0.98 for pronation and from 0.96 to 0.98 for supination, depending on the examiner and the group measured. For the PLG method, intrarater reliability ranged from 0.95 to 0.98 for pronation and from 0.94 to 0.98 for supination. Interrater reliability was 0.91 or above for both methods, regardless of the motion measured (HHP 0.92–0.96; PLG 0.91–0.96).

Other studies have also examined the HHP method of measuring forearm rotation. Cimatti et al.[49] measured forearm pronation and supination ROM in 33 injured (n = 13) and non-injured (n = 20) individuals. Using both the HHP method and the goniometric method described in this text (see Chapter 4). Two experienced examiners performed three measurements each of active forearm pronation and supination range of motion using each of the two methods. Interrater reliability (ICC) was calculated using the means of the three measurements and ranged from a low of 0.76 for measurements of forearm pronation in injured subjects using the HHD method to a high of 0.97 for measurements of forearm supination in both injured and non-injured individuals using the method described in this text (see Table 7.10).

Gajdosik[47] determined the intrarater reliability of three different goniometric methods of measuring active pronation and supination ROM in a group of 31 healthy subjects (21 F, 10 M) aged 19–40 years. Method 1 consisted of measuring forearm rotation using the same HHP method used by Karagiannopoulos et al.[48] Forearm rotation measurements using Method 2 occurred as described in this text (see Chapter 4) while in Method 3, the moving arm of the goniometer was aligned with "a visualized line connecting the distal aspects of the ulna and radius."[47] For all three methods the stationary arm of the goniometer was aligned parallel to the midline of the humerus. Forearm pronation and supination ROM measurements were taken three times each for each method during a single testing session. A second identical testing session took place 1 h later. ICCs were calculated for intrarater reliability both within each session and between the two sessions and ranged from 0.81 to 0.97 (see Table 7.9). An analysis of variance was used to determine differences between the amount of motion measured using each of the methods. The author reported that significantly less pronation and significantly more supination were measured using the HHP method than when using the other two methods. Increases in supination measured using the HHP method were attributed to observed movements of the fourth and fifth metacarpals. The author concluded that while all three methods displayed good intrarater reliability, the HHP method was inappropriate for clinical use because of the questionable validity of supination measurement.

Wrist Flexion/Extension

Passive

LaStayo and Wheeler[50] coordinated a multicenter study that focused on the reliability of three different methods of performing goniometric measurement of passive wrist flexion and extension. They recruited 140 patients aged 6–81 years from eight different clinical sites around the United States. Thirty-two examiners from the eight clinics performed the goniometric measurements. In each of the clinics participating in the study, examiners were randomly paired for purposes of determining interrater reliability. Passive wrist flexion and extension were measured twice in each subject by each member of the randomly chosen pair of examiners, using three different measuring techniques. The three techniques used for measuring passive wrist motion included positioning the goniometer: (1) along the radial side of the forearm, with the stationary arm aligned with the "radial midline of the forearm" and the moving arm

aligned with the "longitudinal axis of the second metacarpal"; (2) along the ulnar side of the forearm, with the stationary arm aligned with the "longitudinal midline of the ulna toward the olecranon" and the moving arm aligned with the "longitudinal axis of the third metacarpal"; and (3) along the dorsal (for flexion) or volar (for extension) surface of the wrist, with the stationary arm aligned with the dorsal or volar surface of the forearm and the moving arm aligned with the "longitudinal axis of the third metacarpal."[50] The ICC was used to analyze the data for both intrarater and interrater reliability. Intrarater reliability ranged from 0.80 for measurements of passive wrist extension using ulnar or radial alignment to 0.92 for measurements of passive wrist flexion using dorsal alignment (Table 7.11). The SEM for wrist flexion within examiners ranged from 5.48 to 9.68 degrees for the radial alignment technique, from 5.52 to 9.10 degrees for the ulnar alignment technique, and from 4.11 to 7.12 degrees for the dorsal alignment technique, depending on the clinic in which the measurements were taken. For wrist extension, the SEM within examiners ranged from 6.60 to 9.98 degrees using the radial alignment technique, from 6.29 to 10.58 degrees using the ulnar alignment technique, and from 3.87 to 9.20 degrees using the volar alignment technique, again depending on the clinic in which the measurements were taken. Interrater reliability ranged from 0.80 for measurements of passive wrist extension using radial or ulnar alignment, to 0.93 for measurements of passive wrist flexion using dorsal alignment. The SEM for wrist flexion between examiners ranged from 4.74 to 9.28 degrees for the radial alignment technique, from 4.67 to 8.85 degrees for the ulnar alignment technique, and from 4.59 to 6.50 degrees for the dorsal alignment technique. For wrist extension, the SEM between examiners ranged from 6.36 to 11.16 degrees using the radial alignment technique, from 6.29 to 11.33 degrees using the ulnar alignment technique, and from 3.53 to 9.20 degrees using the volar alignment technique. As was the case for the SEM within examiners, variations in the SEM were dependent on the clinic in which the measurements were taken. The authors concluded that the dorsal-volar alignment technique was "the most reliable method both within and between testers for measurements of passive wrist flexion and extension."[50]

Carter et al.[51] performed a study similar to the one performed by LaStayo and Wheeler[50] but used cadaver wrists rather than patients. Two experienced examiners, a hand therapist and a hand surgeon, measured passive wrist flexion and extension ROM in 10 cadaver wrists using the same 3 different measuring techniques used in the study by LaStayo and Wheeler.[50] Goniometric measurements were compared with fluoroscopic measurement of wrist position to examine validity of the goniometric measurements. Intrarater and interrater reliability of the goniometric measurements was reported using ICCs. Accuracy of the goniometric

Table 7.11	INTRARATER RELIABILITY: WRIST FLEXION/EXTENSION ROM				

WRIST FLEXION

STUDY	TECHNIQUE	n	SAMPLE	r*	ICC†
Carter et al.[51]	PROM; 3 standardized techniques (radial, ulnar, and dorsal volar goniometer alignment) with forearm in neutral rotation; 2 raters (hand surgeon, hand therapist)	10	Cadaver wrists; no ages provided		0.8–1.0—Ulnar 0.8–0.9—Radial 1.0—Dorsal volar
Costa et al.[39]	AROM; seated with forearm supported and pronated; compared goniometer (G) to inertial sensors (IS); 2 examiners (PTs)	29	Healthy adults (9 F, 20 M) (F $\bar{x}=21.33\pm1.50$, M $\bar{x}=24.10\pm3.86$)		0.93 (G) 0.91–0.93 (IS)
Geertzen et al.[13]	AROM; seated with forearm supported and pronated; standardized technique; affected (A) and nonaffected (NA) extremities tested using digital inclinometer (DI). 2 experienced examiners	29	Adults with reflex sympathetic dystrophy(19 F, 10 M) ($\bar{x}=49.1\pm13.3$ years)		0.93–0.94 (A, DI) 0.66–0.90 (NA, DI)
Greene and Wolf [3]	AROM; technique not described	20	Healthy adults (18–55 years)		0.96
Horger[52]	AROM; nonstandardized technique	48	Patients (18–71 years)		0.96
	PROM; nonstandardized technique	48	Patients (18–71 years)		0.96
Macedo and Magee[6]	PROM; standardized technique; seated with shoulder in 90° abduction, elbow flexed to 90°, forearm neutral and supported with hand over edge of table	12	Healthy Caucasian females (18–59 years) ($\bar{x}=37.2$ years)		0.83
LaStayo and Wheeler[50]	PROM; radial alignment	140	Patients (6–81 years)		0.86
	PROM; ulnar alignment	140	Patients (6–81 years)		0.87
	PROM; dorsal alignment	140	Patients (6–81 years)		0.92
Walker et al.[11]	AROM; AAOS technique	4	Healthy adults; no ages provided	>0.81	

WRIST EXTENSION

STUDY	TECHNIQUE	n	SAMPLE	r*	ICC†
Carter et al.[51]	PROM; 3 standardized techniques (radial, ulnar, and dorsal volar goniometer alignment) with forearm in neutral rotation; 2 raters (hand surgeon, hand therapist)	10	Cadaver wrists; no ages provided		0.5—Ulnar 0.3—Radial 0.9—Dorsal volar
Costa et al.[39]	AROM; seated with forearm supported and pronated; compared goniometer (G) to inertial sensors (IS); 2 examiners (PTs)	29	Healthy adults (9 F, 20 M) (F $\bar{x}=21.33\pm1.50$, M $\bar{x}=24.10\pm3.86$)		0.84–0.89 (G) 0.82–0.89 (IS)
Geertzen et al.[13]	AROM; seated with forearm supported and pronated; standardized technique; affected (A) and nonaffected (NA) extremities tested using digital inclinometer (DI). 2 experienced examiners	29	Adults with reflex sympathetic dystrophy(19 F, 10 M) ($\bar{x}=49.1\pm13.3$ years)		0.87–0.96(A, DI) 0.80–0.86 (NA, DI)
Greene and Wolf [3]	AROM; technique not described	20	Healthy adults (18–55 years)		0.94
Horger[52]	AROM; nonstandardized technique	48	Patients (18–71 years)		0.96
	PROM; nonstandardized technique	48	Patients (18–71 years)		0.96
LaStayo and Wheeler[50]	PROM; radial alignment	140	Patients (6–81 years)		0.80
	PROM; ulnar alignment	140	Patients (6–81 years)		0.80
	PROM; volar alignment	140	Patients (6–81 years)		0.84
Macedo and Magee[6]	PROM; standardized technique; seated with shoulder in 90° abduction, elbow flexed to 90°, forearm neutral and supported with hand over edge of table	12	Healthy Caucasian females (18–59 years) ($\bar{x}=37.2$ years)		0.85
Pandya et al.[23]	PROM; AAOS technique; patient supine	150	Patients with Duchenne muscular dystrophy (<1–20 years)		0.87
Walker et al.[11]	AROM; AAOS technique	4	Healthy adults; no ages provided	>0.81	

AAOS, American Academy of Orthopaedic Surgeons; *AROM,* active ROM; *PROM,* passive ROM.
*Pearson's *r*.
†Intraclass correlation coefficient.

measurements compared with the fluoroscopic measurements was reported using root mean squared error (RMSE) and mean deviation. The authors reported intrarater reliability for goniometric measurements of wrist flexion and extension together and found high intrarater reliability in all three measuring positions, ranging from 0.8 to 0.9 for measurements using radial alignment to 1.0 for measurements using dorsal-volar alignment. Lower values of interrater reliability were reported (0.3–0.9), with the highest reliability again found when using the dorsal-volar alignment technique. However, when reporting accuracy of the three techniques, the dorsal-volar technique yielded slightly higher RMSE values (8 degrees) than did the other two techniques (7 degrees for each).[51]

In an earlier study, Horger[52] compared intrarater and interrater reliability of goniometric measurements of active compared with passive wrist motion. Thirteen examiners, with a range of experience from 2 months to 17 years, participated in the study. Both active and passive wrist motions were measured twice each by two randomly paired examiners in 48 patients aged 18–71 years. No specific method of patient positioning or measuring technique was used during the study. The ICC was used to analyze the data, and results are reported in Tables 7.11 and 7.12. Intrarater reliability was high (0.96) and did not vary regardless of the motion (flexion compared with extension) or type of motion (active compared with passive) measured. The SEM within raters was 3.5 degrees and 4.4 degrees for passive wrist extension and flexion, respectively, whereas the SEM for active motions was 3.7 degrees for extension and 4.5 degrees for flexion. Levels of interrater reliability were slightly lower (0.84–0.91) and tended to be slightly higher for wrist flexion than for wrist extension. The SEM between raters for passive wrist motions was 7.0 degrees for extension and 8.2 degrees for flexion. For active motion, the SEM between raters was 7.0 degrees for extension and 6.6 degrees for flexion.

A fourth group of investigators, whose work has been described previously (see Section "Shoulder Abduction"), examined the reliability of goniometric measurements of passive wrist motion, but this group measured wrist extension and not flexion.[23] Both intrarater and interrater reliability of goniometric measurements of passive wrist extension were investigated in groups of 150 and 21 patients, respectively, with Duchenne muscular dystrophy. Techniques advocated by the AAOS were used in the study, and intrarater reliability was 0.87 (see Table 7.11), while interrater reliability was 0.83 (see Table 7.12).

In another study described previously (see Section "Shoulder Complex and Glenohumeral Flexion/ Extension"), Macdeo and Magee[6] examined intrarater reliability of goniometric measurements of passive wrist flexion and extension. Measurements were taken with the goniometer aligned along the ulnar surface

of the forearm. Intrarater reliability for wrist flexion (ICC = 0.83, SEM = 3.9 degrees, MDC = 10.7 degrees) was slightly lower than for wrist extension (ICC = 0.85, SEM = 2.9 degrees, MDC = 8.1 degrees) (see Table 7.11).

Active

Several groups of investigators in addition to Horger[52] (see Section "Passive Wrist Flexion/Extension") have reported intrarater reliability of active wrist motion measurements. Costa et al.,[39] Walker et al.,[11] Geertzen et al.,[13] and Greene and Wolf[3] have examined the intrarater reliability of goniometric measurements of active wrist flexion and extension. Healthy adults were used as the subjects in the studies by Costa et al.,[39] Walker et al.[11] and Greene and Wolf,[3] while Geertzen et al.[13] examined subjects with a diagnosis of reflex sympathetic dystrophy. All of these studies have been described previously (see Sections "Shoulder Complex and Glenohumeral Flexion/ Extension" and "Elbow Flexion/Extension"). Greene and Wolf[3] reported intrarater reliability levels that were quite similar to those reported by Horger[52] (see Table 7.11), with 95% CIs of 9.0 degrees for wrist flexion and 9.3 degrees for wrist extension. Intrarater reliability levels reported by Walker et al.[11] could not be precisely determined, being cited only as greater than 0.81 (see Table 7.11), with a mean error of 5 degrees. Costa et al.,[39] Geertzen et al.,[13] and Horger[52] reported both intrarater and interrater reliability for wrist flexion and extension. Costa et al.[39] reported intrarater reliability (ICC) of 0.93 with MDC_{90} values of 9–10 degrees for wrist flexion, and from 0.84 to 0.89 with MDC_{90} values of 10–12 degrees for wrist extension (see Table 7.11). For interrater reliability, ICCs ranged from 0.95 to 0.97 with MDC_{90} values of 7–8 degrees for wrist flexion and from 0.92 to 0.94 with MDC_{90} values of 8–9 degrees for wrist extension (see Table 7.12).

The results of the Horger study have been reported previously (see Section "Passive Wrist Flexion/ Extension"). Geertzen et al.[13] measured wrist motion using a digital inclinometer and reported values for intrarater reliability that were higher for the affected (wrist flexion 0.93–94; wrist extension 0.87–0.96) than the nonaffected side (wrist flexion 0.66–0.90; wrist extension 0.80–0.86). Interrater reliability exhibited the same pattern of higher reliability for measurements of the affected (wrist flexion 0.89–0.93; wrist extension 0.82–0.92) than for the nonaffected side (wrist flexion 0.76–0.78; wrist extension 0.68–0.70).

Wrist Abduction/Adduction

Both intrarater and interrater reliability of wrist abduction (radial deviation) and adduction (ulnar deviation) motions have been investigated by Costa et al.[39] and Horger,[52] and Boone et al.[34] have investigated intrarater and interrater reliability of wrist adduction measurements. These studies have been described previously

Table 7.12	INTERRATER RELIABILITY: WRIST FLEXION/EXTENSION ROM				
WRIST FLEXION					
STUDY	**TECHNIQUE**	**n**	**SAMPLE**	**ICC***	
Carter et al.[51]	PROM; 3 standardized techniques (radial, ulnar, and dorsal volar goniometer alignment) with forearm in neutral rotation; 2 raters (hand surgeon, hand therapist)	10	Cadaveric wrists; no ages provided	0.5—Ulnar 0.3—Radial 0.9—Dorsal volar	
Costa et al.[39]	AROM; seated with forearm supported and pronated; compared goniometer (G) to inertial sensors (IS); 2 examiners (PTs)	29	Healthy adults (9 F, 20 M) (F $\bar{x}=21.33\pm1.50$, M $\bar{x}=24.10\pm3.86$)	0.95–0.97 (G) 0.97–0.99 (IS)	
Geertzen et al.[13]	AROM; seated with forearm supported and pronated; standardized technique; affected (A) and nonaffected (NA) extremities tested using digital inclinometer (DI). 2 experienced examiners.	29	Adults with reflex sympathetic dystrophy(19 F, 10 M) ($\bar{x}=49.1\pm13.3$ years)	0.89–0.93 (A, DI) 0.76–0.78 (NA, DI)	
Horger[52]	AROM; nonstandardized technique	48	Patients (18–71 years)	0.91	
	PROM; nonstandardized technique	48	Patients (18–71 years)	0.86	
LaStayo and Wheeler[50]	PROM; radial alignment	140	Patients (6–81 years)	0.88	
	PROM; ulnar alignment	140	Patients (6–81 years)	0.89	
	PROM; volar alignment	140	Patients (6–81 years)	0.93	
WRIST EXTENSION					
Carter et al.[51]	PROM; 3 standardized techniques (radial, ulnar, and dorsal volar goniometer alignment) with forearm in neutral rotation; 2 raters (hand surgeon, hand therapist)	10	Cadaver wrists; no ages provided	0.8–1.0—Ulnar 0.8–0.9—Radial 1.0—Dorsal volar	
Costa et al.[39]	AROM; seated with forearm supported and pronated; compared goniometer (G) to inertial sensors (IS); 2 examiners (PTs)	29	Healthy adults (9 F, 20 M) (F $\bar{x}=21.33\pm1.50$, M $\bar{x}=24.10\pm3.86$)	0.92–0.94 (G) 0.93–0.97 (IS)	
Geertzen et al.[13]	AROM; seated with forearm supported and pronated; standardized technique; affected (A) and nonaffected (NA) extremities tested using digital inclinometer (DI). 2 experienced examiners.	29	Adults with reflex sympathetic dystrophy(19 F, 10 M) ($\bar{x}=49.1\pm13.3$ years)	0.82–0.92 (A, DI) 0.68–0.70 (NA, DI)	
Horger[52]	AROM; nonstandardized technique	48	Patients (18–71 years)	0.85	
	PROM; nonstandardized technique	48	Patients (18–71 years)	0.84	
LaStayo and Wheeler[50]	PROM; radial alignment	140	Patients (6–81 years)	0.80	
	PROM; ulnar alignment	140	Patients (6–81 years)	0.80	
	PROM; volar alignment	140	Patients (6–81 years)	0.84	
Pandya et al.[23]	PROM; AAOS technique; patient supine	21	Patients with Duchenne muscular dystrophy (<1–20 years)	0.83	

AAOS, American Academy of Orthopaedic Surgeons; *AROM*, active ROM; *PROM*, passive ROM.
*Intraclass correlation coefficient.

(see Section "Elbow Flexion/Extension" for Costa et al.,[39] Section "Wrist Flexion/Extension" for Horger,[52] and Section "Shoulder Medial/Lateral Rotation" for Boone et al.[34]) and involved different research protocols. Horger[53] used patients as subjects in her study and employed 13 examiners who measured both active and passive wrist motions without the use of a standardized technique. Boone et al.[34] and Costa et al.[39] used healthy adults as subjects in their studies and employed four and two examiners, respectively.

Costa et al.[39] reported intrarater reliability (ICC) ranging from 0.81 to 0.88 with MDC_{90} values of 8–10 degrees for wrist abduction, and from 0.81 to 0.85 with MDC_{90} values of 10–12 degrees for wrist adduction (see Table 7.13). For interrater reliability, ICCs ranged from 0.92 to 0.97 with MDC_{90} values of 4–6 degrees for wrist abduction and from 0.92 to 0.95 with MDC_{90} values of 6–7 degrees for wrist adduction (see Table 7.14).

Horger[52] reported intrarater reliability coefficients greater than or equal to 0.90 for goniometric measurements of active and passive wrist motions, with the exception of passive wrist adduction, where intrarater reliability was reported as 0.78 (Table 7.13). The SEM within raters reported in the Horger[52] study ranged from 2.6 degrees for active wrist abduction to 3.5 degrees for active wrist adduction. Intrarater reliability for goniometric measurements of active wrist adduction were higher in the Horger[52] study than in the study by Boone et al.[34] (0.92 and 0.76, respectively) (see Table 7.13), and ANOVA reported in the Boone et al.[34] study revealed significant intratester variation for one examiner in measurements of active wrist adduction. Although interrater reliability for measurements of active wrist adduction was similar between the two studies (Table 7.14), the ANOVA reported by Boone et al.[34] revealed significant intertester variation

Table 7.13 INTRARATER RELIABILITY: WRIST ABDUCTION (RADIAL DEVIATION)/WRIST ADDUCTION (ULNAR DEVIATION) ROM

WRIST ABDUCTION (RADIAL DEVIATION)

STUDY	TECHNIQUE	n	SAMPLE	r*	ICC†
Costa et al.[39]	AROM; seated with forearm and palm supported and pronated; compared goniometer (G) to inertial sensors (IS); 2 examiners (PTs)	29	Healthy adults (9 F, 20 M) (F $\bar{x}$ = 21.33 ± 1.50, M $\bar{x}$ = 24.10 ± 3.86)		0.81–0.88 (G) 0.83–0.88 (IS)
Geertzen et al.[13]	AROM; seated with forearm supported and pronated; standardized technique; affected (A) and nonaffected (NA) extremities tested using digital inclinometer (DI). 2 experienced examiners.	29	Adults with reflex sympathetic dystrophy(19 F, 10 M) ($\bar{x}$ = 49.1 ± 13.3 years)		0.65–0.73 (A, DI) 0.57 (NA, DI)
Greene and Wolf [3]	AROM; technique not described	20	Healthy adults (18–55 years)		0.91
Horger[52]	AROM; nonstandardized technique	48	Patients (18–71 years)		0.91
	PROM; nonstandardized technique	48	Patients (18–71 years)		0.90
Macedo and Magee[6]	PROM; standardized technique; seated with shoulder in 90° abduction, elbow flexed to 90°, forearm neutral, wrist neutral, forearm and hand supported	12	Healthy Caucasian females (18–59 years) ($\bar{x}$ = 37.2 years)		0.81
Walker et al.[11]	AROM; AAOS technique	4	Healthy adults; no ages provided	>0.81	

WRIST ADDUCTION (ULNAR DEVIATION)

STUDY	TECHNIQUE	n	SAMPLE	r*	ICC†
Boone et al.[34]	AROM; AAOS technique	12	Adult males (26–54 years)		0.76
Costa et al.[39]	AROM; seated with forearm and palm supported and pronated; compared goniometer (G) to inertial sensors (IS); 2 examiners (PTs)	29	Healthy adults (9 F, 20 M) (F $\bar{x}$ = 21.33 ± 1.50, M $\bar{x}$ = 24.10 ± 3.86)		0.81–0.85 (G) 0.81–0.87 (IS)
Geertzen et al.[13]	AROM; seated with forearm supported and pronated; standardized technique; affected (A) and nonaffected (NA) extremities tested using digital inclinometer (DI). 2 experienced examiners	29	Adults with reflex sympathetic dystrophy(19 F, 10 M) ($\bar{x}$ = 49.1 ± 13.3 years)		0.75–0.87 (A, DI) 0.70–0.73 (NA, DI)
Greene and Wolf[3]	AROM; technique not described	20	Healthy adults (18–55 years)		0.94
Horger[52]	AROM; nonstandardized technique	48	Patients (18–71 years)		0.92
	PROM; nonstandardized technique	48	Patients (18–71 years)		0.78
Macedo and Magee[6]	PROM; standardized technique; seated with shoulder in 90° abduction, elbow flexed to 90°, forearm neutral, wrist neutral, forearm and hand supported	12	Healthy Caucasian females (18–59 years) ($\bar{x}$ = 37.2 years)		0.86
Walker et al.[11]	AROM; AAOS technique	4	Healthy adults; no ages provided	>0.81	

AAOS, American Academy of Orthopedic Surgeons; *AROM,* active ROM; *PROM,* passive ROM.
*Pearson's *r*.
†Intraclass correlation coefficient.

in measurements of wrist adduction between two of the examiners. The SEM between examiners reported by Horger[52] ranged from 3.0 to 5.8 degrees for wrist abduction and adduction motions.

As they did for wrist flexion and extension motions, Greene and Wolf[3] and Walker et al.[11] used healthy adults to examine intrarater reliability of goniometric measurements of active wrist abduction and adduction ROM. Greene and Wolf[3] reported intrarater reliability of 0.91 and a 95% CI of 7.6 degrees for active wrist abduction and a reliability of 0.94 and 95% CI of 8.4 degrees for active wrist adduction. Walker et al.[11] reported reliability only as greater than 0.81, with a mean error of 5 degrees for both measurements (see Table 7.13).

In a study involving healthy adult women, Macedo and Magee[6] reported lower intrarater reliability

and higher SEM levels for passive wrist abduction (ICC = 0.81, SEM = 3.0 degrees, MDC = 8.3 degrees) and adduction (ICC = 0.86, SEM = 7.4 degrees, MDC = 20.6 degrees) than values reported by Horger (passive abduction: ICC = 0.91, SEM = 2.7 degrees; passive adduction: ICC = 0.94, SEM = 3.0 degrees) (see Table 7.13).[52] Geertzen et al.[13] reported intrarater and interrater reliability of active wrist abduction and adduction measurements in patients with reflex sympathetic dystrophy using a digital inclinometer. Intrarater reliability ranged from 0.57 for measurements of wrist abduction on the nonaffected side to 0.87 for measurements of wrist adduction on the affected side. Interrater reliability exhibited the same pattern of higher reliability for measurements of the affected side, with reliability for wrist adduction ranging from 0.60 on the nonaffected

Table 7.14	INTERRATER RELIABILITY: WRIST ABDUCTION (RADIAL DEVIATION)/WRIST ADDUCTION (ULNAR DEVIATION) ROM				
STUDY	**TECHNIQUE**	**n**	**SAMPLE**		**ICC***
Costa et al.[39]	AROM; seated with forearm and palm supported and pronated; compared goniometer (G) to inertial sensors (IS); 2 examiners (PTs)	29	Healthy adults (9 F, 20 M) (F $\bar{x}$ = 21.33 ± 1.50, M $\bar{x}$ = 24.10 ± 3.86)		0.92–0.97 (G) 0.96–0.97 (IS)
Geertzen et al.[13]	AROM; seated with forearm supported and in neutral rotation; standardized technique; affected (A) and nonaffected (NA) extremities tested using digital inclinometer (DI). 2 experienced examiners	29	Adults with reflex sympathetic dystrophy(19 F, 10 M) ($\bar{x}$ = 49.1 ± 13.3 years)		0.55–0.59 (A, DI)
Horger[52]	AROM; nonstandardized technique	48	Patients (18–71 years)		0.86
	PROM; nonstandardized technique	48	Patients (18–71 years)		0.66
WRIST ADDUCTION (ULNAR DEVIATION)					
Boone et al.[34]	AROM; AAOS technique	12	Adult males (26–54 years)		0.73
Costa et al.[39]	AROM; seated with forearm and palm supported and pronated; compared goniometer (G) to inertial sensors (IS); 2 examiners (PTs)	29	Healthy adults (9 F, 20 M) (F $\bar{x}$ = 21.33 ± 1.50, M $\bar{x}$ = 24.10 ± 3.86)		0.92–0.95 (G) 0.95–0.96 (IS)
Geertzen et al.[13]	AROM; seated with forearm supported and in neutral rotation; standardized technique; affected (A) and nonaffected (NA) extremities tested using digital inclinometer (DI). 2 experienced examiners.	29	Adults with reflex sympathetic dystrophy(19 F, 10 M) ($\bar{x}$ = 49.1 ± 13.3 years)		0.73–0.89 (A, DI) 0.60–0.76 (NA, DI)
Horger[52]	AROM; nonstandardized technique	48	Patients (18–71 years)		0.78
	PROM; nonstandardized technique	48	Patients (18–71 years)		0.83

AAOS, American Academy of Orthopedic Surgeons; *AROM*, active ROM; *PROM*, passive ROM.
*Intraclass correlation coefficient.

side to 0.89 on the affected side. (Interrater reliability of wrist abduction on the nonaffected side was not reported.)

Finger Motion

Active

A few studies were found that used statistical analysis to report reliability levels of discrete active ROM of the fingers. Groth et al.[53] investigated interrater reliability and concurrent validity of goniometric measurements of active proximal interphalangeal joint (PIP) and distal interphalangeal joint (DIP) flexion and extension. ROM measurements were taken from a single patient who had slight to significant decreases in motion in several joints of the fingers following a crush injury with multiple fractures. Thirty-nine examiners (29 occupational therapists and 10 physical therapists) with an average of 10 years of experience and 6 years of practice in hand therapy participated in the study. Each examiner measured active flexion and extension of the DIP and PIP joints of the fingers using both dorsal and lateral placements of the goniometer. Interrater reliability was determined by calculating ICCs on a random sample subgroup of 6 raters drawn from the 39 participants. Although reliability for individual joints was not provided, reliability for the two different goniometer placement methods was reported (see Table 7.16). While both measurement methods showed good reliability,

the dorsal method of goniometer placement demonstrated higher interrater reliability (ICC = 0.99) than did the lateral placement method (ICC = 0.86). The investigators were unable to determine concurrent validity because of significant differences in hand positioning used as part of the protocol for measuring ROM and that used during radiographs taken for comparison (gold standard).

Lewis et al.[54] examined intrarater and interrater reliability of active and passive flexion of the metacarpophalangeal (MCP), PIP, and DIP joints of the middle finger in 20 healthy adults with no history of hand or finger injuries. Seven therapists (six occupational therapists and one physical therapist) at a hand clinic served as examiners, with each examiner measuring each subject three times for all motions. Standardized positioning of the subjects was used, and all measurements were taken with the same type of goniometer using a dorsal placement technique. The authors calculated ICCs for each measurement by each examiner (intrarater reliability) and for each measurement across all examiners (interrater reliability). Intrarater reliability was highest for DIP flexion (ICC = 0.72–0.99), followed by PIP flexion (ICC = 0.43–0.94) and then MCP flexion (0.57–0.93) (Table 7.15). Measurements of active flexion were generally more reliable than measurements of passive flexion. Values for interrater reliability were lower than those for intrarater reliability, with interrater ICCs ranging from 0.24 to 0.88 (Table 7.16).

	Table 7.15 INTRARATER RELIABILITY: FINGER ROM			
STUDY	**TECHNIQUE**	**n**	**SAMPLE**	**ICC***
Brown et al.[55]	AROM; total active motion for digit; elbows rested on table, forearm and wrist in neutral.	30	Patients with upper extremity orthopedic injuries (21–66 years)	0.97–0.98[†]
Flowers and LaStayo[56]	PROM; PIP extension Patient position: hand rested, palm up, on the edge of the table with metacarpals and proximal phalanges as flat as possible.	20	Patients with fused PIP joints (18–84 years)	0.98
Lewis et al.[54]	AROM and PROM; MCP, PIP, and DIP flexion; seated, elbow supported forearm neutral, wrist extended 5°–15°; examiners (6 OTs, 1 PT); standardized goniometer placement	20	Adults with no hand or finger injuries (14 F, 6 M) ($\bar{x}$=45±15 years)	0.64–0.93 (AROM, MCP) 0.57–0.84 (PROM, MCP) 0.68–0.94 (AROM, PIP) 0.43–0.93 (PROM, PIP) 0.78–0.99 (AROM, DIP) 0.72–0.99 (PROM, DIP)
Macionis[57]	Static hand positions; dorsal method; used standard finger goniometer (SGn) and paper goniometer (PGn); measured flexion (F) and extension (E) at the MCP, PIP, and DIP of left ring finger; 2–10 examiners.	12	Healthy adults (20–24 years)	0.885–0.89 (MCP, E, SGn) 0.87–0.90 (MCP, E, PGn) 0.90–0.93 (MCP, F, SGn) 0.88–0.90 (MCP, F, PGn) 0.84–0.90 (PIP, E, SGn) 0.82–0.86 (PIP, E, PGn) 0.85–0.89 (PIP, F, SGn) 0.82–0.86 (PIP, F, PGn) 0.865–0.91 (DIP, E, SGn) 0.83–0.89 (DIP, E, PGn) 0.82–0.86 (DIP, F, SGn) 0.77–0.83 (DIP, F, PGn)

AROM, Active ROM; *PIP,* proximal interphalangeal; *PROM,* passive ROM; *UE,* upper extremity.
*Intraclass correlation coefficient.
[†]Three separate examiners.

	Table 7.16 INTERRATER RELIABILITY: FINGER ROM			
STUDY	**TECHNIQUE**	**n**	**SAMPLE**	**ICC***
Brown et al.[55]	AROM; total active motion for digit; elbows rested on table, forearm and wrist in neutral	30	Patients with upper extremity orthopedic injuries (21–66 years)	0.98
Engstrand et al.[58]	AROM; standardized technique; goniometer measurements of MCP flexion and extension, PIP flexion, DIP flexion, and total active flexion (TAF) and extension (TAE) using dorsal placement technique; 8 examiners (OTs with 6 or more years of experience)	13	Adults with Dupuytren disease (2 F, 11 M) ($\bar{x}$=73±7.2 years)	0.952 (MCP ext) 0.973 (PIP ext) 0.960 (DIP ext) 0.832 (MCP flex) 0.920 (PIP flex) 0.909 (DIP flex) 0.949 (TAE) 0.898 (TAF)
Groth et al.[53]	AROM: PIP and DIP flexion and extension; dorsal placement of goniometer	1	Patient with crush injuries to hand	0.99[†]
	AROM: PIP and DIP flexion and extension; lateral placement of goniometer Forearm rested on table in neutral with wrist slightly extended.	1	Patient with crush injuries to hand	0.86[†]
Kato et al.[59]	PROM; PIP flexion; fixed joint position; 3 goniometers and both dorsal and lateral alignment methods used	16	PIP joints of cadaver hands fixed in varying degrees of flexion	0.80–0.82[‡]
Macionis[57]	Static hand positions; dorsal method; used standard finger goniometer (SGn) and paper goniometer (PGn); measured flexion (F) and extension (E) at the MCP, PIP, and DIP of left ring finger; 2–10 examiners	12	Healthy adults (20–24 years)	0.77–0.87 (MCP, E, SGn) 0.77–0.87 (MCP, E, PGn) 0.76–0.88 (MCP, F, SGn) 0.72–0.87 (MCP, F, PGn) 0.69–0.84 (PIP, E, SGn) 0.72–0.83 (PIP, E, PGn) 0.67–0.86 (PIP, F, SGn) 0.62–0.83 (PIP, F, PGn) 0.77–0.88 (DIP, E, SGn) 0.71–0.85 (DIP, E, PGn) 0.61–0.83 (DIP, F, SGn) 0.54–0.78 (DIP, F, PGn)

AROM, Active ROM; *UE,* upper extremity.
*Intraclass correlation coefficient.
[†]Derived from data of random sample of 6 out of 39 examiners participating in study.
[‡]See text for more details.

Only the interrater reliability of active ROM was examined by Engstrand et al.[58] when they measured MCP, PIP, and DIP flexion and extension in a group of 13 adult subjects with Dupuytren disease. Eight occupational therapists with 6 or more years of experience served as the examiners for the study. They used standardized techniques, including subject positioning and instructions, goniometer used, and goniometer placement (dorsal surface of joint). Each examiner measured each motion once in each subject. Interrater reliability was calculated using the ICC, and SEMs also were reported. ICCs ranged from 0.83 for MCP flexion to 0.97 for PIP extension (see Table 7.16). Standard errors of the measurement were 1 degree for all flexion measurements and 2 degrees for all extension measurements.

In a study published in 2000, Brown et al.[55] investigated intrarater and interrater reliability of the finger goniometer compared with the Dexter hand evaluation and therapy system goniometer in measuring total active digit motion. They recruited 30 patients aged 21–66 years with orthopedic injuries of the upper extremity of at least 3 months' duration for the study. Three examiners performed the goniometric measurements, which consisted of measuring the total active flexion and the total active extension of one injured finger and of the corresponding contralateral uninjured finger (not the thumb) of each subject. Each measurement was repeated three times by each examiner using standardized patient positioning and techniques for goniometer placement. Goniometer readings were rounded to the nearest 5 degrees. Both intrarater and interrater reliability were calculated using the ICC. Intrarater reliability using the finger goniometer ranged from 0.97 to 0.98, depending on the examiner performing the measurement (see Table 7.15), whereas interrater reliability was 0.98 (see Table 7.16).

Passive

Several groups of investigators have used inferential statistics to analyze the reliability of goniometric measurement of either passive motion or static position of the digits. Flowers and LaStayo[56] examined the intrarater reliability of goniometric measurements of passive extension of the PIP joint in 20 fused PIP joints in seven patients. This examination of reliability was part of a larger study that investigated the correlation between the time spent in serial casting and the change in ROM in PIP joints of the fingers. The measurement of passive motion in both studies involved placement of the goniometer over the dorsal surface of the joint while a predetermined, controlled extension torque was applied across the PIP joint. After the torque had been applied for 20s, the goniometer was read and the ROM was recorded. Intrarater reliability of this so-called torque passive ROM test[56,60] was reported as 0.98 (ICC) (see Table 7.15). Breger-Lee et al.[60] reported poor

intrarater and interrater reliability using a technique that was similar but with a dial rather than a universal goniometer.

Kato et al.[59] used three examiners to measure the fixed angles of 16 PIP joints in four cadaver hands. Each PIP joint was fixed in a different angle of flexion using Kirschner wires. Examiners (all hand therapists, each with over 10 years of experience) measured each PIP joint with three different goniometers using both lateral and dorsal alignment methods five times per joint. The Pearson's correlation coefficient was used to calculate interrater reliability, which ranged from 0.80 to 0.82 (see Table 7.16), depending on the set of examiners being compared.

Macionis[57] compared intrarater and interrater reliability of traditional goniometry in measuring the static position of MCP, PIP, and DIP joints to diagrammatic recording of finger joint angles. Subjects consisted of 12 healthy adult medical students who were examined by inexperienced examiners (also medical students). Subjects had their hands placed in several different static postures using plastic funnels and wooden tri-square-type guides. Each position was measured twice for each joint by each examiner using both a standard finger goniometer and an "improvised paper goniometer."[57] Reliability was calculated using the ICC, and SEM values also were reported. The authors reported higher intrarater than interrater reliability and higher reliability for MCP joints than for PIP or DIP joints. Intrarater reliability was highest for measurements of MCP flexion using the standard goniometer (ICC=0.91–0.93; SEM=2.4–2.8 degrees) and lowest for measurements of DIP flexion using the paper goniometer (ICC=0.82–0.83; SEM=3.8–4.3 degrees) (see Table 7.15). Interrater reliability showed a similar pattern, with the highest values reported for MCP flexion using the standard goniometer (ICC=0.86–0.88; SEM=3.0–3.5 degrees) and the lowest values for DIP flexion using the paper goniometer (ICC=0.69–0.78; SEM=4.9 degrees) (see Table 7.16).

Burr et al.[61] also compared the reliability of different goniometers in the measurement of static position of the PIP ad DIP joints of a single subject. Forty examiners (13 occupational therapists and 27 physical therapists) used three different goniometers to measure the position of the PIP and DIP joints of the subject's index and middle fingers. The three goniometers used included the Roylan Smith and Nephew hyperextension goniometer, the Electro-Medical Supplies (EMS) goniometer, and the Dexter Computerized Assessment unit. Examiners were provided with a measurement protocol detailing positioning of the subject's wrist and forearm and placement of the goniometer over the dorsal surface of the joint. Each measurement was taken three times by each examiner, and the mean of the three measurements was used to calculate interrater reliability. Reliability (both intrarater and interrater) was reported using 95% CIs and was higher for intrarater reliability using the EMS goniometer (EMS = 5–8 degrees; Smith and Nephew = 6–16 degrees; Dexter = 7–13 degrees). Of note is the fact that 30 of the 40 examiners reported they used the EMS goniometer routinely in their clinical practice.

Thumb Motion

A small number of studies have examined the reliability of goniometric measurements of thumb ROM. De Kraker et al.[62] examined the reliability of six methods (including conventional goniometry) of measuring palmar abduction of the thumb. An experienced (hand therapist) and a novice (plastic surgery resident) examiner measured both active and passive palmar abduction ROM in 25 healthy adults using a universal goniometer, two techniques involving a "Pollexograph" (a protractor-like device), and three additional techniques (intermetacarpal distance, the American Society of Hand Therapists method, and the American Medical Association method). For goniometric measurements, the arms of the goniometer were aligned over the dorsal aspect of the first metacarpal and radial side of the second metacarpal. Reliability was calculated using ICCs, with SEMs and SDDs (equivalent in this case to MDC) also reported. Intrarater reliability was calculated from the measurements of the novice examiner and, for goniometric measurements, were 0.55 (SEM = 4.3 degrees. SDD = 11.8 degrees) for active palmar abduction and 0.76 (SEM = 3.5 degrees, SDD = 9.7 degrees) for passive palmar abduction. Interrater reliability of goniometric measurements was lower (AROM: ICC = 0.31, SEM = 5.2 degrees, SDD = 14.4 degrees; PROM: ICC = 0.37, SEM = 5.9 degrees, SDD = 16.5 degrees). Holzbauer and colleagues[63] also examined intrarater and interrater reliability of six different techniques of measuring thumb abduction range of motion. Like the de Kraker group[62], they included use of the Pollexograph and intermetacarpal distance measurements. However, Holzbauer

and colleagues[63] also measured thumb abduction ROM via thumb-DIP distance and via goniometry using a Moeltgen goniometer. Three different examiners performed the measurements, and the authors reported ICC and SDD (smallest detectable difference) values for both intrarater and interrater reliability. ICC values for intrarater reliability of goniometric measurements ranged from a low of 0.23 to a high of 0.72 (see Table 7.17) and SDD values ranged from 7.6 to 16.2 degrees. ICC values for interrater reliability were low at 0.16 and 0.34 for radial and palmar abduction, respectively (see Table 7.18).

Unlike Holzbauer and colleagues[63] in their study of the interrater reliability of thumb ROM measurements comparing goniometry to the Kapanji Index, Jha et al.[64] reported much higher interrater reliability (ICCs = 0.64–0.73) for CMC radial abduction (extension), although their MDC levels (23°) are higher than the SDD levels (7.6°–16.2°) reported by Holzbauer et al.[63] As part of their study of thumb ROM measurements in patients with CMC osteoarthritis, Jha and colleagues[64] also examined interrater reliability of five other goniometric measurements of the thumb, specifically CMC flexion, MCP extension, MCP flexion, IP extension, and IP flexion. ICC values for interrater reliability ranged from a low of 0.13 for IP flexion to a high of 0.86 for MCP extension (see Table 7.18). Minimal detectable change for these measurements ranged from 21° to 31°.

Finally, McGee and colleagues,[65] in a study in which they measured ROM in healthy thumbs using two different goniometers, reported low interrater reliability for measurements of active and passive CMC flexion (ICCs of 0.01–0.39 and MDC levels of 14.1–16.9 degrees; see Table 7.18). These investigators included measurements of active and passive MP and IP flexion as part of their study. Reliability for those measurements were higher, ranging from ICCs of 0.64 for active IP flexion to 0.82 for active MP flexion (see Table 7.18). Levels for MDC ranged from a low of 8.4° for passive IP flexion to a high of 21.8° for passive MP flexion.[65]

Table 7.17	INTRARATER RELIABILITY: THUMB ROM			
STUDY	**TECHNIQUE**	**n**	**SAMPLE**	**ICC***
de Kraker et al.[62]	AROM and PROM; palmar thumb abduction; seated at a table with elbow flexed to 90° and wrist in neutral; standardized technique; 2 examiners, 1 experienced (EE) and 1 novice (NE); took 2 measurements	25	Right hands of healthy subjects ($\bar{x}$ = 30 ± 7 years)	0.55 (AROM, NE) 0.76 (PROM, NE)
Holzbauer et al.[63]	AROM; used Moeltgen goniometer to measure radial adduction and abduction and palmar abduction; using radius-metacarpal angle (RMA) method with forearm supinated, and intermetacarpal angle (IMA) method with forearm pronated; 3 examiners	29	Healthy adults (16 F, 13 M) (20–34 years)	0.371–0.886 (Radial add, RMA) 0.375–0.768 (Radial add, IMA) 0.800–0.930 (Radial abd, RMA) 0.693–0.810 (Radial abd, IMA) 0.517–0.617 (Palmar abd, RMA) 0.235–0.724 (Palmar abd, IMA)

*Intraclass correlation coefficient.

	Table 7.18	INTERRATER RELIABILITY: THUMB ROM		
STUDY	**TECHNIQUE**	**n**	**SAMPLE**	**ICC***
de Kraker et al.[62]	AROM and PROM; palmar thumb abduction; subject seated at a table with elbow flexed to 90° and wrist in neutral; standardized technique; 2 examiners, 1 experienced (EE) and 1 novice (NE); took 2 measurements	25	Right hands of healthy subjects ($\bar{x}=30\pm7$ years)	0.31 (AROM, NE) 0.37 (PROM, NE)
Holzbauer et al.[63]	AROM; used Moeltgen goniometer to measure radial adduction and abduction and palmar abduction; using radius-metacarpal angle (RMA) method with forearm supinated, and intermetacarpal angle (IMA) method with forearm pronated; 3 examiners	29	Healthy adults (16 F, 13 M) (20–34 years)	0.200 (Radial add, RMA) 0.629 (Radial add, IMA) 0.448 (Radial abd, RMA) 0.817 (Radial abd, IMA) 0.158 (Palmar abd, RMA) 0.339 (Palmar abd, IMA)
Jha et al.[64]	AROM; sitting with forearm and hand supported, wrist neutral, forearm supinated; measured flexion and extension of CMC, MCP and IP joints using clear goniometer; 2 examiners	33 (54 thumbs)	Adults with moderate–severe OA in first CMC joint (82% F, 18% M) (43–80.6 years, $\bar{x}=64.6$ years)	0.642–0.730 (CMC ext) 0.660–0.837 (CMC flex) 0.705–0.860 (MCP ext) 0.557–0.733 (MCP flex) 0.653–0.850 (IP ext) 0.128–0.725(IP flex)
McGee et al.[65]	AROM and PROM; measured CMC joint, MCP joint with IP joint extended, IP joint with MCP joint flexed; compared clear digit goniometer with opaque black digit goniometer; 2 examiners (OT students)	48	Healthy adults (37 F, 11 M) ($\bar{x}=25\pm4.6$ years)	0.18 (AROM, CMC, black) 0.01 (AROM, CMC, clear) 0.39 (PROM, CMC, black) 0.15 (PROM, CMC, clear) 0.77 (AROM, MCP, black) 0.82 (AROM, MCP, clear) 0.81 (PROM, MCP, black) 0.74 (PROM, MCP, clear) 0.78 (AROM, IP, black) 0.64 (AROM, IP, clear) 0.80 (PROM, IP, black) 0.77 (PROM, IP, clear)

*Intraclass correlation coefficient.

RELIABILITY OF MUSCLE LENGTH TESTING

Very little research exists on the reliability of measurement of muscle length of the upper extremity. Five reliability studies are presented related to the sternocleidomastoid (SCM), latissimus dorsi, and pectoralis minor muscles.

Test for Sternocleidomastoid (SCM) Muscle Length

Investigating the muscle length of the SCM muscle in those with and without pain, Cibulka et al.[66] used an inclinometer to examine 51 subjects—37 (23 female, 14 male) with "mild" neck pain and 14 (10 female, 4 male) with no neck pain (mean age = 25.8 ± 4.9 years). The authors reported that intratester reliability ranged from 0.90 to 0.93—pain, no pain, left SCM muscle, right SCM muscle. The authors concluded that "no difference existed comparing left and right sides, nor mild pain vs no pain."

Test for Latissimus Dorsi Muscle Length

As early as 2009, Borstad and Briggs[67] examined the difference between three experienced physical therapists (average of 5 years clinical experience) and three novices, first year physical therapy students, in

the measurement of latissimus dorsi muscle length. Thirty subjects (23 females, 7 males) participated in the study. Both groups of testers showed low intratester reliability—with the experienced group showing reliability of 0.30 and the novice group at 0.15. The authors concluded that "the technique is not recommended for measuring latissimus dorsi length clinically."

Later, a study by Dawood et al.[68] found consistent results with Borstad and Briggs[67]. Using the goniometer, four raters measured the muscle length of the latissimus dorsi muscle in 56 subjects (48 female, 8 male). Results indicated that intratester reliability among the four testers ranged from 0.55 to 0.76. Furthermore, intertester reliability between rater #1 and #2 was 0.48, the same reliability coefficient achieved between rater #3 and #4. The authors concluded that the "poor to moderate" reliability may not make the latissimus dorsi muscle length test "suitable for application in a research study."

Test for Pectoralis Minor Muscle Length

Examining 13 males and three females ($n=16$), Weber et al.[69] used a tape measure to determine the reliability of the measurement of muscle length in the pectoralis minor muscle. Using two testers, reported results indicated intratester reliability of 0.94 and 0.99. Similar results were reported by Lewis and Valentine[70] using a ruler to measure

Table 7.19 INTRATESTER RELIABILITY OF MUSCLE LENGTH OF THE UPPER EXTREMITY			
STUDY	n	SAMPLE	ICC*
Sternocleidomastoid			
Cibulka et al.[66]	37	Mild neck pain ($\bar{x}$=22.8 years)	0.93
	34	Healthy adults ($\bar{x}$=25.8)	0.91
Latissimus Dorsi			
Burstad and Briggs[67]	30	Healthy adults ($\bar{x}$=23.9 years)	0.30 (Experienced)
			0.15 (Novice)
Dawood et al.[68]	56	Healthy adults ($\bar{x}$=22.0 years)	0.60, 0.55, 0.60, 0.76
Pectoralis Minor			
Lewis and Valentine[70]	45	Healthy adults ($\bar{x}$=32.1 years)	0.96 (R)
			0.92 (L)
	45	Symptomatic ($\bar{x}$=42.8 years)	0.95 (R)
			0.97 (L)
Weber et al.[69]	16	Healthy adults ($\bar{x}$=28.6 years)	0.94, 0.99

*Intraclass Correlation Coefficient.

the pectoralis minor muscle length in 45 subjects (23 female, 22 male) with and 45 subjects (24 female, 21 male) without shoulder symptoms. Results indicated intratester reliability above 0.90 for measurement of both the right and left shoulders, irrespective of whether the subject had symptoms. The authors reported that "our findings suggest that the pectoralis minor length test can be used in the clinic to investigate pectoralis minor shortness."

Summary

Table 7.19 summarizes the available research performed on intratester reliability of measurements of upper extremity muscle length. More research is needed in muscle length testing of the upper extremity. The reader is encouraged to use the information on reliability that does exist, as well as the information of each technique presented in Chapter 6, to perform reliability studies to enhance the knowledge base of muscle length testing related to muscles of the upper extremity.

References

1. Riddle DL, Rothstein JM, Lamb RL. Goniometric reliability in a clinical setting. Shoulder measurements. *Phys Ther.* 1987;67(5):668–673.
2. Correll S, et al. Reliability and validity of the halo digital goniometer for shoulder range of motion in healthy subjects. *Int J Sports Phys Ther.* 2018;13:707–714.
3. Greene BL, Wolf SL. Upper extremity joint movement: comparison of two measurement devices. *Arch Phys Med Rehabil.* 1989;70(4):288–290.
4. Hayes K, et al. Reliability of five methods for assessing shoulder range of motion. *Aust J Physiother.* 2001;47(4):289–294.
5. Kolber MJ, Hanney WJ. The reliability and concurrent validity of shoulder mobility measurements using a digital inclinometer and goniometer: a technical report. *Int J Sports Phys Ther.* 2012;7(3):306–313.
6. Macedo LG, Magee DJ. Effects of age on passive range of motion of selected peripheral joints in healthy adult females. *Physiother Theory Pract.* 2009;25(2):145–164.
7. Mullaney MJ, et al. Reliability of shoulder range of motion comparing a goniometer to a digital level. *Physiother Theory Pract.* 2010;26(5):327–333.
8. Muir SW, Corea CL, Beaupre L. Evaluating change in clinical status: reliability and measures of agreement for the assessment of glenohumeral range of motion. *N Am J Sports Phys Ther.* 2010;5(3):98–110.
9. Sabari JS, et al. Goniometric assessment of shoulder range of motion: comparison of testing in supine and sitting positions. *Arch Phys Med Rehabil.* 1998;79(6):647–651.
10. Shin SH, et al. Within-day reliability of shoulder range of motion measurement with a smartphone. *Man Ther.* 2012;17(4):298–304.
11. Walker JM, et al. Active mobility of the extremities in older subjects. *Phys Ther.* 1984;64(6):919–923.
12. Dougherty J, Walmsley S, Osmotherly PG. Passive range of movement of the shoulder: a standardized method for measurement and assessment of intrarater reliability. *J Manipulative Physiol Ther.* 2015;38(3):218–224.
13. Geertzen JH, et al. Variation in measurements of range of motion: a study in reflex sympathetic dystrophy patients. *Clin Rehabil.* 1998;12(3):254–264.
14. Green S, et al. A standardized protocol for measurement of range of movement of the shoulder using the Plurimeter-V inclinometer and assessment of its intrarater and interrater reliability. *Arthritis Care Res.* 1998;11(1):43–52.
15. Hoving JL, et al. How reliably do rheumatologists measure shoulder movement? *Ann Rheum Dis.* 2002;61(7):612–616.
16. Kolber MJ, et al. The reliability and minimal detectable change of shoulder mobility measurements using a digital inclinometer. *Physiother Theory Pract.* 2011;27(2):176–184.
17. Tveitå EK, et al. Range of shoulder motion in patients with adhesive capsulitis; intra-tester reproducibility is acceptable for group comparisons. *BMC Musculoskelet Disord.* 2008;9:49.
18. Valentine RE, Lewis JS. Intraobserver reliability of 4 physiologic movements of the shoulder in subjects with and without symptoms. *Arch Phys Med Rehabil.* 2006;87(9):1242–1249.
19. Escalante A, Lichtenstein MJ, Hazuda HP. Determinants of shoulder and elbow flexion range: results from the San Antonio longitudinal study of aging. *Arthritis Care Res.* 1999;12(4):277–286.
20. de Jong LD, Nieuwboer A, Aufdemkampe G. The hemiplegic arm: interrater reliability and concurrent validity of passive range of motion measurements. *Disabil Rehabil.* 2007;29(18):1442–1448.
21. de Jong LD, et al. Repeated measurements of arm joint passive range of motion after stroke: interobserver reliability and sources of variation. *Phys Ther.* 2012;92(8):1027–1035.
22. Werner BC, et al. Validation of an innovative method of shoulder range-of-motion measurement using a smartphone clinometer application. *J Shoulder Elbow Surg.* 2014;23(11):e275–e282.
23. Pandya S, et al. Reliability of goniometric measurements in patients with Duchenne muscular dystrophy. *Phys Ther.* 1985;65(9):1339–1342.
24. de Winter AF, et al. Inter-observer reproducibility of measurements of range of motion in patients with shoulder pain using a digital inclinometer. *BMC Musculoskelet Disord.* 2004;5:18.
25. Sharma SP, Bærheim A, Kvåle A. Passive range of motion in patients with adhesive shoulder capsulitis, an intertester reliability study over eight weeks. *BMC Musculoskelet Disord.* 2015;16:37.
26. Boon AJ, Smith J. Manual scapular stabilization: its effect on shoulder rotational range of motion. *Arch Phys Med Rehabil.* 2000;81(7):978–983.

27. Lunden JB, et al. Reliability of shoulder internal rotation passive range of motion measurements in the supine versus sidelying position. *J Orthop Sports Phys Ther.* 2010;40(9):589–594.

28. Wilk KE, et al. Glenohumeral internal rotation measurements differ depending on stabilization techniques. *Sports Health.* 2009;1(2):131–136.

29. Cools AM, et al. Measuring shoulder external and internal rotation strength and range of motion: comprehensive intra-rater and inter-rater reliability study of several testing protocols. *J Shoulder Elbow Surg.* 2014;23(10):1454–1461.

30. Fieseler G, et al. Intrarater reliability of goniometry and hand-held dynamometry for shoulder and elbow examinations in female team handball athletes and asymptomatic volunteers. *Arch Orthop Trauma Surg.* 2015;135:1719–1726.

31. Furness J, et al. Assessment of shoulder active range of motion in prone versus supine: a reliability and concurrent validity study. *Physiother Theory Pract.* 2015;31:489–495.

32. Walker H, et al. The reliability of shoulder range of motion measures in competitive swimmers. *Phys Ther Sport.* 2016;21:26–30.

33. Kevern MA, Beecher M, Rao S. Reliability of measurement of glenohumeral internal rotation, external rotation, and total arc of motion in 3 test positions. *J Athl Train.* 2014;49(5):640–646.

34. Boone DC, et al. Reliability of goniometric measurements. *Phys Ther.* 1978;58(11):1355–1360.

35. MacDermid JC, et al. Intratester and intertester reliability of goniometric measurement of passive lateral shoulder rotation. *J Hand Ther.* 1999;12(3):187–192.

36. Mitchell K, et al. Reliability and validity of goniometric iPhone applications for the assessment of active shoulder external rotation. *Physiother Theory Pract.* 2014;30(7):521–525.

37. Armstrong AD, et al. Reliability of range-of-motion measurement in the elbow and forearm. *J Shoulder Elbow Surg.* 1998;7(6):573–580.

38. Chapleau J, et al. Validity of goniometric elbow measurements: comparative study with a radiographic method. *Clin Orthop Relat Res.* 2011;469(11):3134–3140.

39. Costa V, et al. Validity and reliability of inertial sensors for elbow and wrist range of motion assessment. *Peer J.* 2020;8, e9687.

40. Golden DW, et al. Body mass index and elbow range of motion in a healthy pediatric population: a possible mechanism of overweight in children. *J Pediatr Gastroenterol Nutr.* 2008;46(2):196–201.

41. Goodwin J, et al. Clinical methods of goniometry: a comparative study. *Disabil Rehabil.* 1992;14(1):10–15.

42. Rothstein JM, Miller PJ, Roettger RF. Goniometric reliability in a clinical setting. Elbow and knee measurements. *Phys Ther.* 1983;63(10):1611–1615.

43. Blonna D, et al. Accuracy and inter-observer reliability of visual estimation compared to clinical goniometry of the elbow. *Knee Surg Sports Traumatol Arthrosc.* 2012;20(7):1378–1385.

44. Petherick M, et al. Concurrent validity and intertester reliability of universal and fluid-based goniometers for active elbow range of motion. *Phys Ther.* 1988;68(6):966–969.

45. Colaris J, et al. Pronation and supination after forearm fractures in children: reliability of visual estimation and conventional goniometry measurement. *Injury.* 2010;41(6):643–646.

46. Flowers KR, et al. Intrarater reliability of a new method and instrumentation for measuring passive supination and pronation: a preliminary study. *J Hand Ther.* 2001;14(1):30–35.

47. Gajdosik RL. Comparison and reliability of three goniometric methods for measuring forearm supination and pronation. *Percept Mot Skills.* 2001;93(2):353–355.

48. Karagiannopoulos C, Sitler M, Michlovitz S. Reliability of 2 functional goniometric methods for measuring forearm pronation and supination active range of motion. *J Orthop Sports Phys Ther.* 2003;33(9):523–531.

49. Cimatti B, et al. A study to compare two goniometric methods for measuring active pronation and supination range of motion. *Hand Ther.* 2013;18:57–63.

50. LaStayo PC, Wheeler DL. Reliability of passive wrist flexion and extension goniometric measurements: a multicenter study. *Phys Ther.* 1994;74(2):162–174. discussion 174–176.

51. Carter TI, et al. Accuracy and reliability of three different techniques for manual goniometry for wrist motion: a cadaveric study. *J Hand Surg Am.* 2009;34(8):1422–1428.

52. Horger MM. The reliability of goniometric measurements of active and passive wrist motions. *Am J Occup Ther.* 1990;44(4):342–348.

53. Groth GN, et al. Goniometry of the proximal and distal interphalangeal joints, Part II: placement preferences, interrater reliability, and concurrent validity. *J Hand Ther.* 2001;14(1):23–29.

54. Lewis E, Fors L, Tharion WJ. Interrater and intrarater reliability of finger goniometric measurements. *Am J Occup Ther.* 2010;64(4):555–561.

55. Brown A, et al. Validity and reliability of the dexter hand evaluation and therapy system in hand-injured patients. *J Hand Ther.* 2000;13(1):37–45.

56. Flowers KR, LaStayo P. Effect of total end range time on improving passive range of motion. *J Hand Ther.* 1994;7(3):150–157.

57. Macionis V. Reliability of the standard goniometry and diagrammatic recording of finger joint angles: a comparative study with healthy subjects and non-professional raters. *BMC Musculoskelet Disord.* 2013;14:17.

58. Engstrand C, Krevers B, Kvist J. Interrater reliability in finger joint goniometer measurement in Dupuytren's disease. *Am J Occup Ther.* 2012;66(1):98–103.

59. Kato M, et al. The accuracy of goniometric measurements of proximal interphalangeal joints in fresh cadavers: comparison between methods of measurement, types of goniometers, and fingers. *J Hand Ther.* 2007;20(1):12–18. quiz 19.

60. Breger-Lee D, et al. Reliability of torque range of motion: a preliminary study. *J Hand Ther.* 1993;6(1):29–34.

61. Burr N, Pratt AL, Stott D. Inter-rater and intra-rater reliability when measuring interphalangeal joints: comparison between three hand-held goniometers. *Physiotherapy.* 2003;89(11):641–652.

62. de Kraker M, et al. Palmar abduction: reliability of 6 measurement methods in healthy adults. *J Hand Surg Am.* 2009;34(3):523–530.

63. Holzbauer M, et al. Radial and palmar active range of motion measurement: reliability of six methods in healthy adults. *J Plast Surg Hand Surg.* 2021;55:41–47.

64. Jha R, et al. Measuring thumb range of motion in first carpometacarpal joint arthritis: the inter-rater reliability of the kapandji index versus goniometry. *Hand Ther.* 2016;21:45–53.

65. McGee C, et al. Inter-rater and inter-instrument reliability of goniometric thumb active and passive flexion range of motion measurements in healthy hands. *Hand Ther.* 2017;22:110–117.

66. Cibulka MT, et al. The reliability of assessing sternocleidomastoid muscle length and strength in adults with and without mild neck pain. *Physiother Theory Pract.* 2017;33(4):323–330.

67. Borstad JD, Briggs MS. Reproducibility of a measurement for latissimus dorsi muscle length. *Physiother Theory Pract.* 2010;26(3):195–203.

68. Dawood M, et al. Inter- and intra-rater reliability of a technique assessing the length of the Latissimus Dorsi muscle. *S Afr J Physiother.* 2018;74(1), a388.

69. Weber C, et al. Validation of the pectoralis minor length test: a novel approach. *Man Ther.* 2016;22:50–55.

70. Lewis JS, Valentine RE. The pectoralis minor length test: a study of the intra-rater reliability and diagnostic accuracy in subjects with and without shoulder symptoms. *BMC Musculoskelet Disord.* 2007;8:64.

HEAD, NECK, AND TRUNK

8

MEASUREMENT of RANGE of MOTION of the THORACIC and LUMBAR SPINE

William D. Bandy and Chad Lairamore

ANATOMY AND OSTEOKINEMATICS

The following discussion of the thoracic and lumbar spine is a synopsis of information presented in several contemporary sources.[1-3] Although the cervical spine is built for maximum mobility, the thoracic spine and lumbar spine are built for weight bearing and stability. Twelve vertebrae (composed of the superior and inferior vertebral facets, the vertebral bodies, and the discs that are interposed between the vertebral bodies) make up the thoracic spine, and five make up the lumbar spine. A typical lumbar vertebra is pictured in Fig. 8.1, and a typical thoracic vertebra is pictured in Fig. 8.2. The major differences between the two are the long spinous process of the thoracic spine, which is directed downward rather than posteriorly, and the articulation of the thoracic spine with the ribs.

A general overview of the connective tissue of the thoracic and lumbar spine includes the intervertebral disc, which connects the vertebral bodies to form intervertebral cartilaginous joints, and the following supporting ligaments: anterior longitudinal, posterior longitudinal, ligamentum flavum, intraspinous, and supraspinous (Fig. 8.3).

The facet joints of the thoracic spine are formed by the facet surfaces of two vertebrae, which lie in the frontal plane with the inferior facet surface of the superior vertebrae (oriented anteriorly and slightly inferior) articulating with the superior facet surface of the inferior vertebrae (oriented posteriorly and slightly superior). This alignment of facets in the thoracic spine facilitates the main motions of lateral flexion and rotation.

The facet joints of the lumbar spine are formed by combination of the facet surfaces of two vertebrae, which lie in the sagittal plane, with the inferior facet surface of the superior vertebrae (oriented laterally), which articulate with the superior facet surface of the inferior vertebrae (oriented medially). Alignment of facets in the lumbar spine facilitates the main motions of flexion and extension.

Segmental motion in the thoracic and lumbar spine occurs as the top vertebrae slide onto the bottom vertebrae (arthrokinematic movement), whereby the facet joints of the spinal segment contribute to and guide the motion. Although segmental movements at each vertebra are small, combined movement in the entire thoracic and lumbar spine produces a large range of motion (ROM) in the spine. During movement of the thoracic and lumbar spine, the combined movement of all facet joints in the thoracic and lumbar spine (called thoracolumbar movement) or just the lumbar spine is measured because segmental motion is very difficult to measure accurately. Through segmental motion at each vertebra in the thoracic and lumbar spine, osteokinematic movements of flexion and extension occur in the sagittal plane, right and left lateral flexion in the frontal plane, and right and left rotation in the transverse plane.

LIMITATIONS OF MOTION

Six main ligaments, which provide stability and limit motion, are associated with the intervertebral joints. The anterior longitudinal ligament prevents excessive spinal extension, and the posterior longitudinal, ligamentum flavum, interspinous, and supraspinous ligaments limit flexion of the spine. In addition, the spinous processes of the thoracic spine limit extension. The intertransverse ligaments limit lateral flexion. Rotation of the spine is limited by facet orientation. Information on normal ROM for the thoracic and lumbar spine may be found in Appendix B.

FUNCTIONAL RANGE OF MOTION

The amount of lumbar movement required for four functional activities was examined by Hsieh and Pringle[4]: stand-to-sit, sit-to-stand, picking up a small object from the floor, and putting on socks (Figs. 8.4–8.7). The authors examined 48 healthy subjects (mean age, 26.5 ± 4.6 years); instructions were provided to each subject to standardize how each activity was performed. The authors reported that sit-to-stand and stand-to-sit activities required 56% to 66% lumbar flexion. Putting on socks required 90% lumbar flexion.

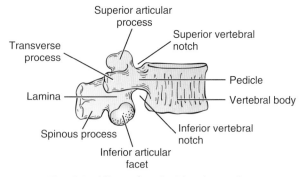

Fig. 8.1   View of typical lumbar spine.

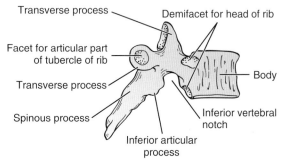

Fig. 8.2   View of typical thoracic spine.

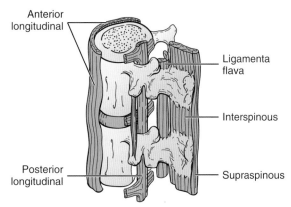

Fig. 8.3   Supporting ligaments of the thoracic and lumbar spine.

Picking up a small object from the floor required almost full lumbar flexion (95%). Therefore, putting on socks and picking up a small object from the floor required almost twice as much lumbar ROM as was required for sit/stand activities. The authors suggested that subjects with less than 79% flexion of the lumbar spine will show compensations during sit/stand activities and will be unable to pick up objects from the floor or put on their socks.

TECHNIQUES OF MEASUREMENT

Tape Measure

The least expensive instrument for measuring spinal movement and perhaps the easiest to use is a tape

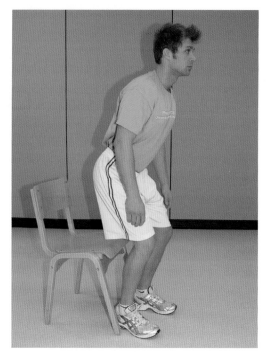

Fig. 8.4   Stand to sit.

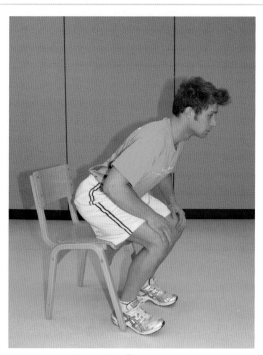

Fig. 8.5   Sit to stand.

measure. Additionally, a tape measure probably has been used in the clinic for measuring ROM of the spine longer than any other measurement device.[5]

Flexion

Schober Method

One of the most common tape measure procedures used to measure lumbar flexion relates to a technique

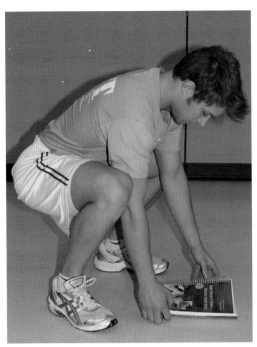

Fig. 8.6   Picking up small object from the floor.

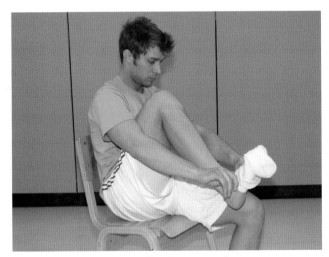

Fig. 8.7   Putting on socks.

originated by Schober and subsequently modified for measurement of spinal flexion. According to Macrae and Wright,[5] in 1937 Schober described the original two-mark method for measuring spinal flexion, in which one mark is made at the lumbosacral junction and a second mark is made 10 cm above the first mark while the subject stands with the spine in a neutral position. After the standing subject bends forward as far as possible, the increase in distance between the first and second marks provides an estimate of the amount of flexion that is present in the spine. Because the tape measure technique relies on stretching or distraction of the skin overlying the spine, this technique (and modifications of the technique) is sometimes referred to as the skin distraction method.

Macrae and Wright[5] modified the original Schober method by introducing a third mark, a measurement mark placed 5 cm below the lumbosacral junction. This modification uses a mark at the lumbosacral junction and other marks 5 cm inferior and 10 cm superior to the lumbosacral junction. The rationale offered by Macrae and Wright[5] for making the modification of the original Schober technique is that when using the Schober technique in their pilot work, the authors observed that skin above and below the lumbosacral spine was distracted during flexion of the lumbar spine, leading to inaccuracies in measurement. Therefore, the technique that Macrae and Wright[5] referred to as the "modified" Schober technique included three marks: (1) the lumbosacral junction, (2) 5 cm inferior to the lumbosacral junction, and (3) 10 cm superior to the lumbosacral junction.

Van Adrichem and van der Korst[6] suggested that using the lumbosacral junction (the base mark used for the Schober technique), which had to be identified by palpation, added difficulty to this method of measurement. Given this information, Williams et al.[7] suggested that the "modified-modified Schober," rather than the Schober or the modified Schober method, should be used. The modified-modified Schober uses two skin landmarks (as opposed to three skin landmarks used with the modified Schober). These two landmarks include a point bisecting a line that connects the two posterior superior iliac spines (PSIS) (baseline) and a mark 15 cm superior to the baseline landmark. Given the ease of palpating the PSIS and the difficulty involved in determining the lumbosacral junction, the baseline for measuring lumbar flexion and thoracolumbar flexion used in this chapter is the bisection of the line that connects the two PSIS, as described by Williams et al.[7] (see Figs. 8.8–8.15).

Fingertip-to-floor method

In an attempt to examine flexion of the spine quickly and reproducibly, some authors have advocated the fingertip-to-floor method.[9,10] The fingertip-to-floor method differs from the Schober method and its modifications in that these measurements are not taken directly over the lumbar spine. The patient simply bends forward, and the distance between the tip of the middle finger and the floor is measured with a tape measure (Figs. 8.16–8.19).

Extension

Schober Method

Moll and Wright[8] suggested that modifications of the Schober technique might be appropriate for examining lumbar extension. These authors suggested measuring the change in skin marks as the marks move closer together during the extension movement. Again, for reasons previously described, the baseline for measuring lumbar extension used in this chapter is the bisection of the line connecting the two PSIS, as described by Williams et al.[7] (see Figs. 8.43–8.44).

Lateral Flexion

Two methods for using a tape measure to examine lateral flexion of the spine have been introduced in the literature, with neither method becoming predominant in clinical use. These two methods include placing marks at the lateral thigh and the fingertip-to-floor method.

Measuring lateral flexion by placing a mark at the location on the lateral thigh that the third fingertip can touch during erect standing and after lateral flexion (see Figs. 8.70–8.72) was first introduced by Mellin.[11] The distance between the two marks represents the range of lateral flexion to that side.

Using the fingertip-to-floor method, the distance from the third fingertip to the floor is measured, first with the patient standing erect and then after the subject laterally flexes the spine.[12] The change in distance from erect standing to lateral flexion is considered the range of lateral flexion (see Fig. 8.73).

Rotation

Using the lateral tip of the ipsilateral acromion and the greater trochanter of the contralateral femur, Frost et al.[12] described a method for measuring rotation in the thoracolumbar spine using a tape measure. See Fig. 8.90–8.93, which illustrates this technique in detail.

Goniometer

The standard goniometer, consisting of two hinged rulers rotating on a protractor (described in detail in Chapter 1), is commonly used for measuring ROM of the spine. Techniques for measurement of flexion (see Figs. 8.20–8.23), extension (see Figs. 8.49–8.52), lateral flexion (see Figs. 8.74–8.77), and rotation (see Figs. 8.94–8.97) are described later in this chapter.

Inclinometer

The American Medical Association (AMA) has published its *Guides to the Evaluation of Permanent Impairment*,[13] in which the use of inclinometers has been stipulated as "a feasible and potentially accurate method of measuring spine mobility." Therefore, it appears that the use of the inclinometer for appropriate measurement of spinal mobility has gained acceptance.

Several options are available for using the inclinometer in measuring spinal movement. Two inclinometers can be used simultaneously to measure spinal movement (referred to as the *double-inclinometer method*), or one inclinometer can be used to measure the same spinal movement (referred to as the *single-inclinometer*

method). In addition, the inclinometer can be held against the subject during the examination of ROM, or the inclinometer can be strapped onto and attached to the individual (back range of motion [BROM] device). All these techniques have been accepted by the AMA[13] as appropriate methods for measuring spinal mobility. This chapter describes the use of the dual-inclinometer technique to measure movement of the lumbar and thoracic spine for flexion (see Figs. 8.24–8.27), extension (see Figs. 8.53–8.56), lateral flexion (see Figs. 8.78–8.81), and rotation (see Figs. 8.98–8.104).

However, Saunders[14] suggests that the protocol for measurement measuring flexion and extension of the lumbar spine proposed by the AMA[13] is "seriously flawed" because the erect standing position is used as the reference, or zero, point. He advocates that the actual measurement at the end of the range of flexion or extension is the important parameter—not the ROM from the erect standing position (in which the individual may be in lordotic, neutral, or kyphotic posture for this initial measurement) to full ROM, as advocated by the AMA.[13] Saunders[14] recommends the use of what he refers to as the "curve angle method," which is presented later in this chapter as an alternative technique for measuring lumbar flexion and extension using the inclinometer.

The BROM device (Performance Attainment Associates, Roseville, MN) was developed using mechanisms based on the inclinometer technique. The BROM device consists of two plastic frames that are secured to the lumbar spine of the subject by two elastic straps. One frame consists of an L-shaped slide arm that is free to move within a notch on the fixed base unit during flexion and extension; ROM is read from a protractor scale. The second frame has two measurement devices attached to it. One attachment is a vertically mounted gravity-dependent inclinometer that measures lateral flexion. The second attachment is a horizontally mounted compass that is used to measure rotation. During measurement of trunk rotation, the device requires that a magnetic yoke be secured to the pelvis. Descriptions and figures showing how to use the BROM device to measure flexion (see Figs. 8.28–8.31), extension (see Figs. 8.57–8.60), lateral flexion (see Figs. 8.82–8.85), and rotation (see Figs. 8.105–8.108) are presented later in this chapter. From a clinical perspective, it remains to be seen whether the BROM will be readily accepted as a device of choice by the AMA in the new revision of its publication *Guides to the Evaluation of Permanent Impairment*.[13]

Smartphone

Sensors and software programs can be added to Smartphones allowing the device to act like an inclinometer to measure joint ROM and muscle length. Adding the ROM application (app) to the Smartphone is inexpensive, easy to use, and requires minimal training. Using the Smartphone to measure ROM of the lumbar spine is presented later in this chapter for flexion (Figs. 8.32–8.35), extension (Figs. 8.61–8.64), and lateral flexion (Figs. 8.86–8.89).

Flexicurve

The draughtsman's flexible curve or Flexicurve is a bendable ruler made of wire covered in plastic that maintains its shape after being positioned. By manually molding the Flexicurve to the contours of the thoracic or lumbar spine and marking specific spinous processes on the bendable ruler, the curvature of the spine and location of spinous processes can be traced onto drafting paper and angles of the thoracic and lumbar spine can be calculated. While this technique is commonly used to assess static thoracic kyphosis,[15] the device can also be used to measure thoracic and lumbar flexion and extension in the sagittal plane.[16–21] While the Flexicurve technique provides angles similar to radiographic assessments, these angles must be calculated after the assessment resulting in a potential clinician burden. This chapter describes the use of the Flexicurve technique to measure angles of the lumbar and thoracic spine in flexion (see Figs. 8.36–8.40) and extension (see Figs. 8.65–8.69).

Flexion—Lumbar Spine: Tape Measure Method (Video 8.1)

Fig. 8.8 Starting position for measurement of lumbar flexion using tape measure method. Bony landmarks for tape measure alignment (midline of spine in line with PSIS, 15 cm above baseline mark) indicated by red line and dots.

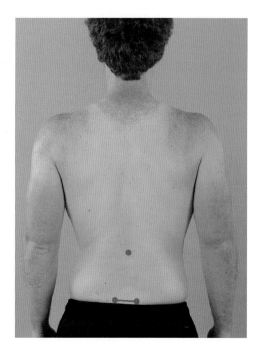

Patient position

Standing, feet shoulder width apart (Fig. 8.8).

Patient action

Patient is instructed in the desired motion. Running both hands down the front of both legs, patient flexes spine as far as possible while keeping knees extended. Patient then returns to starting position. This movement provides an estimate of ROM and demonstrates to patient exact motion desired (Fig. 8.9).

Fig. 8.9 End ROM of lumbar flexion. Bony landmarks for tape measure alignment (midline of spine in line with PSIS, 15 cm above baseline mark) indicated by red line and dots.

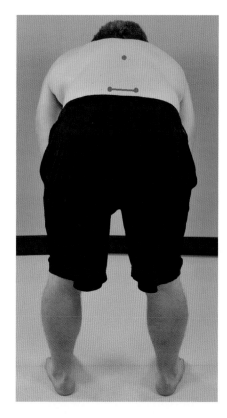

Fig. 8.10 Initial tape measure alignment for measurement of lumbar flexion. Bony landmarks for tape measure alignment (midline of spine in line with PSIS, 15 cm above baseline mark).

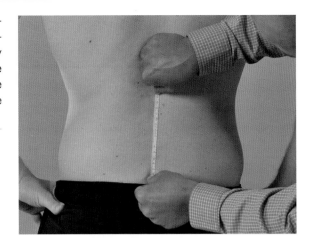

Tape measure alignment	Palpate the bony landmarks (shown in Fig. 8.8) and align tape measure accordingly (Fig. 8.10).
Baseline	Midline of spine in line with PSIS.
Superior	15 cm above baseline landmark.
	Tape measure is aligned with 0 cm at baseline landmark and is maintained against subject's spine (see Fig. 8.10).
Patient/Examiner action	As patient flexes spine through available ROM, examiner allows tape measure to unwind from tape measure case. Tape measure should be held firmly against patient's skin during movement. Examiner records distance between superior and baseline landmarks (Fig. 8.11).
Documentation	Flexion ROM recorded is the difference between original 15-cm measurement and length measured at end of flexion motion. Example: 16.5 cm (measurement at full flexion) − 15 cm (initial measurement) = 1.5 cm of lumbar flexion. Record patient's ROM.

Fig. 8.11 Tape measure alignment at end ROM of lumbar flexion. Bony landmarks for tape measure alignment (midline of spine in line with PSIS, 15 cm above baseline mark).

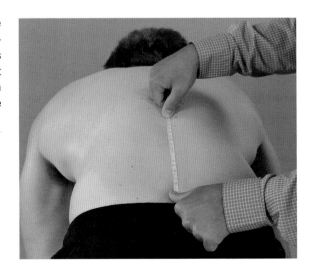

Flexion—Thoracolumbar Spine: Tape Measure Method (Video 8.2)

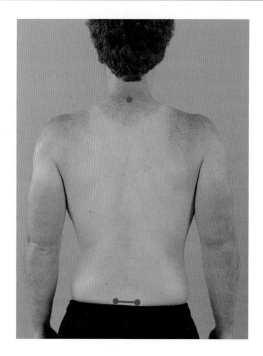

Fig. 8.12 Starting position for measurement of thoracolumbar flexion using tape measure method. Bony landmarks for tape measure alignment (midline of spine in line with PSIS, spinous process of C7 vertebra) indicated by red line and dots.

Patient position	Standing, feet shoulder width apart (Fig. 8.12).
Patient action	Patient is instructed in desired motion. Running both hands down the front of both legs, patient flexes spine as far as possible while keeping knees extended. Patient then returns to starting position. This movement provides an estimate of ROM and demonstrates to patient exact motion desired (Fig. 8.13).
Tape measure alignment	Palpate the bony landmarks (shown in Fig. 8.12) and align tape measure accordingly (Fig. 8.14).
Baseline	Midline of spine in line with PSIS.
Superior	Spinous process of C7 vertebra.

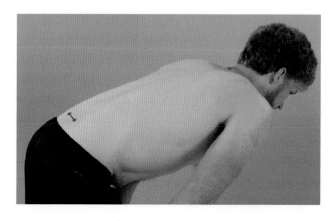

Fig. 8.13 End ROM of thoracolumbar flexion. Bony landmarks for tape measure alignment (midline of spine in line with PSIS, C7 vertebra) indicated by red line and dots.

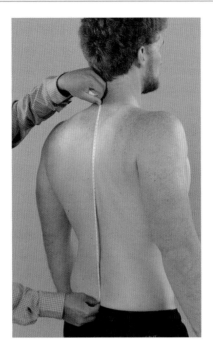

Fig. 8.14 Initial tape measure alignment for measurement of thoracolumbar flexion. Bony landmarks for tape measure alignment (midline of spine in line with PSIS, spinous process of C7 vertebra).

Tape measure is aligned with 0 cm at baseline landmark. Maintaining tape measure against subject's spine, measure distance between the baseline and superior landmark, referred to as initial measurement (see Fig. 8.14).

Patient/Examiner action   As patient flexes spine through available ROM, examiner allows tape measure to unwind from tape measure case. Tape measure should be held firmly against patient's skin during movement. Examiner records distance between superior and baseline landmarks, referred to as final measurement (Fig. 8.15).

Documentation   Flexion ROM recorded is difference between initial and final measurements. Example: 57 cm (final measurement) – 50 cm (initial measurement) = 7 cm of thoracolumbar flexion. Record patient's ROM.

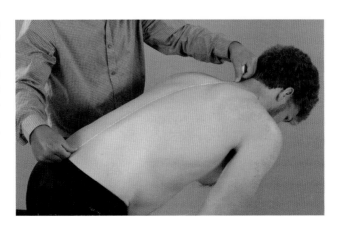

Fig. 8.15 Tape measure alignment at end ROM of thoracolumbar flexion. Bony landmarks for tape measure alignment (midline of spine in line with PSIS, spinous process of C7 vertebra).

Flexion—Lumbar Spine: Fingertip-to-Floor

Fig. 8.16 Starting position for measurement of lumbar flexion using finger-to-floor technique.

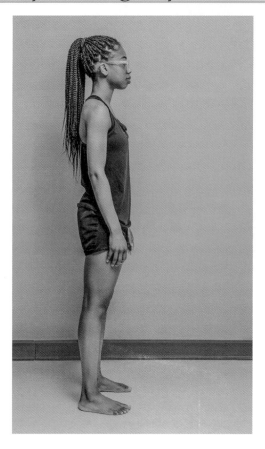

Patient position	Standing, feet shoulder width apart (Fig. 8.16).
Patient action	Patient is instructed in the desired motion. Running both hands down the front of both legs, patient flexes spine as far as possible while keeping the knees extended. Patient then returns to starting position. This movement provides an estimate ROM and demonstrates to patient exact motion desired (Fig. 8.17).

Fig. 8.17 End ROM of lumbar flexion.

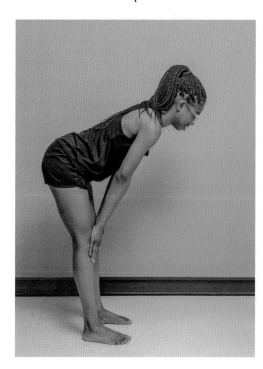

Fig. 8.18 Patient at end ROM of lumbar flexion holding extended arms out in front of trunk perpendicular to the floor.

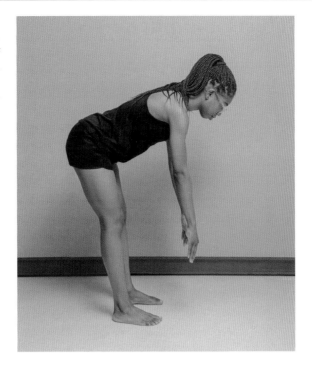

Patient/Examiner action   Running both hands down the front of both legs, patient flexes the spine as far as possible while keeping knees extended. Holding this position, patient reaches extended arms out in front of trunk perpendicular to the floor (Fig. 8.18).

Patient/Examiner action   At maximal flexion, distance from tip of middle finger to the floor is measured (Fig. 8.19).

Documentation   Distance between tip of middle finger and floor is recorded.

Fig. 8.19 Measure distance between middle finger and floor.

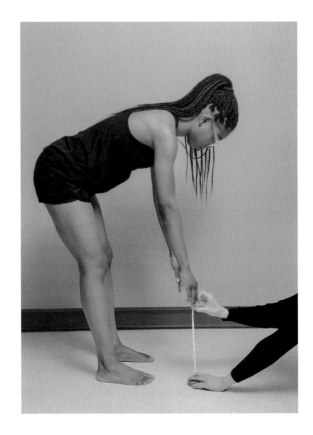

Flexion—Lumbar Spine: Goniometer Technique (Video 8.3)

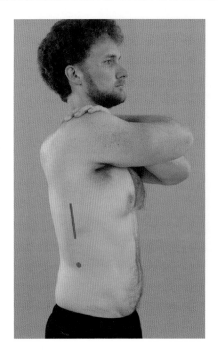

Fig. 8.20 Starting position for measuring lumbar flexion using goniometer technique. Landmarks for goniometric alignment (midaxillary line at level of lowest rib, midaxillary line) indicated by red line and dot.

Patient position	Standing, feet shoulder width apart (Fig. 8.20).
Patient action	Patient is instructed in desired motion. With hands folded across chest, patient flexes spine as far as possible while keeping knees extended. Patient then returns to starting position. This movement provides an estimate of ROM and demonstrates to patient exact motion required (Fig. 8.21).

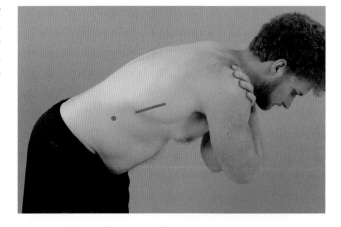

Fig. 8.21 End ROM of lumbar flexion. Landmarks for goniometric alignment (midaxillary line at level of lowest rib, midaxillary line) indicated by red line and dot.

Fig. 8.22 Goniometer alignment at beginning range of
lumbar flexion.

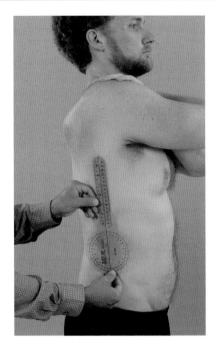

Goniometer alignment	Palpate the landmarks (shown in Fig. 8.20) and align goniometer accordingly (Fig. 8.22).
Stationary arm	Vertical to floor.
Axis	Midaxillary line at level of lowest rib.
Moving arm	Along midaxillary line.
	Read scale of goniometer.
Patient/Examiner action	With arms folded across chest, patient flexes spine as far as possible while keeping knees extended (see Fig. 8.21).
Confirmation of alignment	Repalpate landmarks and confirm proper goniometer alignment at end ROM, correcting alignment as necessary (Fig. 8.23). Read scale of goniometer.
Documentation	Record patient's ROM.

Fig. 8.23 Goniometer alignment at end ROM of lumbar
flexion.

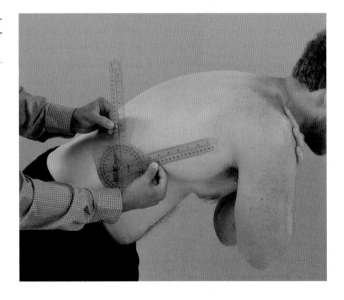

Flexion—Lumbar Spine: Inclinometer Method (Video 8.4)

Fig. 8.24 Starting position for measurement of lumbar flexion using dual-inclinometer (AMA) technique. Bony landmarks for inclinometer alignment (midline of spine in line with PSIS, 15 cm above baseline mark) indicated by red line and dots.

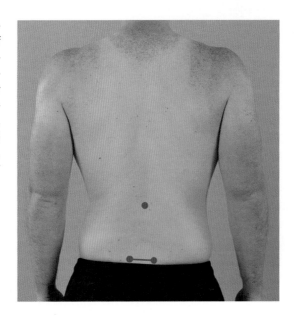

Patient position	Standing, feet shoulder width apart (Fig. 8.24).
Patient action	Patient is instructed in desired motion. Running both hands down the front of both legs, patient flexes spine as far as possible while keeping knees extended. Patient then returns to starting position. This movement provides an estimate of ROM and demonstrates to patient exact motion desired (Fig. 8.25).
Inclinometer alignment	Palpate the bony landmarks (shown in Fig. 8.24) and align inclinometers accordingly (Fig. 8.26). Ensure that inclinometers are set at 0 degrees.
Baseline	Midline of spine in line with PSIS.
Superior	15 cm above baseline landmark.

Fig. 8.25 End ROM of lumbar flexion. Bony landmarks for inclinometer alignment (midline of spine in line with PSIS, 15 cm above baseline mark) indicated by red line and dots.

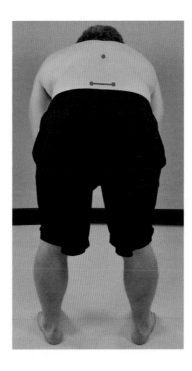

Fig. 8.26 Initial inclinometer alignment for measuring lumbar flexion using dual-inclinometer (AMA) technique. Inclinometers set at 0 degrees.

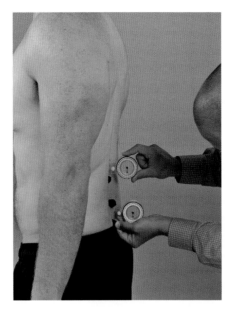

Patient/Examiner action	Holding inclinometers in place as patient flexes spine through available ROM, examiner reads angle on each device (Fig. 8.27). Inclinometer at superior landmark indicates flexion of lumbar spine and hips. Inclinometer at baseline landmark indicates flexion of the hips alone.
Documentation	Flexion ROM recorded is measurement at baseline landmark (after full flexion) subtracted from measurement at superior landmark (after full flexion). Example: 105 degrees (reading at superior landmark) − 45 degrees (reading at baseline landmark) = 60 degrees of lumbar flexion. Record patient's ROM.
Note	Thoracolumbar flexion can be measured using the spinous process of the C7 vertebra as the superior landmark. Fig. 8.12 indicates this superior landmark.

Alternative Technique: The Curve Angle Method

Patient/Examiner action	Patient flexes spine through available ROM. Examiner places *single* inclinometer at baseline landmark at midline of spine in line with PSIS (see Fig. 8.24) and sets the inclinometer at 0 degrees. With patient maintaining full lumbar flexion, examiner then moves *single* inclinometer to superior landmark (see Fig. 8.24).
Documentation	Flexion ROM recorded is the measurement at the superior landmark.

Fig. 8.27 Inclinometer alignment at end ROM of lumbar flexion.

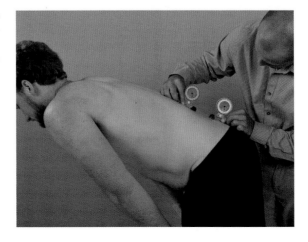

Flexion—Lumbar Spine: BROM Device (Video 8.5)

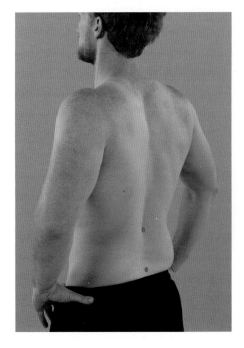

Fig. 8.28 Starting position for measuring lumbar flexion using BROM. Bony landmarks for BROM alignment (spinous process of S1 vertebra, spinous process of T12 vertebra) indicated by red dots.

Patient position	Standing erect, feet shoulder width apart (Fig. 8.28).
Patient action	Patient is instructed in desired motion. Running both hands down the front of both legs, patient flexes spine as far as possible while keeping knees extended. Patient then returns to starting position. This movement provides an estimate of ROM and demonstrates to patient exact motion desired (Fig. 8.29).
BROM alignment	Palpate the bony landmarks (see Fig. 8.28).
Baseline	Spinous process of S1 vertebra.
Superior	Spinous process of T12 vertebra.
Examiner action	Place BROM flexion-extension unit (consisting of base and movable arm) with pivot point on spinous process of S1 vertebra. Hold in place by attaching with Velcro straps to lower abdomen (down-pull of strap is essential to maintain unit against sacrum during flexion and extension) (Fig. 8.30).

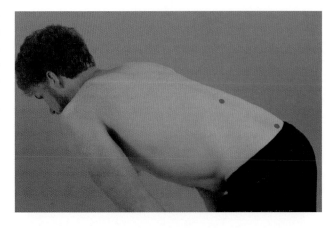

Fig. 8.29 End ROM of lumbar flexion. Bony landmarks for BROM alignment (spinous process of S1 vertebra, spinous process of T12 vertebra) indicated by red dots.

Fig.   8.30 Alignment   of BROM flexion-extension unit at beginning range of lumbar flexion. Bony landmark for alignment of movable arm of BROM (spinous process of T12 vertebra).

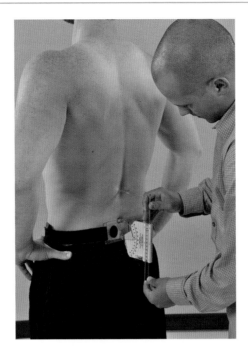

With patient standing erect, examiner places tip of moving arm at level of T12 spinous process. Record reading from unit as initial measurement (see Fig. 8.30).

Patient/Examiner action

Running both hands down the front of the legs, patient flexes spine through available ROM. Examiner places tip of moving arm at level of T12 spinous process. Record reading from unit as full flexion measurement (Fig. 8.31).

Documentation

Flexion ROM is the measurement of initial reading (in erect standing) subtracted from the full flexion reading. Example: 115 degrees (reading at full flexion) − 80 degrees (reading in standing) = 35 degrees of lumbar flexion. Record patient's ROM.

Fig.   8.31 Alignment   of BROM at end ROM of lumbar flexion. Bony landmark for alignment of movable arm of BROM (spinous process of T12 vertebra).

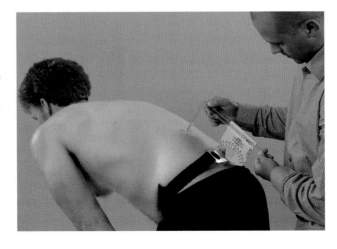

Flexion—Lumbar Spine: Smartphone Method

Fig. 8.32 Starting position for measuring lumbar flexion using Smartphone..

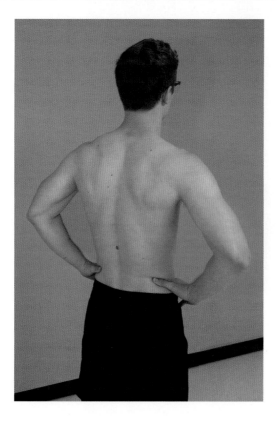

Patient position   Standing, feet shoulder width apart (Fig. 8.32).

Patient action   Patient is instructed in desired motion. Running both hands down the front of both legs, patient flexes spine as far as possible while keeping knees extended. Patient then returns to starting position. This movement provides an estimate of ROM and demonstrates to patient exact motion desired (Fig. 8.33).

Fig. 8.33 End range of lumbar flexion.

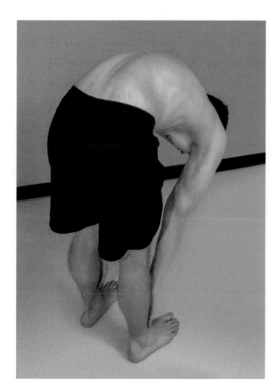

Fig. 8.34 Smartphone alignment at beginning of range of lumbar flexion.

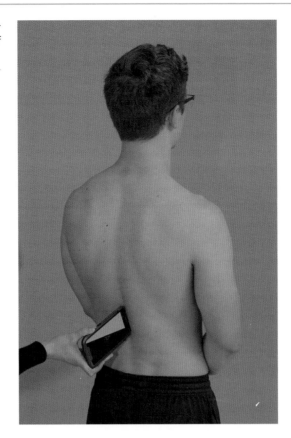

Smartphone alignment

Palpate spinous process of T12 and place border of Smartphone at that location (Fig. 8.34) with Smartphone screen facing toward therapist. Ensure the Smartphone application starts at 0 degrees, cue the patient to adjust trunk as needed.

Patient/Examiner action

Patient flexes lumbar spine through available ROM as examiner reads angle of Smartphone at end of flexion ROM (Fig. 8.35).

Documentation

Record patient's ROM.

Fig. 8.35 Smartphone alignment at end of range of lumbar flexion.

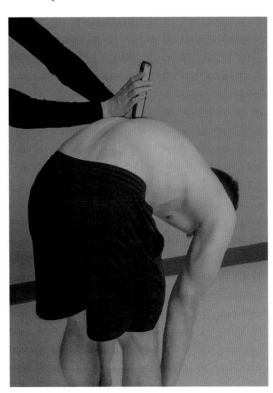

Flexion—Thoracic and Lumbar Spine: Flexicurve Technique

Fig. 8.36 Alignment of Flexicurve in standing neutral posture. Bony landmarks for Flexicurve alignment (spinous process of T1 vertebra, spinous process of T6 vertebra, spinous process of T12 vertebra, spinous process of L4 vertebra, spinous process of S2 vertebra,) indicated by red dots.

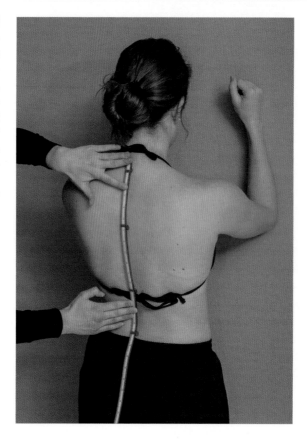

Patient position	The neutral position is assessed with the patient standing erect, feet shoulder width apart, shoulders and elbows flexed to 90 degrees with forearms lightly resting on a wall (Fig. 8.36).
Flexicurve alignment	With patient standing, palpate the bony landmarks and mark with dermographic pencil.
Thoracic	Spinous process of T1 vertebra. Spinous process of T6 vertebra. Spinous process of T12 vertebra.
Lumbar	Spinous process of T12 vertebra. Spinous process of L4 vertebra. Spinous process of S2 vertebra.

Fig. 8.37 After molding Flexicurve to patient in standing, trace contours of Flexicurve onto paper and mark position of spinous processes on paper.

Examiner action

With patient in standing, mold Flexicurve to patient spine and mark spinous processes on the Flexicurve (Fig. 8.36). Trace contours of Flexicurve and position of spinous processes onto paper (Fig. 8.37).

Patient action

Patient is instructed in desired motion. In sitting, patient looks downward, rounds shoulders, and flexes the spine as far as possible while keeping ischia in contact with the seat. Patient then relaxes and returns to a neutral position. This movement demonstrates to patient exact motion desired (Fig. 8.38).

Fig. 8.38 End ROM of thoracolumbar flexion using the Flexicurve.

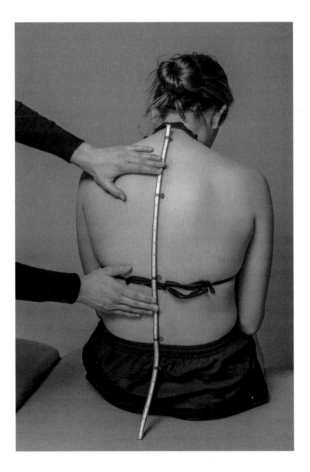

Fig.   8.39   After   molding Flexicurve to subject in prone, trace contours of Flexicurve onto paper and mark position of spinous processes on paper.

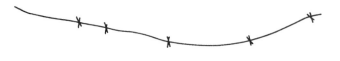

Fig. 8.39 After molding Flexicurve to subject in prone, trace contours of Flexicurve onto paper and mark position of spinous processes on paper.

Patient/Examiner action	Sitting in a chair, patient flexes spine through available ROM keeping ischia on the seat.
	With patient in sitting with back flexed, examiner molds Flexicurve to patient spine and marks spinous processes on the Flexicurve (Fig. 8.38). Examiner traces contours of Flexicurve and position of spinous processes onto paper (Fig. 8.39).
Documentation	Thoracic curvature angles are calculated by drawing line L between the T1 and T12 spinous processes, and line H is constructed so it is perpendicular to Line L at the T6 mid-point bisecting line L creating Line L1 and Line L2 (Fig. 8.40). The angles of the thoracic curve in neutral and in flexion are calculated using the formula [theta] = [arctan(H/L1)] + [arctan(H/L2)] where [theta] represents the magnitude of the thoracic curve. The thoracic angle in full flexion is reported in degrees from the seated measurement. Additionally, the thoracic flexion ROM can be calculated by subtracting the thoracic angle in neutral position (standing) from the thoracic angle in full flexion (seated).

Fig. 8.40 To measure thoracic flexion, mark T1 at the top of the drawing and T12 at the bottom. To measure lumbar flexion, mark T12 at the top of the drawing and S2 at the bottom.

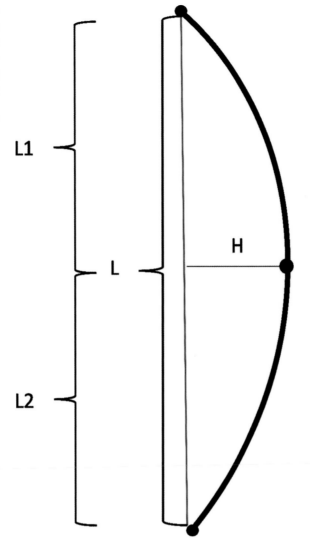

Lumbar curvature angles are calculated by drawing line L between the T12 and S2 spinous processes. Line H is constructed so it bisects and is perpendicular to Line H at the L4 mid-point (Fig. 8.40). The angles of the lumbar curve in neutral and flexion are calculated using the formula [alpha] = 4 X [arctan(2H/L)] where [alpha] represents the magnitude of the lumbar curve. The lumbar angle in full flexion is reported in degrees from the seated measurement. Additionally, lumbar flexion ROM can be calculated by adding the lumbar angle in full flexion (seated) to the lumbar angle in neutral position (standing).

Extension—Lumbar Spine: Tape Measure Method (Video 8.7)

Fig. 8.41 Starting position for measuring lumbar extension using tape measure method. Bony landmarks for tape measure alignment (midline of spine in line with PSIS, 15 cm above baseline mark) indicated by red line and dots.

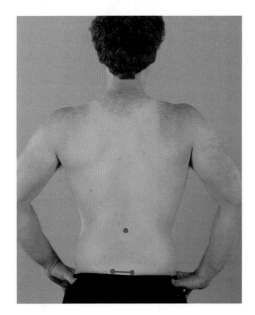

Patient position	Standing, feet shoulder width apart, hands on hips (Fig. 8.41).
Patient action	Patient is instructed in desired motion. Placing hands on waist, patient bends backward as far as possible while keeping knees extended. Patient then returns to starting position. This movement provides an estimate of ROM and demonstrates to patient exact motion desired (Fig. 8.42).
Tape measure alignment	Palpate the bony landmarks (shown in Fig. 8.41) and align tape measure accordingly (Fig. 8.43).
Baseline	Midline of spine in line with PSIS.
Superior	15 cm above baseline landmark.
	Tape measure is aligned with 0 cm at baseline landmark and is maintained against subject's spine (see Fig. 8.43).

Fig. 8.42 End ROM of lumbar extension. Bony landmarks for tape measure alignment (midline of spine in line with PSIS, 15 cm above baseline mark) indicated by red line and dots.

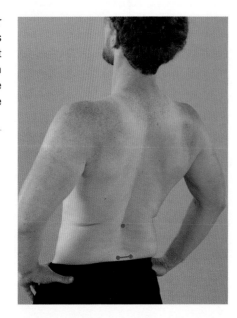

Fig. 8.43 Initial tape measure alignment for measuring lumbar extension. Bony landmarks for tape measure alignment (midline of spine in line with PSIS, 15 cm above baseline mark).

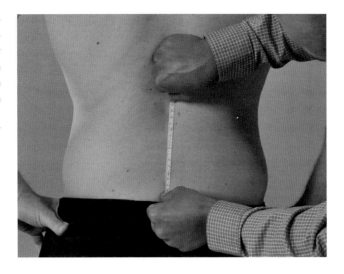

Patient/Examiner action   As patient extends spine through available ROM, examiner allows tape measure to retract into tape measure case. Tape measure should be held firmly against patient's skin during movement. Examiner records distance between superior and baseline landmarks (Fig. 8.44).

Documentation   Extension ROM recorded is difference between original 15 cm measurement and length measured at end of extension motion. Example: 15 cm (initial measurement) – 13 cm (measurement at full extension) = 2 cm of extension. Record patient's ROM.

Fig. 8.44 Tape measure alignment at end ROM of lumbar extension. Bony landmarks for tape measure alignment (midline of spine in line with PSIS, 15 cm above baseline mark).

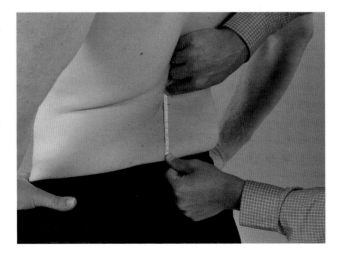

Extension—Lumbar Spine: Tape Measure Method—Prone (Video 8.6)

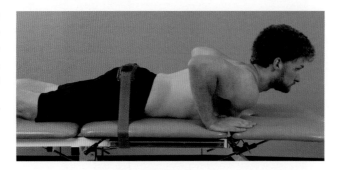

Fig. 8.45 Starting position for measuring lumbar extension in prone position using tape measure method. Note stabilization belt across pelvis.

Patient position

Prone, hands under shoulders. Stabilization belt placed across pelvis at buttocks (Fig. 8.45).

Patient action

Patient is instructed in desired motion. Patient extends elbows and raises trunk as far as possible. Although increased muscle activity will occur appropriately across upper back, patient should relax muscles of lumbar spine.

Patient then returns to starting position. This movement provides an estimate of ROM and demonstrates to patient exact motion desired (Fig. 8.46).

Fig. 8.46 End ROM of lumbar extension in prone position.

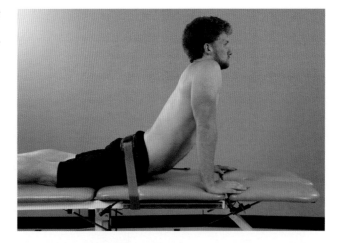

Fig. 8.47 Tape measure alignment at end ROM of lumbar extension in prone position.

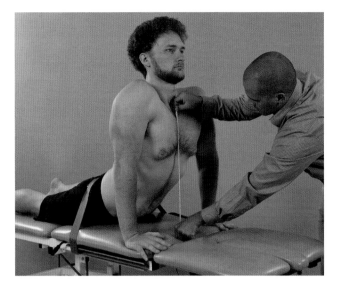

Tape measure alignment	Palpate the landmarks and align tape measure accordingly (Fig. 8.47).
Superior	Sternal notch.
Inferior	Perpendicular to and in contact with support surface.
Patient/Examiner action	At end of ROM in prone extension, examiner measures distance from sternal notch to support surface (see Fig. 8.47).
Documentation	Distance between sternal notch and support surface is recorded.
Precaution	Lifting of pelvis from support surface (Fig. 8.48) should be prevented.

Fig. 8.48 Lifting pelvis from support surface during lumbar extension in prone position because of lack of pelvic stabilization.

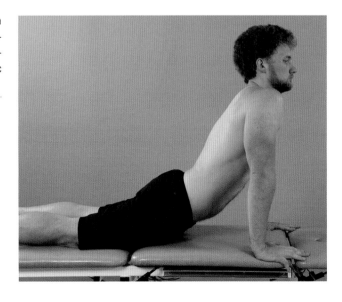

Extension—Lumbar Spine: Goniometer Technique (Video 8.8)

Fig. 8.49 Starting position for measuring lumbar extension using goniometer technique. Landmarks (midaxillary line at level of lowest rib, midaxillary line) indicated by red line and dot.

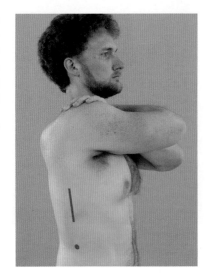

Starting position	Standing, feet shoulder width apart (Fig. 8.49).
Patient action	Patient is instructed in desired motion. Patient crosses arms, placing hands on opposite shoulders, and bends backward as far as possible while keeping knees extended. Patient then returns to starting position. This movement provides an estimate of ROM and demonstrates to patient exact motion desired (Fig. 8.50).
Goniometer alignment	Palpate the landmarks (shown in Fig. 8.49) and align goniometer accordingly (Fig. 8.51).
Stationary arm	Vertical to floor.
Axis	Midaxillary line at level of lowest rib.
Moving arm	Along midaxillary line.
	Read scale of goniometer.

Fig. 8.50 End ROM of lumbar extension. Landmarks (midaxillary line at level of lowest rib, midaxillary line) indicated by red line and dot.

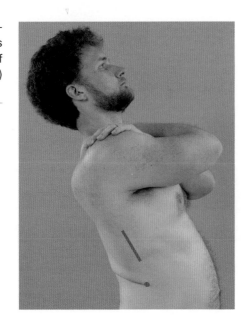

Fig. 8.51 Goniometer alignment at beginning range of
lumbar extension.

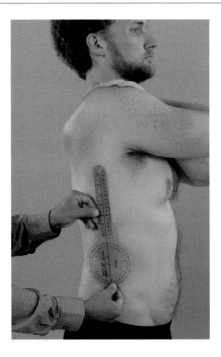

Patient/Examiner action   Patient crosses arms, placing hands on opposite shoulders, and bends backward as
far as possible; full extension of knees should be maintained (see Fig. 8.50).

Confirmation of alignment   Repalpate landmarks and confirm proper goniometer alignment at end ROM, correcting alignment as necessary (Fig. 8.52). Read scale of goniometer.

Documentation   Record patient's ROM.

Fig. 8.52 Goniometer alignment at end ROM of lumbar
extension.

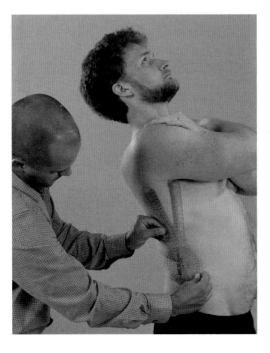

Extension—Lumbar Spine: Inclinometer Method (Video 8.9)

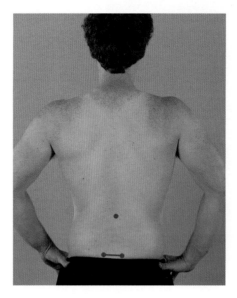

Fig. 8.53 Starting position for measuring lumbar extension using dual-inclinometer (AMA) technique. Bony landmarks for inclinometer alignment (midline of spine in line with PSIS, 15 cm above baseline mark) indicated by red line and dots.

Patient position	Standing, feet shoulder width apart, hands on hips (Fig. 8.53).
Patient action	Patient is instructed in desired motion. Placing hands on hips, patient bends backward as far as possible while keeping knees extended. Patient then returns to starting position. This movement provides an estimate of ROM and demonstrates to patient exact movement desired (Fig. 8.54).
Inclinometer alignment	Palpate the bony landmarks (shown in Fig. 8.53) and align inclinometers accordingly (Fig. 8.55). Ensure that inclinometers are set at 0 degrees.
Baseline	Midline of spine in line with PSIS.
Superior	15 cm above baseline landmark.
Patient/Examiner action	Holding inclinometers in place as patient extends spine through available ROM, examiner reads angle on each device (Fig. 8.56). Inclinometer at superior landmark indicates extension of lumbar spine and hips. Inclinometer at baseline landmark indicates extension of hips alone.

Fig. 8.54 End ROM of lumbar extension. Bony landmarks for inclinometer alignment (midline of spine in line with PSIS, 15 cm above baseline mark) indicated by red line and dots.

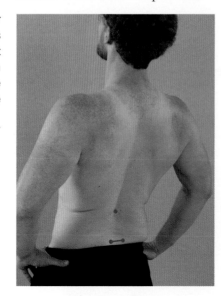

Fig. 8.55 Initial inclinometer alignment for measuring lumbar extension using dual-inclinometer (AMA) technique. Inclinometer set at 0 degrees.

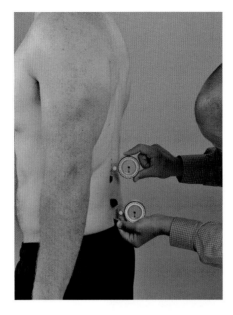

Documentation	Extension ROM recorded is measurement at baseline landmark (after full extension) subtracted from measurement at superior landmark (after full extension). Example: 45 degrees (reading at superior landmark)–20 degrees (reading at baseline landmark)=25 degrees of extension. Record patient's ROM.
Note	Thoracolumbar extension can be measured using the spinous process of C7 vertebra as the superior landmark.

Alternative Technique: The Curve Angle Method

Patient/Examiner action	Patient extends spine through available ROM. Examiner places *single* inclinometer at base landmark at midline of spine in line with PSIS (see Fig. 8.53) and sets the inclinometer at 0 degrees. With patient maintaining full lumbar extension, examiner then moves *single* inclinometer to superior landmark (see Fig. 8.53).
Documentation	Extension ROM recorded is the measurement at the superior landmark.

Fig. 8.56 Inclinometer alignment at end ROM of lumbar extension.

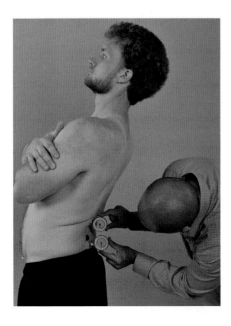

Extension—Lumbar Spine: BROM Device (Video 8.10)

Fig. 8.57 Starting position for measuring lumbar extension using BROM. Bony landmarks for BROM alignment (spinous process of S1 vertebra, spinous process of T12 vertebra) indicated by red dots.

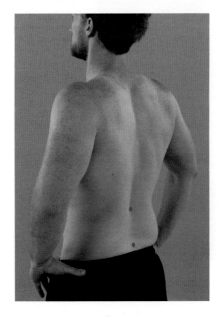

Patient position	Standing erect, feet shoulder width apart (Fig. 8.57).
Patient action	Patient is instructed in desired motion. Placing hands on waist, patient bends backward as far as possible while keeping knees extended. Patient then returns to starting position. This movement provides an estimate of ROM and demonstrates to patient exact motion desired (Fig. 8.58).
BROM alignment	Palpate the bony landmarks (see Fig. 8.57).
Baseline	Spinous process of S1 vertebra.
Superior	Spinous process of T12 vertebra.
Examiner action	Place BROM flexion-extension unit (consisting of base and movable arm) with pivot point on spinous process of S1 vertebra. Hold in place by attaching with Velcro straps to lower abdomen (down-pull of strap is essential to maintain unit against sacrum during flexion and extension) (Fig. 8.59).

Fig. 8.58 End ROM of lumbar extension. Bony landmarks for BROM alignment (spinous process of S1 vertebra, spinous process of T12 vertebra) indicated by red dots.

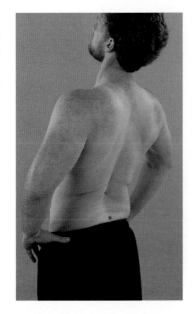

Fig. 8.59 Alignment of BROM flexion-extension unit at beginning of range of lumbar extension. Bony landmark for alignment of movable arm of BROM (spinous process of T12 vertebra).

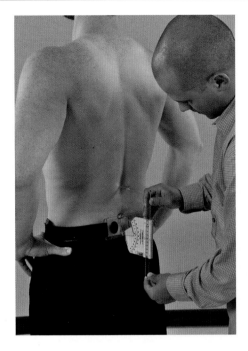

With patient standing erect, examiner places tip of moving arm at level of T12 spinous process (see Fig. 8.59). Record reading from unit as initial measurement.

Patient/Examiner action

Placing hands on waist, patient extends spine through available ROM. Examiner places tip of moving arm at level of T12 spinous process (Fig. 8.60).

Record reading from full extension measurement.

Documentation

Extension ROM is the result of the full extension reading subtracted from initial reading (in erect standing). Example: 85 degrees (initial reading)−75 degrees (reading in full extension)=10 degrees of lumbar extension. Record patient's ROM.

Fig. 8.60 Alignment of BROM at end ROM of lumbar extension.

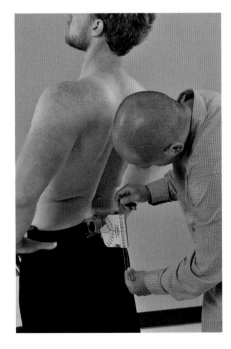

Extension—Lumbar Spine: Smartphone Method

Fig. 8.61 Starting position for measuring lumbar extension using Smartphone.

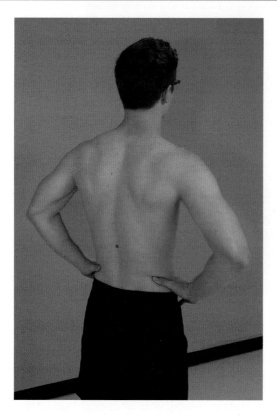

Patient position   Standing, feet shoulder width apart (Fig. 8.61).

Patient motion   Patient is instructed in desired motion. Placing hands on hips, patient bends backward as far as possible while keeping knees extended. Patient then returns to starting position. This movement provides an estimate of ROM and demonstrates to patient exact movement desired (Fig. 8.62).

Fig. 8.62 End range of lumbar extension.

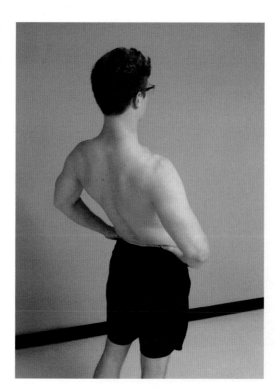

Fig. 8.63 Smartphone alignment at beginning of range of lumbar extension.

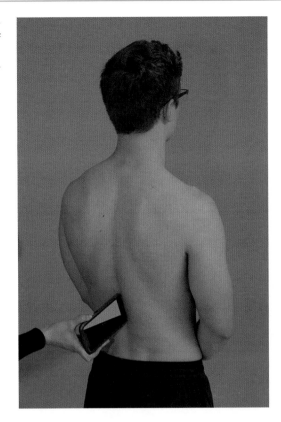

Smartphone alignment

Palpate spinous process of T12 and place border of Smartphone at that location (Fig. 8.63) with Smartphone screen facing toward therapist. Ensure the Smartphone application starts at 0 degrees, cue the patient to adjust trunk as needed.

Patient/Examiner action

Patient extends lumbar spine through available ROM as examiner reads angle of Smartphone at end of extension ROM (Fig. 8.64).

Documentation

Record patient's ROM.

Fig. 8.64 Smartphone alignment at end of range of lumbar extension.

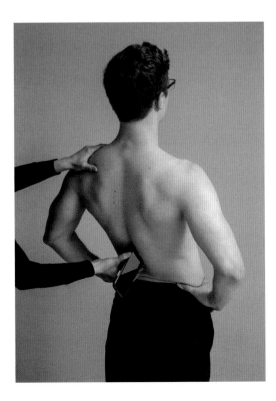

Extension—Thoracic and Lumbar Spine: Flexicurve Technique

Fig.   8.65 Alignment   of Flexicurve in standing neutral posture. Bony landmarks for Flexicurve alignment (spinous process of T1 vertebra, spinous process of T6 vertebra, spinous process of T12 vertebra, spinous process of L4 vertebra, spinous process of S2 vertebra,) indicated by red dots.

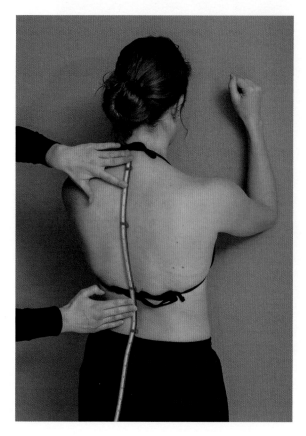

Patient position	The neutral position is assessed with the patient standing erect, feet shoulder width apart, shoulders and elbows flexed to 90 degrees with forearms lightly resting on a wall (Fig. 8.65).
Flexicurve alignment	With patient standing, palpate the bony landmarks and mark with dermographic pencil.
Thoracic	Spinous process of T1 vertebra. Spinous process of T6 vertebra. Spinous process of T12 vertebra.
Lumbar	Spinous process of T12 vertebra. Spinous process of L4 vertebra. Spinous process of S2 vertebra.

Fig. 8.66 After molding Flexicurve to subject in standing, trace contours of Flexicurve onto paper and mark position of spinous processes on paper.

Examiner action

With patient in standing, mold Flexicurve to patient spine and mark spinous processes on the Flexicurve (Fig. 8.65). Trace contours of Flexicurve and position of spinous processes onto paper (Fig. 8.66).

Patient action

Patient is instructed in desired motion. In prone patient places hands on the plinth aligned with their shoulders with the elbows bent, patient extends elbows bending backward as far as possible keeping ASIS in contact with the plinth. Patient then relaxes. This movement demonstrates to patient exact motion desired (Fig. 8.67).

Fig. 8.67 End ROM of thoracolumbar extension using the Flexicurve.

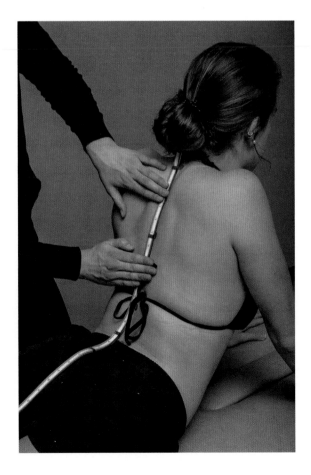

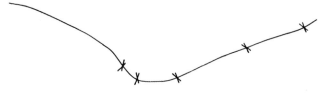

Patient/Examiner action

In prone, patient pushes through arms and extends spine through available ROM. With patient in prone with back extended, examiner molds Flexicurve to patient spine and mark spinous processes (Fig. 8.67). Trace contours of Flexicurve and position of spinous processes onto paper (Fig. 8.68).

Documentation

Thoracic curvature angles are calculated by drawing line L between the T1 and T12 spinous processes, and line H is constructed so it is perpendicular to Line L at the T6 mid-point bisecting line L creating Line L1 and Line L2 (Fig. 8.69). The angles of the thoracic curve in neutral and in extension are calculated using the formula $[\text{theta}] = [\arctan(H/L1)] + [\arctan(H/L2)]$ where [theta] represents the magnitude of the thoracic curve. The thoracic angle in full extension is reported in degrees from the prone measurement. Additionally, the thoracic extension ROM can be calculated by subtracting the thoracic angle in full extension (prone) from the thoracic angle in neutral position (standing).

Fig. 8.69 To measure thoracic extension, mark T1 at the top of the drawing and T12 at the bottom. To measure lumbar extension, mark T12 at the top of the drawing and S2 at the bottom.

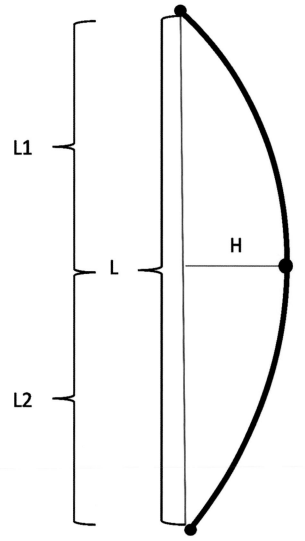

Lumbar curvature angles are calculated by drawing line L between the T12 and S2 spinous processes. Line H is constructed so it bisects and is perpendicular to Line H at the L4 mid-point (Fig. 8.69). The angles of the lumbar curve in neutral and in extension are calculated using the formula [alpha]=4 X [arctan(2H/L)] where [alpha] represents the magnitude of the lumbar curve. The lumbar angle in full extension is reported in degrees from the prone measurement. Additionally, lumbar extension ROM can be calculated by subtracting the lumbar angle in full extension (prone) from the lumbar angle in neutral position (standing).

Lateral Flexion—Thoracolumbar Spine: Tape Measure Method (Video 8.11)

Fig. 8.70 Starting position for measuring thoracolumbar lateral flexion using the tape measure method. Landmark indicated by red dot at level of tip of middle finger.

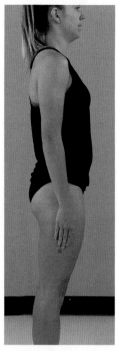

Patient position	Standing, feet shoulder width apart, palm of hand against thigh (Fig. 8.70).
Patient action	Patient is instructed in desired motion. Running hand down the side of the leg, patient laterally flexes spine as far as possible. Patient keeps knees extended and does not bend trunk forward or backward while performing movement.
	Patient then returns to starting position. This movement provides an estimate of ROM and demonstrates to patient exact motion desired (Fig. 8.71).
Landmark	With patient positioned in erect standing, skin mark is placed at thigh level with tip of middle finger (see Fig. 8.70).

Fig. 8.71 End ROM of thoracolumbar lateral flexion. Landmark indicated by red dot at level of tip of middle finger at end ROM.

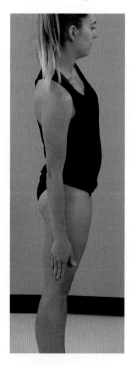

Fig. 8.72 Measuring difference between skin marks on thigh using tape measure.

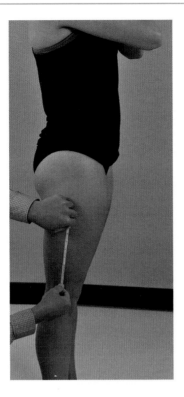

Patient/Examiner action	Patient laterally flexes spine, running hand down the side of the leg as far as possible. At maximal lateral flexion, position of the middle fingertip against thigh is marked again (Fig. 8.71).
Documentation	Lateral flexion ROM is the difference between the skin mark on thigh in erect standing and skin mark on thigh in full lateral flexion (see Fig. 8.72). Record patient's ROM.

Alternative Technique (Video 8.12)

Patient/Examiner action	At maximal lateral flexion, distance from tip of middle finger to floor is measured (Fig. 8.73).
Documentation	Distance between tip of middle finger and floor is recorded.

Fig. 8.73 Tape measure alignment at end ROM of lateral flexion using alternative (distance-to-floor) technique.

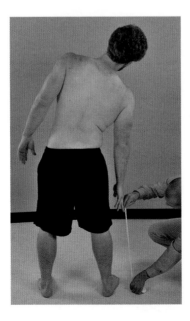

Lateral Flexion—Lumbar Spine: Goniometer Technique (Video 8.13)

Fig. 8.74 Starting position for measuring lumbar lateral flexion using goniometer technique. Landmarks for goniometer alignment (spinous process of S1 vertebra, spinous process of C7 vertebra) indicated by red dots.

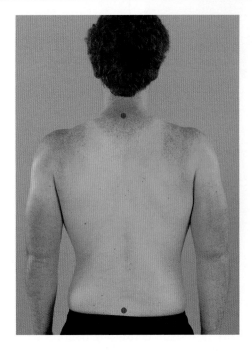

Patient position	Standing, feet shoulder width apart (Fig. 8.74).
Patient action	Patient is instructed in desired motion. Running hand down the side of the leg, patient laterally flexes spine as far as possible. Patient keeps knees extended and does not bend trunk forward or backward while performing movement. Patient then returns to starting position. This movement provides an estimate of ROM and demonstrates to patient exact motion desired (Fig. 8.75).
Goniometer alignment	Palpate the bony landmarks (shown in Fig. 8.74) and align goniometer accordingly (Fig. 8.76).

Fig. 8.75 End ROM of lumbar lateral flexion. Landmarks for goniometer alignment (spinous process of S1 vertebra, spinous process of C7 vertebra) indicated by red dots.

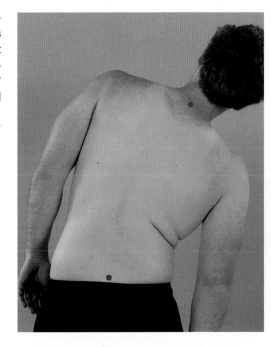

Fig. 8.76 Goniometer alignment at beginning range of lumbar lateral flexion.

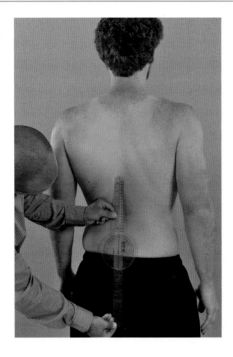

Stationary arm	Vertical to floor.
Axis	Spinous process of S1 vertebra.
Moving arm	Spinous process of C7 vertebra.
	Read scale of goniometer.
Patient/Examiner action	Running hand down the side of the leg, patient laterally flexes spine as far as possible (see Fig. 8.77).
Confirmation of alignment	Repalpate landmarks and confirm proper goniometer alignment at end ROM, correcting alignment as necessary (Fig. 8.77). Read scale of goniometer.
Documentation	Record patient's ROM.

Fig. 8.77 Goniometer alignment at end ROM of lumbar lateral flexion.

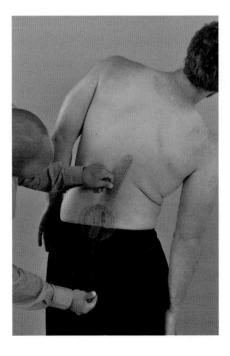

Lateral Flexion—Lumbar Spine: Inclinometer Method (Video 8.14)

Fig. 8.78 Starting position for measuring lumbar lateral flexion using inclinometer method. Bony landmarks for inclinometer alignment (midline of spine at level of PSIS, 15 cm above baseline landmark) indicated by red line and dots.

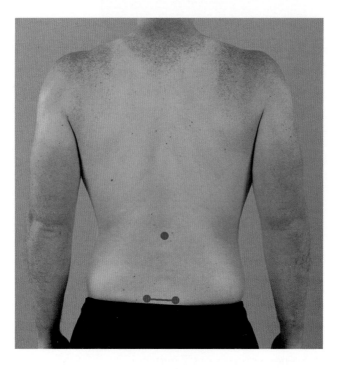

Patient position	Standing, feet shoulder width apart, arms at sides (Fig. 8.78).
Patient action	Patient is instructed in desired motion. Running hand down the side of the leg, patient laterally flexes spine as far as possible. Patient keeps knees extended and does not bend trunk forward or backward while performing movement. Patient then returns to starting position. This movement provides an estimate of ROM and demonstrates to patient exact motion desired (Fig. 8.79).
Inclinometer alignment	Palpate the bony landmarks (shown in Fig. 8.78) and align inclinometers accordingly (Fig. 8.80). Ensure that inclinometers are set at 0 degrees.

Fig. 8.79 End ROM of lumbar lateral flexion. Bony landmarks for inclinometer alignment (midline of spine at level of PSIS, 15 cm above baseline landmark) indicated by red line and dots.

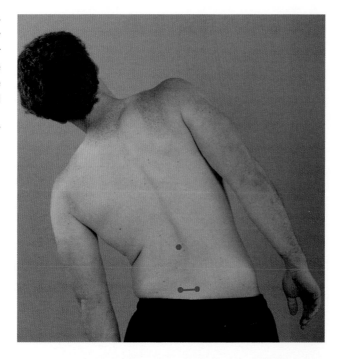

Fig. 8.80 Initial inclinometer alignment for measurement of lumbar lateral flexion. Bony landmarks for inclinometer alignment (midline of spine at level of PSIS, 15 cm above baseline landmark).

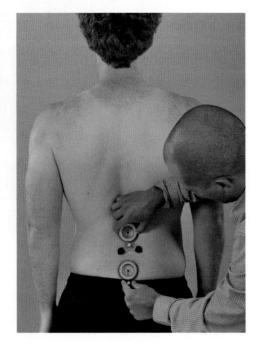

Inferior	Midline of spine in line with PSIS.
Superior	15 cm above baseline landmark.
Patient/Examiner action	Patient laterally flexes spine through available ROM while examiner holds both inclinometers in place. When patient reaches end ROM, examiner reads angle on each device (Fig. 8.81).
Documentation	Lateral flexion ROM recorded is the measurement at the baseline landmark (after full lateral flexion) subtracted from measurement at the superior landmark (after full lateral flexion). Example: 20 degrees (reading at superior landmark) – 0 degrees (reading at baseline landmark) = 20 degrees of lateral flexion. Record patient's ROM.

Fig. 8.81 Inclinometer alignment at end ROM of lumbar lateral flexion. Bony landmarks for inclinometer alignment (midline of spine at level of PSIS, 15 cm above baseline landmark).

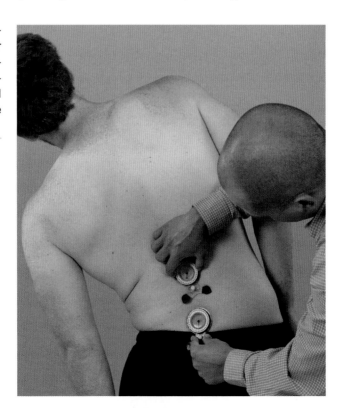

Lateral Flexion—Lumbar Spine: BROM Device

Fig. 8.82 Starting position for measuring lumbar lateral flexion using the BROM. Bony landmark (spinous process of T12 vertebra) indicated by red dot.

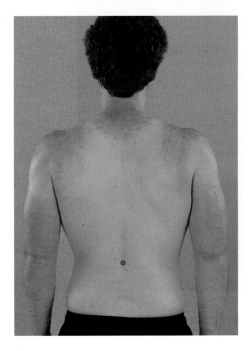

Patient position   Standing erect, feet shoulder width apart (Fig. 8.82).

Patient action   Patient is instructed in desired motion. Running hand down the side of the leg, patient laterally flexes spine as far as possible. Patient keeps knees extended and does not bend trunk forward or backward while performing movement. Patient then returns to starting position. This movement provides an estimate of ROM and demonstrates to patient exact motion desired (Fig. 8.83).

Fig. 8.83 End ROM of lumbar lateral flexion. Bony landmark (spinous process of T12 vertebra) indicated by red dot.

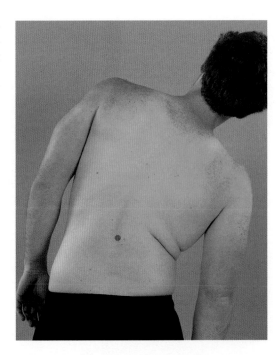

Fig. 8.84 Alignment of BROM at beginning range of lumbar lateral flexion.

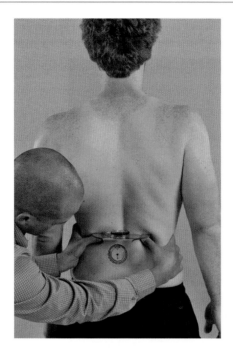

BROM alignment

Palpate spinous process of T12 vertebra (see Fig. 8.82).

Examiner places center of BROM lateral flexion-rotation unit firmly against patient's back so that feet of unit are in line with spinous process of T12. Examiner places thumbs over feet of unit and grasps patient's rib cage with fingers. Position of unit is adjusted on patient's back until inclinometer reads 0 degrees (Fig. 8.84).

Patient/Examiner action

Patient laterally flexes spine through available ROM while examiner holds lateral flexion-rotation unit in place. When patient reaches end ROM, examiner reads inclinometer (Fig. 8.85).

Documentation

Record patient's ROM.

Fig. 8.85 Alignment of BROM at end ROM of lumbar lateral flexion.

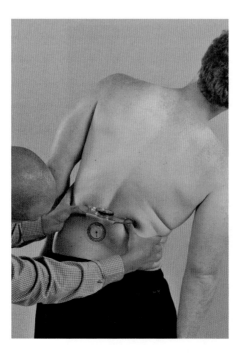

Lateral Flexion—Lumbar Spine: Smartphone Method

Fig. 8.86 Starting position for measuring lateral flexion using Smartphone.

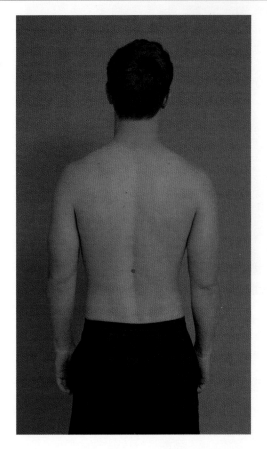

Patient position   Standing, feet shoulder width apart, arms at sides (Fig. 8.86).

Patient action   Patient is instructed in desired motion. Running hand down the side of the leg, patient laterally flexes spine as far as possible. Patient keeps knees extended and does not bend trunk forward or backward while performing movement. Patient then returns to starting position. This movement provides an estimate of ROM and demonstrates to patient exact motion desired (Fig. 8.87).

Fig. 8.87 End of range of lateral flexion.

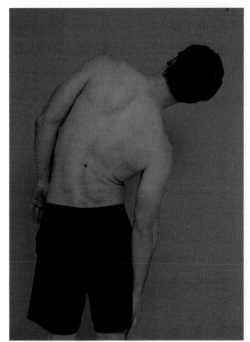

Fig. 8.88 Smartphone alignment at beginning range of lateral flexion.

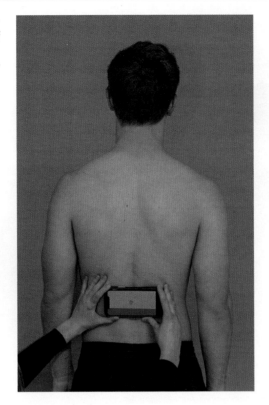

Smartphone Alignment

Palpate spinous process of T12 and place border of Smartphone at that location (Fig. 8.88) with Smartphone screen facing toward therapist. Ensure the Smartphone application starts at 0 degrees, cue the patient to adjust trunk as needed.

Patient/Examiner action   Patient laterally flexes lumbar spine through available ROM as examiner reads angle of Smartphone at end of lateral flexion ROM (Fig. 8.89).

Documentation   Record patient's ROM.

Fig. 8.89 Smartphone alignment at end of range of lateral flexion.

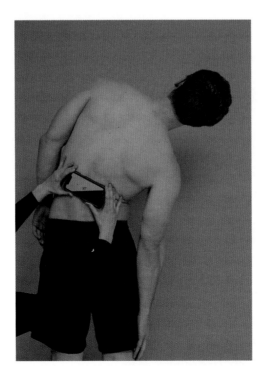

Rotation—Thoracolumbar Spine: Tape Measure Method (Video 8.15)

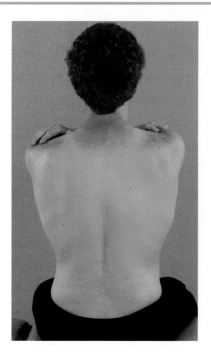

Fig. 8.90 Starting position for measuring thoracolumbar rotation using tape measure method.

Patient position	Sitting erect, arms crossed, and hands on opposite shoulders (Fig. 8.90).
Patient action	Patient is instructed in desired motion. Maintaining neutral position of spine and arms crossed with hands on opposite shoulders, patient rotates spine as far as possible. No lateral flexion should occur during rotation. Patient then returns to starting position. This movement provides an estimate of ROM and demonstrates to patient exact motion desired (Fig. 8.91).
Tape measure alignment	Palpate the bony landmarks and align tape measure accordingly (Fig. 8.92).
Superior	Lateral tip of ipsilateral acromion.

Fig. 8.91 End ROM of thoracolumbar rotation.

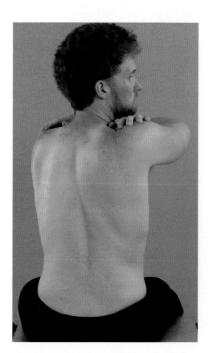

Fig. 8.92 Initial tape measure alignment for measuring thoracolumbar rotation in sitting. *Note:* Patient holds tape measure against superior landmark (lateral tip of ipsilateral acromion).

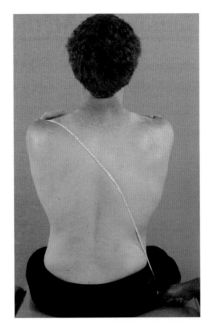

Inferior	Greater trochanter of contralateral femur.
Examiner action	Tape measure is aligned with 0 cm at superior landmark and is maintained against subject's back. After placing tape measure at acromion, examiner asks patient to maintain tape measure at that position. Distance between superior and inferior landmark is measured, referred to as the *initial measurement* (see Fig. 8.92).
Patient/Examiner action	As patient rotates spine through available ROM while holding tape measure on superior landmark, examiner allows tape measure to unwind from tape measure case. Examiner records distance between superior and inferior landmarks, referred to as the *final measurement* (Fig. 8.93).
Documentation	Rotation ROM is difference between length measured at beginning of rotation motion (initial measurement) and length measured at end of rotation motion (final measurement). Example: 86 cm (final measurement) – 80 cm (initial measurement) = 6 cm of rotation. Record patient's ROM.

Fig. 8.93 Tape measure alignment at end ROM of thoracolumbar rotation.

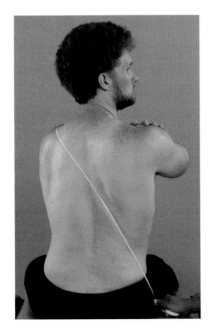

Rotation—Thoracic Spine: Goniometer Method

Fig. 8.94 Starting position for measuring thoracic rotation using goniometer method.

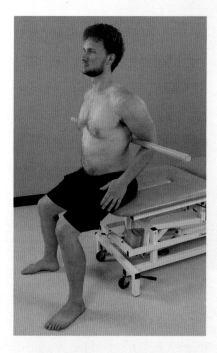

Patient position

Seated, hips and knees at 90 degrees, trunk in an upright and neutral posture. Bar is held behind back in the cubital fossa of the elbows. Palmar aspects of the patient's hands are placed at the hips; fingers do not need to interlock (Fig. 8.94).

Patient action

Patient is instructed in desired motion. Maintaining neutral position of the spine, patient rotates as far as possible. Patient then returns to starting position. This movement provides an estimate of ROM and demonstrates to patient exact motion desired (Fig. 8.95).

Fig. 8.95 End ROM of thoracic rotation in sitting position.

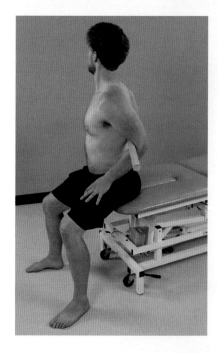

Fig. 8.96 Initial goniometer alignment measuring of thoracic rotation in sitting position.

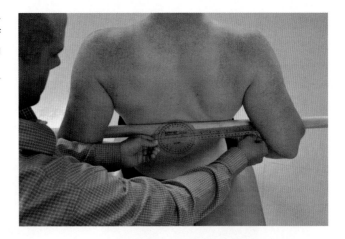

Goniometer alignment	Align the goniometer as follows (Fig. 8.96).
Stationary arm	Parallel to scapula in starting position.
Axis	At the level of the T1-T2 spinous process.
Moving arm	Parallel to bar held behind back.
	Read scale of goniometer.
Examiner action	Standing behind the patient, the subject actively rotates the thoracic spine, keeping the spine in neutral position.
Confirmation of alignment	Confirm proper goniometer alignment at end of ROM, correcting alignment as necessary (Fig. 8.97). Read scale of goniometer.
Documentation	Record patient's ROM.

Fig. 8.97 Goniometer alignment at end ROM of thoracic rotation in sitting position.

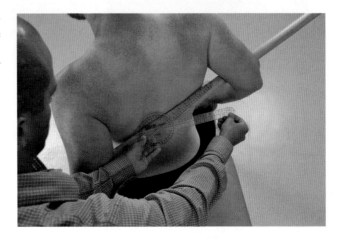

Rotation—Thoracolumbar Spine: Inclinometer Method

Fig. 8.98 Starting position for measuring thoracolumbar rotation in side-lying position using inclinometer method.

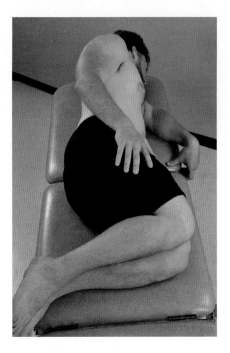

Patient position

Side-lying, hips and knees flexed to 90 degrees. The subject's trunk, scapula, and posterior deltoid muscle (not the lateral shoulder) are in contact with the support surface. The subject places the hand closest to the support surface on the support surface and the hand farthest away from the support surface on the hip (Fig. 8.98).

Patient action

Patient is instructed in desired motion. Maintaining position of hands, patient rotates as far as possible. Patient then returns to starting position. This movement provides an estimate of ROM and demonstrates to patient exact motion desired (Fig. 8.99).

Fig. 8.99 End ROM of thoracolumbar rotation in side-lying position.

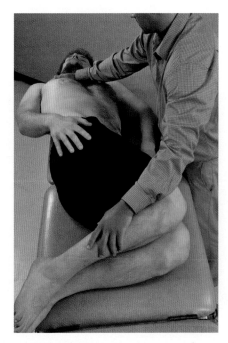

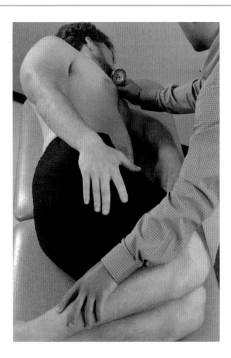

Fig. 8.100 Initial inclinometer alignment for measurement of thoracolumbar rotation in side-lying position.

Inclinometer alignment	The inclinometer is placed across the subject's sternoclavicular joint using the sternoclavicular notch as the reference point. The examiner zeros the inclinometer at the starting point that is perpendicular to the treatment table (Fig. 8.100).
Examiner action	The examiner stands behind the patient and stabilizes the subject by holding calves down and not allowing the knees to separate. The examiner rotates the patient's trunk posteriorly back onto the support surface to approximate the scapula to the surface and the measurement is recorded (Fig. 8.101).
Documentation	Record patient's ROM.

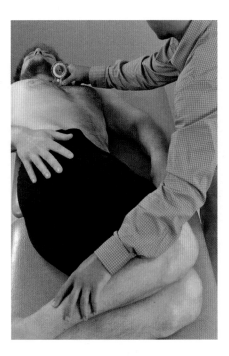

Fig. 8.101 Inclinometer alignment at end ROM of thoracolumbar rotation in side-lying position.

Rotation—Thoracic Spine: Inclinometer Method (Video 8.16)

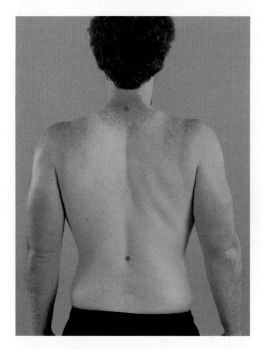

Fig. 8.102 Starting position for measuring thoracic rotation using inclinometer method. Bony landmarks (spinous process of T12 vertebra, spinous process of T1 vertebra) indicated by red dots.

Patient position	Standing, feet shoulder width apart (Fig. 8.102).
Patient action	Patient is instructed in desired motion. Patient forward flexes until thoracic spine is as parallel to floor as possible. In this position, ask subject to rotate the trunk maximally. This movement provides an estimate of ROM and demonstrates to patient exact motion desired.
Inclinometer alignment	Palpate the bony landmarks (shown in Fig. 8.102) and align inclinometers accordingly. With patient flexed so that the thoracic spine is as close to horizontal as possible, one inclinometer is held at the baseline landmark, and one is held at the superior landmark (Fig. 8.103). Ensure that inclinometers are set at 0 degrees.

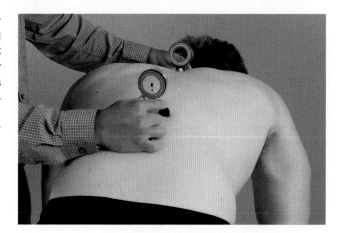

Fig. 8.103 Initial inclinometer alignment for measuring thoracic rotation with patient flexed to horizontal. Bony landmarks (spinous process of T12 vertebra, spinous process of T1 vertebra).

Fig. 8.104 Inclinometer alignment at end ROM of thoracic rotation. Bony landmarks (spinous process of T12 vertebra, spinous process of T1 vertebra).

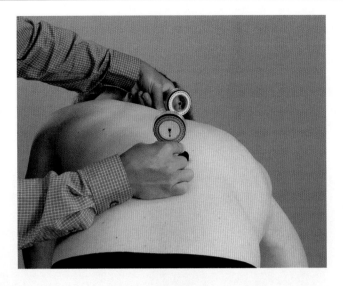

Baseline	Spinous process of T12 vertebra.
Superior	Spinous process of T1 vertebra.
Patient/Examiner action	Holding inclinometers in place as patient rotates spine through available ROM, examiner reads angle on each device (Fig. 8.104).
Documentation	Rotation ROM recorded is the measurement of the angle at the T12 vertebra (after full rotation) subtracted from angle at T1 vertebra (after full rotation). Example: 70 degrees (reading at T1) − 50 degrees (reading at T12) = 20 degrees of rotation. Record patient's ROM.

Rotation—Lumbar Spine: BROM (Video 8.17)

Fig. 8.105 Starting position for measuring lumbar rotation using BROM. Bony landmarks (spinous process of S1 vertebra, spinous process of T12 vertebra) indicated by red dots.

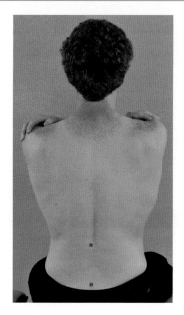

Patient position	Sitting erect on nonrotating stool facing west, feet flat on floor. Patient crosses arms, placing hands on opposite shoulders (Fig. 8.105).
Patient action	Patient is instructed in desired motion. Maintaining neutral position of spine and arms crossed with hands on opposite shoulders, patient rotates spine as far as possible. No lateral flexion should occur during rotation. Patient then returns to starting position. This movement provides an estimate of ROM and demonstrates to patient exact motion desired.
BROM alignment	Palpate the bony landmarks (shown in Fig. 8.105).
Baseline	Spinous process of S1 vertebra.
Superior	Spinous process of T12 vertebra.

To measure rotation, a magnetic reference is used in conjunction with a horizontally placed magnetic inclinometer. Magnetic reference is placed over S1 vertebra and is held in place with Velcro straps (Fig. 8.106).

Fig. 8.106 Addition of magnetic reference.

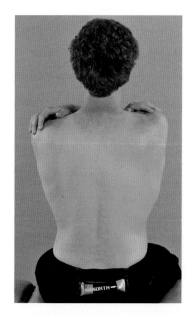

Fig. 8.107 BROM alignment at beginning range of lumbar rotation.

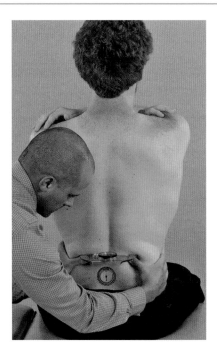

Examiner places center of BROM lateral flexion-rotation unit firmly against patient's back so that the feet of the unit are in line with the spinous process of T12 and sets the horizontal inclinometer at 0 degrees. Examiner then changes hand position, holding rotation unit so examiner's thumbs grasp the feet of the unit and examiner's fingers grasp the patient's rib cage (Fig. 8.107).

Patient/Examiner action

Holding rotation unit in place as patient rotates spine through available ROM, examiner reads number of degrees on inclinometer (Fig. 8.108).

Documentation

Record patient's ROM.

Fig. 8.108 BROM alignment at end ROM of lumbar rotation.

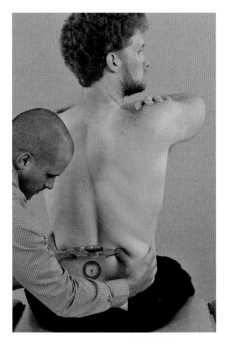

References

1. Grant R, ed. *Physical Therapy of the Cervical and Thoracic Spine.* 3rd ed. New York: Churchill Livingstone; 2002.
2. Levangie PL, Norkin CC. *Joint Structure & Function: A Comprehensive Analysis.* 5th ed. Philadelphia: F.A. Davis Co; 2011.
3. Neumann DA. *Kinesiology of the Musculoskeletal System.* 2nd ed. St. Louis: Mosby, Inc; 2009.
4. Hsieh CJ, Pringle RK. Range of motion of the lumbar spine required for four activities of daily living. *J Manipulative Physiol Ther.* 1994;17:353–358.
5. Macrae IF, Wright V. Measurement of back movement. *Ann Rheum Dis.* 1969;28:584–589.
6. van Adrichem JAM, van der Korst JK. Assessment of the flexibility of the lumbar spine. *Scand J Rheumatol.* 1973;2:87–91.
7. Williams R, Binkley J, R B, et al. Reliability of the modified–modified Schober and double inclinometer methods for measuring lumbar flexion and extension. *Phys Ther.* 1993;73:26–37.
8. Moll JMV, Wright V. Normal range of motion: an objective clinical study. *Ann Rheum Dis.* 1971;30:381–386.
9. Gauvin MG, Riddle DL, Rothstein JM. Reliability of clinical measurements of forward bending using the modified fingertip–to–floor method. *Phys Ther.* 1990;70:443–447.
10. Hyytiainen K, Salminen JJ, Suvitie T, et al. Reproducibility of nine tests to measure spinal mobility and trunk muscle strength. *Scand J Rehabil Med.* 1991;23:3–10.
11. Mellin GP. Accuracy of measuring lateral flexion of the spine with a tape. *Clin Biomech.* 1986;1:85–89.
12. Frost M, Stuckey S, Smalley LA, Dorman G. Reliability of measuring trunk motions in centimeters. *Phys Ther.* 1982;62:1431–1437.
13. American Medical Association. *Guides to the Evaluation of Permanent Impairment.* 6th ed. Chicago: Author; 2007.
14. Saunders HD. *Saunders Digital Inclinometer.* Chaska, MN: Saunders Group; 1998.
15. Barrett E, McCreesh K, Lewis J. Reliability and validity of non-radiographic methods of thoracic kyphosis measurement: a systematic review. *Man Ther.* 2014;19(1):10–17.
16. Burton AK. Regional lumbar sagittal mobility; measurement by flexicurves. *Clin Biomech.* 1986;1(1):20–26.
17. de Oliveira TS, Candotti CT, La Torre M, et al. Validity and reproducibility of the measurements obtained using the flexicurve instrument to evaluate the angles of thoracic and lumbar curvatures of the spine in the sagittal plane. *Rehabil Res Pract.* 2012;2012:1–9.
18. Hart DL, Rose SJ. Reliability of a noninvasive method for measuring the lumbar curve. *J Orthop Sports Phys Ther.* 1986;8(4):180–184.
19. Tillotson KM, Burton AK. Noninvasive measurement of lumbar sagittal mobility an assessment of the flexicurve technique. *Spine.* 1991;16(1):29–33.
20. Valle MB, Dutra VH, Candotti CT, Sedrez JA, Wagner Neto ES, Loss JF. Validity of flexicurve for the assessment of spinal flexibility in asymptomatic individuals. *Fisioterapia em Movimento.* 2020;33.
21. Youdas JW, Suman VJ, Garrett TR. Reliability of measurements of lumbar spine sagittal mobility obtained with the flexible curve. *J Orthop Sports Phys Ther.* 1995;21(1):13–20.

9

MEASUREMENT of RANGE of MOTION of the CERVICAL SPINE and TEMPOROMANDIBULAR JOINT

William D. Bandy

CERVICAL SPINE

ANATOMY AND OSTEOKINEMATICS

The following discussion of the cervical spine is a synopsis of information presented in several contemporary sources.[1-4] The cervical region of the spine is composed of two anatomically and functionally distinct regions: the suboccipital region and the lower cervical region. The bones of the suboccipital region include the occipital bone and the first and second cervical vertebrae (C1–C2); the third through the seventh cervical vertebrae (C3–C7) make up the lower cervical region (Fig. 9.1).

The atlas (C1) has no body or spinous process and is shaped like a ring. Articulation between the two superior facets of the atlas and the two condyles on the occiput of the skull forms the atlantooccipital joint. Movement between the atlas and the occiput (atlantooccipital joint) is primarily a nodding motion in the sagittal plane about a medial–lateral axis. The axis (C2) has a vertical projection called the dens (also known as the odontoid process) that arises from the superior surface of the body (Fig. 9.2). The dens of the axis fits into a ring formed by the anterior arches of the atlas and the transverse (cruciform) ligament so that the atlas pivots around the dens of the axis. Fifty percent of rotation in the cervical spine occurs at the atlantoaxial joint.

The C3–C7 vertebrae have common structural features that are typical for the spine. These features are presented in Fig. 9.3.

A general overview of the connective tissue of the cervical spine includes the intervertebral discs, which connect the vertebral bodies starting with C2–C3 and lower that form intervertebral cartilaginous joints. The supporting ligaments include the anterior longitudinal, posterior longitudinal, ligamentum flavum, interspinous, ligamentum nuchae, and the joint capsules of the facet joints (Fig. 9.4).

The facet joints are located laterally on each side of the spine and are formed by the articulation of the facet surfaces of the two vertebrae. These facet joints occur in pairs in the cervical spine, with the inferior facet of the superior cervical vertebrae (oriented inferiorly and anteriorly) articulating with the superior facet surface of the inferior vertebrae (oriented superiorly and posteriorly) (see Fig. 9.1).

Segmental motion occurs as the top vertebra slides onto the bottom vertebra (arthrokinematic movement), whereby the facet joints of the vertebrae contribute to and guide the motion. The direction of movement between two vertebrae is greatly influenced, in large part, by the orientation of the joint surfaces that make up the facet joints. Although movement at each segment of the cervical spine is somewhat small, the combined movement of all cervical segments produces a large, triaxial/triplanar range of motion (ROM) of the whole cervical spine, including the head. During measurement of cervical movement, the combined motions of all facet joints between the occiput and C7 are measured because segmented motion is very difficult to assess accurately. With the neutral, resting position of the head and neck as a point of reference, these multisegment, osteokinematic movements are called flexion and extension (sagittal plane), right and left lateral flexion (frontal plane), and right and left rotation (transverse plane).

LIMITATIONS OF MOTION: CERVICAL SPINE

Limitation of motion in the first two cervical vertebrae is due to a ligamentous support system specific to this area of the spine. This support structure at the atlantooccipital and atlantoaxial joints includes the tectorial membrane and the atlantoaxial (anterior and posterior), alar, and transverse ligaments. From C2 to C7, the anterior longitudinal ligament and the contact of the spinous processes limit excessive extension. Flexion is limited by the same ligaments that limit flexion in the lumbar spine (the posterior longitudinal, ligamentum flavum, and interspinous ligaments), with the addition of the ligamentum nuchae in the cervical spine. Running along the tips of the spinous processes of the cervical spine, the ligamentum nuchae is actually a continuation of the supraspinous ligament. Lateral flexion is limited by the bony configuration of the saddle-shaped surface

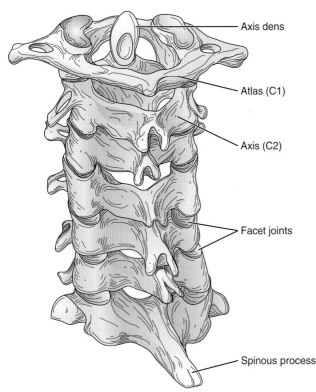

Fig. 9.1   The cervical spine.

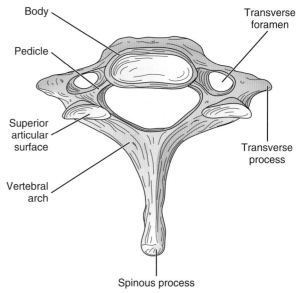

Fig. 9.3   Typical cervical vertebra.

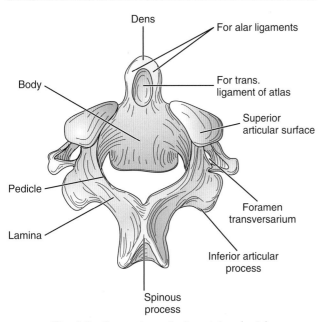

Fig. 9.2   Second cervical vertebra (axis).

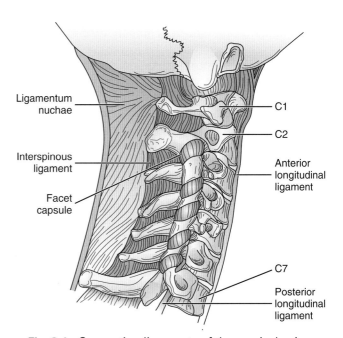

Fig. 9.4   Supporting ligaments of the cervical spine.

of the vertebral body, and rotation is limited by the fibers of the annulus fibrosus of the disc. Appendix B provides information regarding normal ROM of the cervical spine.

FUNCTIONAL RANGE OF MOTION: CERVICAL SPINE

The cervical spine is more mobile than the thoracic and the lumbar spine and is designed to meet the requirements of positioning the head in space and moving it to alter the visual field.[3] Limitations in cervical ROM may restrict the ability of a person to perform those tasks that require full ROM or may cause the person to adapt by using trunk movement. Bennett et al.[5] reported on the amount of cervical ROM required for 13 daily functional tasks in 28 subjects (aged 21–26 years). Activities that required the greatest amount of cervical ROM were reported to be looking over the shoulder when driving a car in reverse (rotation) (Fig. 9.5), placing an object on a high shelf (Fig. 9.6), drinking from a glass (Fig. 9.7), putting on socks (Fig. 9.8), and washing hair in the shower. Cutting with a knife, holding a telephone to the ear, reading a newspaper, rising from a chair, opening a door, pouring from

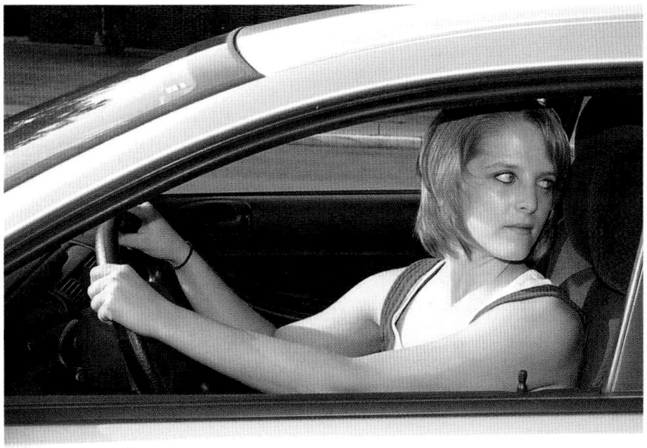

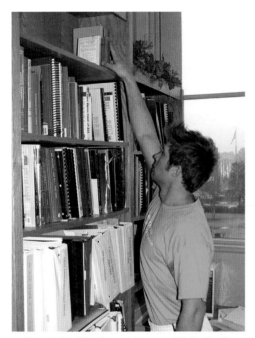

Fig. 9.5   Driving car in reverse.

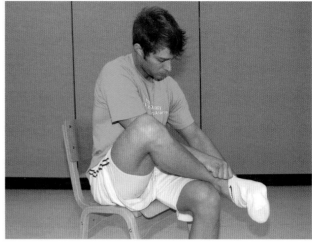

Fig. 9.8   Putting on socks.

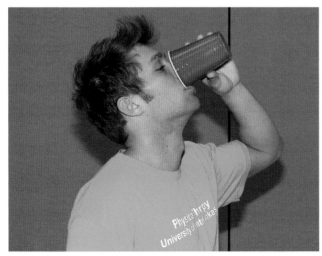

Fig. 9.6   Placing object on high shelf.

a pitcher, writing at a table, and working on a computer did not require much cervical ROM.

TECHNIQUES OF MEASUREMENT: CERVICAL SPINE

Tape Measure and Goniometer

Measurement of ROM of the cervical spine using both the tape measure and the goniometer is common. These measurement devices are easy to use and are relatively inexpensive.

Inclinometer

In Chapter 8, which describes measurement of the thoracic and lumbar spine, it is noted that the American Medical Association (AMA) has accepted the inclinometer as "a feasible and potentially accurate method of measuring spine mobility."[6] This statement was directed not only at examination of the thoracic and lumbar spine but also at measurement of the cervical spine. The use of single and double inclinometers that are held in place manually is specifically included in the *Guides to the Evaluation of Permanent Impairment*.[6]

Attachment of Inclinometer to the Head

The process of attaching an inclinometer to the head to measure cervical ROM has undergone a sort of evolution, beginning with the inclinometer attached to the ears and worn like headphones in the early 1960s and progressing with increasing sophistication to use of the cervical range of motion (CROM) device (Performance Attainment Associates, Roseville, MN) in the late 1990s. This evolution included the "bubble goniometer,"[7] the attachment of the inclinometer to the head with elastic straps,[8] a "cloth helmet,"[9] the use of rigid headgear with three scales calibrated in degrees mounted on a skull cap,[10] the use of an inclinometer mounted on a wood block and placed on the head,[11] the "rangiometer,"[12] and

Fig. 9.7   Drinking from a glass.

finally, the CROM device.[13] Although not included in the *Guides to the Evaluation of Permanent Impairment*,[6] the CROM device has been widely adopted by clinicians.

Smartphone

The Smartphone is a device that is easy to use for measuring ROM. Studies that will be presented in Chapter 10 will indicate that the Smartphone is a reliable device to use clinically in measuring cervical ROM. The use of the Smartphone device will vary between each phone type.

TEMPOROMANDIBULAR JOINT

ANATOMY AND OSTEOKINEMATICS

The temporomandibular joint (TMJ) is unique in that the mandible has two articulations with the temporal bone, forming two separate but solidly connected joints

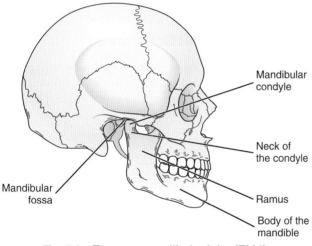

Fig. 9.9   Temporomandibular joint (TMJ).

(Fig. 9.9). The two joints must be considered together in any examination. In addition, each TMJ has a disc that completely divides each joint into two cavities (Fig. 9.10). Movement that occurs in the upper cavity (the joint formed by the temporal bone and the superior surface of the disc) is a gliding or translatory motion, and movement that occurs in the lower cavity (the joint formed by the mandibular condyle and the inferior surface of the disc) is a rotatory or hinge movement.

The primary ligament reinforcing the TMJ is the lateral temporomandibular ligament, which stabilizes the lateral capsule (Fig. 9.11). Medial to the joint capsule, the stylomandibular and sphenomandibular ligaments are accessory ligaments to the capsule (Fig. 9.12).

Movement of the mandible involves bilateral action of the TMJ. Abnormal function of one joint interferes with the function of the other. Movement of the TMJ occurs by a process that combines rotation of the mandible, in which the mandibular condyles roll onto the inferior surface of the disc, and translation of the combination of the mandibular condyle and the disc, which move onto the mandibular fossa of the temporal bone. For a detailed description of the condyle-disc-complex translation, the reader is referred to Levangie and Norkin.[3]

During protrusion, that is, the anterior movement of the mandible in the horizontal plane, the mandibular condyle and the disc translate anteriorly and posteriorly, respectively, on the mandibular fossa of the temporal bone. Lateral deviation (excursion), lateral movement of the mandible in the horizontal plane, occurs with side-to-side translation of the condyle and disc on the mandibular fossa.

During mandibular depression (opening the mouth), movement is slightly different from the translation that occurs during protrusion and lateral deviation. During the opening, the TMJ experiences a combination of rotation and translation between the mandibular condyle, articular disc, and mandibular fossa.

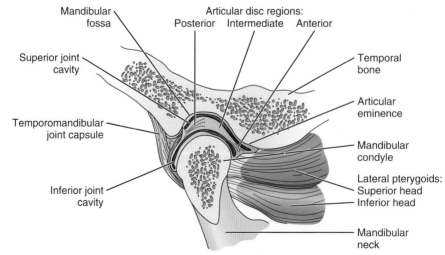

Fig. 9.10   View of TMJ indicating the regions of the disc separating the temporal bone and the mandibular condyle.

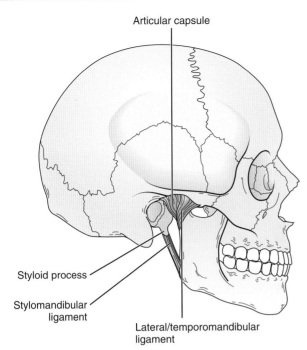

Fig. 9.11   Temporomandibular ligament.

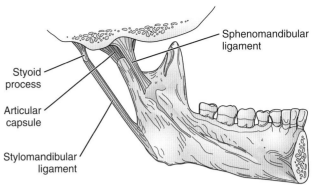

Fig.   9.12   Stylomandibular   and   sphenomandibular ligaments.

LIMITATIONS OF MOTION: TEMPOROMANDIBULAR JOINT

The temporomandibular, or lateral, ligament is a strong ligament that limits mandibular depression, protrusion, and lateral deviation. Protrusion is also limited by the stylomandibular ligament.

FUNCTIONAL RANGE OF MOTION: TEMPOROMANDIBULAR JOINT

Stentpetery[14] defined functional mandibular depression (opening) as the minimal amount of movement needed in the TMJ to eat and speak without problems. This author defined functional mandibular depression as 25–30 mm. Kraus[15] described functional mandibular depression as the "patient's ability to actively open his or her mouth to 40 mm." Magee[16] suggested that "only 25–35 mm of opening is needed for everyday activity." Friedman and Weisberg[17] suggested that the amount of functional opening varies according to the individual's size, and that on average, an individual should be able to place two to two-and-a-half knuckles between the upper and lower incisors.

TECHNIQUES OF MEASUREMENT: TEMPOROMANDIBULAR JOINT

The most frequently used device for measuring ROM of the TMJ is a small ruler. A unique tool that can be used to measure motion at the TMJ is the TheraBite (TheraBite Corp., Newtown Square, PA). Procedures for using these devices are described later in this chapter.

Flexion—Cervical Spine: Tape Measure Method (Video 9.1)

Fig. 9.13 Starting position for measurement of cervical flexion using tape measure method. Bony landmark (sternal notch) indicated by red dot.

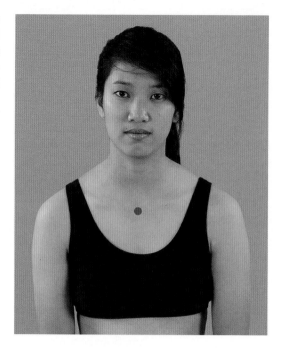

Patient position	Sitting erect (Fig. 9.13).
Patient action	After being instructed in motion desired, patient flexes neck maximally. Patient then returns to starting position. This movement provides an estimate of ROM and demonstrates to patient exact motion desired (Fig. 9.14). If patient is able to touch chin to chest, full flexion ROM is indicated. No further measurement is needed.
Tape measure alignment	Palpate the bony landmarks as shown in Fig. 9.13 and align tape measure accordingly (Fig. 9.15). Tape measure should be aligned with 0 cm at tip of mandible.

Fig. 9.14 End ROM of cervical flexion. Bony landmark (sternal notch) indicated by red dot.

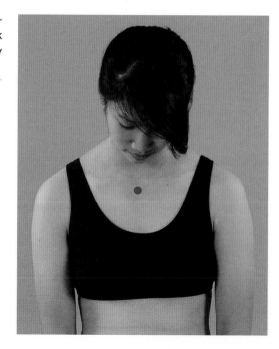

Fig. 9.15 Initial tape measure alignment for measurement of cervical flexion.

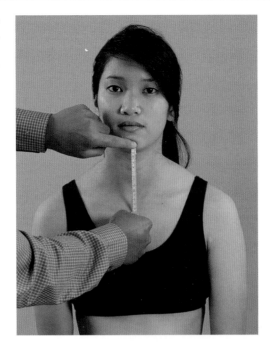

Superior   Tip of mandible (chin).

Inferior   Sternal notch.

Measure distance between sternal notch and tip of mandible, which is referred to as the initial measurement (see Fig. 9.15).

Patient/Examiner action   Patient flexes cervical spine through available ROM. Examiner measures distance between sternal notch and chin, which is referred to as the final measurement (Fig. 9.16).

Documentation   Difference between initial and final measurements is the ROM. Record patient's ROM in centimeters.

Fig. 9.16 Tape measure alignment at end ROM of cervical flexion.

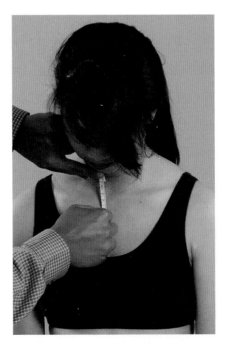

Flexion—Cervical Spine: Goniometer Technique (Video 9.2)

Fig. 9.17 Starting position for measurement of cervical flexion using goniometer technique.

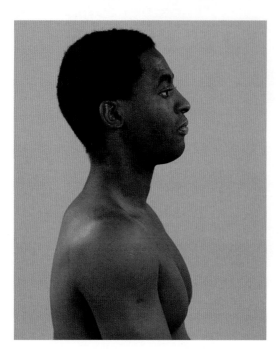

Patient position	Sitting erect (Fig. 9.17).
Patient action	After being instructed in motion desired, patient actively flexes cervical spine. Patient then returns to starting position. This movement provides an estimate of ROM and demonstrates to patient exact motion desired (Fig. 9.18). Patient returns to starting position and is manually positioned so that a line between the ear lobe and the base of the nares is parallel to floor.

Fig. 9.18 End ROM of cervical flexion.

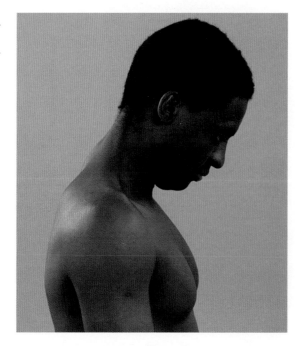

Fig. 9.19 Goniometer alignment at beginning range of cervical flexion.

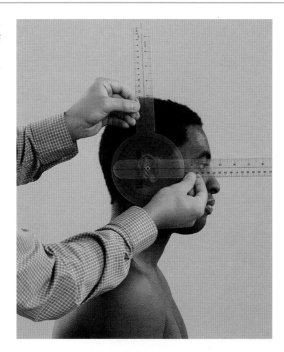

Goniometer alignment	Palpate the following landmarks and align goniometer accordingly (Fig. 9.19).
Stationary arm	Perpendicular to floor.
Axis	Earlobe.
Moving arm	Base of nares.
	Read scale of goniometer.
Patient/Examiner action	Patient performs active cervical flexion (see Fig. 9.18).
Confirmation of alignment	Repalpate landmarks and confirm proper goniometer alignment at end ROM, correcting alignment as necessary (Fig. 9.20). Read scale of goniometer.
Documentation	Record patient's ROM.

Fig. 9.20 Goniometer alignment at end ROM of cervical flexion.

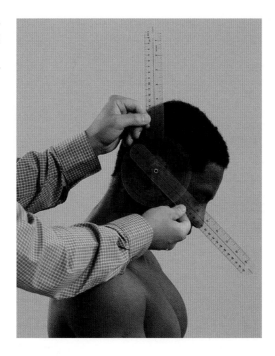

Flexion—Cervical Spine: Inclinometer Method (Video 9.3)

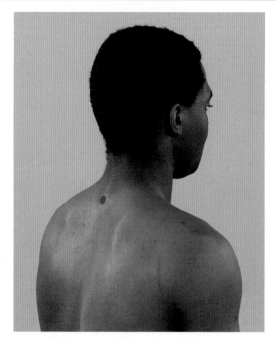

Fig. 9.21 Starting position for measurement of cervical flexion using inclinometer method. Bony landmark (spinous process of T1 vertebra) indicated by red dot.

Patient position	Sitting erect (Fig. 9.21).
Patient action	After being instructed in motion desired, patient flexes neck maximally. Patient then returns to starting position. This movement provides an estimate of ROM and demonstrates to patient exact motion desired (Fig. 9.22).
Inclinometer alignment	Palpate the following bony landmarks (shown in Figs. 9.21 and 9.22) and align inclinometers accordingly (Fig. 9.23). Ensure that inclinometers are set at 0 degrees once they are positioned on patient.
Inferior	Spinous process of T1 vertebra.
Superior	Vertex of skull, defined as half the distance between the glabella (flattened triangular area on forehead, also known as "bridge of nose") and the inion (palpable "bump" at base of occiput).

Fig. 9.22 End ROM of cervical flexion. Bony landmark (spinous process of T1 vertebra) indicated by red dot.

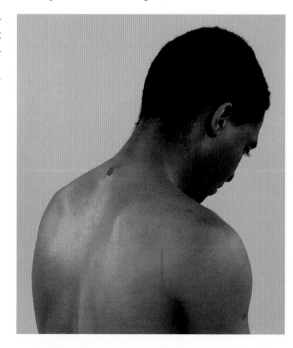

Fig. 9.23 Initial inclinometer alignment for measurement of cervical flexion. Inclinometers set at 0 degrees.

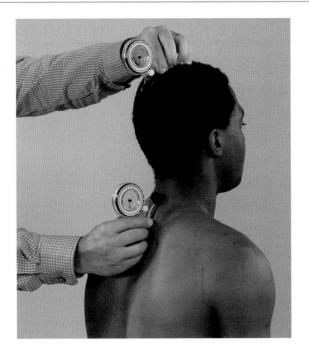

Patient/Examiner action

Patient flexes cervical spine through available ROM as examiner holds inclinometers in place. Examiner reads angle on inclinometers at end of flexion ROM (Fig. 9.24).

Documentation

Flexion ROM recorded is measurement at inferior landmark subtracted from measurement at superior landmark. Example: 45 degrees (reading at superior landmark) – 5 degrees (reading at inferior landmark) = 40 degrees of flexion. Record patient's ROM.

Fig. 9.24 Inclinometer alignment at end ROM of cervical flexion.

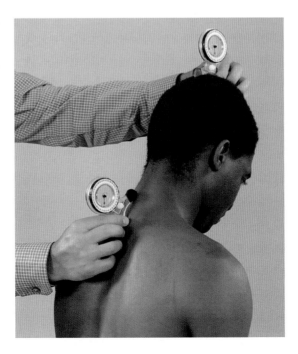

Flexion—Cervical Spine: CROM Device (Video 9.4)

Fig. 9.25 Starting position for measurement of cervical flexion using CROM device.

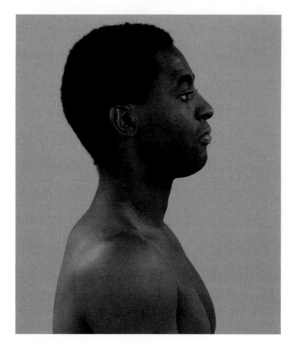

Patient position	Sitting erect (Fig. 9.25).
Patient action	After being instructed in motion desired, patient actively flexes cervical spine. Patient then returns to starting position. This movement provides an estimate of ROM and demonstrates to patient exact motion desired (Fig. 9.26).
CROM alignment	Examiner positions CROM device on bridge of patient's nose and on ears, as one would put on a pair of eyeglasses. Velcro straps are fastened firmly behind head to hold CROM device in place (Fig. 9.27). Record scale of inclinometer on side of patient's head, which is referred to as the initial measurement.

Fig. 9.26 End ROM of cervical flexion.

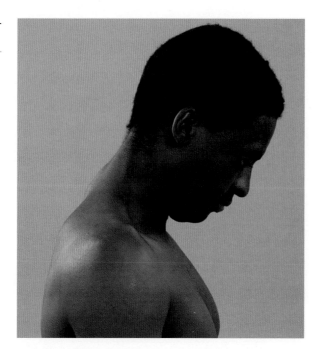

Fig. 9.27 CROM alignment at beginning range of cervical flexion.

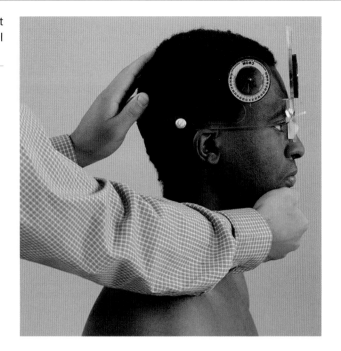

Patient/Examiner action	Patient performs active cervical flexion while maintaining thoracic spine against back of chair (see Fig. 9.26).
Confirmation of alignment	Ensure that CROM device has remained in place at end ROM. Read scale of inclinometer on side of patient's head, which is referred to as the final measurement (Fig. 9.28).
Documentation	Flexion ROM recorded is the initial measurement subtracted from the final measurement. Example: 45 degrees (final measurement) − 0 degrees (initial measurement) = 45 degrees of flexion. Record patient's ROM.

Fig. 9.28 CROM alignment at end ROM of cervical flexion.

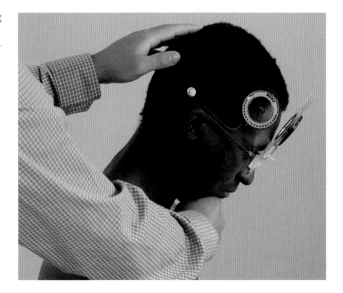

Flexion—Cervical Spine: Smartphone Method

Patient position and examiner action

Fig. 9.29 Starting position for measurement of cervical flexion using Smartphone.

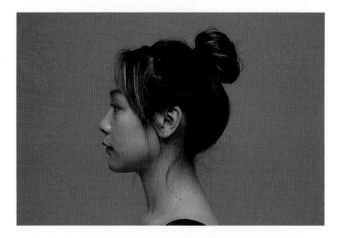

Patient position	Sitting erect (Fig. 9.29).
Patient action	After being instructed in motion desired, patient actively flexes cervical spine. Patient then returns to starting position. This movement provides an estimate of ROM and demonstrates to patient exact motion desired (Fig. 9.30). Patient returns to starting position and is manually positioned so that a line between the ear lobe and the base of the nares is parallel to floor.
Smartphone alignment	Place Smartphone anterior to external auditory meatus, in line with the base of the nose (Fig. 9.31) and face the Smartphone screen toward the therapist. Ensure the Smartphone application starts at 0 degrees before initiating motion, cue the patient to adjust neck as needed.

Fig. 9.30 End ROM of cervical flexion.

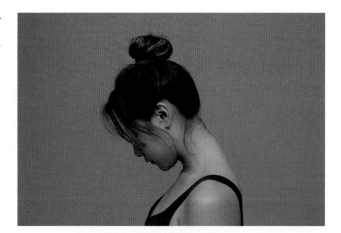

Fig. 9.31 Smartphone alignment at beginning of range of cervical flexion.

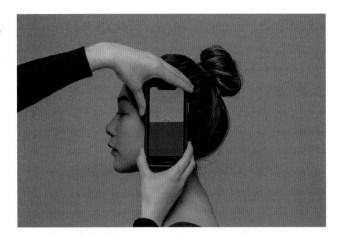

Patient/Examiner action

Patient flexes cervical spine through available ROM as examiner holds Smartphone in place. Examiner reads angles on smartphone at end of flexion ROM (Fig. 9.32).

Documentation

Record patient's ROM.

Fig. 9.32 Smartphone alignment at end of range of cervical flexion.

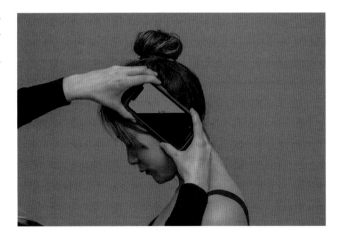

Extension—Cervical Spine: Tape Measure Method (Video 9.5)

Fig. 9.33 Starting position for measurement of cervical extension using tape measure method. Bony landmark (sternal notch) indicated by red dot.

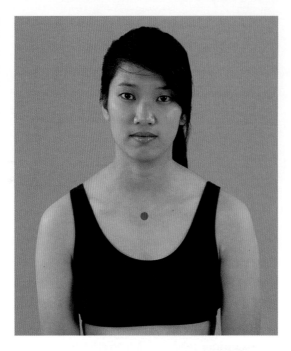

Patient position	Sitting erect (Fig. 9.33).
Patient action	After being instructed in motion desired, patient extends neck as far as possible. Patient then returns to starting position. This movement provides an estimate of ROM and demonstrates to patient exact motion desired (Fig. 9.34).
Tape measure alignment	Palpate the following bony landmarks (shown in Figs. 9.33 and 9.34), and align tape measure accordingly (Fig. 9.35). Tape measure should be aligned with 0 cm at tip of mandible.

Fig. 9.34 End ROM of cervical extension. Bony landmark (sternal notch) indicated by red dot.

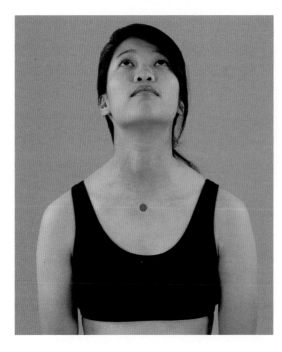

Fig. 9.35 Initial tape measure alignment for measurement of cervical flexion.

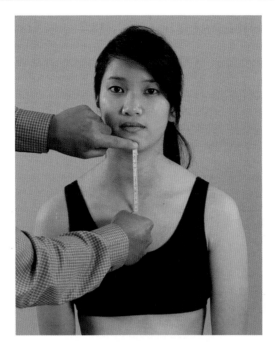

Superior   Tip of mandible (chin).

Inferior   Sternal notch.

Measure distance between sternal notch and tip of mandible, which is referred to as the initial measurement (see Fig. 9.35).

Patient/Examiner action   Patient extends cervical spine through available ROM. Examiner measures distance between sternal notch and chin, which is referred to as the final measurement (Fig. 9.36).

Documentation   Difference between initial and final measurements is the ROM. Record patient's ROM in centimeters.

Fig. 9.36 Tape measure alignment at end ROM of cervical extension.

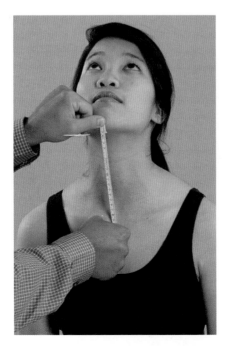

Extension—Cervical Spine: Goniometer Technique (Video 9.6)

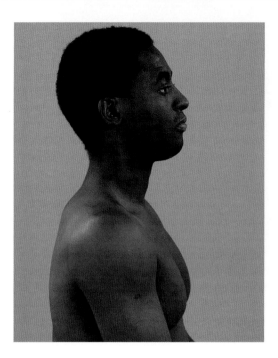

Fig. 9.37 Starting position for measurement of cervical extension using goniometer technique.

Patient position	Sitting erect (Fig. 9.37).
Patient action	After being instructed in motion desired, patient actively extends cervical spine. This movement provides an estimate of ROM and demonstrates to patient exact motion desired (Fig. 9.38). Patient returns to starting position and is manually positioned so that a line between the earlobe and the base of the nares is parallel to the floor.

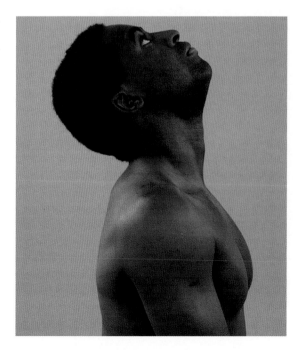

Fig. 9.38 End ROM of cervical extension.

Fig. 9.39 Goniometer alignment at beginning range of cervical extension.

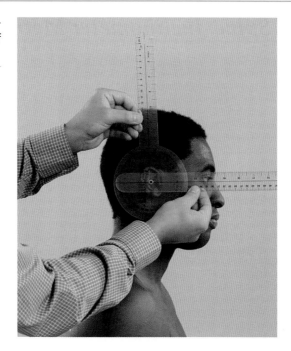

Fig. 9.39 Goniometer alignment at beginning range of cervical extension.

Goniometer alignment	Palpate the following landmarks and align goniometer accordingly (Fig. 9.39).
Stationary arm	Perpendicular to floor.
Axis	Earlobe.
Moving arm	Base of nares.
	Read scale of goniometer.
Patient/Examiner action	Patient performs active cervical extension (see Fig. 9.38).
Confirmation of alignment	Repalpate landmarks and confirm proper goniometer alignment at end ROM, correcting alignment as necessary (Fig. 9.40). Read scale of goniometer.
Documentation	Record patient's ROM.

Fig. 9.40 Goniometer alignment at end ROM of cervical extension.

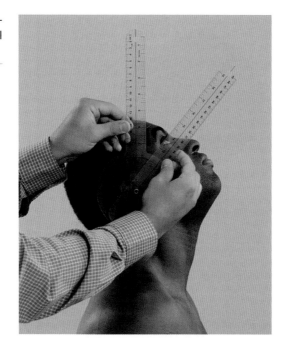

Extension—Cervical Spine: Inclinometer Method (Video 9.7)

Fig. 9.41 Starting position for measurement of cervical extension using inclinometer method. Bony landmark (spinous process of T1 vertebra) indicated by red dot.

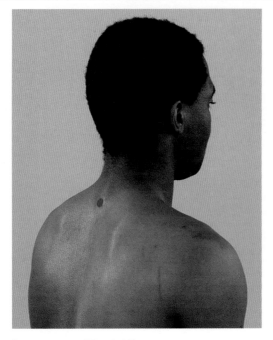

Patient position	Sitting erect (Fig. 9.41).
Patient action	After being instructed in motion desired, patient extends neck as far as possible. Patient then returns to starting position. This movement provides an estimate of ROM and demonstrates to patient exact motion desired (Fig. 9.42).
Inclinometer alignment	Palpate the bony landmarks as shown in Figs. 9.41 and 9.42 and align inclinometers accordingly (Fig. 9.43). Ensure that inclinometers are set at 0 degrees once they are positioned on patient.
Inferior	Spinous process of T1 vertebra.
Superior	Vertex of skull, defined as half the distance between the glabella (flattened triangular area on the forehead, also known as "bridge of nose") and inion (palpable "bump" at base of occiput).

Fig. 9.42 End ROM of cervical extension. Bony landmark (spinous process of T1 vertebra) indicated by red dot.

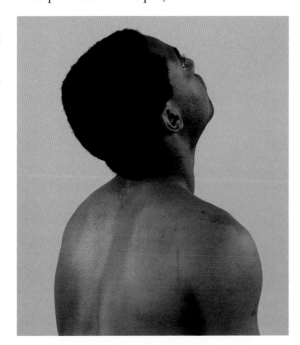

Fig. 9.43 Initial inclinometer alignment for measurement of cervical extension. Inclinometers set at 0 degrees.

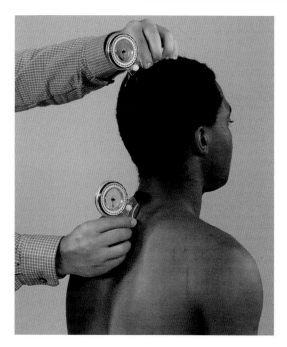

Patient/Examiner action

Patient extends cervical spine through available ROM as examiner holds inclinometers in place. Examiner reads angle on inclinometers at end of extension ROM (Fig. 9.44).

Documentation

Extension ROM recorded is measurement at inferior landmark subtracted from measurement at superior landmark. Example: 30 degrees (reading at superior landmark) – 0 degrees (reading at inferior landmark) = 30 degrees of extension. Record patient's ROM.

Fig. 9.44 Inclinometer alignment at end ROM of cervical extension.

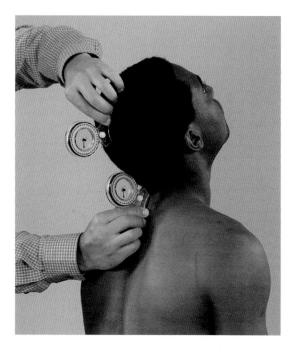

Extension—Cervical Spine: CROM Device (Video 9.8)

Fig. 9.45 Starting position for measurement of cervical extension using CROM device.

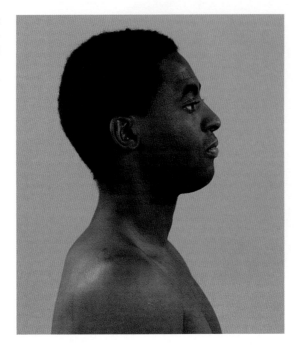

Patient position	Sitting erect (Fig. 9.45).
Patient action	After being instructed in motion desired, patient actively extends cervical spine. Patient then returns to starting position. This movement provides an estimate of ROM and demonstrates to patient exact motion desired (Fig. 9.46).
CROM alignment	Examiner positions CROM device on bridge of patient's nose and on the ears as one would put on a pair of eyeglasses. Velcro straps are fastened firmly behind head to hold CROM device in place (Fig. 9.47). Read scale of inclinometer on side of patient's head, which is referred to as the initial measurement.

Fig. 9.46 End ROM of cervical extension.

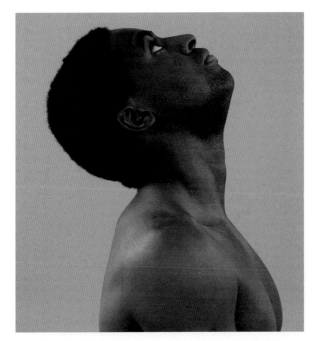

Fig. 9.47 CROM alignment at beginning range of cervical extension.

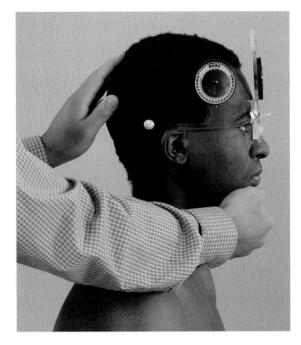

Patient/Examiner action   Patient performs active cervical extension while maintaining thoracic spine against back of chair (see Fig. 9.46).

Confirmation of alignment   Ensure that CROM device has remained in place at end ROM. Read scale of inclinometer on side of patient's head, which is referred to as the final measurement (Fig. 9.48).

Documentation   Extension ROM recorded is the initial measurement subtracted from the final measurement. Example: 25 degrees (final measurement) − 0 degrees (initial measurement) = 25 degrees of extension. Record patient's ROM.

Fig. 9.48 CROM alignment at end ROM of cervical extension.

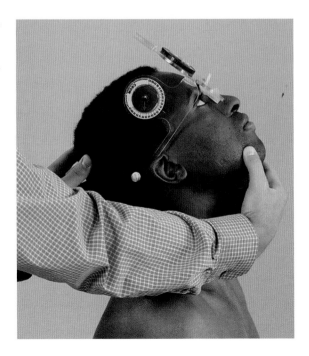

Extension—Cervical Spine: Smartphone Method

Patient position and examiner action

Fig. 9.49 Starting position for measurement of cervical extension using Smartphone.

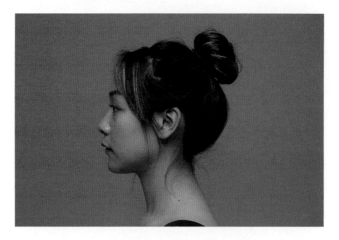

Patient position	Sitting erect (Fig. 9.49).
Patient action	After being instructed in motion desired, patient extends neck as far as possible. Patient then returns to starting position. This movement provides an estimate of ROM and demonstrates to patient exact motion desired (Fig. 9.50).

Fig. 9.50 End ROM of cervical extension.

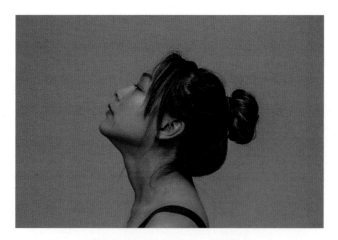

Fig. 9.51 Smartphone alignment at beginning of range of cervical extension.

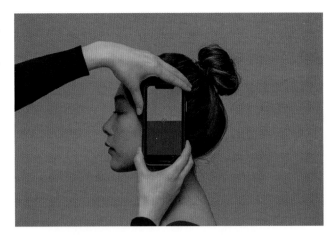

Smartphone alignment

Place border of Smartphone anterior to external auditory meatus, in line with the base of the nose (Fig. 9.51) and face the Smartphone screen toward the therapist. Ensure that Smartphone application starts at 0 degrees, cue the patient to adjust neck as needed.

Patient/Examiner action

Patient extends cervical spine through available ROM as examiner holds Smartphone in place. Examiner reads angle of smartphone at end of cervical extension ROM (Fig. 9.52).

Documentation

Record patient's ROM

Fig. 9.52 Smartphone alignment at end of range of cervical extension.

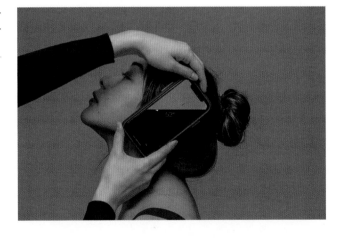

Lateral Flexion—Cervical Spine: Tape Measure Method (Video 9.9)

Fig. 9.53 Starting position for measurement of cervical lateral flexion using tape measure method.

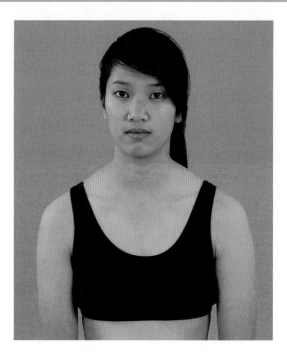

Patient position   Sitting erect (Fig. 9.53).

Patient action   After being instructed in motion desired, patient actively laterally flexes cervical spine, bringing ear as close as possible to shoulder; no rotation, flexion, or extension of cervical spine is allowed. Examiner must ensure that patient does not elevate shoulders during movement. Patient then returns to starting position. This movement provides an estimate of ROM and demonstrates to patient exact motion desired (Fig. 9.54).

Fig. 9.54 End ROM of cervical lateral flexion.

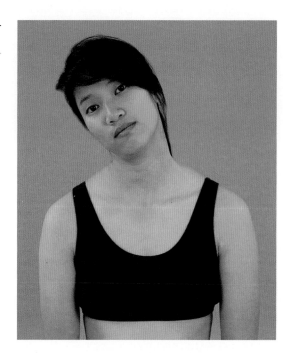

Fig. 9.55 Initial tape measure alignment for measurement of cervical lateral flexion.

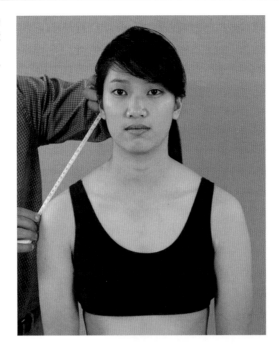

Tape measure alignment	Palpate the following landmarks and align tape measure accordingly (Figs. 9.55 and 9.56). Tape measure should be aligned with 0 cm at tip of mastoid process.
Superior	Tip of mastoid process (behind ear).
Inferior	Lateral tip of acromion process.
	Measure distance between lateral tip of acromion process and tip of mastoid process, which is referred to as the initial measurement (see Fig. 9.55).
Patient/Examiner action	Patient laterally flexes cervical spine toward side of tape measure through available ROM. Examiner measures distance from acromion process to mastoid process, which is referred to as the final measurement (see Fig. 9.56).
Documentation	Difference between initial and final measurements is the ROM. Record patient's ROM in centimeters.

Fig. 9.56 Tape measure alignment at end ROM of cervical lateral flexion.

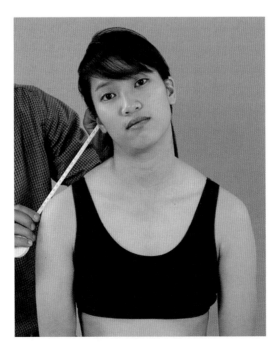

Lateral Flexion—Cervical Spine: Goniometer Technique (Video 9.10)

Fig. 9.57 Starting position for measurement of cervical lateral flexion using goniometer technique. Bony landmark (spinous process of C7 vertebra) indicated by red dot.

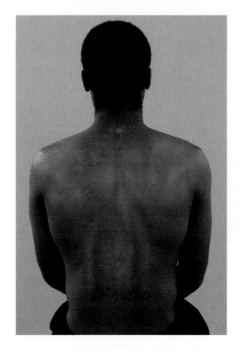

Patient position	Sitting erect (Fig. 9.57).
Patient action	After being instructed in motion desired, patient actively laterally flexes cervical spine, bringing ear as close as possible to shoulder; no rotation, flexion, or extension of cervical spine is allowed. Examiner must ensure that patient does not elevate shoulders during movement. Patient then returns to starting position. This movement provides an estimate of ROM and demonstrates to patient exact motion desired (Fig. 9.58).
Goniometer alignment	Palpate the following landmarks (shown in Figs. 9.57 and 9.58) and align goniometer accordingly (Fig. 9.59).
Stationary arm	Perpendicular to floor.

Fig. 9.58 End ROM of cervical lateral flexion. Bony landmark (spinous process of C7 vertebra) indicated by red dot.

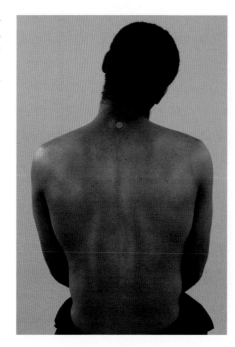

Fig. 9.59 Goniometer alignment at beginning range of cervical lateral flexion.

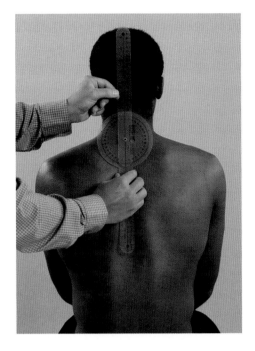

Axis	Spinous process of C7 vertebra.
Moving arm	Posterior midline of skull.
	Read scale of goniometer.
Patient/Examiner action	Patient performs active lateral cervical flexion. Examiner ensures that patient's shoulders do not elevate during movement (see Fig. 9.58).
Confirmation of alignment	Repalpate landmarks and confirm proper goniometer alignment at end ROM, correcting alignment as necessary (Fig. 9.60). Read scale of goniometer.
Documentation	Record patient's ROM.

Fig. 9.60 Goniometer alignment at end ROM of cervical lateral flexion.

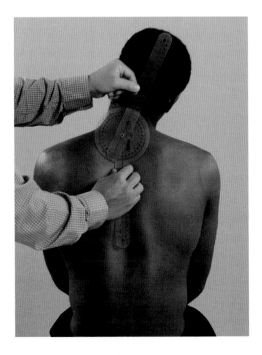

Lateral Flexion—Cervical Spine: Inclinometer Method (Video 9.11)

Fig. 9.61 Starting position for measurement of cervical lateral flexion using inclinometer method. Bony landmark (spinous process of T1 vertebra) indicated by red dot.

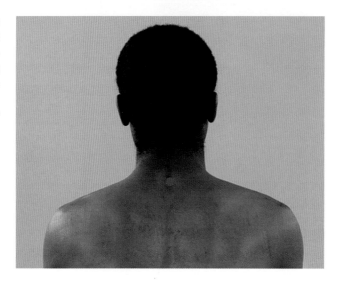

Patient position	Sitting erect (Fig. 9.61).
Patient action	After being instructed in motion desired, patient actively laterally flexes cervical spine, bringing ear as close as possible to shoulder; no rotation, flexion, or extension of cervical spine is allowed. Examiner must ensure that patient does not elevate shoulders during movement. Patient then returns to starting position. This movement provides an estimate of ROM and demonstrates to patient exact motion desired (Fig. 9.62).
Inclinometer alignment	Palpate the following bony landmarks (shown in Figs. 9.61 and 9.62) and align inclinometers accordingly (Fig. 9.63). Ensure that inclinometers are set at 0 degrees once they are positioned on patient.

Fig. 9.62 End ROM of cervical lateral flexion. Bony landmark (spinous process of T1 vertebra) indicated by red dot.

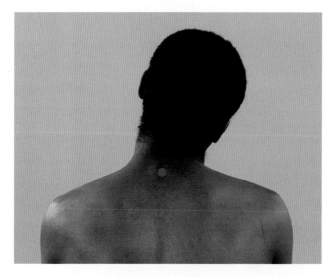

Fig. 9.63 Initial inclinometer alignment for measurement of cervical lateral flexion. Inclinometers set at 0 degrees.

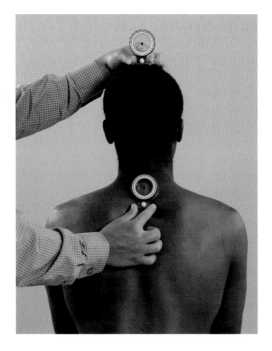

Inferior	Spinous process of T1 vertebra.
Superior	Vertex of skull, defined as half the distance between the glabella (flattened triangular area on forehead, also known as "bridge of nose") and inion (palpable "bump" at base of occiput).
Patient/Examiner action	Patient laterally flexes cervical spine through available ROM as examiner holds inclinometers in place. Examiner reads angle on inclinometers at end of lateral flexion ROM (Fig. 9.64).
Documentation	Lateral flexion ROM recorded is measurement at the inferior landmark subtracted from measurement at superior landmark. Example: 30 degrees (reading at superior landmark) − 5 degrees (reading at inferior landmark) = 25 degrees of lateral flexion. Record patient's ROM.

Fig. 9.64 Inclinometer alignment at end ROM of cervical lateral flexion.

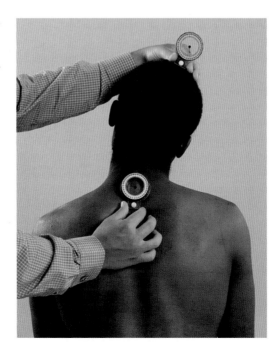

Lateral Flexion—Cervical Spine: CROM Device (Video 9.12)

Fig. 9.65 Starting position for measurement of cervical lateral flexion using CROM device.

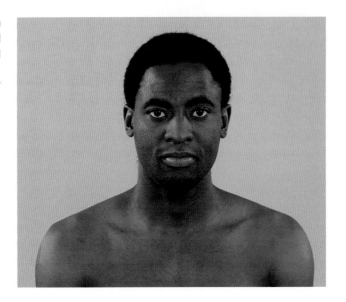

Patient position	Sitting erect (Fig. 9.65).
Patient action	After being instructed in motion desired, patient actively laterally flexes cervical spine, bringing ear as close as possible to shoulder; no rotation, flexion, or extension of cervical spine is allowed. Examiner must ensure that patient does not elevate shoulders during movement. Patient then returns to starting position. This movement provides an estimate of ROM and demonstrates to patient exact motion desired (Fig. 9.66).
CROM alignment	Examiner positions CROM device on bridge of patient's nose and on the ears as one would put on a pair of eyeglasses. Velcro straps are fastened firmly behind head to hold CROM device in place (Fig. 9.67). Read scale of inclinometer on patient's forehead, which is referred to as the initial measurement.

Fig. 9.66 End ROM of cervical lateral flexion.

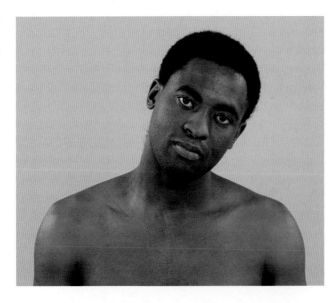

Fig. 9.67 CROM alignment at beginning range of cervical lateral flexion.

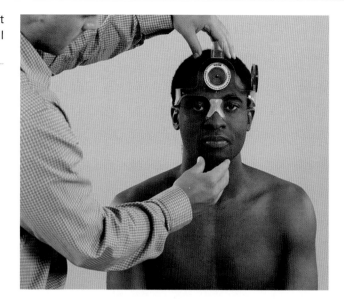

Patient/Examiner action

Patient performs active lateral cervical flexion. Examiner ensures that patient's shoulders do not elevate during movement.

Confirmation of alignment

Ensure that CROM device has remained in place at end ROM. Read scale of inclinometer on patient's forehead, which is referred to as the final measurement (Fig. 9.68).

Documentation

Lateral flexion ROM recorded is the initial measurement subtracted from the final measurement. Example: 40 degrees (final measurement) − 0 degrees (initial measurement) = 40 degrees of lateral flexion. Record patient's ROM.

Fig. 9.68 CROM alignment at end ROM of cervical lateral flexion.

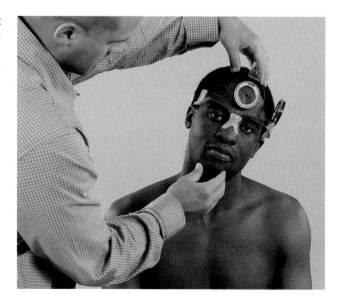

Lateral Flexion—Cervical Spine: Smartphone Method

Fig. 9.69 Starting position for measurement of cervical lateral flexion using Smartphone.

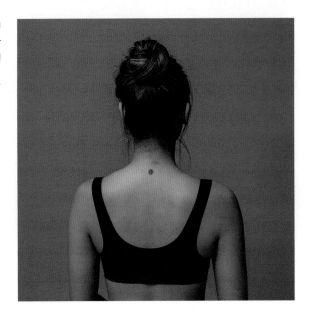

Patient position	Sitting erect (Fig. 9.69).
Patient action	After being instructed in motion desired, patient actively laterally flexes cervical spine, bringing ear as close as possible to shoulder; no rotation, flexion, or extension of cervical spine is allowed. Examiner must ensure that patient does not elevate shoulders during movement. Patient then returns to starting position. This movement provides an estimate of ROM and demonstrates to patient exact motion desired (Fig. 9.70).

Fig. 9.70 End ROM of cervical lateral flexion.

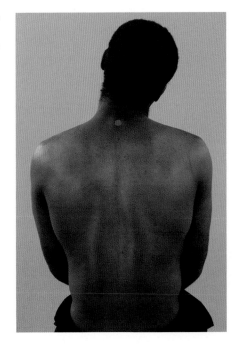

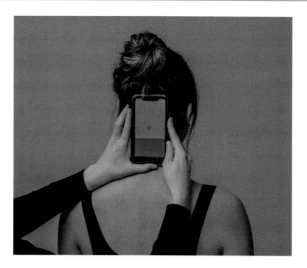

Fig. 9.71 Smartphone alignment at beginning of range of cervical lateral flexion.

Smartphone alignment

Palpate spinous process of C7 and align border of Smartphone accordingly (Fig. 9.71) with Smartphone screen facing toward the therapist. Ensure the Smartphone application starts at 0 degrees before beginning motion, cue the patient to adjust neck as needed.

Patient/Examiner action

Patient laterally flexes cervical spine through available ROM as examiner holds smartphone in place. Examiner reads angle of smartphone at end of lateral flexion ROM (Fig. 9.72).

Documentation

Record patient's ROM.

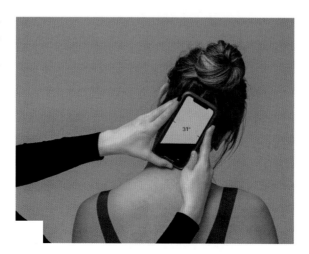

Fig. 9.72 Smartphone alignment at end of range of cervical lateral flexion.

Rotation—Cervical Spine: Tape Measure Method (Video 9.13)

Fig. 9.73 Starting position for measurement of cervical rotation using tape measure method.

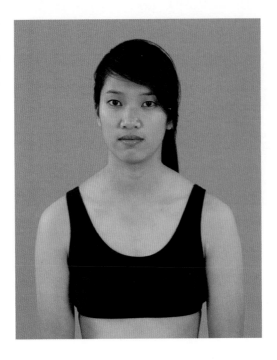

Patient position	Sitting erect (Fig. 9.73).
Patient action	After being instructed in motion desired, patient actively rotates cervical spine; no flexion, extension, or lateral flexion of cervical spine is allowed. Examiner must ensure that patient does not rotate trunk during movement. Patient then returns to starting position. This movement provides an estimate of ROM and demonstrates to patient exact motion desired (Fig. 9.74).

Fig. 9.74 End ROM of cervical rotation.

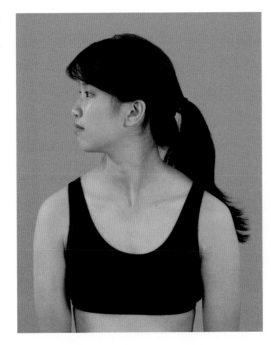

Fig. 9.75 Initial tape measure alignment for measurement of cervical rotation.

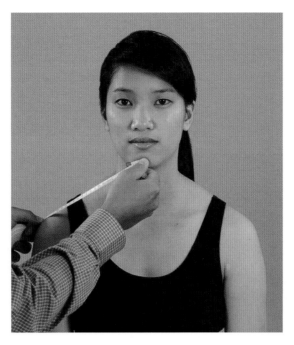

Tape measure alignment	Palpate the following landmarks and align tape measure accordingly (Figs. 9.75 and 9.76). Tape measure should be aligned with 0 cm at tip of mandible.
Superior	Tip of mandible (chin).
Inferior	Lateral tip of acromion process.
	Measure distance between lateral tip of acromion process and tip of mandible, which is referred to as the initial measurement (see Fig. 9.75).
Patient/Examiner action	Patient rotates cervical spine through available ROM toward side of tape measure. Examiner ensures that patient's trunk does not rotate during movement and measures distance from lateral tip of acromion process to tip of mandible, which is referred to as the final measurement (see Fig. 9.76).
Documentation	Difference between initial and final measurements is the ROM. Record patient's ROM in centimeters.

Fig. 9.76 Tape measure alignment at end ROM of cervical rotation.

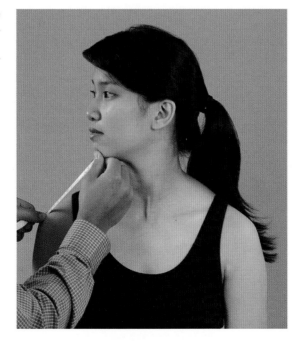

Rotation—Cervical Spine: Goniometer Technique (Video 9.14)

Fig. 9.77 Starting position for measurement of cervical rotation using goniometer technique.

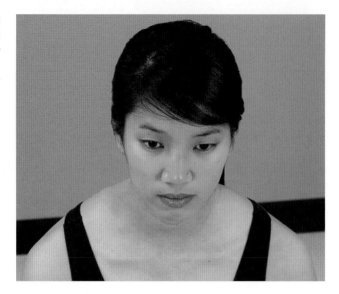

Patient position	Sitting erect (Fig. 9.77).
Patient action	After being instructed in motion desired, patient actively rotates cervical spine; no flexion, extension, or lateral flexion of cervical spine is allowed. Examiner must ensure that patient does not rotate trunk during movement. Patient then returns to starting position. This movement provides an estimate of ROM and demonstrates to patient exact motion desired (Fig. 9.78).

Fig. 9.78 End ROM of cervical rotation.

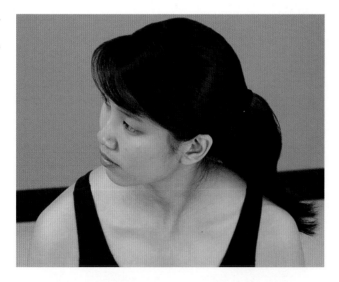

Fig. 9.79 Goniometer alignment at beginning range of cervical rotation.

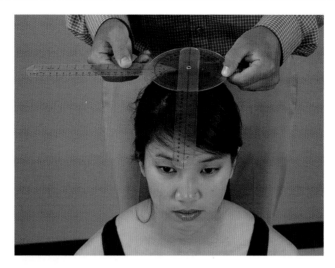

Goniometer alignment	Palpate the following landmarks, and align goniometer accordingly (Figs. 9.79 and 9.80). (*Note:* Measurement occurs from the top of the patient's head.)
Stationary arm	Imaginary line connecting patient's two acromion processes.
Axis	Top of subject's head.
Moving arm	Nose.
	Read scale of goniometer.
Patient/Examiner action	Patient rotates cervical spine through available ROM. Examiner ensures that patient's trunk does not rotate (see Fig. 9.78).
Confirmation of alignment	Repalpate landmarks and confirm proper goniometer alignment at end ROM, correcting alignment as necessary (see Fig. 9.80). Read scale of goniometer.
Documentation	Record patient's ROM.

Fig. 9.80 Goniometer alignment at end ROM of cervical rotation.

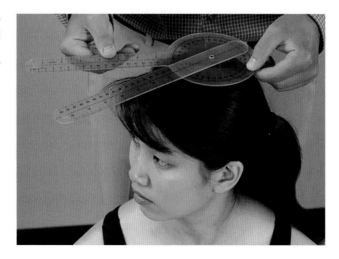

Rotation—Cervical Spine: Inclinometer Method (Video 9.15)

Fig. 9.81 Starting position for measurement of cervical rotation using inclinometer method. Bony landmark (base of forehead) indicated by red dot.

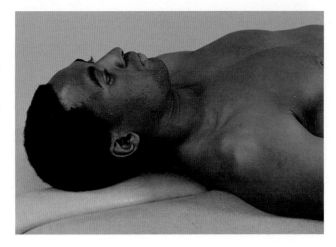

Patient position

Supine, with top of patient's head slightly over end of table, nose pointing to ceiling (Fig. 9.81).

Patient action

After being instructed in motion desired, patient actively rotates cervical spine as far as possible; no flexion, extension, or lateral flexion of cervical spine is allowed. Examiner must ensure that patient does not rotate trunk during movement. Patient then returns to starting position. This movement provides an estimate of ROM and demonstrates to patient exact motion desired (Fig. 9.82).

Fig. 9.82 End ROM of cervical rotation. Bony landmark (base of forehead) indicated by red dot.

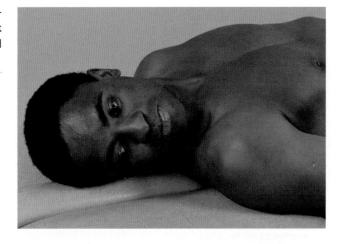

Fig. 9.83 Initial inclinometer alignment for measurement of cervical rotation. Inclinometer set at 0 degrees.

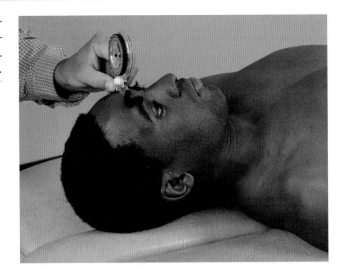

Inclinometer alignment

Palpate base of forehead (see Fig. 9.81), and align inclinometer accordingly (Fig. 9.83). Ensure that inclinometer is set at 0 degrees.

Patient/Examiner action

Patient rotates cervical spine through available ROM as examiner holds inclinometer in place. Examiner reads angle on inclinometer at end of rotation ROM (Fig. 9.84).

Documentation

Record patient's ROM.

Fig. 9.84 Inclinometer alignment at end ROM of cervical rotation.

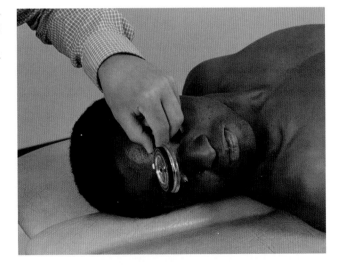

Rotation—Cervical Spine: CROM Device (Video 9.16)

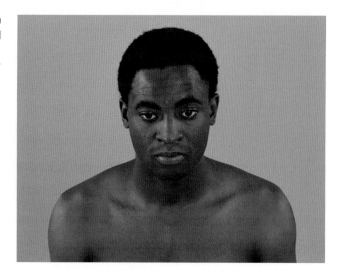

Fig. 9.85 Starting position for measurement of cervical rotation using CROM device.

Patient position	Sitting erect, facing west (Fig. 9.85).
Patient action	After being instructed in motion desired, patient actively rotates cervical spine as far as possible; no flexion, extension, or lateral flexion of cervical spine is allowed. Examiner must ensure that patient does not rotate trunk during movement. Patient then returns to starting position. This movement provides an estimate of ROM and demonstrates to patient exact motion desired (Fig. 9.86).
CROM alignment	To obtain accurate measurement, determine which direction is north. Place magnetic yoke on subject's shoulders with arrow pointing north (Fig. 9.87). Examiner should add rotation arm to the CROM device. Examiner positions CROM device on bridge of patient's nose and on ears, as one would put on a pair of eyeglasses. Velcro straps are fastened firmly behind head to hold CROM device in place (see Fig. 9.87). As subject faces straight ahead, meter on top of subject's head is set to 0 degrees.
Patient/Examiner action	Patient performs active cervical rotation (see Fig. 9.86).
Confirmation of alignment	Ensure that CROM device has remained in place at end ROM.

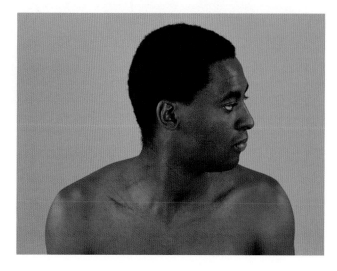

Fig. 9.86 End ROM of cervical rotation.

Fig. 9.87 CROM alignment at beginning range of cervical rotation; note placement of magnetic yoke pointing north. Inclinometer over vertex of skull set at 0 degrees.

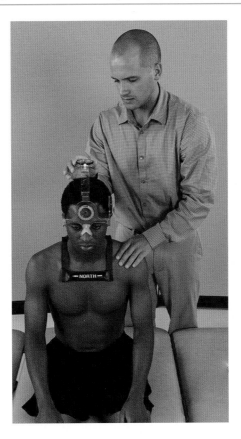

Read scale of inclinometer at the top of the head (Fig. 9.88).

Documentation   Record patient's ROM.

Fig. 9.88 CROM alignment at end ROM of cervical rotation.

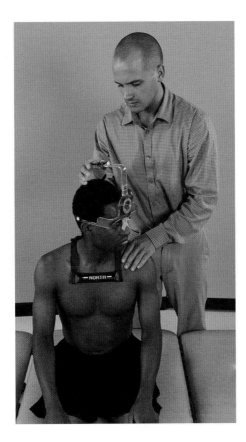

Rotation—Cervical Spine: Smartphone Method

Fig. 9.89 Starting position for measurement of cervical rotation using Smartphone.

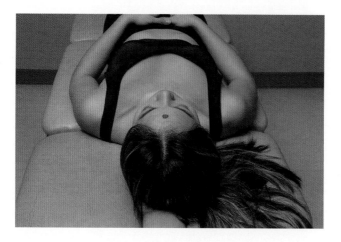

Patient position	Supine, with top of patient's head slightly over end of table, nose pointing to ceiling (Fig. 9.89).
Patient action	After being instructed in motion desired, patient actively rotates cervical spine as far as possible; no flexion, extension, or lateral flexion of cervical spine is allowed. Examiner must ensure that patient does not rotate trunk during movement. Patient then returns to starting position. This movement provides an estimate of ROM and demonstrates to patient exact motion desired (Fig. 9.90).

Fig. 9.90 End ROM of cervical rotation.

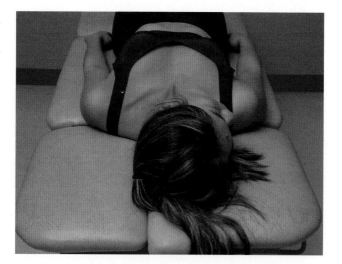

Fig. 9.91 Initial smartphone alignment for measurement of cervical rotation.

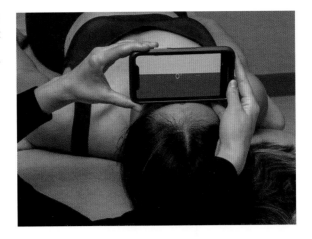

Fig. 9.91 Initial smartphone alignment for measurement of cervical rotation.

Smartphone alignment

Palpate base of forehead and align smartphone accordingly (Fig. 9.91) with Smartphone screen facing therapist. Ensure the Smartphone application starts at 0 degrees before initiating motion, cue the patient to adjust neck as needed.

Patient/Examiner action

Patient rotates cervical spine through available ROM as examiner holds smartphone in place. Examiner reads angle of smartphone at end of cervical rotation ROM (Fig. 9.92).

Documentation

Record patient's ROM.

Fig. 9.92 Smartphone alignment at end of range of cervical rotation.

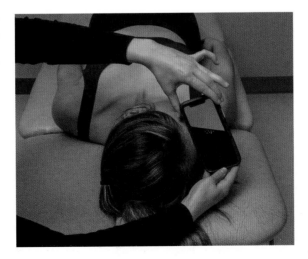

Mandibular Depression (Opening)—Temporomandibular Joint: Ruler Method (Video 9.17)

Fig. 9.93 End ROM of mandibular depression.

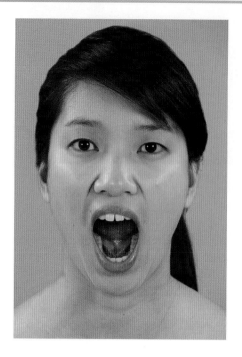

Patient position	Sitting erect.
Patient action	Patient opens mouth as wide as possible. This movement provides an estimate of ROM and demonstrates to patient exact motion desired (Fig. 9.93).
Patient/Examiner action	Tips of right (or left) maxillary and mandibular central incisors are used as reference points. As patient maximally opens mouth, distance between tips of right (or left) maxillary and mandibular central incisors is measured with a ruler (Fig. 9.94).
Documentation	Distance between tips of central incisors is recorded.

Fig. 9.94 Ruler alignment at end ROM of mandibular depression.

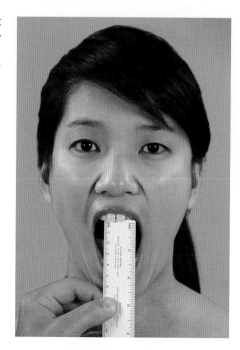

Mandibular Depression (Opening)—Temporomandibular Joint: TheraBite Range of Motion Scale (Video 9.18)

Fig. 9.95 End ROM of mandibular depression.

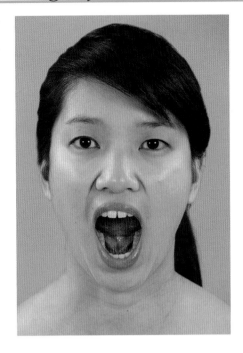

Patient position	Sitting erect.
Patient action	Patient opens mouth as wide as possible. This movement provides an estimate of ROM and demonstrates to patient exact motion desired (Fig. 9.95).
Patient/Examiner action	Tips of right (or left) maxillary and mandibular central incisors are used as reference points. As patient maximally opens mouth, the TheraBite device (TheraBite Corp.) is used. Notch of TheraBite rests on tip of right (or left) mandibular central incisor, and scale is rotated until TheraBite contacts top of right (or left) maxillary central incisor (Fig. 9.96).
Documentation	Measurement at point of contact on tip of maxillary central incisor is recorded.

Fig. 9.96 TheraBite alignment at end ROM of mandibular depression.

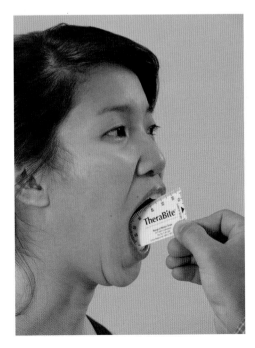

Protrusion—Temporomandibular Joint (Video 9.19)

Fig. 9.97 End ROM of man-dibular protrusion.

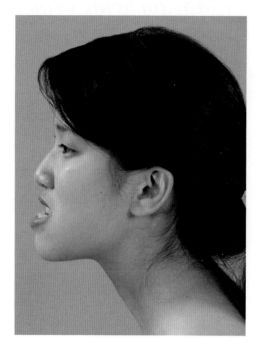

Patient position	Sitting erect.
Patient action	Patient opens mouth slightly (just enough to eliminate tooth contact) and protrudes or juts the lower jaw anteriorly past the upper teeth. This movement provides an estimate of ROM and demonstrates to patient exact motion desired (Fig. 9.97).

Fig. 9.98 Ruler alignment at end ROM of mandibular protrusion.

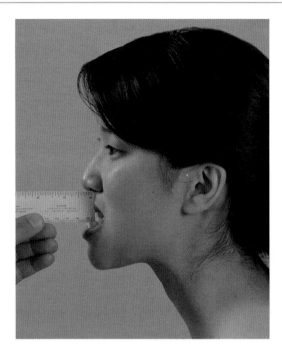

Patient/Examiner action Tips of right (or left) maxillary and mandibular central incisors are used as reference points. As patient protrudes lower jaw, distance that tip of right (or left) mandibular central incisor moves horizontally past tip of right (or left) maxillary central incisor is measured with a ruler (Fig. 9.98).

Documentation Distance between tips of central incisors is recorded.

Note One edge of TheraBite device contains a ruler that can be used for measuring protrusion.

Lateral Deviation (Excursion)—Temporomandibular Joint (Video 9.20)

Fig. 9.99 End ROM of mandibular lateral deviation.

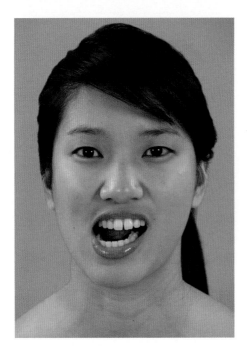

Patient position	Sitting erect.
Patient action	Patient opens mouth slightly (just enough to eliminate tooth contact) and moves mandible laterally in horizontal plane, first to one side and then to other side. This movement provides an estimate of ROM and demonstrates to patient exact motion desired (Fig. 9.99).
Patient/Examiner action	Space between maxillary central incisors and space between mandibular central incisors (interproximal space) are used as reference points for initial measurement with a ruler (Fig. 9.100). At beginning of ROM, ruler is placed in front of central

Fig. 9.100 Ruler alignment at beginning range of mandibular lateral deviation. (Note that space between mandibular central incisors is aligned with 5-cm mark of ruler.)

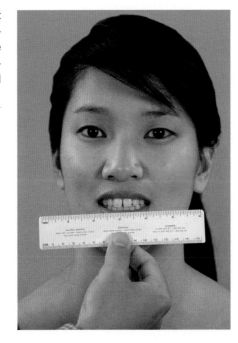

Fig. 9.101 Ruler alignment at end ROM of mandibular lateral deviation. (Note that space between mandibular central incisors lines up with 4.3 cm, indicating 0.7 cm of mandibular lateral deviation.)

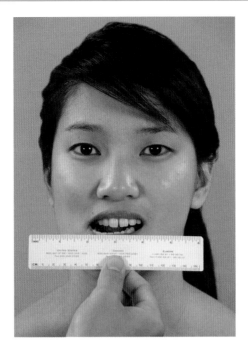

incisors, and distance from space between maxillary central incisors to space between mandibular central incisors is measured, referred to as the initial measurement. In Fig. 9.100, the spaces between both maxillary and mandibular central incisors line up with the 5-cm mark on the ruler, so the initial measurement equals 0 cm. As patient laterally deviates the jaw, distance from space between maxillary central incisors to space between mandibular central incisors is measured with ruler and referred to as the final measurement (Fig. 9.101).

Documentation

Difference between initial and final measurements is ROM. Record patient's ROM in centimeters.

Note

One edge of TheraBite device contains a ruler that can be used for measuring lateral deviation.

References

1. Grant R. *Physical Therapy of the Cervical and Thoracic Spine.* 3rd ed. New York: Churchill Livingstone; 2002.
2. Iglarsh A, Snyder-Mackler L. Temporomandibular joint and the cervical spine. In: Richardson JK, Iglarsh ZA, eds. *Clinical Orthopaedic Physical Therapy.* 2nd ed. Philadelphia: WB Saunders; 2006.
3. Levangie PL, Norkin CC. *Joint Structure & Function: A Comprehensive Analysis.* 3rd ed. Philadelphia: F.A. Davis Co; 2001.
4. Neumann DA. *Kinesiology of the Musculoskeletal System.* 2nd ed. St. Louis: Mosby, Inc; 2009.
5. Bennett SE, Schenk RJ, Simmons ED. Active range of motion utilized in the cervical spine to perform daily functional tasks. *J Spinal Disord Tech.* 2002;15:307–311.
6. American Medical Association. *Guides to the Evaluation of Permanent Impairment.* 6th ed. Chicago: AMA; 2007.
7. Bennett JG, Bergmanis LE, Carpenter JK, Skowlund HV. Range of motion of the neck. *Phys Ther.* 1963;43:45–47.
8. Balogun JA, Abereoje OK, Olaogun MO, Obajuluwa VA. Inter- and intratester reliability of measuring neck motions with tape measure and Myrin gravity–reference goniometer. *J Orthop Sports Phys Ther.* 1989;10:248–253.
9. Alaranta H, Hurri H, M H, et al. Flexibility of the spine: normative values of goniometric and tape measurements. *Scand J Rehabil Med.* 1994;26:147–154.
10. Kadir N, Grayson MF, Goldberg AAJ, Swain M. A new neck goniometer. *Rheumatol Rehabil.* 1981;20:219–226.
11. Tucci SM, Hicks JE, Gross EG, et al. Cervical motion assessment: a new, simple and accurate method. *Arch Phys Med Rehabil.* 1986;67:225–230.
12. Zachman ZJ, Traina AD, Keating JC, et al. Interexaminer reliability and concurrent validity of two instruments for the measurement of cervical ranges of motion. *J Manipulative Physiol Ther.* 1989;12:205–210.
13. Youdas JW, Garrett TR, Suman VJ, et al. Normal range of motion of the cervical spine: an initial goniometric study. *Phys Ther.* 1992;72:770–780.
14. Stentpetery A. Clinical utility of mandibular movement ranges. *J Orofac Pain.* 1993;7:163–168.
15. Kraus SL. Evaluation and management of temporomandibular disorders. In: Saunders HD, Saunders R, eds. *Evaluation, Treatment and Prevention of Musculoskeletal Disorders.* 4th ed. Chaska, MN: The Saunders Group; 2004.
16. Magee DJ. *Orthopedic Physical Assessment.* 5th ed. Philadelphia: W.B. Saunders; 2007.
17. Freidman MH, Weisberg J. Application of orthopedic principles in evaluation of the temporomandibular joint. *Phys Ther.* 1982;62:597–603.

RELIABILITY and VALIDITY of MEASUREMENT of RANGE of MOTION of the SPINE and TEMPOROMANDIBULAR JOINT

William D. Bandy and Chad Lairamore

Chapters 8 and 9 described techniques for measurement of the spine and the temporomandibular joint. The purpose of this chapter is to present information on the reliability and validity of these techniques for measuring the spine. After an extensive review of published literature, each study related to reliability and validity was screened. Inclusion in this chapter was dependent on the study comprising appropriate statistical analyses that included the use of an intraclass correlation coefficient (ICC) or Pearson product–moment correlation coefficient (Pearson's r) with appropriate follow-up procedures (refer to Chapter 2 for further discussion of reliability and validity). In a few instances in which only one study was performed using a specific technique, an article that did not meet the established criteria was nevertheless included in this chapter, but exceptions to the criteria were rare and are specifically noted in the text.

No attempt was made to rate one measurement technique as better or worse than another technique. As was indicated previously, the purpose of this chapter is to present information on the accuracy and reproducibility of measurement techniques for the spine. This information, with the accompanying tables, will enable the reader to make an educated decision as to the most appropriate measurement technique for a particular clinical situation.

THORACIC AND LUMBAR SPINE

TAPE MEASURE

Flexion

Schober Method

Methods for using the tape measure for measuring range of motion of the lumbar spine are numerous. The earliest technique used was the Schober method, in which the distance between the lumbosacral junction and a point 10 cm above the lumbosacral junction was measured before and after the patients flexed and extended the spine.[1,2] The original Schober method has been modified by changing the landmarks used when range of motion of the spine is measured. These changes in landmarks include measuring the distance between points 5 cm inferior and 10 cm superior to the lumbosacral junction (known as the modified Schober[1]) and measuring from a point in the center of a line connecting the two posterior superior iliac spines to a mark 15 cm superior to this baseline landmark (the modified-modified Schober).[3] Chapter 8 provides detailed descriptions of these measurement techniques.

In a study that examined lumbar range of motion of 172 individuals, Fitzgerald et al.[4] used the original Schober method. Before data collection, reliability of the Schober technique was determined by two independent testers who used as subjects 17 college-age students not involved in the larger study. Interrater reliability of the original Schober technique was reported to be 1.0 (Pearson's r). Although no follow-up statistical test was performed after the Pearson correlation analysis, as is appropriate (refer to Chapter 2), this study was included in this chapter because it is the only reliability study performed using the original Schober technique.

Before collecting values on back mobility in 282 children without disability, Haley et al.[5] established reliability in a pilot study. In one of the few studies conducted to examine intrarater reliability of the modified Schober test, one tester measured six children between the ages of 5 and 9 years. Intrarater reliability was analyzed statistically by using an ICC, yielding a result of 0.83. The authors reported that the test was not only accurate but was "relatively easy and quick to perform on young children."

Interrater reliability of the modified Schober technique for measuring lumbar flexion was reported by Burdett et al.,[6] who measured 23 individuals between the ages of 20 and 40 years. The authors reported interrater reliability of 0.72 using an ICC and 0.71 using Pearson's r. Follow-up testing with an analysis of variance (ANOVA) indicated no significant difference between testers.

A comprehensive study by Hyytiainen et al.[7] provided intrarater and interrater reliability of the modified Schober test administered to measure lumbar flexion. After examining 30 males using the modified Schober method, the authors reported intrarater reliability of 0.88 and interrater reliability of 0.87 (Pearson's r). Follow-up testing using a paired t-test indicated no significant difference related to intrarater or interrater reliability. The authors concluded that the tape measure "was easy to use and required no expensive equipment." Examining a group of 159 adults with ankylosing spondylosis, Haywood et al.[8] reported reliability of the modified Schober technique as 0.90 for intratester (n = 26) and 0.94 for intertester (n = 51).

Williams et al.[3] examined the intrarater and interrater reliability of the modified-modified Schober method for measuring lumbar flexion by using three clinicians whose clinical experience ranged from 3 to 12 years. Examination of 15 patients with low back pain resulted in intrarater reliability using Pearson correlation coefficients of 0.89 for clinician No. 1, 0.78 for clinician No. 2, and 0.83 for clinician No. 3. An ICC performed across all three clinicians resulted in an overall intertester reliability coefficient of 0.72.

Also examining the intratester reliability and validity of the modified-modified Schober, Tousignant et al.[9] examined 31 adults with low back pain. Results indicated intratester reliability for two testers to be 0.79 and 0.81; intertester reliability between the two testers was 0.91. Examining validity by establishing the relationship of the range found by the modified-modified Schober and X-ray examination, a Pearson's correlation of 0.67 was found. (*Note:* This study is included despite the fact that only a Pearson correlation was performed because there are a few studies about the validity of the Schober technique.)

Macrae and Wright[1] tested their contention that the modified Schober was a better test than the original Schober by comparing the correlations of lumbar flexion measurements obtained by both methods vs measurements obtained radiographically (X-rays). The correlation coefficient (Pearson's r) between the original Schober and the X-ray (validity) was 0.90 (standard error = 6.2 degrees), and between the modified Schober technique and the X-ray (validity), 0.97 (standard error = 3.3 degrees). Although data on test–retest

reliability were not obtained, the authors concluded that "the proposed modification was an improvement over the original Schober's."

In a second study that compared the modified Schober versus radiographic examination of lumbar flexion in an attempt to determine validity, Portek et al.[10] evaluated 11 subjects. The reliability correlation between the modified Schober technique and X-ray (validity) was reported as 0.43 (Pearson's r). However, a t-test revealed no significant difference between measures obtained with the modified Schober and with X-rays. In contrast to the study by Macrae and Wright,[1] this study demonstrated little correlation between clinical and radiographic techniques. The authors concluded that the modified Schober "only gave indices of back movement which did not reflect true intervertebral movement."

Summary: Tape Measure for Measurement of Lumbar Flexion

Tables 10.1–10.3 provide a summary of reviewed studies that related to the reliability and validity of using a tape measure to measure lumbar flexion. As is indicated in these tables, intrarater reliability ranged from 0.78 to 0.89 (see Table 10.1), and interrater reliability ranged from 0.71 to 1.0 (see Table 10.2) for all techniques in which a tape measure was used. Correlation between measurements made with a tape measure using either the Schober or the modified Schober technique and radiographic examination yielded reliability coefficients of greater than 0.90 for one study and less than 0.70 for two additional studies (see Table 10.3).

Extension

After a modification of the Schober technique was used to measure extension in two studies, Williams et al.[3] examined the intrarater reliability of three clinicians using the modified–modified Schober technique on 15 subjects with low back pain, reporting correlation coefficients ranging from 0.69 to 0.91 (Pearson's r and ICC). Using a similar measurement technique in the examination of 100 patients with low back pain and

				CORRELATION	
STUDY	**TECHNIQUE**	**n**	**SAMPLE**	**ICC***	**r†**
Haley et al.[5]	Modified Schober	6	Healthy children (5–9 years)	0.83	
Hyytiainen et al.[7]	Modified Schober	30	Healthy adults (35–44 years)		0.88
Haywood et al.[8]	Modified Schober	26	Patient with ankylosing spondylitis	0.94	
Williams et al.[3]	Modified-Modified Schober	15	Low back pain adults (25–53 years; $\bar{x}$ = 35.7)		0.89, 0.78, 0.83‡
Tousignant et al.[9]	Modified-Modified Schober	31	Adults with low back pain ($\bar{x}$ = 44 years)	0.79, 0.81	

Table 10.1 TAPE MEASURE: INTRATESTER RELIABILITY FOR LUMBAR FLEXION

*Intraclass correlation coefficient.
†Pearson's r.
‡Three testers performed measurements.

100 individuals without low back pain, Beattie et al.[11] reported slightly higher intrarater reliability than was reported by Williams et al.[3] Test–retest reliability for individuals with low back pain was 0.93, and for those without low back pain, reliability was 0.90 (ICC). Beattie et al.[11] also examined intertester reliability in 11 subjects without low back pain, reporting a correlation coefficient of 0.94 (ICC).

Using a technique that was slightly different from the Schober method, Frost et al.[12] used a tape measure to examine the changed distance between the spinous process of C7 and the posterior superior iliac spine during spinal extension. After examining 24 subjects, Frost et al.[12] reported an intrarater reliability of 0.78 and an interrater reliability of 0.79 (Pearson's r). ANOVA

performed to analyze the difference between first and second measurements (intrarater) indicated no significant difference. However, ANOVA performed to analyze the difference between examiners (interrater) revealed that a significant difference existed ($P < 0.05$).

Tables 10.4 and 10.5 provide a summary of reliability studies that used the tape measure to examine extension of the spine. As is indicated in these tables, intrarater reliability ranged from 0.69 to 0.93 (see Table 10.4), and interrater reliability was reported as 0.79 and 0.94 (see Table 10.5).

A unique method for using a tape measure to measure lumbar extension range of motion was investigated by Bandy and Reese.[13] By using a prone press-up and measuring the perpendicular distance from the sternal

Table 10.2   TAPE MEASURE: INTERTESTER RELIABILITY FOR LUMBAR FLEXION

STUDY	TECHNIQUE	n	SAMPLE	CORRELATION ICC*	$r^\dagger$
Fitzgerald et al.[4]	Schober	17	Healthy adults (20–82 years)		1.0
Burdett et al.[6]	Modified Schober	23	Healthy adults (20–40 years)	0.72	0.71
Hyytiainen et al.[7]	Modified Schober	30	Healthy adults (35–44 years)		0.87
Haywood et al.[8]	Modified Schober	51	Patient with ankylosing spondylitis ($\bar{x}=49.0$ years)	0.90	
Williams et al.[3]	Modified-Modified Schober	15	Low back pain adults (25–53 years; $\bar{x}=35.7$)	0.72‡	
Tousignant et al.[9]	Modified-Modified Schober	31	Adults with low back pain ($\bar{x}=44$ years)	0.91	

*Intraclass correlation coefficient.
†Pearson's r.
‡Three testers performed measurements.

Table 10.3   TAPE MEASURE: VALIDITY FOR LUMBAR FLEXION

STUDY	TECHNIQUE	n	SAMPLE	CORRELATION*
Macrae and Wright[1]	Schober vs. Modified Schober		Not able to determine	Schober: 0.90 Modified: 0.97
Portek et al.[10]	Modified Schober	11	Healthy adults (25–36 years; $\bar{x}=29.5$)	0.43
Tousignant et al.[9]	Modified-Modified Schober	31	Adults with low back pain ($\bar{x}=44$ years)	0.67

*Pearson's r.

Table 10.4   TAPE MEASURE: INTRATESTER RELIABILITY FOR LUMBAR EXTENSION

STUDY	TECHNIQUE	n	SAMPLE	CORRELATION ICC*	$r^\dagger$
Frost et al.[12]	PSIS/C7	24	Healthy adults (20–55 years; $\bar{x}=33.8$)		0.78
Williams et al.[3]	Modified-Modified Schober	15	Low back pain adults (25–53 years; $\bar{x}=35.7$)	0.76	0.79, 0.91, 0.69‡
Beattie et al.[11]	Modified Schober	100	Healthy adults (20–76 years; $\bar{x}=32.4$)	0.93	
		(B) 100	Low back pain adults (16–65 years; $\bar{x}=37.6$)	0.90	

*Intraclass correlation coefficient.
†Pearson's r.
‡Three testers performed measurements.

Table 10.5   TAPE MEASURE: INTERTESTER RELIABILITY FOR LUMBAR EXTENSION

STUDY	TECHNIQUE	n	SAMPLE	CORRELATION ICC*	$r^\dagger$
Frost et al.[12]	PSIS/C7	24	Healthy adults (20–55 years; $\bar{x}=33.8$)		0.79
Beattie et al.[11]	Modified Schober	11	Healthy adults (20–76 years; $\bar{x}=32.4$)	0.94	

*Intraclass correlation coefficient.
†Pearson's r.

				CORRELATION	
STUDY	**TECHNIQUE**	**n**	**SAMPLE**	**ICC***	**r†**
Hyytiainen et al.[7]	Marks at lateral thigh	30	Healthy adults (35–44 years)		0.85
Rose[14]	Marks at lateral thigh	18	Healthy adults (x̄ = 19.5 years)		0.78 (left)
					0.89 (right)
Haley et al.[5]	Marks at lateral trunk	6	Healthy children (5–9 years)	0.89 (right)	
				0.77 (left)	
Frost et al.[12]	Finger to floor	24	Healthy adults (20–55 years; x̄ = 33.8)		0.91
Haywood et al.[8]	Finger to floor	26	Patients with ankylosing spondylitis (x̄ = 49.0 years)	0.98	
Haywood et al.[8]	Marks at lateral hip	26	Patients with ankylosing spondylitis (x̄ = 49.0 years)	0.98 (right)	
				0.95 (left)	

Table 10.6 TAPE MEASURE: INTRATESTER RELIABILITY FOR LUMBAR LATERAL FLEXION

*Intraclass correlation coefficient.
†Pearson's r.

notch and the support surface, the authors found that the technique was reliable, irrespective of whether or not the examiner was experienced. Intrarater reliability for the experienced examiner was 0.90 and 0.82 for the inexperienced examiner. Interrater reliability between the experienced and the inexperienced examiners was 0.85. The authors included that the "prone press up appears to be a reliable method to measure lumbar extension."

Lateral Flexion

Fingertip to Floor

The fingertip-to-floor method measures the distance from the third fingertip to the floor after the patient laterally flexes the spine (a detailed description is presented in Chapter 8). Frost et al.[12] examined right lateral flexion in 24 individuals using the fingertip-to-floor method. Both intrarater reliability and interrater reliability were reported as 0.91. However, follow-up ANOVA revealed a significant difference ($P < 0.01$) between measurements for both intrarater and interrater reliability. In their examination of adults with ankylosing spondylosis, Haywood et al.[8] reported intrarater and interrater reliability of the finger-to-floor method as 0.98 and 0.96, respectively.

Marks at Lateral Thigh

A second technique for measuring lateral flexion is to place marks at the points on the lateral thigh that the third fingertip touches in an individual standing erect and after lateral flexion (a detailed description is presented in Chapter 8). After measuring 18 subjects, Rose[14] reported intrarater reliability of 0.89 for right lateral flexion and 0.78 for left lateral flexion (Pearson's r). The least significant difference (defined as the extent to which repeated measures must differ for significant difference to occur) was reported as 3.0 cm and 4.0 cm for right and left lateral flexion, respectively.

Hyytiainen et al.[7] examined 30 subjects and reported intrarater reliability of 0.85 and interrater reliability of 0.86 (Pearson's r). Follow-up testing using an ANOVA for both intrarater and interrater reliability revealed no significant differences between measurements taken. Slightly higher intertester reliability was reported by Alaranta et al.,[15] who reported a correlation of 0.91 (Pearson's r) in the measurement of 24 individuals. Follow-up testing in which a paired t-test was used revealed no significant differences between testers. Using the ICC, Haywood et al.[8] reported reliability as follows: intrarater reliability (n = 26) of 0.95 to the left and 0.98 to the right and interrater reliability (n = 51) of 0.95 to the left and 0.98 to the right.

Marks at Lateral Trunk

A third method of measuring lateral flexion is to place two marks on the lateral trunk and measure the change in distance between these two marks before and after lateral flexion. Using marks on the lateral trunk to measure lateral flexion in six children between the ages of 5 and 9 years, Haley et al.[5] reported intratester reliability correlations of 0.89 and 0.77 for right and left lateral flexion, respectively (ICC).

Summary: Tape Measure for Measurement of Lateral Flexion

A summary of studies investigating the reliability of examination of lateral flexion using a tape measure is presented in Tables 10.6 and 10.7. As indicated, intratester reliability across all methods ranged from 0.77 to 0.91 (see Table 10.6), and intertester reliability ranged from 0.85 to 0.91 (see Table 10.7).

Rotation

A unique method of measuring rotation of the thoracolumbar spine using a tape measure was described by Frost et al.,[12] who measured the distance between the ipsilateral acromion and the contralateral greater

Table 10.7   TAPE MEASURE: INTERTESTER RELIABILITY FOR LUMBAR LATERAL FLEXION

STUDY	TECHNIQUE	n	SAMPLE	CORRELATION (r*)
Frost et al.[12]	Finger to floor	24	Healthy adults (20–55 years; $\bar{x}=33.8$)	0.91
Haywood et al.[8]	Finger to floor	51	Patients with ankylosing spondylitis ($\bar{x}=49.0$ years)	0.96
Hyytiainen et al.[7]	Marks at lateral thigh	30	Healthy adults (35–44 years)	0.85
Alaranta et al.[15]	Marks at lateral thigh	24	Healthy adults	0.91[†]
Haywood et al.[8]	Marks at lateral hip	51	Patients with ankylosing spondylitis ($\bar{x}=49.0$ years)	0.98 (right) 0.95 (left)

*Pearson's r.
[†]Total = left and right lateral flexion combined.

trochanter before and after the subject rotated the spine (a detailed description is presented in Chapter 8). Only one study has attempted to document the use of the tape measure to examine the amount of spinal rotation. Frost et al.[12] not only provided a description but also determined the reliability of the rotation technique using the tape measure. Intratester reliability on 24 subjects was reported as 0.71; intertester reliability was extremely low, with a reliability coefficient of 0.13. Follow-up testing using ANOVA indicated no significant difference between measurements related to intrarater reliability, but there was a significant difference ($P < 0.05$) between testers related to intertester reliability. The authors indicated that the inability of the two testers to define the landmarks accurately was a limiting factor in this measurement technique and was the cause of the low correlation for interrater reliability.

GONIOMETER

Goniometry is a relatively quick and easy method of measuring spinal mobility. In addition, goniometers are readily accessible to the clinician and are commonly used.[4]

Flexion and Extension

Burdett et al.[6] examined intertester reliability by using goniometry to measure flexion and extension in 23 subjects. These authors reported intertester reliability coefficients of 0.85 (ICC and Pearson's r) for flexion and 0.75 (ICC) and 0.77 (Pearson's r) for extension. Testing using ANOVA indicated no significant difference between testers for measurements of lumbar flexion or extension.

Although similar results for intertester correlation coefficients were reported by Nitschke et al.,[16] the authors' interpretation of the findings was very different. After examining intertester reliability in measuring flexion and extension in 34 patients with low back pain, Nitschke et al.[16] reported correlations of 0.84 (ICC) and 0.90 (Pearson's r) for flexion. The 95% confidence interval (CI) for flexion was 30.37 degrees, and the t-test showed no significant difference. For extension, the correlation reported was 0.63 (ICC) and 0.76 (Pearson's r)

Table 10.8   GONIOMETER: INTRATESTER RELIABILITY FOR FLEXION AND EXTENSION OF LUMBAR SPINE

STUDY	n	SAMPLE	CORRELATION	
			ICC*	r[†]
Flexion				
Nitschke et al.[16]	34	LBP (20–65 years)	0.92	0.92
Extension				
Nitschke et al.[16]	34	LBP (20–65 years)	0.81	0.82

LBP, Low back pain.
*Intraclass correlation coefficient.
[†]Pearson's r.

Table 10.9   GONIOMETER: INTERTESTER RELIABILITY FOR FLEXION AND EXTENSION OF LUMBAR SPINE

STUDY	n	SAMPLE	CORRELATION	
			ICC*	r[†]
Flexion				
Burdett et al.[6]	23	Healthy adults (20–40 years)	0.85	0.85
Nitschke et al.[16]	34	LBP	0.84	0.90
Extension				
Burdett et al.[6]	23	Healthy adults (20–40 years)	0.75	0.77
Nitschke et al.[16]	34	LBP (20–65 years)	0.63	0.76

LBP, Low back pain.
*Intraclass correlation coefficient.
[†]Pearson's r.

(95% CI = 18.34 degrees; t-test not significant). In addition, this study examined these 34 patients for test–retest intrarater reliability, reporting correlations of 0.92 (ICC and Pearson's r) for flexion (95% CI = 29.12 degrees; t-test not significant), and 0.81 (ICC) and 0.82 (Pearson's r) for extension (95% CI = 17.15 degrees; t-test not significant). Nitschke et al.[16] suggested that although the t-test that was performed did not indicate systematic error, the large 95% CI indicated the presence of random error, revealing that "the measurement with a long arm goniometer had poor reliability."

Tables 10.8 and 10.9 present a summary of studies related to use of the goniometer to measure lumbar flexion and extension. As indicated in the tables, only one study reported intratester reliability (see Table 10.8), and intertester reliability ranged from 0.63 to 0.90 (see Table 10.9).

Lateral Flexion

Fitzgerald et al.[4] examined intertester reliability for lateral flexion using two testers and 17 subjects. Intertester correlations reported were 0.76 for right lateral flexion and 0.91 for left lateral flexion (Pearson's r). Although the Pearson correlation was not followed up with an appropriate test to analyze random or systematic error (refer to Chapter 2), this study was included because only one other study explored the reliability of the goniometer in measuring lateral flexion. The authors suggested that the goniometer was "an objective and reliable method for measuring spinal range of motion."

Nitschke et al.[16] also established intertester reliability for lateral flexion as part of their study, which was previously described. Intertester reliability correlations were 0.62 (ICC and Pearson's r) for right lateral flexion (95% CI = 14.23 degrees; t-test not significant) and 0.80 (ICC and Pearson's r) for left lateral flexion (95% CI = 10.33 degrees; t-test not significant). In addition to examining intertester reliability, Nitschke et al.[16] examined these same 34 patients with low back pain to establish intratester reliability. The authors reported intratester reliabilities of 0.76 (ICC and Pearson's r) for right lateral flexion (95% CI = 10.91 degrees; t-test not significant) and 0.84 (ICC and Pearson's r) for left lateral flexion (95% CI = 9.43 degrees; t-test not significant). On the basis of these results, the authors suggested that the use of the goniometer for measurement of spinal range of motion "is inadequate."

A summary of intertester reliabilities for use of the goniometer for measurement of lateral flexion is presented in Table 10.10. As indicated in the table, intertester reliability ranged from 0.62 to 0.91.

Rotation

A unique method of measuring thoracolumbar rotation using a goniometer was presented by Johnson et al.[17] using a rod held behind the back at the level of the elbows. Testing 46 subjects (31 males, 15 females), the authors reported intratester reliability of 0.85 with rotation to the right and then, again, to the left. Intertester reliability was reported as 0.84 when rotating to the right and 0.87 when rotating to the left. Furness et al.[18] used a similar technique for measuring lumbar rotation, this time the subjects held the bar in front of them, in 30 subjects (10 females, 20 males). The authors reported reliabilities for left and right rotation above 0.94 for intratester reliability and above.87 for intertester reliability, thereby, reporting reliability very similar to those reported by Johnson et al.[17] (Tables 10.11 and 10.12). Using a goniometer while holding a rod behind the patient to measure thoracolumbar spine appears to have provided "good reliability and low levels of measurement error."[17]

Table 10.10   GONIOMETER: INTERTESTER RELIABILITY FOR LATERAL FLEXION OF LUMBAR SPINE

STUDY	n	SAMPLE	CORRELATION	
			ICC*	r[†]
Fitzgerald et al.[4]	17	Healthy adults (20–82 years)		0.76 (right) 0.91 (left)
Nitschke et al.[16]	34	Low back pain (20–65 years)	0.62 (right) 0.80 (left)	0.62 (right) 0.80 (left)

*Intraclass correlation coefficient.
[†]Pearson's r.

Table 10.11   GONIOMETER: INTRATESTER RELIABILITY OF ROTATION OF LUMBAR SPINE

STUDY	n	SAMPLE	CORRELATION*(ICC)	
			ROTATION RIGHT	ROTATION LEFT
Johnson et al.[17]	46	Healthy Adults ($\bar{x}$ = 23.6 years)	0.87	0.87
Furness et al.[18]	30	Healthy Adults ($\bar{x}$ = 29.8 years)	0.97, 0.97	0.98, 0.94

*ICC = Intraclass correlation coefficient.

Table 10.12   GONIOMETER: INTERTESTER RELIABILITY OF ROTATION OF LUMBAR SPINE

STUDY	n	SAMPLE	CORRELATION*(ICC)	
			ROTATION RIGHT	ROTATION LEFT
Johnson et al.[17]	46	Healthy Adults ($\bar{x}$ = 23.6 years)	0.84	0.87
Furness et al.[18]	30	Healthy Adults ($\bar{x}$ = 29.8 years)	0.84	0.84

*ICC = Intraclass correlation coefficient.

INCLINOMETER

Expressing the concern that "joint movements in the spine are still being assessed largely by clinical observation and subjective impression" and not by objective measurement, Loebl[19] in 1967 described the use of the inclinometer, which he referred to as "a new, simple method for accurate clinical measure of spinal posture and movement." Although his study was descriptive in nature, with no reliability data to support any contention of accuracy, Loebl[19] was one of the first to describe the use of the inclinometer.

Since Loebl's[19] article appeared, much needed research has been published on the reliability and validity of the inclinometer in measuring spinal mobility. In contrast to the reliability reported for the tape measure procedures, which is relatively consistent and high, the reliability of the accuracy of measurement using the inclinometer reported in the literature varies widely.

Flexion and Extension

Several studies used a test–retest design, with one tester performing the inclinometer technique to determine intrarater reliability for measurements of flexion and extension. Other studies used two testers to perform the inclinometer technique, comparing the results obtained by the two testers to determine interrater reliability. Because of the number of publications related to the reliability of using inclinometers to measure flexion and extension, this section is divided into the following subsections for clarity: studies dealing with intrarater reliability, investigations related to intertester reliability, and research comparing results obtained with the inclinometer versus data derived from radiographic (X-ray) examination (validity).

Techniques used for each study vary, with some authors placing the inclinometer at locations similar to those used with the Schober technique, as previously described in the tape measure section of Chapter 8. This inclinometer technique involves designated measurement of lumbar flexion and extension. Other authors placed one inclinometer at the sacral base and a second inclinometer at the level of the C7-T1 spinous process. This measurement is designated as thoracolumbar flexion and extension.

Finally, some studies reported not only reliability of flexion and extension, but also reliability of "total" movement. Total movement is the measurement of maximal flexion added to maximal extension, with a correlation performed on the sum.

Intratester Reliability

Using an inclinometer, Mellin[20] reported intrarater reliability coefficients in the examination of 10 subjects as 0.86 for lumbar flexion, 0.93 for thoracolumbar flexion, 0.93 for extension, and 0.98 for thoracolumbar extension (Pearson's *r*). However, matched *t*-tests comparing the first measure versus the second measure for each motion indicated that a significant difference ($P < 0.05$) existed for each motion. A second study, in which Mellin was involved, provided somewhat different results. Mellin et al.[21] examined 27 subjects, resulting in an intratester reliability of 0.91 for lumbar flexion, 0.94 for thoracolumbar flexion, 0.79 for lumbar extension, and 0.87 for thoracolumbar extension (Pearson's *r*). In this study, a matched *t*-test comparing the first measurement versus the second measurement resulted in no significant difference. The authors concluded that "the accuracy of the methods described (inclinometer) makes them useful for measurement of thoracolumbar mobility."

Nitschke et al.[16] and Rondinelli et al.[22] reported reliability coefficients similar to those reported in the studies just presented but came to different conclusions in their analysis of data. Measuring lumbar flexion and extension in 34 individuals with low back pain, Nitschke et al.[16] reported correlations of 0.90 (Pearson's *r* and ICC) for flexion and 0.70 (ICC) and 0.71 (Pearson's *r*) for extension. Although no systematic error was found (as determined by *t*-tests between measurements that were not significant), the authors suggested that the large random error (95% CI = 28.46 degrees for flexion, 16.52 degrees for extension) indicated "poor intrarater reliability." Establishing the intrarater reliability of two testers using three different inclinometer techniques, Rondinelli et al.[22] measured flexion in eight subjects. The authors reported correlations ranging from 0.70 to 0.90 for intrarater reliability for flexion (ICC) and concluded that "these findings appear to undermine the expectations that clinicians can reliably apply surface inclinometry."

Establishing intratester reliability, Williams et al.[3] examined lumbar flexion and extension in 15 patients with low back pain using three testers. Results for intratester reliability for each examiner ranged from 0.13 to 0.87 for flexion and from 0.28 to 0.66 for extension (ICC). The conclusion reached by the authors was that the "inclinometer technique needs improvement."

Higher reliability than that found by Williams et al.[3] was reported by Ng et al.[23], Pourahmadi et al.[24], Kolder et al.[25], and, to some extent, Lee et al.[26] Examining test–retest intratester reliability in 12 adults with back pain, Ng et al.[23] reported reliability of 0.87 for flexion and 0.92 for extension for each of the two examiners. Pourahmadi et al.[24] also used 2 examiners to measure 30 subjects across three sessions. The authors reported intratester reliability of 0.87 and 0.84 for each tester for flexion; and 0.91 and 0.85 for each tester in extension.

Very similar results were described by Lee et al.,[26] who reported intratester reliability of 0.84 and 0.88 in

Table 10.13　INCLINOMETER: INTRATESTER RELIABILITY FOR LUMBAR FLEXION

STUDY	TECHNIQUE	n	SAMPLE	CORRELATION ICC*	CORRELATION $r^†$
Mellin[20]	Single	10	Healthy adults ($\bar{x}$=31.3 years)		0.86 0.93 (T-L‡)
Mellin et al.[21]	Single	27	Healthy adults (24–50 years; $\bar{x}$=30.6)		0.91 0.94 (T-L‡)
Williams et al.[3]	Double	15	LBP adults (25–53 years; $\bar{x}$=35.7)	0.60	0.87, 0.76, 0.13§
Nitschke et al.[16]	Double	34	LBP adults (20–65 years)	0.90	0.90
Breum et al.[27]	BROM¶¶	47	Healthy adults (18–38 years; $\bar{x}$=25.8)	0.91	
Madson et a[28]	BROM	40	Healthy adults (20–40 years; $\bar{x}$=25.5)	0.67	
Rondinelli et al.[22]	Single, double, BROM	8	Healthy adults (18–30 years)	0.85, 0.86 (single)¶ 0.70, 0.81 (double)¶ 0.81, 0.90 (BROM)¶	
Ng et al.[23]	Single	12	Adult low back pain (23–62 years; $\bar{x}$=28.0)	0.87	0.87
Kolber et al.[25]	Single	30	Healthy adults ($\bar{x}$=25.6 years)	0.83	
Pourahmadi et al.[24]	Single	30	Healthy adults ($\bar{x}$=27.9 years)	0.87, 0.84	
Lee et al.[26]	Single	35	Healthy adults ($\bar{x}$=27.2 years)	0.84, 0.88¶	
Kachingwe and Phillips[29]	BROM	91	Adult low back pain ($\bar{x}$=28.0 years)	0.84, 0.79¶	

LBP, Low back pain.

*Intraclass correlation coefficient.

†Pearson's *r*.

‡Thoracolumbar range of motion.

§Three testers performed measurement.

¶¶Back range of motion device (Performance Attainment Associates, Roseville, MN).

¶Two testers performed measurement.

the measurement of flexion in 35 healthy adults measured by two examiners. However, Lee et al.[26] did not find the inclinometer to be as accurate for the measurement of extension, reporting intratester reliability among the two examiners at 0.79 and 0.48.

The back range of motion (BROM) device is a specialized measurement tool that consists of two separate plastic frames that are secured to the individual with elastic straps. Within the plastic frames, inclinometers are mounted, allowing measurement of flexion, extension, lateral flexion, and rotation. A detailed description of the BROM device is presented in Chapter 8. Using the BROM device to analyze intrarater reliability in two testers who measured lumbar flexion in eight subjects, Rondinelli et al.[22] reported reliability correlations of 0.81 and 0.90 (ICC). Expanding the study by Rondinelli et al.[22] to include not only flexion but also measurement of intratester reliability for extension in 47 subjects, Breum et al.[27] reported correlation coefficients (ICC) of 0.91 for flexion and 0.63 for extension. They concluded that the "BROM was found to be a reliable instrument in the measurement of lumbar mobility." Using the same basic design as was employed in the study by Breum et al.,[27] Madson et al.[28] analyzed the reliability of the BROM device in measuring lumbar range of motion in 40 subjects. Intrarater reliability was 0.67 for flexion and 0.78 for extension. The 95% CI was 5.0 degrees for both flexion and extension measurements. After examining 91 adults with low back pain, Kachingwe and Phillips[29] reported intratester reliability of 0.84 and 0.79 for flexion in two examiners. However, Lee et al.[26] did

not find the inclinometer to be as accurate for the measurement of extension, reporting intratester reliability of two examiners as 0.79 and 0.48.

Tables 10.13 and 10.14 provide a summary of studies investigating intratester reliability for the measurement of flexion and extension using the inclinometer. As indicated, reliability coefficients across all studies ranged from 0.13 to 0.94 for measurement of flexion (see Table 10.13) and from 0.28 to 0.98 for measurement of extension (see Table 10.14).

Intertester Reliability

Several groups of investigators who examined intrarater reliability also studied interrater reliability of measuring spinal flexion and extension using the inclinometer. Mellin[20] examined intertester reliability in 15 subjects, reporting correlation coefficients of 0.97 for lumbar flexion, 0.95 for thoracolumbar flexion, and 0.89 for both lumbar and thoracolumbar extension (Pearson's *r*). Matched *t*-tests comparing the first tester vs the second tester for each motion indicated that a significant difference ($P < 0.001$) existed for each motion. Nitschke et al.[16] examined 34 patients with low back pain and by using the inclinometer reported intertester reliability of 0.52 (ICC) and 0.67 (Pearson's *r*) for flexion (95% CI=28.46 degrees; *t*-test=significant difference at $P < 0.05$) and 0.35 (ICC and Pearson's *r*) for extension (95% CI=16.52 degrees; *t*-test not significant). In their study examining 35 healthy adults, Lee et al.[26] reported interrater reliability of 0.83 for flexion and 0.75 for extension.

Table 10.14   INCLINOMETER: INTRATESTER RELIABILITY FOR LUMBAR EXTENSION

STUDY	TECHNIQUE	n	SAMPLE	CORRELATION ICC*	CORRELATION $r^†$
Mellin[20]	Single	10	Healthy adults ($\bar{x}=31.3$ years)		0.93 0.98 (T-L[‡])
Mellin et al.[21]	Single	27	Healthy adults (24–50 years; $\bar{x}=30.6$)		0.79 0.87 (T-L)
Williams et al.[3]	Double	15	LBP (25–53 years; $\bar{x}=35.7$)	0.48	28, 0.66, 0.55[§]
Nitschke et al.[16]	Double	34	LBP (20–65 years)	0.70	0.71
Breum et al.[27]	BROM[¶]	47	Healthy adults (18–38 years; $\bar{x}=25.8$)	0.63	
Madson et al.[28]	BROM	40	Healthy adults (20–40 years; $\bar{x}=25.5$)	0.78	
Ng et al.[23]	Single	12	Adult low back pain (23–62 years; $\bar{x}=28.0$)	0.92	0.92
Kolber et al.[25]	Single	30	Healthy adults ($\bar{x}=25.6$ years)	0.88	
Pourahmadi et al.[24]	Single	30	Healthy adults ($\bar{x}=27.9$ years)	0.91, 0.85	
Lee et al.[26]	Single	35	Healthy adults ($\bar{x}=27.2$ years)	0.79, 0.48	
Kachingwe and Phillips[29]	BROM	91	Adult low back pain ($\bar{x}=28.0$ years)	0.60, 0.74	

LBP, Lowback pain.

*Intraclass correlation coefficient.

[†]Pearson's *r.*

[‡]Thoracolumbar range of motion.

[§]Three testers performed measurements.

[¶]Back range of motion device (Performance Attainment Associates, Roseville, MN).

Pourahmadi et al.[24] and Kolber et al.[25] also expanded their studies on intratester reliability, both providing similar results. The investigation by Pourahmadi et al.[24] reported reliability of 0.77 for lumbar flexion and 0.87 for extension, while the reliabilities of 0.81 for flexion and 0.91 for extension were reported by Kolber et al.[25]

Intertester reliability in measuring eight subjects was reported by Rondinelli et al.[22] as correlations (ICC) of 0.76 for lumbar flexion using a single inclinometer, 0.69 using a double inclinometer, and 0.77 when the BROM device was used. Very similar correlations (0.77) to those of Rondinelli et al.[22] were reported by Breum et al.[27] for intertester reliability of the BROM device in measuring lumbar flexion in a study of 40 subjects (ICC). The reliability correlation reported when lumbar extension was measured with the BROM device was 0.35 (ICC). Also with the BROM, similar results to those of Breum et al.[27] were described by Kachingwe and Phillips,[29] who reported that intertester reliability (ICC) for flexion was 0.74 and for extension was 0.55. The conclusions and opinions proposed by the authors of these studies about the use of various types of inclinometers for the measurement of flexion and extension based on their data collection are exactly the same as the information already presented in the previous section, which discusses intratester reliability.

Other groups of investigators examined only intertester reliability of spinal measurements with use of the inclinometer. Burdett et al.[6] reported reliability coefficients of 0.91 (ICC) and 0.93 (Pearson's *r*) for lumbar flexion and 0.71 (ICC) and 0.72 (Pearson's *r*) for lumbar extension in their single-inclinometer examination of 23 subjects. Follow-up testing using ANOVA indicated

no significant difference between testers in interrater reliability for extension, but a significant difference between testers for flexion ($P < 0.05$).

Slightly lower results were reported in a study performed by Chiarello and Savidge[30] of 12 subjects without back pain and 6 patients with back pain. Correlations (ICC) were reported as 0.74 for lumbar flexion for subjects without back pain, 0.64 for lumbar flexion for patients with low back pain, 0.65 for lumbar extension for subjects without back pain, and 0.83 for lumbar extension for patients with low back pain. The authors concluded that these results indicated "acceptable reliability," and that use of the inclinometer "in a clinical setting to document lumbar spine range of motion represents a vast improvement over observational methods."

Newton and Waddell[31] examined intertester reliability for lumbar flexion and extension in 20 patients with low back pain. Reported reliability correlations (ICC) were good (0.98) for flexion but relatively poor (0.48) for extension. After examining 24 normal individuals for intertester reliability of lumbar flexion, Alaranta et al.[15] reported a correlation of 0.61 (Pearson's *r*). A *t*-test between measurements by the two testers indicated a significant difference ($P < 0.05$). In a study investigating interrater reliability in only flexion of the spine, Sullivan et al.[32] reported test–retest reliability of 0.75.

Tables 10.15 and 10.16 summarize studies performed on intra and intertester reliability for the use of the inclinometer in measuring flexion and extension. As indicated, intertester reliability ranged from 0.52 to 0.98 (see Table 10.15) for flexion and from 0.35 to 0.89 for extension (see Table 10.16).

Table 10.15	INCLINOMETER: INTERTESTER RELIABILITY FOR LUMBAR FLEXION					
				CORRELATION		
STUDY	TECHNIQUE	n	SAMPLE	ICC*	r†	
Burdett et al.[6]	Single	23	Healthy adults (20–40 years)	0.91	0.93	
Mellin[20]	Single	15	Healthy adults ($\bar{x}$=31.3 years)		0.97	
					0.95 (T-L‡)	
Newton and Waddell[31]	Single	20	Healthy adults (20–55 years)	0.98		
Chiarello and Savidge[30]	Single	12	Healthy adults (23–55 years; $\bar{x}$=25.5)	0.74		
		6	LBP (24–37 years; $\bar{x}$=32.7)	0.64		
Alaranta et al.[15]	Double	24	Healthy adults (35–54 years)		0.61	
Nitschke et al.[16]	Double	34	LBP (20–65 years)	0.52	0.67	
Pourahmadi et al.[24]	Single	30	Healthy adults ($\bar{x}$=27.9 years)	0.77		
Kolber et al.[25]	Single	30	Healthy adults ($\bar{x}$=25.6 years)	0.81		
Rondinelli et al.[22]	Single, double, BROM§	8	Healthy adults (18–30 years)	0.76 (single) 0.69 (double) 0.77 (BROM)		
Breum et al.[27]	BROM	47	Healthy adults (18–38 years; $\bar{x}$=25.8)	0.77		
Sullivan et al.[32]	Double	36	Adult low back pain	0.75		
Lee et al.[26]	Single	35	Healthy adults ($\bar{x}$=27.2 years)	0.83		
Kachingwe and Phillips[29]	BROM	91	Adult low back pain ($\bar{x}$=28.0 years)	0.74		

LBP, Low back pain.

*Intraclass correlation coefficient.

†Pearson's *r.*

‡Thoracolumbar range of motion.

§Back range of motion device (Performance Attainment Associates, Roseville, MN).

Table 10.16	INCLINOMETER: INTERTESTER RELIABILITY FOR LUMBAR EXTENSION				
				CORRELATION	
STUDY	TECHNIQUE	n	SAMPLE	ICC*	r†
Burdett et al.[6]	Single	23	Healthy adults (20–40 years)	0.71	0.72
Mellin[20]	Single	15	Healthy adults ($\bar{x}$=31.3 years)		0.89
					0.89 (T-L‡)
Newton and Waddell[31]	Single	20	Healthy adults (20–55 years)	0.48	
Chiarello and Savidge[30]	Single	12	Healthy adults (23–55 years; $\bar{x}$=25.5)	0.65	
		6	LBP (24–37 years; $\bar{x}$=32.7)	0.83	
Nitschke et al.[16]	Double	34	LBP (20–65 years)	0.35	0.35
Pourahmadi et al.[24]	Single	30	Healthy adults ($\bar{x}$=27.9 years)	0.87	
Kolber et al.[25]	Single	30	Healthy adults ($\bar{x}$=25.6 years)	0.91	
Breum et al.[27]	BROM§	47	Healthy adults ($\bar{x}$=25.8 years)	0.35	
Lee et al.[29]	Single	35	Healthy adults ($\bar{x}$=27.2 years)	0.75	
Kachingwe and Phillips[29]	BROM	91	Adult low back pain ($\bar{x}$=28.0 years)	0.55	

LBP, Low back pain.

*Intraclass correlation coefficient.

†Pearson's *r.*

‡Thoracolumbar range of motion.

§Back range of motion device (Performance Attainment Associates, Roseville, MN).

Validity

In an effort to establish the validity of the use of the inclinometer to measure lumbar flexion and extension, investigators compared results of their examination with the inclinometer versus results of examination by radiographic (X-ray) assessment. Mayer et al.[33] examined flexion in 12 patients with low back pain with an inclinometer (both single and double) and by X-ray. Results indicated no significant difference (ANOVA) between the X-ray examination and either the single- or the double-inclinometer method. The authors concluded

that "inclinometer measurement of range of motion is a simple, effective, quantitative technique for assessing disability and measuring progress in rehabilitation."

Additional studies have examined the validity of the inclinometer. After examining flexion in 27 subjects with the inclinometer and after comparing these results versus those obtained with examination by X-ray, Burdett et al.[6] reported a correlation coefficient of 0.73 for lumbar flexion and 0.15 for extension (Pearson's *r*). An ANOVA indicated no significant difference between inclinometer and X-ray measurement techniques for

Table 10.17 VALIDITY: X-RAY VERSUS INCLINOMETER FOR FLEXION OF LUMBAR SPINE					
				CORRELATION	
STUDY	**TECHNIQUE**	**n**	**SAMPLE**	**ICC***	**r†**
Portek et al.[10]	Single	11	Healthy adults (25–36 years; $\bar{x}=29.5$)		0.42
Burdett et al.[6]	Single	23	Healthy adults (20–40 years)		0.73
Newton and Waddell[31]	Single	20	Healthy adults (20–55 years)	0.76	
Mayer et al.[33]	Single, double	12	Low back pain (19–51 years; $\bar{x}=31.0$)	No significant difference between X-ray and single inclinometer, or between X-ray and double inclinometer (total)‡	
Williams et al.[34]	Double	18	Adults with back pain (23–62 years; $\bar{x}=41.2$)	0.67	

*Intraclass correlation coefficient.
†Pearson's r.
‡Total = extension and flexion range of motion combined; analysis of variance with repeated measures was statistical analysis performed.

Table 10.18 VALIDITY: X-RAY VERSUS INCLINOMETER FOR EXTENSION OF LUMBAR SPINE				
STUDY	**TECHNIQUE**	**n**	**SAMPLE**	**CORRELATION (r*)**
Portek et al.[10]	Single	11	Healthy adults (25–36 years; $\bar{x}=29.5$)	0.55
Burdett et al.[6]	Single	27	Healthy adults (20–40 years)	0.15
Mayer et al.[33]	Single, double	12	Low back pain (20–59 years; $\bar{x}=34.0$)	No significant difference between X-ray and single inclinometer, or between X-ray and double inclinometer (total)†

*Pearson's r.
†Total = extension and flexion range of motion combined; analysis of variance with repeated measures was statistical analysis performed.

flexion or extension. Newton and Waddell[31] examined flexion in only 20 patients with low back pain, reporting a correlation of 0.76 between results obtained with the use of an inclinometer and by X-ray (ICC).

Lower correlations between radiologic examination and the inclinometer were reported by Williams et al.[34] and Portek et al.[10] After examining 18 subjects with low back pain, Williams et al.[34] reported the relationship between the inclinometer and X-ray for flexion to be 0.67. After measuring flexion and extension in 11 healthy subjects, Portek et al.[10] reported correlations of 0.42 for flexion and 0.55 for extension (Pearson's r). No significant difference was found between inclinometer and radiographic examination (t-test). Because of the poor correlations, the authors concluded that "comparison with the radiologic technique showed that the clinical measure only gave indices of back movement." A summary of the results of validity studies that compared results obtained by the inclinometer and by X-ray examination is presented in Tables 10.17 and 10.18.

Lateral Flexion

Although research on the use of the inclinometer for measurement of flexion and extension of the spine is relatively common, investigations reporting the reliability of the inclinometer in the measurement of lateral fewer are less in number. Mellin et al.[21] used the inclinometer to examine intratester reliability for measurement of lateral flexion in 27 subjects, measuring right and left

lateral lumbar flexion (inclinometer placed both at and 20 cm superior to the posterior superior iliac spine) and right and left lateral thoracolumbar flexion (inclinometer placed at the posterior superior iliac spine and at the spinous process of T1). Reported correlations for intratester reliability were as follows: right lateral lumbar flexion 0.84, left lateral lumbar flexion 0.86, right lateral thoracolumbar flexion 0.81, and left lateral thoracolumbar flexion 0.85 (Pearson's r). Matched t-tests analyzing differences between measurements were not significant for any motion examined.

After investigating intratester reliability of two examiners who measured lateral flexion in 12 subjects with low back pain, Ng et al.[22] reported reliability to be greater than 0.90 for movement in both directions for both examiners. Studies by both Kolber et al.[25] and Lee[26] examined intratester and intertester reliability for measuring lateral flexion using the inclinometer. Measuring 30 subjects, Kolber et al.[25] reported intratester reliability of 0.88 and 0.83 for right and left lateral flexion, respectively. Related to intertester reliability, the authors reported reliability to be 0.88 for right lateral flexion and 0.84 when laterally flexing to the left. Lee et al.[26] also examined both intra and intertester reliability using the inclinometer to measure lateral flexion in 35 subjects.

Although the author reported intratester reliability of greater than 0.80 for two examiners for right and left lateral flexion, intertester reliability was lower (0.79 to the left and 0.45 to the right). Newton and Waddell[31] reported similar correlations for intertester reliability in

Table 10.19 INCLINOMETER: INTRATESTER RELIABILITY FOR LUMBAR LATERAL FLEXION

STUDY	TECHNIQUE	n	SAMPLE	CORRELATION ICC*	CORRELATION r[†]
Mellin et al.[21]	Single	27	Healthy adults (24–50 years; x̄ = 30.6)		0.84 (right) 0.86 (left) 0.81 (right T-L) [‡] 0.85 (left T-L)
Nitschke et al.[16]	Double	34	Healthy adults (20–65 years)	0.90 (right) 0.89 (left)	0.90 (right) 0.89 (left)
Breum et al.[27]	BROM[§]	47	Healthy adults (18–38 years; x̄ = 25.8)	0.89 (right) 0.92 (left)	
Madson et al.[28]	BROM	40	Healthy adults (20–40 years; x̄ = 25.5)	0.91 (right) 0.95[38] (left)	
Ng et al.[23]	Single	12	Adult low back pain (23–62 years; x̄ = 28.0)	0.96 (right) 0.92 (left)	0.96 (right) 0.94 (left)
Kolber et al.[25]	Single	30	Healthy adults (x̄ = 25.6 years)	0.88 (right) 0.83 (left)	
Lee et al.[26]	Single	35	Healthy adults (x̄ = 27.2 years)	0.84 (right) 0.86 (left)	0.84 (right) 0.78 (left)
Kachingwe and Phillips[29]	BROM	91	Adult low back pain (x̄ = 28.0 years)	0.85, 0.84 (right) 0.83, 0.85 (left)	

*Intraclass correlation coefficient.
[†]Pearson's r.
[‡]Thoracolumbar range of motion.
[§]Back range of motion device (Performance Attainment Associates, Roseville, MN).

the measurement of 20 patients with low back pain. The correlation for right lateral flexion was 0.78 and for left lateral flexion, 0.84.

Nitschke et al.[16] examined both intrarater and interrater reliability of lateral flexion measurements in 34 subjects. Results of analysis of intrarater reliability were reported at 0.90 (95% CI = 10.26 degrees; t-test not significant) for right lateral lumbar flexion and 0.89 (95% CI = 10.77 degrees; t-test not significant) for left lateral lumbar flexion, irrespective of the correlation analysis used (ICC or Pearson's r). However, data for interrater reliability were far less than acceptable; right lateral lumbar flexion was 0.18 (ICC) and 0.62 (Pearson's r) (95% CI = 15.79 degrees; t-test was significant at $p < 0.05$), and left lateral lumbar flexion was 0.13 (ICC) and 0.55 (Pearson's r) (95% CI = 16.76 degrees; t-test was significant at $p < 0.05$). Nitschke et al.[16] suggested that because of "systematic and random error," their findings indicate that use of the inclinometer for "spinal range of motion measurements is inadequate."

Madson et al.[28], Breum et al.[27], and Kachingwe and Phillips[29] used the BROM device to investigate the reliability of measuring lateral flexion. Examining only intratester reliability, Madson et al.[28] reported correlations (Pearson's r) on 40 subjects of 0.91 for right lateral flexion and 0.95 for left lateral flexion (95% CI = 5 degrees). Results of intrarater reliability on 47 subjects for right lateral flexion and left lateral flexion were reported by Breum et al.[27] to be 0.89 and 0.92, respectively (ICC). Interrater reliability was reported as 0.89 for right lateral flexion and 0.81 for left lateral flexion (ICC). Similar intratester reliability was described by

Kachingwe and Phillips[29] when using the BROM; they reported test–retest reliability in two examiners to range from 0.83 to 0.85 for right and left lateral flexion. However, intertester reliability was 0.79 for right and 0.64 for left lateral flexion, indicating lower intertester reliability than was seen in previous studies. Tables 10.19 and 10.20 provide a summary of reviewed studies related to the reliability of measurement of lateral flexion with use of an inclinometer.

In addition to collecting reliability data on flexion, extension, and lateral flexion, Lee et al.[26] examined the validity of the use of the inclinometer for the measurement of lateral flexion. After comparing inclinometer results on 15 subjects taken by two examiners versus X-rays taken in full lateral flexion to the left and the right, the author reported validity correlation ranging from 0.43 to 0.66.

Rotation

Few studies have been performed on the reliability of the inclinometer in measuring rotation. In the most extensive study investigating intertester reliability of the inclinometer in the measurement of lumbar rotation, Boline et al.[35] measured 25 subjects without back pain and 25 patients with low back pain using a technique in which the subject fully flexes the lumbar spine and then rotates maximally. Reliability correlations (ICC and Pearson's r) for right rotation, left rotation, and total range of motion (sum of left and right rotation combined) for subjects (n = 25), patients (n = 25), and all individuals combined (n = 50) ranged from 0.52 to 0.86.

Table 10.20   INCLINOMETER: INTERTESTER RELIABILITY FOR LUMBAR LATERAL FLEXION

STUDY	TECHNIQUE	n	SAMPLE	CORRELATION ICC*	$r^†$
Newton and Waddell[31]	Single	20	Healthy adults (20–55 years)	0.78 (right) 0.84 (left)	
Nitschke et al.[16]	Double	34	Healthy adults (20–65 years)	0.18 (right) 0.13 (left)	0.62 (right) 0.55 (left)
Breum et al.[27]	BROM‡	47	Healthy adults (18–38 years; $\bar{x}=25.8$)	0.89 (right) 0.81 (left)	
Kolber et al.[25]	Single	30	Healthy adults ($\bar{x}=25.6$ years)	0.88 (right) 0.84 (left)	
Lee et al.[26]	Single	35	Healthy adults ($\bar{x}=27.2$ years)	0.45 (right) 0.79 (left)	
Kachingwe and Phillips[29]	BROM	91	Adult low back pain ($\bar{x}=28.0$ years)	0.79 (right) 0.64 (left)	

*Intraclass correlation coefficient.
†Pearson's *r*.
‡Back range of motion device (Performance Attainment Associates, Roseville, MN).

Using a different inclinometer technique for measuring rotation, Alaranta et al.[15] measured rotation with subjects seated. Using the mean of the total range of motion of right and left rotation, the authors reported an intertester reliability correlation of 0.79 (Pearson's *r*). Paired *t*-tests between testers indicated no significant difference. Ng et al.[23] measured rotation in standing position and provided pelvic stabilization by using a metal frame. Intratester reliability for two examiners was greater than 0.94 across both examiners for right and left rotation. Iveson et al.[33] measured 10 subjects in side-lying and reported intratester reliability of 0.94 for both left and right rotation and intertester reliability of 0.89 to the right and 0.87 to the left.

Breum et al.[27] examined the reliability of the BROM device in measuring rotation. Intrarater reliability for right rotation was 0.57 and for left rotation was 0.56 (ICC). Interrater reliability was quite low, with the authors reporting a correlation of 0.35 for right rotation and 0.37 for left rotation (ICC). Madson et al.[28] reported a much higher intratester reliability than Breum et al.,[27] using the BROM device: 0.88 for right rotation and 0.93 for left rotation (ICC). In a study of intratester and intertester reliability, Kachingwe and Phillips[29] reported reliability of the BROM in the measurement of rotation that was lower than in previous studies. The authors reported intrarater reliability for two examiners ranging from 0.58 to 0.69. Interrater reliability was equally as low, with reliability reported as 0.60 for right rotation and 0.64 for left rotation. Tables 10.21 and 10.22 summarize the studies presented in this section.

FLEXICURVE

Use of a Draughtman's flexible curve for measuring the flexion and extension of the spine was first proposed by Israel[37] in 1959. He proposed this method as it was analogous to the method used by survey engineers at the time to measure curves of a road. While the study only provided descriptive data, Israel[37] was one of the first to describe the use of the Flexicurve technique for measuring spinal curves.

Since Israel's article several research studies have been published on the reliability and validity of the Flexicurve technique for measuring spinal curves in flexion and extension. The Flexicurve technique has been demonstrated to accurately measure spinal angles when compared to radiographic assessment[38-40] and three-dimensional videography.[41] The reliability of lumbar measurements using the Flexicurve technique reported in the literature is also consistently high.[39,40,42-44]

Spinous process landmarks used for each study vary, but the most common landmarks for assessing the curvature of the lumbar spine are T12 & S2, and the most common landmarks for assessing the curvature of the thoracic spine are T1 & T12. For this text, these common spinous process landmarks were used for both lumbar and thoracic assessments. The L4 spinous process of the lumbar spine and the T6 spinous process of the thoracic spine were also used as landmarks to obtain a standardized midpoint of the curve when creating tracings to calculate spinal angles.

This section is divided into the following subsections for clarity: studies dealing with reliability of lumbar measurements, studies dealing with the reliability of thoracic measurement, and validity studies that compare results obtained with the Flexicure to data derived from radiographic (X-ray) examination or three-dimensional videography.

Reliability for Lumbar Measurements

Use of the Flexicurve technique to assess lumbar flexion and extension has resulted in consistently high intratester reliability. Hart and Rose[39] reported

Table 10.21   INCLINOMETER: INTRATESTER RELIABILITY FOR LUMBAR ROTATION

				CORRELATION	
STUDY	TECHNIQUE	n	SAMPLE	ICC*	r†
Breum et al.[27]	Sitting (BROM)‡	47	Healthy adults (18–38 years; x̄ = 25.8)	0.57 (right) 0.56 (left)	
Madson et al.[28]	Sitting (BROM)	40	Healthy adults (20–40 years; x̄ = 25.5)	0.88 (right) 0.93 (left)	
Ng et al.[23]	Single	12	Adult low back pain (23–62 years; x̄ = 28.0)	0.96 (right) 0.95 (left)	0.96 (right) 0.94 (left)
Kachingwe and Phillips[29]	BROM	91	Adult low back pain (x̄ = 28.0 years)	0.68, 0.76 (right) 0.58, 0.69 (left)	
Iveson et al.[36]	Single (side-lying)	10	Adult low back pain (17–24 years)	0.94 (right), 0.94 (left)	

*Intraclass correlation coefficient.
†Pearson's r.
‡Back range of motion device (Performance Attainment Associates; Roseville, MN).

Table 10.22   INCLINOMETER: INTERTESTER RELIABILITY FOR LUMBAR ROTATION

				CORRELATION	
STUDY	TECHNIQUE	n	SAMPLE	ICC*	r†
Boline et al.[35]	Full flexion and rotate, single	50	25 healthy adults (x̄ = 33.0 years) 25 low back pain (x̄ = 28.0 years)	0.67 0.84 0.53 0.71 0.53 0.71 0.75 0.78 0.70	0.69 R rot (all‡) 0.86 R rot (LBP§) 0.54 R rot (norm¶¶) 0.72 L rot (all) 0.52 L rot (LBP) 0.73 L rot (norm) 0.75 Total¶ rot (all) 0.79 Total rot (LBP) 0.70 Total rot (norm)
Alaranta et al.[15]	Sitting (single)	24	Healthy adults (35–54 years)		0.79 (mean)**
Breum et al.[27]	Sitting (BROM††)	47	Healthy adults (18–38 years; x̄ = 25.8)	0.35 (right) 0.37 (left)	
Kachingwe and Phillips[29]	Sitting (BROM)	91	Adult low back pain (x̄ = 28.0 years)	0.60 (right) 0.64 (left)	
Iveson et al.[36]	Single (sidelying)	10	Adult low back pain (17–24 years)	0.89 (right) 0.87 (left)	

LBP, Low back pain; *L rot*, left rotation; *R rot*, right rotation.
*Intraclass correlation coefficient.
†Pearson's r.
‡All subjects.
§Subgroup of subjects with low back pain.
¶¶Subgroup of subjects with no low back pain.
¶Left and right rotation range of motion combined.
**Mean of the total range of right and left rotation.
††Back range of motion device (Performance Attainment Associates, Roseville, MN).

intratester reliability coefficients in the examination of six subjects of 0.97 (ICC) for 23 pairs of neutral standing assessments and 66 pairs of lumbar flexion assessments. A study by Burton[42] examined 15 subjects and resulted in an intratester reliability of 0.95 for upper lumbar flexion, 0.97 for lower lumbar flexion, 0.96 for upper lumbar extension, and 0.97 for lower lumbar extension (coefficients of correlation). Stokes et al.[43] reported intratester reliability of 0.98 in 10 subjects for total lumbar motion. A study by Tillotson and Burton[40] assessed intratester reliability in 16 subjects and demonstrated correlation coefficients of 0.98 for upper lumbar flexion, 0.96 for lower

lumbar flexion, 0.95 for upper lumbar extension, and 0.82 for lower lumbar extension. In 10 subjects, Youdas et al.[44] reported intratester reliability was high when comparing single measurements over time: 0.84 for seated lumbar flexion, 0.97 for prone lumbar extension, and 0.87 for neutral standing lumbar lordosis. Youdas et al.[44] also found the intratester reliability is increased when the average of two measurement are compared over time: 0.91 for lumbar flexion, 0.98 for lumbar extension, and 0.93 for neutral spine position (ICC); however, the authors stated "the reliability of a single measurement of lumbar spine sagittal mobility would not be improved enough to warrant

Table 10.23 FLEXICURVE: INTRATESTER RELIABILITY FOR FLEXION

STUDY	n	SAMPLE	CORRELATION	
			ICC*	r†
Burton[42]	15	Healthy adults (no age reported)	0.95–0.97	
Hart and Rose[39]	6	Healthy adults (no age reported)	0.97	
Tillotson and Burton[40]	16	Healthy adults (no age reported)		0.96–0.98
Youdas et al.[44]	10	Healthy adults (23–37 years; $\bar{x}$= 24.9 years)	0.84	

*Intraclass correlation coefficient.
†Pearson's r.

Table 10.24 FLEXICURVE: INTRATESTER RELIABILITY FOR EXTENSION

STUDY	n	SAMPLE	CORRELATION	
			ICC*	r†
Burton[42]	15	Healthy adults (no age reported)	0.96–0.97	
Tillotson and Burton[40]	16	Healthy Adults (no age reported)		0.82–0.95
Youdas et al.[44]	10	Healthy adults (23–37 years; $\bar{x}$= 24.9 years)	0.97	

*Intraclass correlation coefficient.
†Pearson's r.

spending the extra time with a patient to make a second measurement."

Tables 10.23 and 10.24 provide a summary of studies investigating intratester reliability for the measurement of flexion and extension using the Flexicurve technique. As indicated, reliability coefficients across all studies ranged from 0.84 to 0.98 for measurement of flexion (see Table 10.23) and from 0.82 to 0.97 for measurement of extension (see Table 10.24).

Limited research exists on the interrater reliability of the Flexicurve technique for assessing lumbar range of motion. Burton[42] reported intertester reliability of 0.90 for upper lumbar flexion, 0.88 for lower lumbar flexion, 0.99 for upper lumbar extension, and 0.82 for lower lumbar extension when comparing among two raters in 10 subjects. While the interrater reliability was good in the aforementioned study, additional research is needed to corroborate these findings.

Reliability for Thoracic Measurements

Two studies have demonstrated the reliability of the Flexicurve technique for assessing static thoracic kyphosis when standing in a neutral position;[38,45]

and limited research exists on the reliability of using this technique for assessing thoracic flexion and extension range of motion. Until further research is completed to determine the intra and intertester reliability of using the Flexicurve technique for assessing thoracic flexion and extension, caution should be used when comparing measurements over time or between raters.

Validity

Validity of the Flexicure technique to accurately measure thoracic and lumbar flexion, extension, and neutral spine has been established by investigators comparing results of their examination with the Flexicurve to results of their examination by radiographic (X-ray) assessment[38–40] and three-dimensional videography.[41] Hart and Rose[39] examined lumbar flexion, extension, and neutral position in six patients using a Flexicurve and X-ray. Results indicated a good correlation $r=0.87$ between the X-ray vertebral angle measure and the Flexicurve measure. The authors concluded "the flexible ruler allows clinicians to record relative curvature of the patient's lumbar spine … and the flexible ruler measurement may be compared directly to the measures from a roentegenograph."[39]

After examining flexion and extension in eight subjects with the Flexicurve and comparing these results to those obtained with examination by X-ray, Tillotson and Burton[40] reported a correlation coefficient of 0.93. The authors concluded that "…lumbar sagittal mobility can be estimated from flexicurve records of back surface curvature."[40] Somewhat lower correlations between radiologic examination and the Flexicurve were reported by deOliveira et al.[38] when a standing neutral posture was assessed. After examining 47 subjects, the authors reported the relationship between the Flexicurve and X-ray Cobb angle for the thoracic spine to be 0.70 and relationship for the lumbar spine to be 0.60.[38]

Valle et al.[41] compared Flexicurve measurements to three-dimensional videography in 39 subjects and found results indicating a good correlation for thoracic flexion 0.75, thoracic extension 0.81, and lumbar flexion 0.85, and moderate correlation for lumbar extension 0.61. The authors concluded "the Flexicurve proved to be valid in assessing maximum flexion and extension of the thoracic spine and maximum flexion of the lumbar spine" and "suggest caution when assessing maximum extension of the lumbar spine."[41]

A summary of the results of validity studies that compared results obtained using the Flexicurve technique and X-ray examination or three-dimensional videography is presented in Tables 10.25 for the lumbar spine and Table 10.26 for the thoracic spine.

Table 10.25   VALIDITY: X-RAY OR 3-D VIDEOGRAPHY VERSUS FLEXICURVE FOR LUMBAR SPINE

				CORRELATION	
STUDY	TECHNIQUE	n	SAMPLE	ICC*	r†
deOliveira et al.[38]	X-ray	47	Adults with prescription for X-ray 44.9 (19.4) years;		0.60
Hart and Rose[39]	X-ray	6	Healthy adults (no age reported)	0.87	
Tillotson and Burton[40]	X-ray	20	Health adults (no age reported)		0.93
Valle et al.[41]	3-D videography	39	Healthy adults (18–50 years)	Flexion 0.85 Extension 0.61	

*Intraclass correlation coefficient.
†Pearson's r.

Table 10.26   VALIDITY: X-RAY OR 3-D VIDEOGRAPHY VERSUS FLEXICURVE FOR THORACIC SPINE

				CORRELATION	
STUDY	TECHNIQUE	n	SAMPLE	ICC*	r†
deOliveira et al.[38]	X-ray	47	Adults with prescription for X-ray 44.9 (19.4) years		0.70
Valle et al.[41]	3-D videography	39	Healthy adults (18–50 years)	Flexion 0.75 Extension 0.81	

*Intraclass correlation coefficient.
†Pearson's r.

SMARTPHONE

The number of cell phones used by the public has increased dramatically in the past decade. Most Smartphones are now equipped with inexpensive sensors to allow the phone to measure range of motion (ROM).[46] Chapter 8 has provided descriptions of suggested techniques for measuring ROM of the lumbar spine.

Flexion, Extension, Lateral Flexion

Intratester Reliability

Using the Smartphone, three investigations studied the test–retest (intratester) reliability of four movements of the lumbar spine—flexion, extension, and left and right lateral flexion.[25,47,48] Macedo et al.[47] examined 20 subjects (11 females, 9 males) and reported excellent intratester reliability above 0.90 for all four measurements. Similar reliability was provided in studies by Kolber et al.[25] who reported test–retest reliability ranging from 0.80 to 0.88 in 30 subjects (18 females, 12 males). The only exception to the good reliability found among these three studies was that Boudreau al[48] reported intratester reliability ranging from 0.67 to 0.90 for flexion, extension, and lateral flexion. While examining 29 subjects (18 female, 11 males), Boudreau et al.[48] presented reliability ranging from 0.75 to 0.90 for right and left lateral flexion, but the intratester reliability for flexion (0.86,0.69) and extension (0.76, 0.67) was lower than the other studies of ROM of the lumbar spine using the Smartphone.

Research by Pourahmadi et al.[24] and Bedekar et al.[49] provide additional data that indicates that measurement of lumbar flexion and extension by the Smartphone is appropriate and offsets the moderate to poor reliability presented by Boudreau et al.[48] Using the Smartphone to investigate only lumbar flexion and extension to 30 individuals (15 female, 15 male), Pourahmadi et al.[24] reported intratester reliability among two testers of 0.87 and 0.90 for flexion and 0.85 and 0.90 for extension ROM. Similar support for good intratester reliability in the measurement of lumbar flexion (0.92) was reported by Bedekar et al.,[49] while investigating 30 subjects (25 females, 5 males).

In summary, the results of these studies on intratester reliability provide evidence that the Smartphone can be used to accurately assess lumbar flexion, extension, and lateral flexion ROM. Table 10.27 Presents data related to the intratester reliability of using the Smartphone to measure flexion, extension, and lateral flexion of the lumbar spine.

Intertester Reliability

Expanding on the research completed on intratester reliability related to the Smartphone for measuring lumbar flexion, extension, and lateral flexion; four studies examined the reliability between two different examiners (intertester reliability) using the same group of subjects.[24,25,48,49] Most of the studies reported intertester reliability above 0.80. Table 10.28 provides information about intertester reliability of the measurement of these motions with the Smartphone. Boudreau et al.[48] suggested "our results provide evidence that the Smartphone can be used to assess lumbar ROM for all lumbar measurements.

Table 10.27 SMARTPHONE: INTRATESTER RELIABILITY FOR LUMBAR FLEXION, EXTENSION, AND LATERAL FLEXION

STUDY	n	SAMPLE	CORRELATION* (ICC)			
			FLEXION	EXTENSION	LATERAL FLEXION RIGHT	LATERAL FLEXION LEFT
Kolber et al.[25]	30	Healthy Adults ($\bar{x}$ = 25.6 years)	0.88	0.80	0.82	0.84
Boudreau et al.[48]	29	Healthy Adults ($\bar{x}$ = 21. years)	0.86, 0.69	0.76, 0.67	0.89, 0.90	0.75, 0.85
Macedo et al.[47]	30	Healthy Adults ($\bar{x}$ = 24.0 years)	0.96	0.92	0.91	0.91
Pourahmadi et al.[24]	30	Healthy Adults ($\bar{x}$ = 27.9 years)	0.87, 0.90	0.90, 0.85	–	–
Bedekar et al.[49]	30	Healthy Adults ($\bar{x}$ = 21.47 years)	0.92	–	–	–

*ICC = Intraclass correlation coefficient.

Table 10.28 SMARTPHONE: INTERTESTER RELIABILITY FOR LUMBAR FLEXION, EXTENSION, AND LATERAL FLEXION

STUDY	n	SAMPLE	CORRELATION* (ICC)			
			FLEXION	EXTENSION	LATERAL FLEXION RIGHT	LATERAL FLEXION LEFT
Kolber et al.[25]	30	Healthy Adults ($\bar{x}$ = 25.6 years)	0.88	0.81	0.93	0.90
Boudreau al[48]	29	Healthy Adults ($\bar{x}$ = 21. years)	0.71	0.84	0.88	0.89
Pourahmadi et al.[24]	30	Healthy Adults ($\bar{x}$ = 27.9 years)	0.89	0.89	–	–
Bedekar et al.[49]	30	Healthy Adults ($\bar{x}$ = 21.47 years)	0.81	–	–	–

*ICC = Intraclass correlation coefficient.

Table 10.29 VALIDITY: SMARTPHONE TO INCLINOMETER FOR LUMBAR FLEXION, EXTENSION, AND LATERAL FLEXION

STUDY	n	SAMPLE	CORRELATION* (ICC)			
			FLEXION	EXTENSION	LATERAL FLEXION RIGHT	LATERAL FLEXION LEFT
Kolber et al.[25]	30	Healthy Adults ($\bar{x}$ = 25.6 years)	0.87	0.91	0.94	0.91
Boudreau et al.[48]	29	Healthy Adults ($\bar{x}$ = 21. years)	0.70	0.64	0.85	0.89
Macedo et al.[47]	30	Healthy Adults ($\bar{x}$ = 24.0 years)	0.94	0.94	0.82	0.88
Pourahmadi et al.[24]	30	Healthy Adults ($\bar{x}$ = 27.9 years)	0.85	0.91	–	–

*ICC = Intraclass Correlation Coefficient.

Validity—Phone to Inclinometer

Four studies examined the criterion validity using the Smartphone (target test) for measuring lumbar ROM and compared the Smartphone data to data collected on the inclinometer (gold standard).[24,25,47,48] [As described in Chapter 2, by using a target test (Smartphone) and comparing it to the gold standard (inclinometer), such measurement for criterion validity assumes that the use of an inclinometer as a gold standard was appropriate.] Overall, the criterion validity between the Smartphone and the inclinometer was very good (Table 10.29). Authors of all studies related to the validity of the Smartphone compared to the gold standard of the inclinometer (criterion validity) tended to agree with Kolber et al.[25] who concluded that the "Smartphone application may offer clinical utility comparable to inclinometer for quantifying mobility of the lumbar spine.

Rotation

Reliability

Although previous studies have examined using the inclinometer and goniometer for the intra and intertester reliability of measuring lumbar rotation, only one study has examined the measurement of lumbar rotation using the Smartphone. Performing a study in which 30 subjects (10 females, 20 males) held a bar in front of their body as they rotated to the left and right, Furness et al.[18] examined the intra and inter tester reliability of the Smartphone. Results indicated that the test–retest reliability for two testers was 0.97, 0.96 and 0.98, 0.97 for right and left rotation, respectfully. Additionally, intertester reliability between the two testers was 0.87 for right rotation and 0.89 for left rotation. Based on the results of their research, Furness et al.[18] suggested "clinicians may find the Smartphone offers greater convenience and efficiency than other measurement devices, meaning that it could be introduced into practice with confidence that it provides reliable measurements both within and between raters."

CERVICAL SPINE

TAPE MEASURE

A study by Hsieh and Yeung[50] evaluated the intratester reliability of two different clinicians who used a tape measure to examine six cervical motions in 34 subjects. As indicated in Table 10.30, intratester reliability ranged from 0.78 to 0.95. The authors concluded that the tape measure method "is a reliable means for clinicians to assess neck range of motion."

Haywood et al.[8] examined 26 patients with ankylosing spondylitis on the interrater reliability of measuring rotation using a tape measure. The authors found high reliability similar to that of Hsieh and Yeung,[50] reporting ICC values of 0.94 for rotation to the right and 0.95 to the left.

GONIOMETER

In addition to studies on the reliability of the goniometer that have been published in the literature related to the lumbar spine, studies also have been performed to test intratester and intertester reliability in use of the goniometer to measure the cervical spine. This section presents information on reliability studies related to cervical flexion, extension, lateral flexion, and rotation.

Procedures for measuring cervical range of motion of flexion, extension, lateral flexion, and rotation

using goniometry techniques similar to those described in Chapter 8 were examined by several authors.[51–55] Youdas et al.[51] reported on the examination of 20 patients with cervical spine pain. Intratester reliability correlations (ICC) ranged from 0.78 to 0.90, and intertester reliability (ICC) ranged from 0.54 to 0.79. Pourahmadi et al.[55] also measured both intra and intertester reliability. Examining 40 subjects, the authors reported intratester reliability ranging from 0.71 to 0.78, which was similar to what was reported for intertester reliability ranging from 0.70 to 0.75.

Reporting only the results of intertester reliability, Pringle[53] examined 27 healthy adults with a goniometer and reported intertester reliability ranging from 0.90 to 0.97. Zachman et al.[52] and Whitcroft et al.[54] also examined intertester reliability in 24 subjects and 100 subjects, respectively. Reliability correlations ranged from 0.43 to 0.87. These authors suggested that range of motion measurements made by the different physical therapists have medium to high reliability.

Using one of the more unique adaptations to a goniometer, Defibaugh[56] examined intratester and intertester reliability in 15 subjects. The device used, which was a "head goniometer," consisted of a mouthpiece (made of ⅛-inch plastic, 2 in. wide and 1½ inches long) attached to a pendulum goniometer (consisting of a 3-in. plastic protractor). Flexion, extension, lateral flexion, and rotation range of motion of the cervical spine were measured while the subject held the device in the mouth. Intratester reliability correlation (Pearson's r) ranged from 0.71 to 0.86, and intertester reliability ranged from 0.80 to 0.94 (see Tables 10.31–10.38). Using a Fisher t statistic, Defibaugh[56] reported no significant differences between measurements (intratester reliability) or testers (intertester reliability). Although unique and "moderately to highly reliable," no other research has appeared in the literature on the use of this device.

Another adaptation for the measurement of lateral flexion was suggested by Pellecchia and Bohannon[57] and consisted of modifying the goniometer by adding a paper clip through the axis of rotation. The paper clip acted as a free-swinging pendulum and served as a pointer. In measuring lateral flexion, both arms of the goniometer were aligned with the base of the subject's nose at the end range of lateral flexion. The paper clip was used to read the measurement scale of the goniometer. Using this technique and measuring 100 subjects, the authors reported an intratester reliability correlation (ICC) of 0.94 for right lateral flexion and 0.91 for left lateral flexion Further analysis of 35 subjects to examine intertester reliability indicated correlations (ICC) of 0.86 for right lateral flexion and 0.65 for left lateral flexion .

Tables 10.31 through 10.34 provide details of the studies investigating intratester reliability of the goniometer to measure cervical ROM. Information as to intertester reliability of the goniometer are presented in Tables 10.35–10.38.

Table 10.30 TAPE MEASURE: INTRATESTER RELIABILITY FOR RANGE OF MOTION OF CERVICAL SPINE

STUDY	n	SAMPLE	CORRELATION (r*)
Flexion			
Hsieh and Yeung[50]	34	Healthy adults (14–31 years; $\bar{x}$ = 18.2)	0.86, 0.95[†]
Extension			
Hsieh and Yeung[50]	34	Healthy adults (14–31 years $\bar{x}$ = 18.2)	0.79, 0.94[†]
Lateral Flexion			
Hsieh and Yeung[50]	34	Healthy adults (14–31 years; $\bar{x}$ = 18.2)	0.91, 0.88 (right)[†] 0.86, 0.87 (left)
Rotation			
Hsieh and Yeung[50]	34	Healthy adults (14–31 years; $\bar{x}$ = 18.2)	0.78, 0.88 (right)[†] 0.81, 0.81 (left)

*Pearson's r.
†Two testers performed measurements.

Table 10.31   GONIOMETER: INTRATESTER RELIABILITY FOR FLEXION OF CERVICAL SPINE

STUDY	n	SAMPLE	CORRELATION ICC*	r†
Defibaugh[56]	15	Healthy adults (20–40 years)		0.77
Youdas et al.[51]	20	Cervical pain (21–84 years; $\bar{x}$=59.1)	0.83	
Pringle[53]	27	Healthy adults (21–41 years; $\bar{x}$=27.6)	0.90‡	

*Intraclass correlation coefficient.
†Pearson's r.
‡Flexion and extension combined.

Table 10.32   GONIOMETER: INTRATESTER RELIABILITY FOR EXTENSION OF CERVICAL SPINE

STUDY	n	SAMPLE	CORRELATION ICC*	r†
Defibaugh[56]	15	Healthy adults (20–40 years)		0.86
Youdas et al.[51]	20	Cervical pain (21–84 years; $\bar{x}$=59.1)	0.86	
Pringle[53]	27	Healthy adults (21–41 years; $\bar{x}$=27.6)	0.90‡	

*Intraclass correlation coefficient.
†Pearson's r.
‡Flexion and extension combined.

Table 10.33   GONIOMETER: INTRATESTER RELIABILITY FOR LATERAL FLEXION OF CERVICAL SPINE

STUDY	n	SAMPLE	CORRELATION ICC*	r†
Defibaugh[56]	15	Healthy adults (20–40 years)		0.83 (right) 0.81 (left)
Youdas et al.[51]	20	Cervical pain (21–84 years; $\bar{x}$=59.1)	0.85 (right) 0.84 (left)	
Pellecchia and Bohannon[57]	100	Healthy adults (14–95 years)	0.94 (right) 0.91 (left)	
Pringle[53]	27	Healthy adults (21–41 years; $\bar{x}$=27.6)	0.97 (combined)	

*Intraclass correlation coefficient.
†Pearson's r.

Table 10.34   GONIOMETER: INTRATESTER RELIABILITY FOR ROTATION OF CERVICAL SPINE

STUDY	n	SAMPLE	CORRELATION ICC*	r†
Defibaugh[56]	15	Healthy adults (20–40 years)		0.81 (right) 0.71 (left)
Youdas et al.[51]	20	Cervical pain (21–84 years; $\bar{x}$=59.1)	0.90 (right) 0.78 (left) 0.97 (combined)	
Pringle[53]	27	Healthy adults (21–41 years; $\bar{x}$=27.6)		

*Intraclass correlation coefficient.
†Pearson's r.

Table 10.35   GONIOMETER: INTERTESTER RELIABILITY FOR FLEXION OF CERVICAL SPINE

STUDY	n	SAMPLE	CORRELATION ICC*	r†
Defibaugh[56]	15	Healthy adults (20–40 years)		0.80
Zachman et al.[52]	24	Healthy subjects (6–51 years)		0.54
Youdas et al.[51]	20	Cervical pain (21–84 years; $\bar{x}$=59.1)	0.57	

*Intraclass correlation coefficient.
†Pearson's r.

Table 10.36   GONIOMETER: INTERTESTER RELIABILITY FOR EXTENSION OF CERVICAL SPINE

STUDY	n	SAMPLE	CORRELATION ICC*	r†
Defibaugh[56]	15	Healthy adults (20–40 years)		0.90
Zachman et al.[52]	24	Healthy subjects (6–51 years)		0.85
Youdas et al.[51]	20	Cervical pain (21–84 years; $\bar{x}$=59.1)	0.79	

*Intraclass correlation coefficient.
†Pearson's r.

Table 10.37   GONIOMETER: INTERTESTER RELIABILITY FOR LATERAL FLEXION OF CERVICAL SPINE

STUDY	n	SAMPLE	CORRELATION ICC*	r†
Defibaugh[56]	15	Healthy adults (20–40 years)		0.85 (right) 0.86 (left)
Zachman et al.[52]	24	Healthy subjects (6–51 years)		0.43 (right) 0.61 (left)
Youdas et al.[51]	20	Cervical pain (21–84 years; $\bar{x}$=59.1)	0.72 (right) 0.79 (left)	
Pellecchia and Bohannon[57]	35	Healthy adults (14–95 years)	0.86 (right) 0.65 (left)	

*Intraclass correlation coefficient.
†Pearson's r.

Table 10.38   GONIOMETER: INTERTESTER RELIABILITY FOR ROTATION OF CERVICAL SPINE

STUDY	n	SAMPLE	CORRELATION ICC*	r†
Defibaugh[56]	15	Healthy adults (20–40 years)		0.87 (right) 0.94 (left)
Zachman et al.[52]	24	Healthy subjects (6–51 years)		0.52 (right) 0.47 (left)
Youdas et al.[51]	20	Cervical pain (21–84 years; $\bar{x}$=59.1)	0.62 (right) 0.54 (left)	

*Intraclass correlation coefficient.
†Pearson's r.

INCLINOMETER

Single Inclinometer (Hand-Held)

Another technique for the measurement of cervical flexion, extension, lateral flexion, and rotation is the use of a single inclinometer (hand-held). Hole et al.[58] examined test–retest reliability in 30 healthy subjects and reported intrarater and interrater reliability ranging from 0.76 to 0.86. After collecting data on intratester and intertester reliability of cervical ROM in 32 subjects with cervical pain, Hoving et al.[59] reported reliability ranging from 0.93 to 0.97 when one person provided the measurements, and from 0.77 to 0.88 when the results of two testers were compared. Measuring intrarater reliability in

30 subjects, Prushansky et al.[60] reported reliability ranging from 0.82 to 0.91. Love et al.[61] measured reliability of the single inclinometer for only flexion and extension of the cervical spine in 27 subjects and reported 0.91 for both flexion and extension for intrarater reliability and 0.89 and 0.80 for flexion and extension, respectively, for interrater reliability. Using a different research design, Bush et al.[62] investigated the reliability of 34 examiners who measured three subjects using a single inclinometer. Bush et al.[62] reported intertester reliability greater than 0.91 for all cervical movements. Each of these authors indicated that the single inclinometer appears to provide consistent results. These studies are summarized in Tables 10.39–10.46.

Table 10.39 INCLINOMETER (NOT CROM*): INTRATESTER RELIABILITY FOR FLEXION OF CERVICAL SPINE

				CORRELATION	
STUDY	TECHNIQUE	n	SAMPLE	ICC[†]	r[‡]
Mayer et al.[63]	Double	58	Healthy adults (17–62 years)		0.99
Hole et al.[58]	Single	30	Healthy adults (21–48 years; $\bar{x}$=28.7)	0.94[§]	
Hoving et al.[59]	Single	32	Cervical pain (18–70 years; $\bar{x}$=45)	0.96, 0.97[§]	
Love et al.[61]	Single	27	Healthy adults ($\bar{x}$=38.6 years)	0.91	
Prushansky et al.[60]	Single	30	Healthy adults ($\bar{x}$=24.2 years)	0.91	

*Cervical range of motion device (Performance Attainment Associates, Roseville, MN).
[†]Intraclass correlation coefficient.
[‡]Pearson's r.
[§]Flexion and extension combined.

Table 10.40 INCLINOMETER (NOT CROM*): INTRATESTER RELIABILITY FOR EXTENSION OF CERVICAL SPINE

				CORRELATION	
STUDY	TECHNIQUE	n	SAMPLE	ICC[†]	r[‡]
Mayer et al.[63]	Double	58	Healthy adults (17–62 years)		0.99
Hole et al.[58]	Single	30	Healthy adults (21–48 years; $\bar{x}$=28.7)	0.94[§]	
Hoving et al.[59]	Single	32	Cervical pain (18–70 years; $\bar{x}$=45)	0.96, 0.97[§]	
Love et al.[61]	Single	27	Healthy adults ($\bar{x}$=38.6 years)	0.90	
Prushansky et al.[60]	Single	30	Healthy adults ($\bar{x}$=24.2 years)	0.94	

*Cervical range of motion device (Performance Attainment Associates, Roseville, MN).
[†]Intraclass correlation coefficient.
[‡]Pearson's r.
[§]Flexion and extension combined.

Table 10.41 INCLINOMETER (NOT CROM*): INTRATESTER RELIABILITY FOR LATERAL FLEXION OF CERVICAL SPINE

				CORRELATION	
STUDY	TECHNIQUE	n	SAMPLE	ICC[†]	r[‡]
Mayer et al.[63]	Double	58	Healthy adults (17–62 years)		0.97 (right) 0.98 (left)
Hole et al.[58]	Single	30	Healthy adults (21–48 years; $\bar{x}$=28.7)	0.94 (right) 0.88 (left)	
Hoving et al.[59]	Single	32	Cervical pain (18–70 years; $\bar{x}$=45)	0.93, 0.93 (combined)	
Prushansky et al.[60]	Single	30	Healthy adults ($\bar{x}$=24.2 years)	0.90 (right) 0.82 (left)	

*Cervical range of motion device (Performance Attainment Associates, Roseville, MN).
[†]Intraclass correlation coefficient.
[‡]Pearson's r.

Table 10.42   INCLINOMETER (NOT CROM*): INTRATESTER RELIABILITY FOR ROTATION OF CERVICAL SPINE

STUDY	TECHNIQUE	n	SAMPLE	ICC[†]	r[‡]
Mayer et al.[63]	Double	58	Healthy adults (17–62 years)		0.98 (right) 0.99 (left)
Guth[65]	Inclinometer "attached by an elastic band to top of head"	8	Healthy adolescents (14–17 years)	0.90–0.96[§]	
Hole et al.[58]	Single	30	Healthy adults (21–48 years; $\bar{x}=28.7$)	0.93 (right) 0.84 (left)	
Hoving et al.[59]	Single	32	Cervical pain (18–70 years; $\bar{x}=45$)	0.96, 0.96 (combined)	
Prushansky et al.[60]	Single	30	Healthy adults ($\bar{x}=24.2$ years)	0.92 (right), 0.84 (left)	

*Cervical range of motion device (Performance Attainment Associates, Roseville, MN).
[†]Intraclass correlation coefficient.
[‡]Pearson's r
[§]Refer to text for explanation.

Table 10.43   INCLINOMETER (NOT CROM*): INTERTESTER RELIABILITY FOR FLEXION OF CERVICAL SPINE

STUDY	TECHNIQUE	n	SAMPLE	ICC[†]	r[‡]
Tucci et al.[66]	Gravity goniometer (with "wooden head" adapter)	10	Healthy adults	0.84	
Zachman et al.[52]	Pendulum goniometer fastened to headpiece (called "rangiometer")	24	Healthy subjects (6–51 years).		0.64
Alaranta et al.[15]	Inclinometer attached to "cloth helmet"	24	Healthy adults		0.69
Hole et al.[58]	Single	30	Healthy adults (21–48 years; $\bar{x}=28.7$)	0.84[§]	
Bush et al.[62]	Single	3 subjects;	N/A	Single, 0.92	
	Double	34 testers		Double, 0.89	
Pringle[53]	Double	27	Healthy adults (21–41 years; $\bar{x}=27.6$)		0.87[§]
Hoving et al.[59]	Single	32	Cervical pain (18–70 years; $\bar{x}=45.0$)	0.89[§]	
Love et al.[61]	Single	27	Healthy adults ($\bar{x}=38.6$ years)	0.89	

*Cervical range of motion device (Performance Attainment Associates, Roseville, MN).
[†]Intraclass correlation coefficient.
[‡]Pearson's r.
[§]Flexion and extension combined.

Table 10.44   INCLINOMETER (NOT CROM*): INTERTESTER RELIABILITY FOR EXTENSION OF CERVICAL SPINE

STUDY	TECHNIQUE	n	SAMPLE	ICC[†]	r[‡]
Tucci et al.[66]	Gravity goniometer (with "wooden head" adapter)	10	Healthy adults	0.86	
Zachman et al.[52]	Pendulum goniometer fastened to headpiece (called "rangiometer")	24	Healthy subjects (6–51 years).		0.89
Alaranta et al.[15]	Inclinometer attached to "cloth helmet"	24	Healthy adults		0.69
Hole et al.[58]	Single	30	Healthy adults (21–48 years; $\bar{x}=28.7$)	0.84[§]	
Bush et al.[62]	Single	3 subjects;	N/A	Single, 0.91	
	Double	34 testers		Double, 0.93	
Pringle[53]	Double	27	Healthy adults (21–41 years; $\bar{x}=27.6$)		0.87[§]
Hoving et al.[59]	Single	32	Cervical pain (18–70 years; $\bar{x}=45.0$)	0.89[§]	
Love et al.[61]	Single	27	Healthy adults ($\bar{x}=38.6$ years)	0.80	

*Cervical range of motion device (Performance Attainment Associates, Roseville, MN).
[†]Intraclass correlation coefficient.
[‡]Pearson's r.
[§]Flexion and extension combined.

Table 10.45	INCLINOMETER (NOT CROM*): INTERTESTER RELIABILITY FOR LATERAL FLEXION OF CERVICAL SPINE				CORRELATION	
STUDY	TECHNIQUE	n	SAMPLE	ICC[†]	r[‡]
Tucci et al.[66]	Gravity goniometer (with "wooden head" adapter)	10	Healthy adults	0.87 (right) 0.82 (left)	
Zachman et al.[52]	Pendulum goniometer fastened to headpiece (called "rangiometer")	24	Healthy subjects (6–51 years).		0.84 (right) 0.79 (left)
Alaranta et al.[15]	Inclinometer attached to "cloth helmet"	24	Healthy adults		0.79 (mean)[§]
Hole et al.[58]	Single	30	Healthy adults (21–48 years; $\bar{x}=28.7$)	0.82 (right) 0.81 (left)	
Bush et al.[62]	Single Double	3 subjects; 34 testers	N/A	Single right, 0.9 Single left, 0.92 Double right, 0.9 Double left, 0.94	
Pringle[53]	Double	27	Healthy adults (21–41 years; $\bar{x}=27.6$)	0.83 (combined)	
Hoving et al.[59]	Single	32	Cervical pain (18–70 years; $\bar{x}=45.0$)	0.77 (combined)	

*Cervical range of motion device (Performance Attainment Associates, Roseville, MN).
[†]Intraclass correlation coefficient.
[‡]Pearson's r.
[§]Mean of the total range of right and left lateral flexion.

Table 10.46	INCLINOMETER (NOT CROM*): INTERTESTER RELIABILITY FOR ROTATION OF CERVICAL SPINE				CORRELATION	
STUDY	TECHNIQUE	n	SAMPLE	ICC[†]	r[‡]
Tucci et al.[66]	Gravity goniometer (with "wooden head" adapter)	10	Healthy adults	0.91 (right) 0.87 (left)	
Zachman et al.[52]	Pendulum goniometer fastened to headpiece (called "rangiometer")	24	Healthy subjects (6–51 years)		0.62 (right) 0.69 (left)
Alaranta et al.[15]	Inclinometer attached to "cloth helmet"	24	Healthy adults		0.86 (mean)[§]
Guth[65]	Inclinometer "attached by an elastic band to top of head"	8	Healthy adolescents (14–17 years)	0.88–0.96[¶]	
Bush et al.[62]	Single Double	3 subjects; 34 testers	N/A	0.91 (combined)	
Pringle[53]	Double	27	Healthy adults (21–41 years; $\bar{x}=27.6$)	0.92 (combined)	
Hoving et al.[59]	Single	32	Cervical pain (18–70 years; $\bar{x}=45.0$)	0.88 (combined)	

*Cervical range of motion device (Performance Attainment Associates, Roseville, MN).
[†]Intraclass correlation coefficient.
[‡]Pearson's r.
[§]Mean of the total range of right and left rotation.
[¶]Refer to text for explanation.

Double Inclinometer (Hand-Held)

The use of a double inclinometer (hand-held) to measure cervical flexion, extension, lateral flexion, and rotation was investigated by Mayer et al.,[63] Pringle,[53] and Bush.[62] In the first part of this study, Mayer et al.[63] examined intratester reliability using a test–retest design on 58 subjects. Excellent reliability (Pearson's r) was reported, with all correlations being greater than 0.97 (see Tables 10.39–10.42). (Although after a Pearson correlation is performed, follow-up testing for random and systematic error is appropriate [refer to Chapter 2], Mayer et al.[63] did not perform any such tests. However, this study is included in this chapter because it is one of only three published investigations on the reliability of

dual inclinometers for measuring cervical range of motion.) The second study that used a double-inclinometer approach to measure cervical range of motion was that of Pringle,[53] who reported intertester reliability ranging from 0.83 to 0.92 in the measurement of 27 healthy adults. Finally, Bush et al.[62] reported interrater reliability of the double inclinometer to be greater than 0.89 for all cervical movements (except that rotation was not measured) (see Tables 10.39–10.46).

Attachment of Inclinometer to the Head

One of the first studies in which an inclinometer-type device was attached to the head was a study by Bennett et al.[62], which used a "bubble goniometer" that was held in place by rubber straps to measure flexion and extension of the cervical spine. Two testers measured the same subject, and "the variation was ±5 degrees." No other statistical analysis of the reliability of this first attempt to attach an inclinometer to the head was provided.

By applying more sophisticated research designs, other researchers took one step further the method proposed by Bennett et al.[64] of attaching the inclinometer to the head with elastic straps. In a study that compared cervical rotation range of motion of swimmers with that of healthy nonswimmers, Guth[65] used an inclinometer attached to the top of the head with an elastic band. The author reported correlations of 0.90 to 0.96 for intratester reliability (see Table 10.42) and of 0.88 to 0.96 for intertester reliability (see Table 10.46); however, why a range of correlations was reported was not clear. The author reported no significant difference between measurements (intratester) or testers (intertester) when a t-test was used.

Differing slightly from previous studies, Alaranta et al.[15] used an inclinometer attached to a "cloth helmet." Instead of reporting the reliability of each motion, the authors used the sum of flexion and extension, the mean of right and left lateral flexion, and the mean of right and left rotation. Intertester reliability correlations ranged from 0.69 to 0.86 (see Tables 10.43–10.46).

Instead of using elastic straps to secure the inclinometer to the head, as was previously described, Tucci et al.[66] placed an inclinometer on head gear constructed from a wood block with an arc cut into it, which then was padded and placed on the head of the subject and held in place with elastic straps. With use of this device on 10 subjects, interrater reliability

resulted in reliability correlations (ICC) ranging from 0.82 to 0.91 (see Tables 10.43–10.46), leading the authors to conclude that the device is "simple, inexpensive, and highly accurate."

In what appears to be a headpiece similar to instruments proposed by Tucci et al.,[66] Zachman et al.[52] introduced the "rangiometer," rigid head gear with an inclinometer mounted on top. After using the device to examine cervical range of motion in 24 subjects, Zachman et al.[52] reported intertester reliability coefficients (Pearson's r) ranging from 0.62 to 0.89 (standard errors of the estimate ranged from 5 to 11 degrees); these values were considered by the authors to be "moderately reliable" (see Tables 10.43–10.46).

Cervical Range of Motion (CROM) Device

The cervical range of motion (CROM) device consists of inclinometers mounted on a plastic frame that is placed over the subject's head and aligned on the bridge of the nose and ears. A detailed description is provided in Chapter 9. Several studies have examined the intertester and intratester reliability of the CROM device used for essentially the same procedures for measurement of cervical flexion, extension, right and left lateral flexion, and right and left rotation. Results are summarized in Tables 10.47–10.54.

Youdas et al.[51] examined 20 patients with cervical pain, reporting correlation coefficients (ICC) ranging from 0.84 to 0.95 for intratester reliability and from 0.73 to 0.90 for intertester reliability. Similar results were found by Capuano-Pucci et al.,[67] who examined 20 subjects without cervical pain using two testers. Intrarater reliability for each tester ranged from 0.62 to 0.91 (Pearson's r). Two separate testing sessions were

Table 10.47 CROM*: INTRATESTER RELIABILITY FOR FLEXION OF CERVICAL SPINE

STUDY	n	SAMPLE	CORRELATION ICC[†]	r[‡]
Youdas et al[69]	20	Healthy adults (21–84 years; x̄ = 59.1)	0.95	
Capuano-Pucci et al.[67]	20	Healthy adults (x̄ = 23.5 years)		0.63, 0.91[§]
Youdas et al.[51]	6	Healthy adults (22–56 years; x̄ = 27.2)	0.64, 0.76, 0.23 0.88, 0.84[¶¶]	
Nilsson[70]	14	Healthy adults (23–45 years)		0.76
Hole et al.[58]	30	Healthy adults (21–48 years; x̄ = 28.7)	0.96	
Olson et al.[71]	12	Healthy adults (21–47 years)	0.88	
Peolsson et al.[72]	30	Healthy adults (20–64 years; x̄ = 32.3)	0.89, 0.91[¶]	
Lindell et al.[73]	50	Cervical pain; 30, Healthy, 20 (20–63 years)	0.86	
Fletcher and Bandy[74]	25	Healthy adults (22–52 years; x̄ = 26.0)	0.87	
	22	Cervical pain (21–55 years; x̄ = 33.0)	0.88	
Love et al.[61]	27	Healthy adults (x̄ = 38.6 years)	0.97	
Audette et al.[75]	20	Healthy adults (x̄ = 37.0 years)	0.89	
Williams et al.[76]	38	Healthy adults (x̄ = 38.0 years)	0.99	

*Cervical range of motion device (Performance Attainment Associates, Roseville, MN).
[†]Intraclass correlation coefficient.
[‡]Pearson's r.
[§]Two testers performed measurements.
[¶¶]Five testers performed measurements; ICC was performed for this study.
[¶]Flexion and extension combined.

			CORRELATION	
Table 10.48 CROM*: INTRATESTER RELIABILITY FOR EXTENSION OF CERVICAL SPINE				
STUDY	**n**	**SAMPLE**	**ICC†**	**r‡**
Youdas et al.[69]	20	Healthy adults (21–84 years; $\bar{x}=59.1$)	0.90	
Capuano-Pucci et al.[67]	20	Healthy adults ($\bar{X}=23.5$ years)		0.90, 0.82§
Youdas et al.[51]	6	Healthy adults (22–56 years; $\bar{x}=27.2$)	0.96, 0.89, 0.96, 0.94, 0.93¶¶	
Nilsson[70]	14	Healthy adults (23–45 years)	0.85	
Hole et al.[58]	30	Healthy adults (21–48 years; $\bar{x}=28.7$)	0.96¶	
Olson et al.[71]	12	Healthy adults (21–47 years)	0.97	
Peolsson et al.[72]	30	Healthy adults (20–64 years; $\bar{x}=32.3$)	0.89, 0.91¶	
Lindell et al.[73]	50	Cervical pain; 30, Healthy 20 (20–63 years)	0.98	
Fletcher and Bandy[74]	25	Healthy adults (22–52 years; $\bar{x}=26.0$)	0.90	
	22	Cervical pain (21–55 years; $\bar{x}=33.0$)	0.92	
Love et al.[61]	27	Healthy adults ($\bar{x}=38.6$ years)	0.97	
Audette et al.[75]	20	Healthy adults ($\bar{x}=37.0$ years)	0.98	
Williams et al.[76]	38	Healthy adults ($\bar{x}=38.0$ years)	0.99	

*Cervical range of motion device (Performance Attainment Associates, Roseville, MN).
†Intraclass correlation coefficient.
‡Pearson's r.
§Two testers performed measurements.
¶¶Five testers performed measurements; ICC was performed for this study.
¶Flexion and extension combined.

			CORRELATION	
Table 10.49 CROM*: INTRATESTER RELIABILITY FOR LATERAL FLEXION OF CERVICAL SPINE				
STUDY	**n**	**SAMPLE**	**ICC†**	**r‡**
Youdas et al.[69]	20	Healthy adults (21–84 years; $\bar{x}=59.1$)	0.92 (right) 0.84 (left)	
Capuano-Pucci et al.[67]	20	Healthy adults ($\bar{X}=23.5$ years)		0.79, 0.89 (right)§ 0.84, 0.90 (left)
Youdas et al.[51]	6	Healthy adults (22–56 years; $\bar{x}=27.2$)	0.75, 0.60, 0.94, 0.88, 0.85¶ (right) 0.77, 0.87, 0.90, 0.86, 0.67 (left)	
Nilsson[70]	14	Healthy adults (23–45 years)		0.61 (right) 0.68 (left)
Hole et al.[58]	30	Healthy adults (21–48 years; $\bar{x}=28.7$)	0.96 (right) 0.96 (left)	
Olson et al.[71]	12	Healthy adults (21–47 years)	0.98 (right) 0.98 (left)	
Peolsson et al.[72]	30	Healthy adults (20–64 years; $\bar{x}=32.3$)	0.88, 0.90 (combined)	
Fletcher and Bandy[74]	25	Healthy adults (22–52 years; $\bar{x}=26.0$)	0.92 (right)	
	22	Cervical pain (21–55 years; $\bar{x}=33.0$)	0.92 (left) 0.93 (right) 0.89 (left)	
Audette et al.[75]	20	Healthy adults ($\bar{x}=37.0$ years)	0.97 (right) 0.97 (left)	
Williams et al.[76]	38	Healthy adults ($\bar{x}=38.0$ years)	0.98 (right) 0.98 (left)	

*Cervical range of motion device (Performance Attainment Associates, Roseville, MN).
†Intraclass correlation coefficient.
‡Pearson's r.
§Two testers performed measurements.
¶Five testers performed measurements; ICC was performed for this study.

performed to measure interrater reliability between the two testers. Reliability correlations ranged for the first session from 0.80 to 0.87, and for the second session from 0.74 to 0.85 (Pearson's r). Paired t-tests analyzing the differences between measurements (intratester) and testers (intertester) revealed no significant difference across all measurements. Rheault et al.[68] reported equally high correlations, but they examined only intertester reliability. After examining 22 subjects, the authors reported intertester reliability correlations ranging from 0.76 to 0.98 (ICC). Each of these authors agreed with the conclusion that the CROM was "a reliable and useful tool for assessing cervical range of motion."[67]

Table 10.50 CROM*: INTRATESTER RELIABILITY FOR ROTATION OF CERVICAL SPINE

STUDY	n	SAMPLE	CORRELATION	
			ICC[†]	r[‡]
Youdas et al.[69]	20	Healthy adults (21–84 years; x̄=59.1)	0.93 (right) 0.90 (left)	
Capuano-Pucci et al.[67]	20	Healthy adults (x̄=23.5 years)		0.85, 0.62 (right) 0.85, 0.89 (left)
Youdas et al.[51]	6	Healthy adults (22–56 years; x̄=27.2)	0.80, 0.58, 0.99, 0.82, 0.71[§] (right) 0.83, 0.84, 0.92, 0.95, 0.81 (left)	
Nilsson[70]	14	Healthy adults (23–45 years)		0.75 (right) 0.68 (left)
Hole et al.[58]	30	Healthy adults (21–48 years; x̄=28.7)	0.92 (right) 0.92 (left)	
Olson et al.[71]	12	Healthy adults (21–47 years)	0.98 (right) 0.99 (left)	
Peolsson et al.[72]	30	Healthy adults (20–64 years; x̄=32.3)	0.93, 0.87 (combined)	
Lindell et al.[73]	50	Cervical; 30, Healthy, 20 (20–63 years)	0.94 (right) 0.86 (left)	
Fletcher and Bandy[74]	25 22	Healthy adults (22–52 years; x̄=26.0) Cervical pain (21–55 years; x̄=33.0)	0.90 (right) 0.94 (left) 0.92 (right) 0.96 (left)	
Audette et al.[75]	20	Healthy adults (x̄=37.0 years)	0.98 (right) 0.99 (left)	
Williams et al.[76]	38	Healthy adults (x̄=38.0 years)	0.92 (right) 0.95 (left)	

*Cervical range of motion device (Performance Attainment Associates, Roseville, MN).
[†]Intraclass correlation coefficient.
[‡]Pearson's r.
[§]Five testers performed measurements; ICC was performed for this study.

Table 10.51 CROM*: INTERTESTER RELIABILITY FOR FLEXION OF CERVICAL SPINE

STUDY	n	SAMPLE	CORRELATION	
			ICC[†]	r[‡]
Youdas et al.[69]	20	Healthy adults (21–84 years; x̄=59.1)	0.86	
Capuano-Pucci et al.[67]	20	Healthy adults (x̄=23.5 years)		0.80 and 0.77[§]
Rheault et al.[68]	22	Healthy adults (x̄=37.4 years)	0.76	
Youdas et al.[51]	6	Healthy adults (22–56 years; x̄=27.2)	0.83[¶¶]	
Nilsson[70]	14	Healthy adults (23–45 years)		0.71
Hole et al.[58]	30	Healthy adults (21–48 years; x̄=28.7)	0.94[¶]	
Olson et al.[71]	12	Healthy adults (21–47 years)	0.58	
Nyland and Johnson[77]	10	Healthy adults (15–19 years)	0.87–0.96**	
Peolsson et al.[72]	30	Healthy adults (20–64 years; x̄=32.3)	0.90[¶]	
Tousignant et al.[78]	31	Healthy adults (18–45 years)	0.99	
Love et al.[61]	27	Healthy adults (x̄=38.6 years)	0.96	
Whitcroft[54]	100	Healthy adults (x̄=32.0 years)	0.93	
Williams et al.[76]	19	Healthy adults (x̄=41.0 years)	0.83	

*Cervical range of motion device (Performance Attainment Associates, Roseville, MN).
[†]Intraclass correlation coefficient.
[‡]Pearson's r.
[§]Intertester reliability was examined across two sessions.
[¶¶]Intertester reliability analyzed using one ICC performed across five testers.
[¶]Flexion and extension combined.
**Intertester reliability using three testers.

In a study designed to provide normative data for cervical range of motion across 9 decades of age, Youdas et al.[51] established reliability in two pilot studies before collecting data on 337 subjects. For intrarater reliability, five testers measured six subjects twice. The authors reported the median ICCs for intratester reliability as "fair" for cervical flexion (ICC=0.76), "high" for cervical extension (ICC=0.94), and "good" for left lateral cervical flexion (ICC=0.86), right lateral cervical flexion (ICC=0.85), left cervical rotation (ICC=0.84), and right cervical rotation (ICC=0.80). For intertester reliability, a "random, unique triplet of testers" was used

Table 10.52	CROM*: INTERTESTER RELIABILITY FOR EXTENSION OF CERVICAL SPINE				
				CORRELATION	
STUDY	n	SAMPLE	**ICC†**	**r‡**	
Youdas et al.[69]	20	Healthy adults (21–84 years; $\bar{x}$=59.1)	0.86		
Capuano-Pucci et al.[67]	20	Healthy adults ($\bar{X}$=23.5 years)		0.83, 0.76§	
Rheault et al.[68]	22	Healthy adults ($\bar{X}$=37.4 years)	0.98		
Youdas et al.[51]	6	Healthy adults (22–56 years; $\bar{x}$=27.2)	0.90¶¶		
Nilsson[70]	14	Healthy adults (23–45 years)		0.71 0.85	
Hole et al.[58]	30	Healthy adults (21–48 years; $\bar{x}$=28.7)	0.94¶		
Olson et al.[71]	12	Healthy adults (21–47 years)	0.97		
Nyland and Johnson[77]	10	Healthy adults (15–19 years)	0.92–0.98**		
Peolsson et al.[72]	30	Healthy adults (20–64 years; $\bar{x}$=32.3)	0.90¶		
Tousignant et al.[78]	31	Healthy adults (18–45 years)	0.99		
Love et al.[61]	27	Healthy adults ($\bar{x}$=38.6 years)	0.97		
Whitcroft[54]	100	Healthy adults ($\bar{x}$=32.0 years)	0.93		
Williams et al.[76]	19	Healthy adults ($\bar{x}$=41.0 years)	0.88		

*Cervical range of motion device (Performance Attainment Associates, Roseville, MN).
†Intraclass correlation coefficient.
‡Pearson's r.
§Intertester reliability was examined across two sessions.
¶¶Intertester reliability analyzed using one ICC performed across five testers.
¶Flexion and extension combined.
**Intertester reliability using three testers.

Table 10.53	CROM*: INTERTESTER RELIABILITY FOR LATERAL FLEXION OF CERVICAL SPINE				
				CORRELATION	
STUDY	n	SAMPLE	**ICC†**	**r‡**	
Youdas et al.[69]	20	Healthy adults (21–84 years; $\bar{x}$=59.1)	0.88 (right) 0.73 (left)		
Capuano-Pucci et al.[67]	20	Healthy adults ($\bar{x}$=23.5 years)		0.84, 0.85 (right)§ 0.87, 0.74 (left)	
Rheault et al.[68]	22	Healthy adults ($\bar{x}$=37.4 years)	0.87 (right) 0.86 (left)		
Youdas et al.[51]	6	Healthy adults (22–56 years; $\bar{x}$=27.2)	0.87 (right)¶¶ 0.89 (left)		
Nilsson[70]	14	Healthy adults (23–45 years)		0.58 (right)	
Hole et al.[58]	30	Healthy adults (21–48 years; $\bar{x}$=28.7)	0.94 (right) 0.88 (left)	0.58 (left)	
Olson et al.[71]	12	Healthy adults (21–47 years)	0.96 (right) 0.94 (left)		
Nyland and Johnson[77]	10	Healthy adults (15–19 years)	0.89–0.94¶ (combined)		
Peolsson et al.[72]	30	Healthy adults (20–64 years; $\bar{x}$=32.3)	0.90 (combined)		
Whitcroft[54]	100	Healthy adults ($\bar{x}$=32.0 years)	0.66 (right) 0.80 (left)		
Williams et al.[76]	19	Healthy adults ($\bar{x}$=41.0 years)	0.82 (right) 0.88 (left)		

*Cervical range of motion device (Performance Attainment Associates, Roseville, MN).
†Intraclass correlation coefficient.
‡Pearson's r.
§Intertester reliability was examined across two sessions.
¶¶Intertester reliability analyzed using one ICC performed across five testers.
¶Intertester reliability using three testers.

for a sample of 20 subjects. Intertester reliability (ICC) ranged from 0.66 to 0.90. The authors concluded that "measurement of the cervical spine with the CROM instrument demonstrates good intratester and intertester reliability."[51]

In a study conducted to determine how age and sex affect cervical mobility, Hole et al.[58] examined intrarater and interrater reliability by measuring healthy adults.

Results indicated correlation greater than 0.85 for all measurements except for the intertester reliability of left cervical rotation (0.84). Love et al.[61] examined 27 healthy adults and reported intrarater and interrater reliability for cervical flexion and extension to be greater than 0.96 for all measurements.

Since 2000, nine studies have examined the reliability of the CROM.[9,54,71–77] In the vast majority of

			CORRELATION	
STUDY	n	SAMPLE	ICC[†]	r[‡]
Youdas et al.[69]	20	Healthy adults (21–84 years; x̄ = 59.1)	0.90 (right) 0.82 (left)	
Capuano-Pucci et al.[67]	20	Healthy adults (x̄ = 23.5 years)		0.84, 0.82 (right)[§] 0.84, 0.79 (left)
Rheault et al.[68]	22	Healthy adults (x̄ = 37.4 years)	0.81 (right) 0.82 (left)	
Youdas et al.[51]	6	Healthy adults (22–56 years; x̄ = 27.2)	0.82 (right)[¶¶] 0.66 (left)	
Nilsson[70]	14	Healthy adults (23–45 years)		0.66 (right) 0.29 (left)
Hole et al.[58]	30	Healthy adults (21–48 years; x̄ = 28.7)	0.93 (right) 0.84 (left)	
Olson et al.[71]	12	Healthy adults (21–47 years)	0.96 (right) 0.98 (left)	
Nyland and Johnson[77]	10	Healthy adults (15–19 years)	0.91–0.93[¶] (combined)	
Peolsson et al.[72]	30	Healthy adults (20–64 years; x̄ = 32.3)	0.75 (combined)	
Whitcroft[54]	100	Healthy adults (x̄ = 32.0 years)	0.67 (right) 0.82 (left)	
Williams et al.[76]	19	Healthy adults (x̄ = 41.0 years)	0.92 (right) 0.87 (left)	

Table 10.54   CROM*: INTERTESTER RELIABILITY FOR ROTATION OF CERVICAL SPINE

*Cervical range of motion device (Performance Attainment Associates, Roseville, MN).
[†]Intraclass correlation coefficient.
[‡]Pearson's r.
[§]Intertester reliability was examined across two sessions.
[¶¶]Intertester reliability analyzed using one ICC performed across five testers.
[¶]Intertester reliability using three testers.

measurements, the intratester and intertester test–retest reliability of using the CROM to measure cervical flexion, extension, lateral flexion, and rotation were found to be quite consistent; similar to the results reported from earlier studies. Before performing a study to ensure the relationship between palpation tenderness, visual analog scales, and active cervical ROM, Olson et al.[71] established intrarater and interrater reliability on flexion, extension, right and left lateral flexion, and right and left rotation on 12 subjects (aged 21–47 years). Results indicated reliability greater than 0.85 for intratester reliability and greater than 0.94 for all measurements except flexion (0.58) for intertester reliability.

Similar to Olson et al.,[71] Peolsson et al.[72] performed a reliability study of the CROM before data were collected for another purpose—to learn the effects of age and sex on cervical range of motion. After examining reliability of the CROM in 30 healthy adults, Peolsson et al.[72] reported reliability ranging from 0.87 to 0.93 for all measurements for intratester reliability and 0.90 or greater for intertester reliability for all measurements except combined left and right rotation (0.75).

In an effort to examine the validity of the CROM in measuring flexion and extension, Tousignant et al.[9] first assessed intertester reliability. After measuring 31 healthy subjects, the authors reported intertester reliability to be 0.99 for both flexion and extension. Results of the validity study are presented in the next section of this chapter.

Before a study was conducted in which CROM of collegiate and high school football players was compared, Nyland and Johnson[77] reported the interrater reliability of three testers who used the CROM in measuring 10 subjects. Results indicated reliability ranging from 0.87 to 0.98 for the measurements of flexion, extension, lateral flexion (combined), and rotation (combined).

In a unique study conducted to determine whether a research assistant could be as accurate as an experienced clinician in using the CROM to measure cervical flexion, extension, and rotation range of motion, Lindell et al.[73] examined the intratester and intertester reliability of these two individuals when measuring 31 healthy adults. Data revealed that the research assistant's intrarater reliability was far less than that of the experienced clinician. Therefore reliability data on only the experienced clinician are presented in this text. Results of intratester reliability of the experienced clinician ranged from 0.86 to 0.98. (*Note*: Intratester reliability of the research assistant ranged from 0.62 to 0.82.)

Fletcher and Bandy[74] examined intrarater reliability in 25 subjects with cervical pain and in 22 subjects with cervical pain. The CROM was found to be reliable, irrespective of cervical pain; reliability for flexion, extension, lateral flexion, and rotation ranged from 0.87 to 0.94 for those without neck pain and from 0.88 to 0.92 for those with neck pain. Audette et al.[75] also limited their study to intrarater reliability but examined healthy individuals. The authors also reported reliability greater than 0.88 for measurement of flexion, extension, lateral flexion, and rotation of the cervical spine.

A study by Williams et al.[76] reported on the intrarater (n = 38) and interrater reliability (n = 19) in cervical flexion, extension, lateral flexion, and rotation. Results indicated that reliability was greater than 0.98 for all movements for intrarater reliability and ranging from 0.82 to 0.92 for interrater reliability. Whitcroft et al.[54] examined only interrater reliability of the cervical motions and reported reliability ranging from 0.82 to 0.93. Summaries of research related to use of the CROM in measuring cervical range of motion are presented in Tables 10.47–10.54.

In the only study undertaken to use the CROM to measure *passive* flexion, extension, lateral flexion, and rotation range of motion of the cervical spine, Nilsson[70] examined 14 subjects. The author reported intrarater reliability (Pearson's r) of *passive* motion of the cervical spine ranging from 0.61 to 0.85, and interrater reliability (Pearson's r) ranging from 0.29 to 0.85 (see Tables 10.47–10.54). Follow-up testing using a paired t-test indicated no significant differences between measurements (intratester) for all measurements of cervical range of motion. However, the paired t-test revealed significant differences between testers (intertester) when measuring the cervical motion of flexion (P < 0.05), extension (P < 0.05), and lateral flexion (P < 0.05). (*Note:* No significant difference between testers was found for cervical rotation.) Given the lower correlations with intertester reliability compared with intratester reliability, as well as the significant t-tests reported with interrater reliability, the author concluded that the CROM "has an acceptable reliability as long as all measurements are carried out by the same examiner."

Validity

Herrmann[79] examined total range of motion (flexion and extension combined) in 11 subjects by using an inclinometer attached to a headband and compared these measurements to those attained by radiographic examination. The correlation between the inclinometer and the X-ray was 0.98 (ICC and Pearson's r), and no significant difference was found between measurements taken by the two devices (Fisher's t-test). On the basis of the statistics, the authors concluded that the method was a "valid tool for measuring neck flexion and extension range of motion."

In the second part of their study, Mayer et al.[63] examined consistency of measurement of cervical flexion between the double inclinometer and radiographic examination in three subjects; they reported a correlation of 0.99 (Pearson's r). As was indicated previously, no follow-up statistical analysis to the Pearson correlation was performed, and this study is included only because no other study on the reliability and validity of double-inclinometer measurement of cervical range of motion has been published.

When investigating validity, Ordway et al.[80] measured cervical flexion and extension in 20 subjects, using the CROM device and X-ray examination. Statistical analysis using ANOVA indicated no significant differences between measurements when the CROM device versus the X-ray was used. In a study by Tousignant et al.,[9] which was presented previously in the CROM section, the authors also examined the validity of the CROM compared with radiographs for measurement of cervical flexion and extension in 31 healthy individuals. Using Pearson's correlation coefficient, the authors reported validity to be 0.97 for flexion and 0.98 for extension. (As was indicated in the Mayer et al.[63] study on validity with the double inclinometer, given that the study by Tousignant et al.[9] is the only investigation that explored the validity of the CROM, the study is included in this review of evidence-based research.) These results support the contention that the CROM device is a valid instrument for measuring cervical flexion and extension range of motion. Table 10.55 provides information on studies conducted to investigate the validity of measurement of cervical range of motion using inclinometers.

Table 10.55   INCLINOMETER (INCLUDING CROM*): VALIDITY FOR FLEXION AND EXTENSION OF CERVICAL SPINE

STUDY	TECHNIQUE	n	SAMPLE	CORRELATION ICC[†]	r[‡]
Herrmann[79]	Pendulum goniometer attached to "head band"	11	Healthy adults (21–68 years)	0.98 (total)	0.98[§]
Mayer et al.[63]	Double	3	Healthy adults (17–62 years)		0.99[¶¶]
Ordway et al.[80]	CROM*	20	Healthy adults (20–49 years; $\bar{x}$ = 31.0)	No significant difference in range of motion between CROM and X-ray (flexion, extension)[¶]	
Tousignant et al.[78]	CROM*	31	Healthy adults (18–45 years)	0.97 flexion 0.98 extension	

*Cervical range of motion device (Performance Attainment Associates, Roseville, MN).
[†]Intraclass correlation coefficient.
[‡]Pearson's r.
[§]Flexion only.
[¶¶]Total = flexion and extension combined.
[¶]Analysis of variance with repeated measures.

SMARTPHONE

Flexion, Extension, Lateral Flexion, and Rotation

As indicated previously, adding the ROM application to the Smartphone provides the user of the phone an inexpensive device for measuring the position of the joint.[46] Chapter 9 suggested that using the Smartphone requires some training; but, overall, the measurement techniques presented are easy to learn and use.

Intratester Reliability

Four studies have utilized the Smartphone to measure the test–retest (intratester) reliability, with four investigations examining cervical flexion, extension, lateral flexion, and rotation. Rodriguez-Sanz et al.[81] and Monreal et al.[82] reported excellent reliability, while studies by Tousignant-Laflamme et al.[83] and Pourahmadi et al.[55] were not able to replicate the good results by these authors.

Twenty-five subjects (14 female, 11 male) with neck pain were measured with the Smartphone by Rodriguez-Sanz et al.,[81] with the authors reporting intratester reliability ranging from 0.90 to 0.96. Similar results were obtained by Monreal et al.[82] while investigating healthy individuals after measuring 50 subjects (35 females, 15 males). These researchers reported reliability of 0.80 to. 93 for every cervical movement except 0.72 for cervical flexion.

Slightly lower results related to intratester reliability were reported by Tousignant-Laflamme et al.[83] and Pourahmadi et al.[55] Measuring 28 subjects (19 females, 9 males). Tousignant-Laflamme et al.[83] reported

reliability generally ranging from 0.66 to.84.for all cervical movements, except for the reliability for right and left rotation measuring 0.17 and 0.28, respectively, for one tester. Pourahmadi et al.[55] measured 40 subjects (20 females, 20 males) and reported reliability ranging from 0.70 to 0.78 for all movements.

In general, the authors all agreed that the, related to intratester reliability, these "findings suggest that the Smartphone might be a reliable, simple tool measuring cervical ROM."[55] A summary of the results of intratester reliability for the Smartphone are presented in Table 10.56.

Intertester Reliability

Of those studies measuring intratester reliability, three investigators expanded their work to examine intertester reliability of cervical flexion, extension, lateral flexion, and rotation using the same subjects.[81–83] The study by Rodriguez-Sanz[81] was the only one of the three studies reporting good intertester reliability, with all measurements above 0.90. Tousignant-Laflamme et al.[83] and Pourahmadi et al.[55] reported intertester reliability ranging from 0.40 to 0.79, with Tousignant-Laflamme et al.[83] reporting reliabilities as low as 0.09 and 0.07 for the measurement of right and left rotation, respectively (Table 10.57).

Validity — Phone to Goniometer

Rodriguez-Sanz et al.[81] and Pourahmadi et al.[55] attempted to determine concurrent validity between the target measurement, Smartphone, compared to the

			CORRELATION* (ICC)			
STUDY	n	SAMPLE	FLEXION	EXTENSION	LATERAL FLEXION (R)IGHT (L)EFT	LATERAL ROTATION (R)IGHT (L)EFT
Tousignant Laflamme et al.[83]	28	Healthy Adults ($\bar{x}=23.0$ years)	0.78, 0.68	0.84, 0.68	(R) 0.77, 0.68 (L) 0.78, 0.68	(R) 0.74, 0.17 (L) 0.66, 0.28
Pourahmadi et al.[55]	40	Healthy Adults ($\bar{x}=31.1$ years)	0.76	0.76	(R) 0.69 (L) 0.69	(R) 0.70 (L) 0.62
Monreal et al.[82]	50	Healthy Adults ($\bar{x}=21.5$ years)	0.72	0.80	(R) 0.92 (L) 0.93	(R) 0.87 (L) 0.89
Rodriguez-Sanz et al.[81]	25	Healthy Adults ($\bar{x}=25.0$ years)	0.90	0.94	(R) 0.83 (L) 0.88	(R) 0.89 (L) 0.96

Table 10.56   SMARTPHONE: INTRATESTER RELIABILITY FOR CERVICAL FLEXION, EXTENSION, LATERAL FLEXION, AND ROTATION

*ICC = Intraclass Correlation Coefficient.

			CORRELATION* (ICC)			
STUDY	n	SAMPLE	FLEXION	EXTENSION	LATERAL FLEXION (R)IGHT (L)EFT	LATERAL ROTATION (R)IGHT (L)EFT
Tousignant Laflamme et al.[85]	28	Healthy Adults ($\bar{x}=23.0$ years)	0.48	0.49	(R) 0.54 (L) 0.40	(R) 0.09 (L) 0.07
Pourahmadi et al.[55]	40	Healthy Adults ($\bar{x}=31.1$ years)	0.65	0.67	(R) 0.76 (L) 0.71	(R) 0.79 (L) 0.76
Rodriguez-Sanz et al.[81]	25	Healthy Adults ($\bar{x}=25.0$ years)	0.90	0.98	(R) 0.88 (L) 0.87	(R) 0.86 (L) 0.94

Table 10.57   INTERTESTER RELIABILITY FOR CERVICAL FLEXION, EXTENSION, LATERAL FLEXION, AND ROTATION

*ICC = Intraclass Correlation Coefficient.

Table 10.58 VALIDITY: SMARTPHONE TO GONIOMETER FOR CERVICAL FLEXION, EXTENSION, LATERAL FLEXION, AND ROTATION						
				CORRELATION* (ICC)		
STUDY	n	SAMPLE	FLEXION	EXTENSION	LATERAL FLEXION (R)IGHT (L)EFT	LATERAL ROTATION (R)IGHT (L)EFT
Pourahmadi et al.[55]	40	Healthy Adults ($\bar{x}$=31.1 years)	0.63	0.81	(R) 0.79 (L) 0.72	(R) 0.78 (L) 0.72
Rodriguez-Sanz et al.[81]	25	Healthy Adults ($\bar{x}$=25.0 years)	0.98	0.98	(R) 0.92 (L) 0.96	(R) 0.93 (L) 0.96

*ICC = Intraclass Correlation Coefficient.

gold standard, goniometer, for the measurements of cervical flexion, extension, lateral flexion, and rotation. [As indicated earlier when discussing validity data for lumbar motions—and described in Chapter 2—by using a target test (Smartphone) and comparing it to the gold standard (goniometer), such measurement for criterion validity assumes that the use of a goniometer as a gold standard was appropriate.] Rodriguez-Sanz et al.[81] reported validity ranging from 0.93 to 0.98, while Pourahmadi et al.[55] reported lower validity ranging from 0.63 to 0.81. Table 10.58 presents the data on concurrent validity for the measurement of cervical ROM.

TEMPOROMANDIBULAR JOINT

Iglarsh and Snyder-Mackler[84] have suggested that mandibular depression (opening), protrusion, and lateral deviation are important range of motion parameters of the temporomandibular joint (TMJ) that should be measured at initial examination, and, if impairment is noted, they should be measured before and after each intervention. Although several references support Iglarsh and Snyder-Mackler's[84] suggestion of the importance of examining range of motion of the TMJ and providing descriptions of the measurement procedure,[85–91] few studies could be found in which reliability of any of these measurements was investigated.

Most studies that examined the reliability of measurement of movement occurring at the TMJ were precursors to a study conducted to investigate something else. In a study that did determine reliability and discriminant validity (whether a test is valid in differentiating between patients with and without TMJ dysfunction), Walker et al.[92] tested two groups: 15 subjects with TMJ dysfunction (mean age=35.2 years) and 15 subjects without TMJ problems (mean age=42.9 years). The author examined two testers using ICCs on the measurement of opening, left and right lateral deviation, and protrusion with a ruler. Results indicated that intratester reliability varied from 0.70 to 0.99, and that intertester reliability ranged from 0.90 to 1.0. Additionally, only mouth opening was found to be valid in discriminating between patients with and without TMJ dysfunction, as those with TMJ dysfunction had significantly less ROM than did those without pain.

In a study undertaken to determine differences in the amount of mandibular opening during three different head positions (head forward, neutral, and retracted) by using a ruler to measure the distance between incisors, Higbie et al.[93] determined intrarater and interrater reliability before the actual time of data collection, using ICCs. Intrarater reliability for the two testers in measuring mandibular opening across all three positions was 0.92 and above; intertester reliability between the two testers was 0.92 and above for all three positions.

In a study that examined interrater reliability in the assessment of a number of clinical signs commonly associated with TMJ dysfunction (including maximal opening in those with and without pain, occlusal relationships, TMJ sounds, pain with function, and pain with palpation), Dworkin et al.[94] examined 24 subjects (aged 20–40 years; a "balanced sample of asymptomatic and symptomatic persons") and reported interrater reliability among three dentists in the measurement of mandibular opening with a ruler in subjects without pain of 0.90. Intertester reliability for lateral deviation and protrusion was reported to be lower, at 0.68 and 0.70, respectively.

References

1. Macrae IF, Wright V. Measurement of back movement. *Ann Rheum Dis.* 1969;28:584–589.
2. Moll JMV, Wright V. Normal range of motion: an objective clinical study. *Ann Rheum Dis.* 1971;30:381–386.
3. Williams R, Binkley J, Bloch R, et al. Reliability of the modified-modified Schober and double inclinometer methods for measuring lumbar flexion and extension. *Phys Ther.* 1993;73:26–37.
4. Fitzgerald GK, Wynveen KJ, Rheault W, Rothschild B. Objective assessment with establishment of normal values for lumbar spinal range of motion. *Phys Ther.* 1983;63:1776–1781.
5. Haley SM, Tada WL, Carmichael EM. Spinal mobility in young children. *Phys Ther.* 1986;66:1697–1703.
6. Burdett RG, Brown KE, Fall MP. Reliability and validity of four instruments for measuring lumbar spine and pelvic positions. *Phys Ther.* 1986;66:677–684.
7. Hyytiainen K, Salminen JJ, Suvitie T, et al. Reproducibility of nine tests to measure spinal mobility and trunk muscle strength. *Scand J Rehab Med.* 1991;23:3–10.
8. Haywood KL, Garatt AM, Jordan K, Dziedzic K, Dawes PT. Spinal mobility in ankylosing spondylitis: reliability, validity and responsiveness. *Rheumatology.* 2004;43:750–757.
9. Tousignant M, Poulin L, Marhcand S, Viau A, Place C. The modified-modified Schober test for range of motion assessment of lumbar flexion in patients with low back pain: a study of criterion validity, intra- and inter-rater reliability and minimum metrically detectable changes. *Disabil Rehabil.* 2005;27:553–559.
10. Portek I, Pearcy MJ, Reader GP, Mowat AG. Correlation between radiographic and clinical measurement of lumbar spine movement. *Br J Rheumatol.* 1983;22:197–205.
11. Beattie P, Rothstein JM, Lamb RL. Reliability of the attraction method for measuring lumbar spine backward bending. *Phys Ther.* 1987;67:364–369.

12. Frost M, Stuckey S, Smalley LA, Dorman G. Reliability of measuring trunk motions in centimeters. *Phys Ther.* 1982;62:1431–1437.

13. Bandy W, Reese NB. Strapped versus unstrapped technique of the prone press-up for measurement of lumbar extension using a tape measure: differences in magnitude and reliability of measurements. *Arch Phys Med Rehabil.* 2004;85:99–103.

14. Rose MJ. The statistical analysis of the intra-observer repeatability of four clinical measurement techniques. *Physiotherapy.* 1991;77:89–91.

15. Alaranta H, Hurri H, Heliovaara M, et al. Flexibility of the spine: normative values of goniometric and tape measurements. *Scand J Rehab Med.* 1994;26:147–154.

16. Nitschke J, Nattrass C, Disler P, et al. Reliability of the American Medical Association guides' model for measuring spinal range of motion. *Spine.* 1999;24:262–268.

17. Johnson K, Kim K, Yu B, Saliba S, Grindstaff T. Reliability of thoracic spine rotation range-of-motion measurements in healthy adults. *J Athl Train.* 2012;47:52–60.

18. Furness J, Schram B, Cox AJ, et al. Reliability and concurrent validity of the iPhone® compass application to measure thoracic rotation range of motion (ROM) in healthy participants. *Peer J.* 2018;6, e4431.

19. Loebl WY. Measurement of spinal posture and range of spinal motion. *Ann Phys Med.* 1967;9:103–110.

20. Mellin GP. Measurement of thoracolumbar posture and mobility with a Myrin inclinometer. *Spine.* 1986;11:759–762.

21. Mellin GP, Kiiski R, Weckstrom A. Effects of subject position on measurements of flexion, extension, and lateral flexion of the spine. *Spine.* 1991;16:1108–1110.

22. Rondinelli R, Murphy J, Esler A, et al. Estimation of normal lumbar flexion with surface inclinometry. *Am J Phys Med Rehabil.* 1992;71:219–224.

23. Ng JKF, Kippers V, Richardson C, Parnianpour M. Range of motion and lordosis of the lumbar spine. *Spine.* 2001;26:53–59.

24. Pourahmadi MR, Taghipour M, Jannati E, et al. Reliability and validity of an iPhone application for the measurement of lumbar spine flexion and extension range of motion. *Peer J.* 2016;4, e2355.

25. Kolber MJ, Pizzini M, Robinson A, et al. The reliability and concurrent validity of measurements used to quantify lumbar spine mobility: an analysis of an iphone application and gravity based inclinometry. *Int J Sports Phys Ther.* 2013;8:129–137.

26. Lee CN, Robbins DP, Roberts HJ, et al. Reliability and validity of single inclinometer measurements for thoracic spine range of motion. *Physiother Can.* 2003;55:73–78.

27. Breum J, Wiberg J, Bolton JE. Reliability and concurrent validity of the BROM II for measuring lumbar mobility. *J Manipulative Physiol Ther.* 1995;18:497–502.

28. Madson TJ, Youdas JW, Suman VJ. Reproducibility of lumbar spine range of motion measurements using the back range of motion device. *J Orthop Sports Phys Ther.* 1999;29:470–477.

29. Kachingwe AF, Phillips BJ. Inter- and intra-rater reliability of a back range of motion instrument. *Arch Phys Med Rehabil.* 2005;86:2347–2353.

30. Chiarello CM, Savidge R. Interrater reliability of the Cybex EDI-320 and fluid goniometer in normals and patients with low back pain. *Arch Phys Med Rehabil.* 1993;74:32–37.

31. Newton M, Waddell G. Reliability and validity of clinical measurement of the lumbar spine in patients with chronic low back pain. *Physiotherapy.* 1991;77:796–800.

32. Sullivan MS, Shoaf LD, Riddle DL. The relationship of lumbar flexion to disability in patients with low back pain. *Phys Ther.* 2000;80:240–250.

33. Mayer TG, Tencer AF, Kristoferson S, Mooney V. Use of noninvasive techniques for quantification of spinal range-of-motion in normal subjects and chronic low-back dysfunction patients. *Spine.* 1984;9:588–595.

34. Williams RM, Goldsmith CH, Minuk T. Validity of the double inclinometer method for measuring lumbar flexion. *Physiother Can.* 1998;50:147–152.

35. Boline PD, Keating JC, Haas M, Anderson AV. Interexaminer reliability and discriminant validity of inclinometric measurement of lumbar rotation in chronic low-back pain patients and subjects without low-back pain. *Spine.* 1992;17:335–338.

36. Iveson BD, McLaughlin SL, Todd RH, Gerber JP. Reliability and exploration of the side-lying thoraco-lumbar rotation measurement (STRM). *N Am J Sports Phys Ther.* 2010;5:201–207.

37. Israel M. A quantitative method of estimating flexion and extension of the spine; a preliminary report. *Mil Med.* 1959;124:181–186.

38. de Oliveira TS, Candotti CT, La Torre M, et al. Validity and reproducibility of the measurements obtained using the flexicurve instrument to evaluate the angles of thoracic and lumbar curvatures of the spine in the sagittal plane. *Rehabil Res Pract.* 2012;2012:1–9. 186156.

39. Hart DL, Rose SJ. Reliability of a noninvasive method for measuring the lumbar curve. *J Orthop Sports Phys Ther.* 1986;8:180–184.

40. Tillotson KM, Burton AK. Noninvasive measurement of lumbar sagittal mobility an assessment of the flexicurve technique. *Spine.* 1991;16:29–33.

41. Valle MB, Dutra VH, Candotti CT, Sedrez JA, Wagner Neto ES, Loss JF. Validity of flexicurve for the assessment of spinal flexibility in asymptomatic individuals. *Fisioterapia em Movimento.* 2020;33.

42. Burton AK. Regional lumbar sagittal mobility; measurement by flexicurves. *Clin Biomech.* 1986;1:20–26.

43. Stokes IA, Bevins TM, Lunn RA. Back surface curvature and measurement of lumbar spinal motion. *Spine.* 1987;12:355–361.

44. Youdas JW, Suman VJ, Garrett TR. Reliability of measurements of lumbar spine sagittal mobility obtained with the flexible curve. *J Orthop Sports Phys Ther.* 1995;21:13–20.

45. Barrett E, McCreesh K, Lewis J. Reliability and validity of non-radiographic methods of thoracic kyphosis measurement: a systematic review. *Man Ther.* 2014;19:10–17.

46. Guidetti L, Placentino U, Baldari C. Reliability and criterion validity of the smartphone inclinometer application to quantify cervical spine mobility. *Clin Spine Surg.* 2017;30:e1359–e1366.

47. Macedo LB, Borges DT, Melo SA, et al. Reliability and concurrent validity of a mobile application to measure thoracolumbar range of motion in low back pain patients. *J Back Musculoskelet Rehabil.* 2020;33:145–151.

48. Boudreau N, Brochu FO, Dubreuil LM, et al. Reliability and criterion validity of the "gyroscope" application of the iPod for measuring lumbar range of motion. *J Back Musculoskelet Rehabil.* 2020;33:685–692.

49. Bedekar N, Suryawanshi M, Rairikar S, et al. Inter and intra-rater reliability of mobile device goniometer in measuring lumbar flexion range of motion. *J Back Musculoskelet Rehabil.* 2014;27:161–166.

50. Hsieh C, Yeung B. Active neck motion measurements with a tape measure. *J Orthop Sports Phys Ther.* 1986;8:88–92.

51. Youdas JW, Garrett TR, Suman VJ, et al. Normal range of motion of the cervical spine: an initial goniometric study. *Phys Ther.* 1992;72:770–780.

52. Zachman ZJ, Traina AD, Keating JC, et al. Interexaminer reliability and concurrent validity of two instruments for the measurement of cervical ranges of motion. *J Manipulative Physiol Ther.* 1989;12:205–210.

53. Pringle RK. Intra-instrument reliability of four goniometers. *J Chiropr Med.* 2003;2:91–95.

54. Whitcroft K, Massouh L, Amirfeyz R, Bannister G. Comparison of methods of measuring active cervical range of motion. *Spine.* 2010;35:E976–E980.

55. Pourahmadi MR, Bagheri R, Taghipour M, et al. A new iPhone application for measuring active craniocervical range of motion in patients with non-specific neck pain: a reliability and validity study. *Spine J.* 2018;18:447–457.

56. Defibaugh JJ. Part II: an experimental study of head motion in adult males. *Phys Ther.* 1964;44:163–168.

57. Pellecchia GL, Bohannon RW. Active lateral neck flexion range of motion measurements obtained with a modified goniometer: reliability and estimates of normal. *J Manipulative Physiol Ther.* 1998;21:443–447.

58. Hole DE, Cook JM, Bolton JE. Reliability and concurrent validity of two instruments for measuring cervical range of motion: effects of age and gender. *Man Ther.* 1995;1:36–42.

59. Hoving JL, Pool JJM, van Mameren H, et al. Reproducibility of cervical range of motion in patients with neck pain. *BMC Musculoskelet Disord.* 2005;6:59–66.

60. Prushansky T, Deryi O, Jabarreen B. Reproducibility and validity of digital inclinometry for measuring cervical range of motion in normal subjects. *Physiother Res Int.* 2010;15:42–48.

61. Love S, Gringmuth RH, Kazemi M, Cornacchia P, Schmolke M. Interexaminer and intraexaminer reliability of cervical passive range of motion using the CROM and Cybex 320 EDI. *J Can Chiropr Assoc.* 1998;42:222–228.

62. Bush KW, Collins N, Portman L, Tillett N. Validity and intertester reliability of cervical range of motion using inclinometer measurements. *J Man Manipulative Ther.* 2000;8:52–61.

63. Mayer T, Brady S, Bovasso E, et al. Noninvasive measurement of cervical tri-planar motion in normal subjects. *Spine.* 1993;18:2191–2195.

64. Bennett JG, Bergmanis LE, Carpenter JK, Skowlund HV. Range of motion of the neck. *Phys Ther.* 1963;43:45–47.

65. Guth EH. A comparison of cervical rotation in age-matched adolescent competitive swimmers and healthy males. *J Orthop Sports Phys Ther*. 1995;21:21–27.

66. Tucci SM, Hicks JE, Gross EG, et al. Cervical motion assessment: a new, simple and accurate method. *Arch Phys Med Rehabil*. 1986;67:225–230.

67. Capuano-Pucci D, Rheault W, Aukai J, et al. Intratester and intertester reliability of the cervical range of motion device. *Arch Phys Med Rehabil*. 1991;72:338–340.

68. Rheault W, Albright B, Byers C, et al. Intertester reliability of the cervical range of motion device. *J Orthop Sports Phys Ther*. 1992;15:147–150.

69. Youdas JW, Carey TR, Garrett TR. Reliability of measurement of cervical spine range of motion–comparison of three methods. *Phys Ther*. 1991;71:98–104.

70. Nilsson N. Measuring passive cervical motion: a study of reliability. *J Manipulative Physiol Ther*. 1995;18:293–297.

71. Olson SL, O'Connor DP, Birmingham G, et al. Tender point sensitivity, range of motion, and perceived disability in subjects with neck pain. *J Ortho Sports Phys Ther*. 2000;30:13–20.

72. Peolsson A, Hedlund R, Ertzgaard S, Oberg B. Intra- and intertester reliability and range of motion of the neck. *Physiother Can*. 2000;52:233–242.

73. Lindell O, Eriksson L, Strender LE. The reliability of a 10-test package for patients with prolonged back and neck pain: could an examiner without formal medical education be used without loss of quality? A methodological study. *BMC Musculoskelet Disord*. 2007;8:31–42.

74. Fletcher JP, Bandy WD. Intrarater reliability of CROM measurement of cervical active range of motion in persons with and without neck pain. *J Orthop Sports Phys Ther*. 2008;38:640–645.

75. Audette I, Dumas J, Côté J, De Serres S. Validity and between-day reliability of the cervical range of motion (CROM) device. *J Orthop Sports Phys Ther*. 2001;40:318–323.

76. Williams M, Williamson E, Gates S, Cooke M. Reproducibility of the cervical range of motion (CROM) device for individuals with subacute whiplash associated disorders. *Eur Spine J*. 2012;21:872–878.

77. Nyland J, Johnson D. Collegiate football players display more active cervical spine mobility than high school football players. *J Athl Train*. 2004;39:146–150.

78. Tousignant M, de Bellefeuille L, O'Donoughue S, Grahovac S. Criterion validity of the cervical range of motion (CROM) goniometer for cervical flexion and extension. *Spine*. 2000;25:324–330.

79. Herrmann DB. Validity study of head and neck flexion-extension motion comparing measurements of a pendulum goniometer and roentgenograms. *J Orthop Sports Phys Ther*. 1990;11:414–418.

80. Ordway NR, Seymour R, Donelson RG, et al. Cervical sagittal range-of-motion analysis using three methods. *Spine*. 1997;22:501–508.

81. Rodriguez-Sanz J, Carrasco-Uribarren A, Cabanillas-Barea S, et al. Validity and reliability of two smartphone applications to measure the lower and upper cervical spine range of motion in subjects with chronic cervical pain. *J Back Musculoskelet Rehabil*. 2019;32:619–627.

82. Monreal C, Luinstra L, Larkins L, May J. Validity and intrarater reliability using a smartphone clinometer application to measure active cervical range of motion including rotation measurements in supine. *J Sport Rehabil*. 2020;30:680–684.

83. Tousignant-Laflamme Y, Boutin N, Dion AM, Vallee CA. Reliability and criterion validity of two applications of the iPhone to measure cervical range of motion in healthy participants. *J Neuroeng Rehabil*. 2013;10:69.

84. Iglarsh A, Snyder-Mackler L. Temporomandibular joint and the cervical spine. In: Richardson JK, Iglarsh ZA, eds. *Clinical Orthopaedic Physical Therapy*. 2nd ed. Philadelphia: WB Saunders; 2006.

85. Agerberg G. Maximal mandibular movements in young men and women. *Swed Dent J*. 1974;67:81–100.

86. Bell WE. *Temporomandibular Disorders*. 4th ed. Chicago: Yearbook Medical Publishers; 1990.

87. Freidman MH, Weisberg J. The temporomandibular joint. In: Gould JA, ed. *Orthopaedic and Sports Physical Therapy*. 2nd ed. St. Louis: Mosby; 1990:575–598.

88. Kaplan AS. Examination and diagnosis. In: Kaplan AS, Assael LA, eds. *Temporomandibular Disorders*. Philadelphia: WB Saunders; 1991:chapter 4.

89. Lewis R, Buschang P, Throckmorton G. Sex differences in mandibular movements during opening and closing. *Am J Orthod Dentofac*. 2001;120:294–303.

90. Magee DJ. *Orthopedic Physical Assessment*. 5th ed. Philadelphia: WB Saunders; 2007.

91. Mezitis M, Rallis G, Zachariades N. The normal range of mouth opening. *J Oral Maxillofac Surg*. 1989;47:1028–1029.

92. Walker N, Bohannon R, Cameron D. Discriminant validity of temporomandibular joint range of motion measurements obtained with a ruler. *J Ortho Sports Phys Ther*. 2000;30:484–492.

93. Higbie E, Seidel-Cobb D, Taylor, et al. Effect of head position on vertical mandibular opening. *J Ortho Sports Phys Ther*. 1999;29:127–130.

94. Dworkin S, LeResche L, DeRouen T, et al. Assessing clinical signs of temporomandibular disorders: reliability of clinical examiners. *J Prosthet Dent*. 1990;63:574–579.

LOWER EXTREMITY

11

MEASUREMENT of RANGE of MOTION of the HIP

Nancy Berryman Reese

ANATOMY

The hip is a ball-and-socket joint that consists of an articulation between the convex head of the femur and the concave acetabulum of the pelvis, or hip bone (Fig. 11.1). All three bones that make up the pelvis (ilium, ischium, and pubis) contribute to the acetabulum, which provides a deep, cup-shaped receptacle for the spherically shaped femoral head. A fibrocartilaginous rim, the acetabular labrum, attaches to the margin of the acetabulum, further increasing its depth.[1,2] Thus, the hip, unlike the glenohumeral joint, has a great deal of inherent bony stability and is less dependent on muscular and ligamentous structures for support. The articular capsule of the hip joint is strong and is crossed by three ligaments that provide additional reinforcement. The iliofemoral ligament is shaped like an inverted Y and reinforces the anterior joint capsule (Fig. 11.2). The stem of the iliofemoral ligament is attached to the anterior inferior spine of the ilium, and its two branches are attached along the whole length of the intertrochanteric line of the femur.[1] The pubofemoral ligament lies along the medial and inferior part of the joint capsule, running from the superior ramus of the pubis and the pubic portion of the acetabular rim to the neck of the femur (see Fig. 11.2). Reinforcing the posterior aspect of the joint capsule is the ischiofemoral ligament (Fig. 11.3). This ligament arises from the ischial portion of the acetabulum and spirals upward across the posterior aspect of the femoral neck to insert into its superior aspect, just medial to the root of the greater trochanter.[2-4]

OSTEOKINEMATICS

Movement at the hip, which occurs in all three of the cardinal planes, consists of flexion, extension, abduction, adduction, medial rotation, and lateral rotation. These motions may be achieved by movement of the femur on the pelvis or by movement of the pelvis on the femur. The pelvic movements of anterior and posterior tilting produce flexion and extension of the hip, respectively. Tilting of the pelvis laterally produces hip adduction on the high side and hip abduction on the lower side of the pelvis. Rotation of the pelvis in the transverse plane results in lateral rotation of the hip ipsilateral to the more

anteriorly displaced pelvis and medial rotation of the contralateral hip. An additional motion, circumduction, has been described as occurring at the hip joint. This motion is a sequence of flexion, abduction, extension, and adduction and is not normally measured with a goniometer.[1,5,6]

ARTHROKINEMATICS

During motions of the hip, the convex femoral head moves within the concave acetabulum. A pure spin of the femoral head within the acetabulum occurs during flexion and extension of the hip.[6] Other motions of the hip produce a combined roll and glide of the femoral head in the opposite direction of the distal femur.

LIMITATIONS OF MOTION: HIP JOINT

Most of the motions at the hip are limited by the ligaments (iliofemoral, ischiofemoral, and pubofemoral) and muscles that surround the joint, as well as by the hip joint capsule. The primary exception to this rule is hip flexion, which frequently is limited by approximation of the soft tissue between the anterior thigh and the abdomen when the knee is flexed. Hip flexion and extension range of motion (ROM) are dependent on the position of the knee during movement. Full hip flexion is obtained only with the knee flexed. If the hip is flexed with the knee extended, tension in the hamstring muscles limits the motion. Likewise, full hip extension requires that the knee is extended, and in this position, motion is limited by tension in the iliofemoral ligament.[1,3] Extending the hip with the knee fully flexed typically decreases the available hip extension ROM subsequent to tension in the rectus femoris muscle.

Adduction of the hip is limited by contact with the contralateral limb and by tension in the lateral portions of the iliofemoral ligament and the hip abductor muscles.[7] Hip abduction is limited by tension in the pubofemoral ligament. Medial rotation of the hip is limited by tension in the ischiofemoral ligament, the posterior aspect of the articular capsule, and the lateral rotator muscles.[4] Lateral rotation is limited by the medial and lateral fibers of the iliofemoral ligament, as well as by tension in the tensor fasciae latae and the

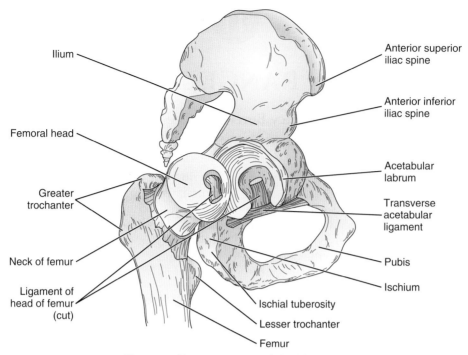

Ilium

Anterior superior
iliac spine

Anterior inferior
iliac spine

Femoral head

Acetabular
labrum

Transverse
acetabular
ligament

Greater
trochanter

Pubis

Neck of femur

Ischium

Ligament of
head of femur
(cut)

Ischial tuberosity

Lesser trochanter

Femur

Fig. 11.1 Bony anatomy of the hip joint.

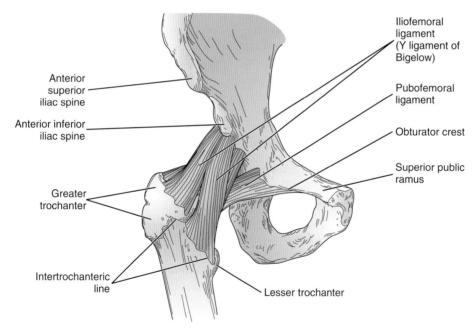

Anterior
superior
iliac spine

Iliofemoral
ligament
(Y ligament of
Bigelow)

Anterior inferior
iliac spine

Pubofemoral
ligament

Obturator crest

Superior public
ramus

Greater
trochanter

Intertrochanteric
line

Lesser trochanter

Fig. 11.2 Ligamentous reinforcement of the hip joint—anterior view.

iliotibial band.[1,6] Information on normal ranges of motion for all motions of the hip is found in Appendix B.

END-FEEL

Normal end-feels for hip extension, abduction, adduction, medial rotation, and lateral rotation are firm, as a result of capsular and ligamentous limitations of motion. The normal end-feel for hip flexion with the knee flexed is soft (soft-tissue approximation), whereas the normal end-feel for hip flexion with the knee extended is firm, because of muscular tension in the hamstring group.[1,5]

CAPSULAR PATTERN

Experts have expressed slight disagreement when describing the capsular pattern in the hip. Cyriax[8] states that flexion, abduction, and medial rotation are all "grossly" limited; extension is less limited than flexion, abduction, and medial rotation; and lateral rotation has no limitation. Although Kaltenborn[9] agrees that lateral

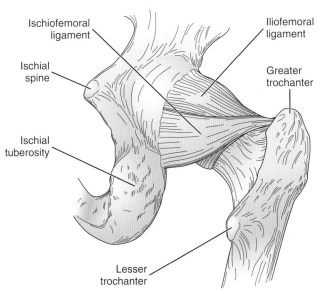

Fig. 11.3   Ligamentous reinforcement of the hip joint— posterior view.

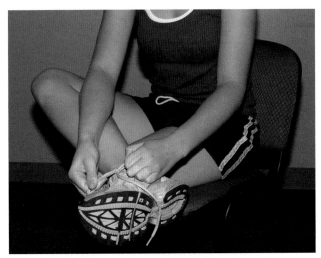

Fig. 11.5   Hip ROM needed to tie shoes.

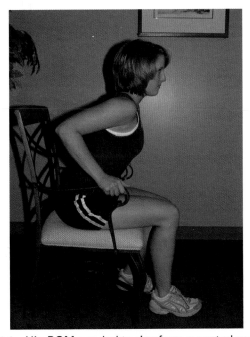

Fig. 11.4   Hip ROM needed to rise from a seated position.

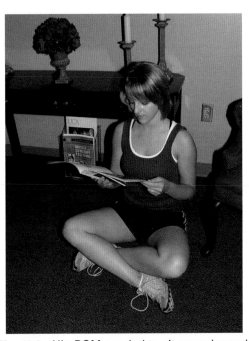

Fig. 11.6   Hip ROM needed to sit cross-legged.

rotation is the least limited, he states that medial rotation is most limited, followed by limitations in extension, then abduction and flexion.

RANGE OF MOTION AND FUNCTIONAL ACTIVITY

Several studies investigating motion of the hip joint during functional activities are described in the literature. Research has involved the examination of a variety of functional activities, including walking on level surfaces,[10–18] ascending and descending stairs,[9,19,20] sitting onto and rising from a chair (Fig. 11.4),[9,21,22]

lifting an object from the floor, dressing and bathing (Fig. 11.5),[9,23] and transitioning from a kneeling to a standing position.[24] A few authors also have examined hip motion in so-called high ROM activities such as kneeling, squatting, and sitting cross-legged (Fig. 11.6).[9,25–27]

A summary of hip range of motion as it relates to various functional activities is shown in Table 11.1. Most of the studies from which data were derived were performed in healthy adults, although some investigations included elderly and pediatric subjects. Essentials of the study populations and instrumentation used are included in the table. Caution should be used in extrapolating these data to the general population because the sample sizes for all studies were small. For more in-depth information on each study, the reader is referred to the reference list at the end of this chapter.

Table 11.1 HIP ROM DURING FUNCTIONAL ACTIVITIES

FUNCTIONAL ACTIVITY	FLEXION	EXTENSION	ABDUCTION	ADDUCTION	EXTERNAL ROTATION	INTERNAL ROTATION	COMMENTS
Ambulation—Level Ground							
Diamond et al.[17]	38°±7°	11°±6°	7°±3°	10°±4°	11°±4°	1°±6°	Measured 15 subjects with symptomatic femoroacetabular impingement and 14 control subjects (mean age 27.1±4.5 years) using Vicon 12-camera motion analysis system (only data from control subjects presented here)
Eitzen et al.[16]	30°±7°	18°±7°					Measured 48 subjects with hip OA and 22 control subjects (mean age 58.5±9 years) using a Qualisys motion analysis system (only data from control subjects presented here)
Han et al.[18]	35°±3°						Measured 40 healthy Chinese adults; mean age 21 years (20F, 20M) using Optotrak system
Jacobsen et al.[15]		13°±5°					Measured 32 subjects with hip dysplasia and 32 control subjects (mean age 33 years) using a Qualisys motion analysis system (only data from control subjects presented here)
Johnston and Smidt[10]	37°±5°	15°±6°	7°±3°	5°±2°	9°±4°	4°±3°	Measured 33 males aged 23–55 years using electrogoniometer
Ostrosky et al.[12]	26°±8° (young) 29°±8° (older)	10°±9° (young) 8°±6° (older)					Measured peak ROM during free speed walking using Expert Vision motion analysis system in 60 subjects divided into two groups according to age. Young group (n=30; 15F, 15M) aged 20–40 years; Older group (n=30; 15F, 15M) aged 60–80 years
Ranchos Los Amigos[14]	25°	20°					Undefined subject group and methodology
Ambulation—Ascending Stairs							
Johnston and Smidt[10]	67°±6°						Measured 33 males aged 23–55 years using electrogoniometer; stair rise height 18 cm
Livingston et al.[19] 20.3 cm stair rise height 20.3 cm stair rise height 12.7 cm stair rise height	59°±7° to 66°±1° 48°±2° to 56°±5° 47°±1° to 60°±2°	−7°±1° to 15°±4° 6°±1° to 11°±2° 1°±1° to 6°±1°					Used cinematographic analysis to measure 15 healthy F aged 19–26 years. Divided into three groups according to height. Taller subjects used ↓ hip flexion and ↑ hip extension compared with shorter subjects on identical steps
Protopapadaki et al.[20]	65°±7°						Measured 33 healthy adults aged 18–39 years (16M, 17F); stair rise height 18 cm
Ambulation—Descending Stairs							
Johnston and Smidt[10]	36°						Measured 33 males aged 23–55 years using electrogoniometer; stair rise height 18 cm
Livingston et al.[19] 20.3 cm stair rise height 20.3 cm stair rise height 12.7 cm stair rise height	37°±1° to 44°±5° 31°±1° to 45°±2° 26°±1° to 35°±3°	−1°±3° to 12°±2° −1°±4° to 12°±4° −1°±3° to 12°±2°					Used cinematographic analysis to measure 15 healthy F aged 19–26 years. Divided into three groups according to height.
Protopapadaki et al.[20]	91°±7°						Measured 33 healthy adults aged 18–39 years (16M, 17F); stair rise height 18 cm
Entering Bath Hyodo et al.[23]	78°±12° to 87°±8°	2°±3° to 8°±8°	25°±7° to 31°±7°	6°±3° to 12°±7°	28°±12° to 37°±13°	19°±16° to 31°±15°	Measured 26 healthy adults aged 20±1 years (13F, 13M) using Fastrak system
Exiting Bath Hyodo et al.[23]	73°±14° to 99°±10°	−1°±6° to 2°±5°	13°±6° to 21°±8°	9°±5° to 12°±6°	26°±13° to 27°±10°	15°±11° to 20°±13°	Measured 26 healthy adults aged 20±1 years (13F, 13M) using Fastrak system
Putting on Pants (in sitting) Hyodo et al.[23]	86°±10°	−35°±8°	14°±10°	11°±7°	30°±14°	19°±11°	Measured 26 healthy adults aged 20±1 years (13F, 13M) using Fastrak system

Activity / Study							Description
Putting on Pants (in standing)							
Hyodo et al.[23]	86°±9°	4°±5°	13°±7°	12°±6°	29°±14°	24°±13°	Measured 26 healthy adults aged 20±1 years (13F, 13M) using Fastrak system
Putting on Shoes (Foot on ankle)							
Hyodo et al.[23]	82°±7°	−43°±8°	18°±8°	0°±8°	61°±12°	6°±11°	Measured 26 healthy adults aged 20±1 years (13F, 13M) using Fastrak system
Putting on Shoes (Foot on knee)							
Hyodo et al.[23]	85°±10°	−45°±8°	4°±7°	17°±9°	26°±14°	7°±11°	Measured 26 healthy adults aged 20±1 years (13F, 13M) using Fastrak system
Rising from a Chair							
Ikeda et al.[21]	101°±9° (young group) 98°±9° (older group)						Measured ROM using Selspot data acquisition system in 9 older subjects aged 61–74 years (6M, 3F) and compared with previous data on 9 healthy F aged 25–36yrs.; chair height 80% of each subjects knee height
Johnston and Smidt[10]	112°±1°						Measured 33 males aged 23–55 years using electrogoniometer; chair height 46cm
Tully et al.[22]	99°±7°	−2°±7°					Measured ROM using 2-dimensional Peak Motus system in 47 healthy subjects (27F, 20M) aged 18–30yrs.; seat height adjusted to length of subject's leg
Sitting onto Chair							
Johnston and Smidt[10]	104°±11°						Measured 33 males aged 23–55 years using electrogoniometer; chair height 46cm
Lifting Object from Floor							
Johnston and Smidt[10]	125°±10°						Measured 33 males aged 23–55 years using electrogoniometer
Tying Shoes							
Johnston and Smidt[10] (foot on floor) (foot on contralateral thigh)	129°±9° 115°±13°		18°±10°		13°±7°		Measured 33 males aged 23–55 years using electrogoniometer
Hyodo et al.[23]	−53°±10° to 54°±11°	89°±10° to 90°±11°	2°±7° to 11°±9°	−3°±8° to 5°±8°	9°±8° to 18°±8°	−4°±8° to 2°±10°	Measured 26 healthy adults aged 20±1 years (13F, 13M) using Fastrak system
Kneeling							
Hemmerich et al.[25] (ankle dorsiflexed) (ankle plantar flexed)	74°±33° 62°±16°		21°±12° 27°±9°		16°±13° 25°±23°		Measured ROM in 30 Indian subjects, average age 48 years (10F, 20M) using Fastrack system
Knee-to-Stand							
Vander Linden and Wilhelm[24]	89°±4°	3°±6°					Measured ROM during kneel-to-stand movement in 10 healthy children aged 5–7 years (6F, 4M) using cinematography
Sitting Cross-Legged							
Hemmerich et al.[25]	84°±36°		34°±15°		37°±18°		Measured ROM in 30 Indian subjects, average age 48 years (10F, 20M) using Fastrack system
Kapoor et al.[26]	91°±3°		39°±6°		49°±6°		Measured ROM in 44 Indian subjects (31M, 13F) aged 21–80 years using universal goniometer
Squatting							
Johnston and Smidt[10] Han et al.[18]	114°±10° 118°±15° (F) 121°±13° (M)						Measured 33 males aged 23–55 years using electrogoniometer Measured 40 healthy Chinese adults; mean age 21 years (20F, 20M) using Optotrak system
Hemmerich et al.[25] (heels down) (heels up)	95°±27° 91°±19°		26°±12° 30°±13°		17°±11° 19°±11°		Measured ROM in 30 Indian subjects, average age 48 years (10F, 20M) using Fastrack system

Vicon Motion Analysis System by Vicon, MX, Oxford, UK. Qualisys Motion Analysis System by Qualisys AB, Gothenburg, Sweden. Optotrak System by NDI, Waterloo, Ontario Canada. Expert Vision Motion Analysis System by Motion Analysis Corp, Santa Rosa, CA. Selspot Data Acquisition System by Selective Electronic Company (SELCOM), Molndal, Sweden. Peak Motus System by Vicon Peak, Centennial, CO. Fastrack System by Polhemus 3Space, Colchester, VT.

TECHNIQUES OF MEASUREMENT: HIP FLEXION/EXTENSION

A variety of techniques have been employed to measure hip flexion. Measurements have been taken with the patient in the supine position with the contralateral hip flexed or extended (Figs. 11.7 and 11.8)[28,29] and with the patient in a side-lying position, using the Mundale[30] (Fig. 11.9) or the pelvifemoral angle technique[31] (Fig. 11.10). These techniques vary in terms of patient positioning, specific landmarks used for goniometric alignment, and the degree to which each method controls for pelvic motion. Values for the normal maximum amount of hip flexion that are provided in the literature vary widely (see www.wb-saunders.com/SIMON/Reese/joint/). Such discrepancies in standards for the normal hip appear to be caused by the technique used and the degree to which each of the different techniques controls for pelvic motion. Of the techniques provided in the preceding list, the one recommended by the American Academy of Orthopaedic Surgeons (AAOS) and the American Medical Association (AMA) places the least emphasis on controlling pelvic motion.[28,29]

Motions of the pelvis on the lumbar spine during measurement of hip flexion or extension can artificially inflate the range of motion measurement obtained. To control for this phenomenon, one should use landmarks on the pelvis to eliminate the possibility of including lumbar spine motion in the measurement, or one should manually ensure that the pelvis remains in a neutral position at the beginning and end of the range of motion measurement. The neutral position of the pelvis has been described as the position in which a line drawn through the anterior superior iliac spines (ASIS) and the symphysis pubis is vertical and lies in the frontal plane.[32,33] With the pelvis in this position, a line connecting the anterior and posterior superior iliac spines of the pelvis is horizontal and lies in the transverse plane.[5]

According to the Mundale technique,[30] the line through the iliac spines is used as the pelvic reference for hip flexion and extension goniometry, and the stationary arm of the goniometer is positioned perpendicular to this line (see Fig. 11.9). Using the pelvis for alignment of the stationary arm of the goniometer eliminates the possibility of including motion of the lumbar spine in goniometric measurements of hip flexion and extension. A second technique, which uses landmarks on the pelvis for alignment of the stationary arm of the goniometer, is the pelvifemoral angle technique.[34] When using this technique, the examiner aligns the stationary arm of the goniometer parallel to a line that extends from the ASIS through the ischial tuberosity of the pelvis (see Fig. 11.10). When the Mundale or the pelvifemoral angle technique is used, the moving arm of the goniometer is aligned along the midline of the

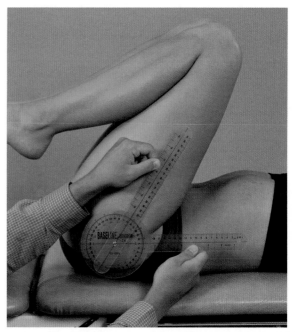

Fig. 11.7 Hip flexion measured with contralateral hip flexed; recommended by AAOS and AMA; allows little control of pelvic motion.

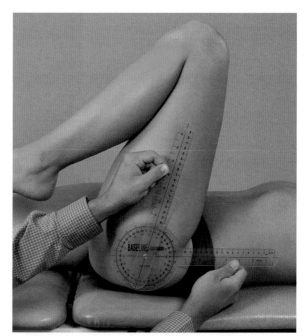

Fig. 11.8 Hip flexion measured with contralateral hip extended, providing greater pelvic stability.

femur toward the lateral femoral epicondyle, while the axis is placed on the greater trochanter.[30,34] With either technique, the patient is placed in a side-lying position to allow the examiner access to the indicated bony landmarks.

Other techniques recommended for measuring hip flexion and extension use landmarks on the trunk or

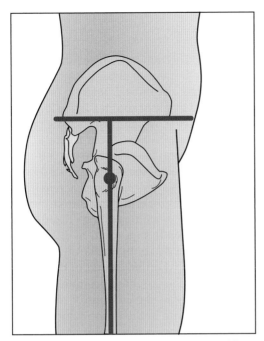

Fig. 11.9   Mundale technique for measuring hip motion. Goniometer is aligned as follows: Stationary arm perpendicular to a line through the iliac spines; axis over greater trochanter; moving arm along lateral midline of femur toward lateral femoral epicondyle. (Modified from Reese NB: *Muscle and Sensory Testing*. 2nd ed. Philadelphia, Saunders/Elsevier, 2005, with permission.)

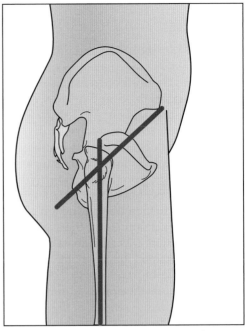

Fig. 11.10   Pelvifemoral angle technique for measuring hip motion. Goniometer is aligned as follows: Stationary arm parallel to a line extending from the ASIS through the ischial tuberosity; axis over the greater trochanter; moving arm along lateral midline of femur toward lateral femoral epicondyle. (Modified from Reese NB: *Muscle and Sensory Testing,* 2nd ed. Philadelphia, Saunders/Elsevier, 2005, with permission.)

the examining table for alignment of the stationary arm of the goniometer.[28,29,35] The danger in using these landmarks is the possibility that lumbar motion may be included in measurements of hip motion, thus creating unreliable goniometric measurements. However, if the pelvis is maintained in a neutral position (see the previous description), then a line through the midline of the trunk will parallel a line connecting the ASIS and the pubic symphysis, thus providing a reliable reference for the stationary arm of the goniometer. The use of such a reference is advantageous because it allows the patient to be placed in a supine (flexion) or a prone (extension) position during the measurement, thus providing greater stability of the pelvis. Additionally, the need for marking lines on, or taping, the patient is avoided. Whenever landmarks on the trunk are used for alignment of the goniometer's stationary arm, extreme care must be taken, as indicated previously, to maintain the pelvis in a neutral position through manual monitoring of pelvic motion and patient positioning. Both the AAOS and the AMA direct that the patient's contralateral hip should be flexed during measurements of ipsilateral hip flexion,[28,29] but maintaining the contralateral thigh against the examining table is necessary to minimize pelvic motion during the measurement.[5] Therefore, the technique of measuring hip flexion

described in this text recommends extension of the contralateral hip during the measurement.

Measurement of hip extension range of motion also can be accomplished using the Mundale and pelvifemoral angle techniques. Additionally, the AAOS describes two methods of measuring hip extension, both of which use a proximal goniometer alignment that is parallel to the tabletop and to a line through the lateral midline of the trunk.[29] The patient is placed in the prone position for both AAOS techniques; the only difference in the two techniques is that the patient's contralateral hip is extended in one technique and is flexed over the end of the examining table in the other. Some examiners also use the Thomas technique (used for measuring hip flexion contracture; see Chapter 14) to measure hip extension.[36] In a comparison of four of these techniques, Bartlett et al.[36] reported the highest intrarater and interrater reliabilities for the AAOS (contralateral hip flexed) and Thomas techniques in children with myelomeningocele and spastic diplegia (see Chapter 15). Although the contralateral hip may be extended or flexed during measurements of hip extension ROM, fewer patients may have difficulty extending the hip while lying prone than while standing and leaning over an examining table.

TECHNIQUES OF MEASUREMENT: HIP ABDUCTION/ADDUCTION

Measurement of hip abduction and adduction is most commonly done with the patient positioned supine and the ipsilateral hip positioned in 0 degrees of extension. The hip is maintained in 0 degrees of extension throughout the measurement.[28,29,35] However, hip abduction occasionally is measured with the ipsilateral hip maintained in 90 degrees of flexion throughout the measurement.[29] This technique appears to be used primarily in the pediatric population and may be less reliable than measurement of hip abduction with the hip extended.[37] Hip abduction and adduction also may be measured with an inclinometer if the subject is placed in a side-lying position. Measurements of iliotibial (IT) band tightness, obtained through this method, have been shown to have high reliability.[38] Although measurement of hip abduction and adduction with the inclinometer is not demonstrated in this chapter, measurement of IT band tightness using this technique may be found in Chapter 14.

TECHNIQUES OF MEASUREMENT: HIP MEDIAL-LATERAL ROTATION

Rotation of the hip is generally measured with the patient's hip in 90 degrees of flexion (patient seated) or with the hip in the anatomical position of 0 degrees of extension (patient prone or supine). In the literature, disagreement exists over which position, if either, allows the greater amount of hip rotation. Haley[39] reported a decrease in medial and lateral active hip rotation in the supine, compared with the seated position, whereas Simoneau et al.[40] reported increased active hip lateral, but not medial, rotation when measured in the prone compared with the seated position. Results reported by Simoneau et al. were supported by Bierma-Zeinstra et al.[41] who reported that both medial and lateral hip rotation were greater when measured in the prone, compared with the supine or seated position. Ellison et al.[42] found no difference in the amount of medial and lateral rotation of the hip in the prone compared with the seated position, although this group measured passive but not active hip rotation.

Additionally, the amount of motion measured at the hip may differ depending on the measurement tool used. Bierma-Zeinstra et al.[41] found significantly higher measurements of hip external rotation ROM when they measured movement with the goniometer compared with measurements obtained with an inclinometer. Conversely, the inclinometer yielded significantly greater measurements of hip flexion and extension than did the goniometer. Unfortunately, most sources reporting standards for hip rotation ROM (e.g., AAOS, AMA) do not include descriptions of the position in which rotation of the hip was measured, nor do many describe the instrument used to measure the motion. Available data for normal ranges of hip rotation are reported in Appendix B.

Because there appears to be no difference in the reliability of measurements of hip rotation taken with the hip flexed or extended[40] and because information is mixed regarding whether the inclinometer or the goniometer is most reliable for measuring hip rotation ROM,[41] the examiner may choose either method or instrument for performing measurements of this motion. However, care should be taken as always to use identical techniques whenever repeated measures are taken, in that the amount of motion may vary depending on patient position and the instrument chosen.[39-41] The techniques described in this text for measuring hip rotation include those in both seated and prone positions with the goniometer and the inclinometer.

Hip Flexion (Video 11.1)

Fig. 11.11 Starting position for measurement of hip flexion. Bony landmarks for goniometer alignment (lateral midline of pelvis/trunk, greater trochanter, lateral femoral epicondyle) indicated by red line and dots.

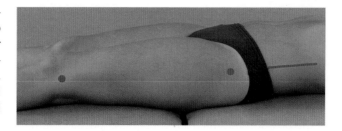

Normal ROM = 120 to 135 degrees.[43-49]

MDC for hip flexion goniometry measured by a single examiner = 8 degrees in normal and 8 to 11 degrees in pathological hips.[46,50,51]

Patient position	Supine, with lower extremities in anatomical position (Fig. 11.11).
Stabilization	Over anterior aspect of ipsilateral pelvis (Fig. 11.12).
Examiner action	After instructing patient in motion desired, stabilize ipsilateral pelvis with one hand and flex patient's hip through available ROM with other hand. Ipsilateral knee should be allowed to flex as well. Hip should not be flexed past the point at which pelvic motion begins to occur (as detected by superior movement of ipsilateral ASIS under examiner's stabilizing hand). Return limb to starting position. Performing passive movement yields an estimate of the ROM and demonstrates to patient exact motion desired (see Fig. 11.12).
Goniometer alignment	Palpate following bony landmarks (shown in Fig. 11.11), and align goniometer accordingly (Fig. 11.13).
Stationary arm	Lateral midline of pelvis and trunk.[*]

---

[*]Lateral midline of pelvis should parallel midline of trunk as long as pelvic motion is prevented and neutral pelvis is maintained (see description of neutral pelvis in Techniques of Measurement: Hip Flexion/Extension).

Fig. 11.12 End of hip flexion ROM, showing proper hand placement for stabilizing pelvis and detecting pelvic motion. Bony landmarks for goniometer alignment (lateral midline of pelvis/trunk, greater trochanter, lateral femoral epicondyle) indicated by red line and dots.

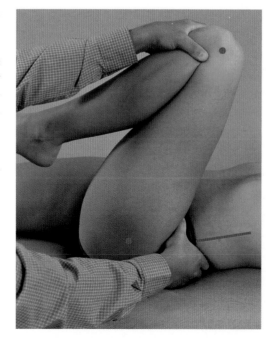

Fig. 11.13 Starting position for measurement of hip flexion, demonstrating proper initial alignment of goniometer.

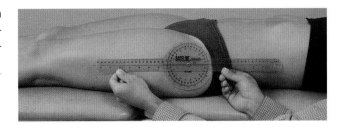

Axis	Greater trochanter of femur.
Moving arm	Lateral midline of femur toward lateral femoral epicondyle.
	Read scale of goniometer.
Patient/Examiner action	Perform passive, or have patient perform active, hip flexion (Fig. 11.14). In either case, hip flexion should not be allowed to continue past point at which pelvic motion is detected (see Examiner action).
Confirmation of alignment	Repalpate landmarks and confirm proper goniometric alignment at end of ROM, correcting alignment as necessary (see Fig. 11.14). Read scale of goniometer.
Documentation	Record patient's ROM.
Precaution	If the hip is allowed to flex past point at which pelvic motion begins to occur, motion measured will include both hip and lumbar flexion. To isolate hip flexion, pelvic motion must not be permitted.
Alternative patient position	Side-lying; stabilization of pelvis is more difficult in this position. Goniometer alignment remains the same.

Fig. 11.14 End of hip flexion ROM, demonstrating proper alignment of goniometer at end of range.

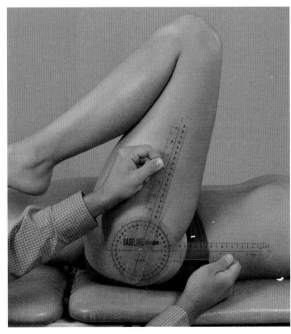
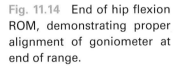

Hip Extension (Video 11.2)

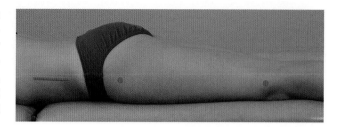

Fig. 11.15 Starting position for measurement of hip extension. Bony landmarks for goniometer alignment (lateral midline of pelvis/trunk, greater trochanter, lateral femoral epicondyle) indicated by red line and dots.

Normal ROM = 10 to 20 degrees.[44–49]

MDC for hip extension goniometry measured by a single examiner = 6 degrees in normal and 11 degrees in pathological hips.[46,51]

Patient position

Prone, with lower extremities in anatomical position (Fig. 11.15).

Stabilization

Over posterolateral aspect of ipsilateral pelvis with palm of hand while fingers palpate ASIS (Fig. 11.16).

Examiner action

After instructing patient in motion desired, stabilize ipsilateral pelvis with one hand and extend patient's hip through available ROM with other hand. Ipsilateral knee should be kept extended to avoid limitation of hip extension by tight rectus femoris muscle. Hip should not be extended past the point at which pelvic motion begins to occur (as detected by inferior movement of ipsilateral ASIS under examiner's stabilizing hand). Return limb to starting position. Performing passive movement provides an estimate of the ROM and demonstrates to patient exact motion desired (see Fig. 11.16).

Goniometer alignment

Palpate following bony landmarks (shown in Fig. 11.15), and align goniometer accordingly (Fig. 11.17).

Stationary arm

Lateral midline of pelvis and trunk.*

Axis

Greater trochanter of femur.

---

*Lateral midline of pelvis should parallel midline of trunk as long as pelvic motion is prevented and neutral pelvis is maintained (see description of neutral pelvis in Techniques of Measurement: Hip Flexion/Extension).

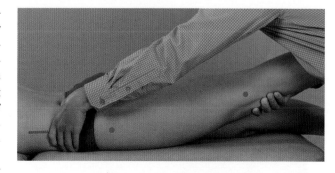

Fig. 11.16 End of hip extension ROM, showing proper hand placement for stabilizing pelvis and detecting pelvic motion. Bony landmarks for goniometer alignment (lateral midline of pelvis/trunk, greater trochanter, lateral femoral epicondyle) indicated by red line and dots.

Fig. 11.17 Starting position for measurement of hip extension, demonstrating proper initial alignment of goniometer.

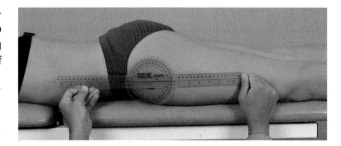

Moving arm	Lateral midline of femur toward lateral femoral epicondyle.
	Read scale of goniometer.
Patient/Examiner action	Perform passive, or have patient perform active, hip extension (Fig. 11.18). In either case, hip extension should not be allowed to continue past point at which pelvic motion is detected (see Examiner action).
Confirmation of alignment	Repalpate landmarks and confirm proper goniometric alignment at end of ROM, correcting alignment as necessary (see Fig. 11.18). Read scale of goniometer.
Documentation	Record patient's ROM.
Precaution	Should hip be allowed to extend past point at which pelvic motion begins to occur, motion measured will include both hip and lumbar extension. To isolate hip extension, pelvic motion must not be permitted.
Alternative patient position	Side-lying; stabilization of pelvis is more difficult in this position. Goniometer alignment remains the same.

Fig. 11.18 End of hip extension ROM, demonstrating proper alignment of goniometer at end of range.

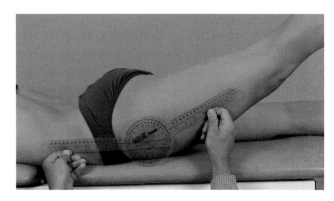

Hip Abduction (Video 11.3)

Fig. 11.19 Starting position for measurement of hip abduction. Bony landmarks for goniometer alignment (ipsilateral ASIS, contralateral ASIS, midline of patella) indicated by red dots and line.

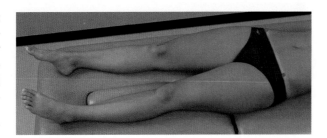

Normal ROM = 40 to 50 degrees.[44,45,47,48,52,53]

MDC for hip abduction goniometry measured by a single examiner = 7 to 9 degrees in normal and 7 degrees in pathological hips.[46,50,51]

Patient position	Supine, with lower extremities in anatomical position (Fig. 11.19).
Stabilization	Over anterior aspect of ipsilateral pelvis (Fig. 11.20).
Examiner action	After instructing patient in motion desired, abduct patient's hip through available ROM, avoiding hip rotation. Return limb to starting position. Performing passive movement provides an estimate of the ROM and demonstrates to patient exact motion desired (see Fig. 11.20).
Goniometer alignment	Palpate following bony landmarks as shown in Fig. 11.19 and align goniometer accordingly (Fig. 11.21).
Stationary arm	Toward contralateral ASIS.

Fig. 11.20 End of hip abduction ROM, showing proper hand placement for stabilizing pelvis. Bony landmarks for goniometer alignment (ipsilateral ASIS, contralateral ASIS, midline of patella) indicated by red dots and line.

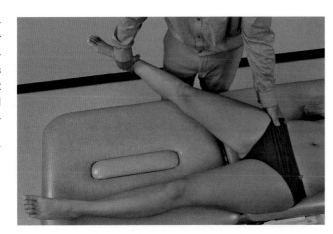

Fig. 11.21 Starting position for measurement of hip abduction, demonstrating proper initial alignment of goniometer.

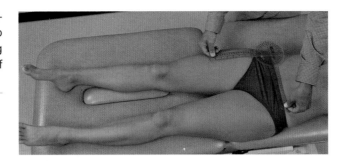

Axis	Ipsilateral ASIS.
Moving arm	Anterior midline of ipsilateral femur, using midline of patella as reference.
	Read scale of goniometer.
Patient/Examiner action	Perform passive, or have patient perform active, hip abduction (Fig. 11.22).
Confirmation of alignment	Repalpate landmarks and confirm proper goniometric alignment at end of ROM, correcting alignment as necessary (see Fig. 11.22) (see Note).
	Read scale of goniometer.
Documentation	Record patient's ROM.
Note	Confirmation of alignment of stationary arm is critical to avoid including lateral pelvic tilting in hip abduction ROM.

Fig. 11.22 End of hip abduction ROM, demonstrating proper alignment of goniometer at end of range.

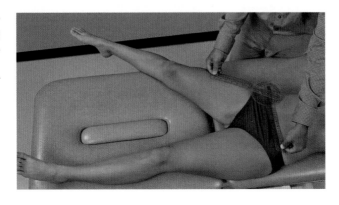

Hip Adduction (Video 11.4)

Fig. 11.23 Starting position for measurement of hip adduction. Contralateral hip is abducted to allow room for adduction of ipsilateral hip. Bony landmarks for goniometer alignment (ipsilateral ASIS, contralateral ASIS, midline of patella) indicated by red dots and line.

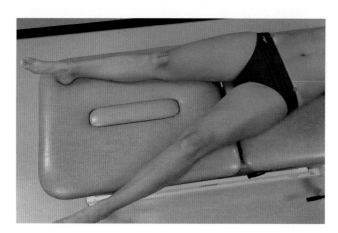

Normal ROM = 120 to 140 degrees.[43–49,53]

MDC for hip adduction goniometry measured by a single examiner = 4 to 7 degrees in normal and 7 degrees in pathological hips.[46,50]

Patient position	Supine with ipsilateral lower extremity in anatomical position; contralateral hip abducted (Fig. 11.23).
Stabilization	Over anterior aspect of ipsilateral pelvis (Fig. 11.24).
Examiner action	After instructing patient in motion desired, adduct patient's hip through available ROM, avoiding hip rotation. Return limb to starting position. Performing passive movement provides an estimate of the ROM and demonstrates to patient exact motion desired (see Fig. 11.24).
Goniometer alignment	Palpate following bony landmarks as shown in Fig. 11.23 and align goniometer accordingly (Fig. 11.25).
Stationary arm	Toward contralateral ASIS.

Fig. 11.24 End of hip adduction ROM, showing proper hand placement for stabilizing pelvis. Bony landmarks for goniometer alignment (ipsilateral ASIS, contralateral ASIS, midline of patella) indicated by red dots and line.

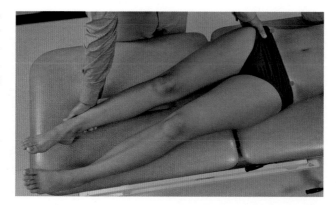

Fig. 11.25 Starting position for measurement of hip adduction, demonstrating proper initial alignment of goniometer.

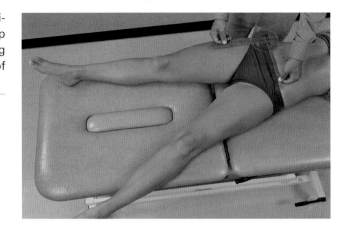

Axis	Ipsilateral ASIS.
Moving arm	Anterior midline of femur, using midline of patella as reference.
	Read scale of goniometer.
Patient/Examiner action	Perform passive, or have patient perform active, hip adduction (Fig. 11.26).
Confirmation of alignment	Repalpate landmarks and confirm proper goniometric alignment at end of ROM, correcting alignment as necessary (see Fig. 11.26) (see Note). Read scale of goniometer.
Documentation	Record patient's ROM.
Note	Confirmation of alignment of stationary arm is critical to avoid including lateral pelvic tilting in hip adduction ROM.

Fig. 11.26 End of hip adduction ROM, demonstrating proper alignment of goniometer at end of range.

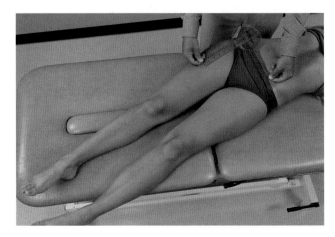

Hip Lateral Rotation With Hip Flexed—Goniometer (Video 11.5)

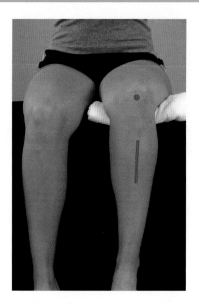

Fig. 11.27 Starting position for measurement of hip lateral rotation in seated position. Weight is distributed evenly over both ischial tuberosities. Towel roll is placed under ipsilateral thigh to position femur in horizontal plane. Bony landmarks for goniometer alignment (midpoint of patella, tibial crest) indicated by red dot and line.

Normal ROM = 30 to 50 degrees.[39,40,45–48,53,54]

MDC for hip lateral rotation goniometry measured by a single examiner = 6 to 7 degrees in normal and 7 to 8 degrees in pathological hips[46,50,51].

Patient position	Seated, with hip and knee flexed to 90 degrees and folded towel under thigh, with weight equally distributed over both ischial tuberosities (Fig. 11.27).
Stabilization	None needed; pelvis is stabilized by patient's weight.
Examiner action	After instructing patient in motion desired, laterally rotate patient's hip through available ROM by keeping the thigh stationary and moving the leg, foot, and ankle medially. Return limb to starting position. Performing passive movement provides an estimate of the ROM and demonstrates to patient exact motion desired (Fig. 11.28).
Goniometer alignment	Palpate following bony landmarks as shown in Fig. 11.27 and align the goniometer accordingly (Fig. 11.29).

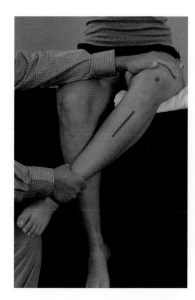

Fig. 11.28 End of hip lateral rotation ROM. Examiner's hand stabilizes thigh against table. Bony landmarks for goniometer alignment (midpoint of patella, tibial crest) indicated by red dot and line.

Fig. 11.29 Starting position for measurement of hip lateral rotation in seated position, demonstrating proper initial alignment of goniometer.

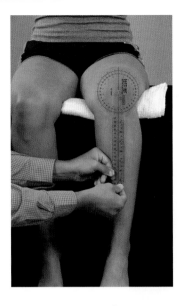

Stationary arm	Perpendicular to floor.
Axis	Midpoint of patella.
Moving arm	Anterior midline of tibia, along tibial crest.
	Read scale of goniometer.
Patient/Examiner action	Perform passive, or have patient perform active, hip lateral rotation. Patient should be instructed to maintain equal weight on both ischial tuberosities (Fig. 11.30).
Confirmation of alignment	Repalpate landmarks and confirm proper goniometric alignment at end of ROM, correcting alignment as necessary (see Fig. 11.30). Read scale of goniometer.
Documentation	Record patient's ROM.
Precaution	Do not allow patient to laterally flex trunk to ipsilateral side or to lift ipsilateral thigh from table during measurement because doing so will result in a falsely increased ROM.
Alternative position	Supine with hip and knee flexed 90 degrees. Stationary arm of goniometer is aligned parallel to anterior midline of trunk. Alignment of rest of goniometer remains the same.

Fig. 11.30 End of hip lateral rotation ROM, demonstrating proper alignment of goniometer at end of range.

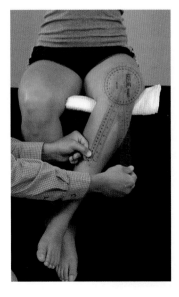

Hip Medial Rotation With Hip Flexed—Goniometer (Video 11.6)

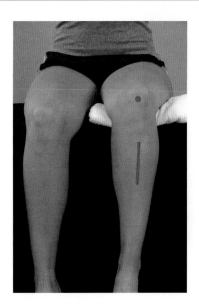

Fig. 11.31 Starting position for measurement of hip medial rotation in seated position. Weight is distributed evenly over both ischial tuberosities. Towel roll is placed under ipsilateral thigh to position femur in horizontal plane. Bony landmarks for goniometer alignment (midpoint of patella, tibial crest) indicated by red dot and line.

Normal ROM = 30 to 50 degrees[39,40,44–48,52,53].

MDC for hip medial rotation goniometry measured by a single examiner = 6 to 9 degrees in normal and 7 to 8 degrees in pathological hips.[46,50,51,55]

Patient position	Seated, with hip and knee flexed to 90 degrees and folded towel under thigh, with weight equally distributed over both ischial tuberosities (Fig. 11.31).
Stabilization	None needed; pelvis is stabilized by patient's weight.
Examiner action	After instructing patient in motion desired, medially rotate patient's hip through available ROM by keeping the thigh stationary and moving the leg, foot, and ankle laterally. Return limb to starting position. Performing passive movement provides an estimate of the ROM and demonstrates to patient exact motion desired (Fig. 11.32).
Goniometer alignment	Palpate following bony landmarks as shown in Fig. 11.31 and align goniometer accordingly (Fig. 11.33).

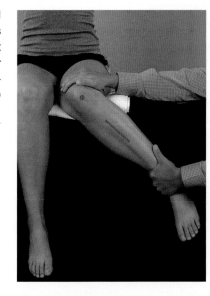

Fig. 11.32 End of hip medial rotation ROM. Examiner's hand stabilizes thigh against table. Bony landmarks for goniometer alignment (midpoint of patella, tibial crest) indicated by red dot and line.

Fig. 11.33 Starting position for measurement of hip medial rotation in seated position, demonstrating proper initial alignment of goniometer.

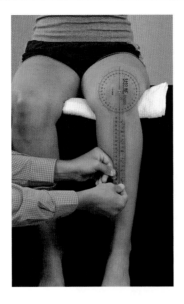

Stationary arm	Perpendicular to floor.
Axis	Midpoint of patella.
Moving arm	Anterior midline of tibia, along tibial crest.
	Read scale of goniometer.
Patient/Examiner action	Perform passive, or have patient perform active, hip medial rotation. Patient should be instructed to maintain equal weight on both ischial tuberosities (Fig. 11.34).
Confirmation of alignment	Repalpate landmarks and confirm proper goniometric alignment at end of ROM, correcting alignment as necessary (see Fig. 11.34). Read scale of goniometer.
Documentation	Record patient's ROM.
Precaution	Do not allow patient to laterally flex trunk to contralateral side or lift ipsilateral thigh from table during measurement, as doing so will result in a falsely increased ROM.
Alternative patient position	Supine with hip and knee flexed to 90 degrees. Stationary arm of goniometer is aligned parallel to anterior midline of trunk. Alignment of rest of goniometer remains the same.

Fig. 11.34 End of hip medial rotation ROM, demonstrating proper alignment of goniometer at end of range.

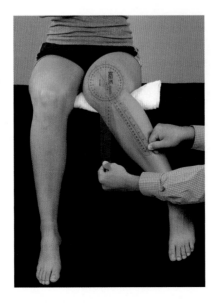

Hip Lateral Rotation With Hip Flexed—Inclinometer (Video 11.7)

Fig. 11.35 Starting position for measurement of hip lateral rotation in seated position. Weight is distributed evenly over both ischial tuberosities. Towel roll is placed under ipsilateral thigh to position femur in horizontal plane.

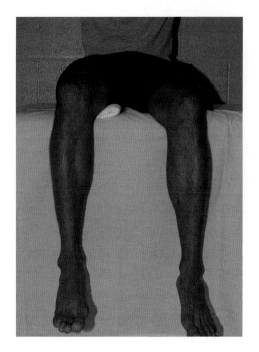

Normal ROM = 30 to 50 degrees.[39,40,45–48,53,54]

Patient position	Seated, with hip and knee flexed to 90 degrees and folded towel under thigh, with weight equally distributed over both ischial tuberosities (Fig. 11.35).
Stabilization	None needed; pelvis is stabilized by patient's weight.
Examiner action	After instructing patient in motion desired, laterally rotate patient's hip through available ROM by keeping the thigh stationary and moving the leg, foot, and ankle medially. Return limb to starting position. Performing passive movement provides an estimate of the ROM and demonstrates to patient exact motion desired (Fig. 11.36).

Fig. 11.36 End of hip lateral rotation ROM. Examiner's hand stabilizes thigh against table.

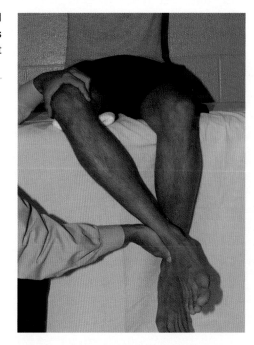

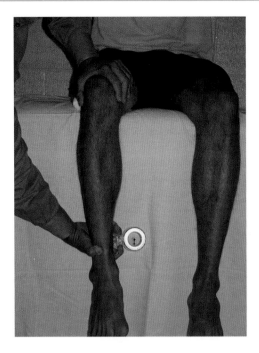

Fig. 11.37 Starting position for measurement of hip lateral rotation in seated position, demonstrating proper initial alignment of inclinometer.

Inclinometer alignment   On medial aspect of lower leg, proximal to the medial malleolus. Ensure that the inclinometer is set to 0 degrees once it is positioned on patient (Fig. 11.37).

Patient/Examiner action   Perform passive, or have patient perform active, hip lateral rotation. Patient should be instructed to maintain equal weight on both ischial tuberosities (Fig. 11.38).

Confirmation of alignment   Ensure that feet of inclinometer remain in firm contact with medial aspect of lower leg. Read scale of inclinometer (see Fig. 11.38).

Documentation   Record patient's ROM.

Precaution   Do not allow patient to laterally flex trunk to ipsilateral side or to lift ipsilateral thigh from table during measurement, as doing so will result in a falsely increased ROM.

Fig. 11.38 End of hip lateral rotation ROM, demonstrating proper alignment of inclinometer at end of range.

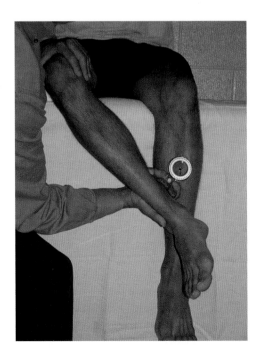

Hip Medial Rotation With Hip Flexed—Inclinometer (Video 11.8)

Fig. 11.39 Starting position for measurement of hip medial rotation in seated position. Weight is distributed evenly over both ischial tuberosities. Towel roll is placed under ipsilateral thigh to position femur in horizontal plane.

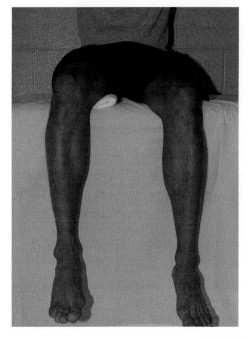

Normal ROM = 30 to 50 degrees.[39,40,44–48,52,53]

MDC for hip medial rotation inclinometry measured by a single examiner = 5 to 9 degrees for active and passive ROM, respectively.[56]

Patient position

Seated, with hip and knee flexed to 90 degrees and folded towel under thigh, with weight equally distributed over both ischial tuberosities (Fig. 11.39).

Stabilization

None needed; pelvis is stabilized by patient's weight.

Examiner action

After instructing patient in motion desired, medially rotate patient's hip through available ROM by keeping the thigh stationary and moving the leg, foot, and ankle laterally. Return limb to starting position. Performing passive movement provides an estimate of the ROM and demonstrates to patient exact motion desired (Fig. 11.40).

Fig. 11.40 End of hip medial rotation ROM. Examiner's hand stabilizes thigh against table.

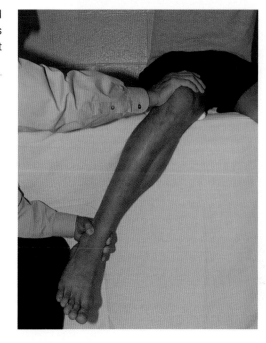

Fig. 11.41 Starting position for measurement of hip medial rotation in seated position, demonstrating proper initial alignment of inclinometer.

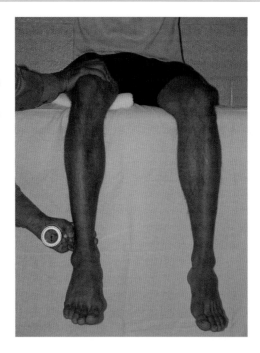

Inclinometer alignment	On lateral aspect of lower leg, proximal to the lateral malleolus. Ensure that the inclinometer is set to 0 degrees once it is positioned on patient (Fig. 11.41).
Patient/Examiner action	Perform passive, or have patient perform active, hip medial rotation. Patient should be instructed to maintain equal weight on both ischial tuberosities (Fig. 11.42).
Confirmation of alignment	Ensure that feet of inclinometer remain in firm contact with lateral aspect of lower leg. Read scale of inclinometer (see Fig. 11.42).
Documentation	Record patient's ROM.
Precaution	Do not allow patient to laterally flex trunk to contralateral side or to lift ipsilateral thigh from table during measurement, as doing so will result in a falsely increased ROM.

Fig. 11.42 End of hip medial rotation ROM, demonstrating proper alignment of inclinometer at end of range.

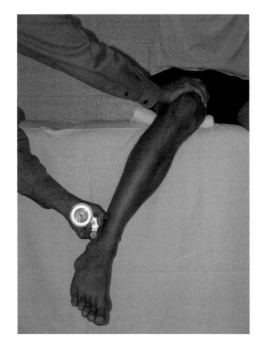

Hip Lateral Rotation With Hip Flexed—Smartphone Method

Fig. 11.43 Starting position for measurement of hip lateral rotation in seated position. Weight is distributed evenly over both ischial tuberosities. Towel roll is placed under ipsilateral thigh to position femur in horizontal plane.

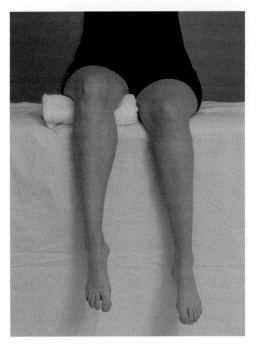

Normal ROM = 30 to 50 degrees[39,40,45–48,53,54].

Patient position	Seated, with hip and knee flexed to 90 degrees and folded towel under thigh, with weight equally distributed over both ischial tuberosities (Fig. 11.43).
Stabilization	None needed; pelvis is stabilized by patient's weight.
Examiner action	After instructing patient in motion desired, laterally rotate patient's hip through available ROM by keeping the thigh stationary and moving the leg, foot, and ankle medially. Return limb to starting position. Performing passive movement provides an estimate of the ROM and demonstrates to patient exact motion desired (Fig. 11.44).

Fig. 11.44 End of hip lateral rotation ROM. Examiner's hand stabilizes thigh against table.

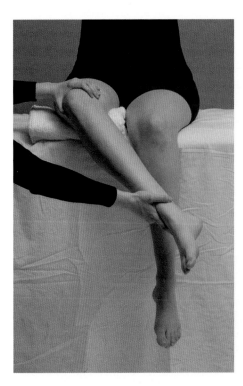

Fig. 11.45 Starting position for measurement of hip lateral rotation in seated position, demonstrating proper initial alignment of smartphone.

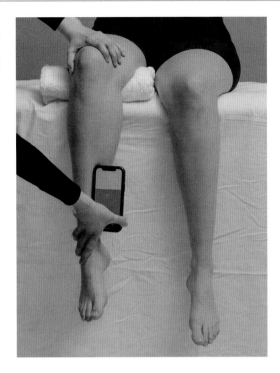

Smartphone alignment	On medial aspect of lower leg, proximal to the medial malleolus. Ensure that measurement app on Smartphone reads 0 degrees once it is positioned on patient (Fig. 11.45).
Patient/Examiner action	Perform passive, or have patient perform active, hip lateral rotation. Patient should be instructed to maintain equal weight on both ischial tuberosities (Fig. 11.46). Read angle on Smartphone at end of ROM.
Documentation	Record patient's ROM.
Precaution	Do not allow patient to laterally flex trunk to ipsilateral side or to lift ipsilateral thigh from table during measurement, as doing so will result in a falsely increased ROM.

Fig. 11.46 End of hip lateral rotation ROM, demonstrating proper alignment of smartphone at end of range.

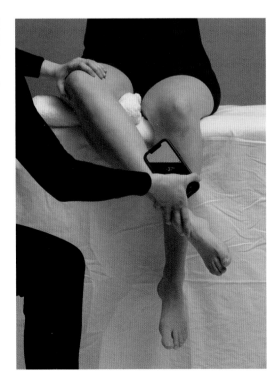

Hip Medial Rotation With Hip Flexed—Smartphone Method

Fig. 11.47 Starting position for measurement of hip medial rotation in seated position. Weight is distributed evenly over both ischial tuberosities. Towel roll is placed under ipsilateral thigh to position femur in horizontal plane.

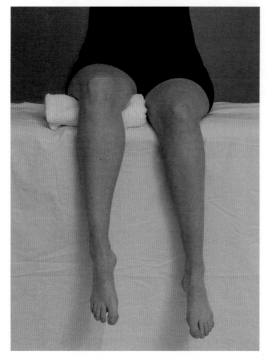

Normal ROM = 30 to 50 degrees.[39,40,44–48,52,53]

Patient position	Seated, with hip and knee flexed to 90 degrees and folded towel under thigh, with weight equally distributed over both ischial tuberosities (Fig. 11.47).
Stabilization	None needed; pelvis is stabilized by patient's weight.
Examiner action	After instructing patient in motion desired, medially rotate patient's hip through available ROM by keeping the thigh stationary and moving the leg, foot, and ankle laterally. Return limb to starting position. Performing passive movement provides an estimate of the ROM and demonstrates to patient exact motion desired (Fig. 11.48).

Fig. 11.48 End of hip medial rotation ROM. Examiner's hand stabilizes thigh against table.

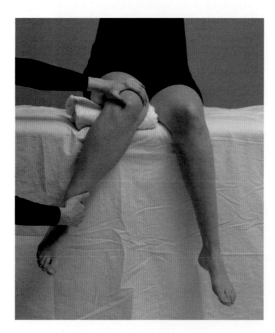

Fig. 11.49 Starting position for measurement of hip medial rotation in seated position, demonstrating proper initial alignment of smartphone.

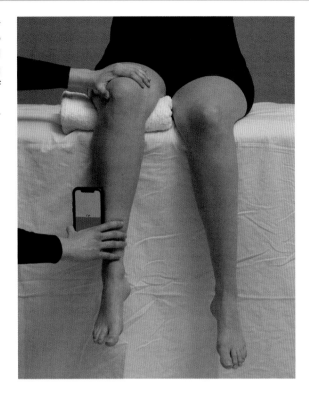

Smartphone alignment

On lateral aspect of lower leg, proximal to the lateral malleolus. Ensure that measurement app on Smartphone reads 0 degrees once it is positioned on patient (Fig. 11.49).

Patient/Examiner action

Perform passive, or have patient perform active, hip medial rotation. Patient should be instructed to maintain equal weight on both ischial tuberosities (Fig. 11.50).Read angle on Smartphone at end of ROM.

Documentation

Record patient's ROM.

Precaution

Do not allow patient to laterally flex trunk to contralateral side or to lift ipsilateral thigh from table during measurement, as doing so will result in a falsely increased ROM.

Fig. 11.50 End of hip medial rotation ROM, demonstrating proper alignment of smartphone at end of range.

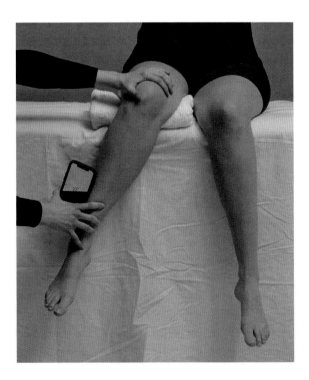

Hip Lateral Rotation With Hip Extended—Goniometer (Video 11.9)

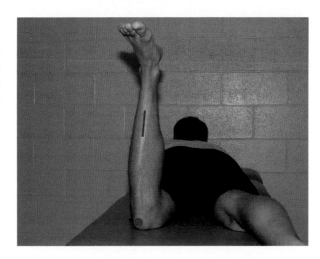

Fig. 11.51 Starting position for measurement of hip lateral rotation in prone position. Bony landmarks for goniometer alignment (midpoint of patella, tibial crest) indicated by red dot and line.

Patient position	Prone, with knees at end of table, knee of lower extremity being measured is flexed to 90 degrees; contralateral lower extremity is slightly abducted (Fig. 11.51).
Stabilization	None needed; pelvis and thigh are stabilized by patient's weight.
Examiner action	After instructing patient in motion desired, laterally rotate patient's hip through available ROM by keeping the thigh stationary and moving the leg, foot, and ankle medially. Return limb to starting position. Performing passive movement provides an estimate of the ROM and demonstrates to patient exact motion desired (Fig. 11.52).
Goniometer alignment	Palpate following bony landmarks as shown in Fig. 11.44 and align goniometer accordingly (Fig. 11.53).
Stationary arm	Perpendicular to floor.
Axis	Midpoint of patella.

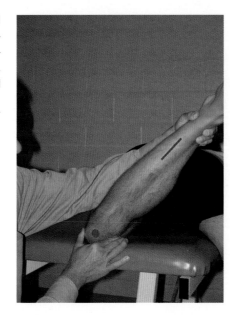

Fig. 11.52 End of hip lateral rotation ROM. Bony landmarks for goniometer alignment (midpoint of patella, tibial crest) indicated by red dot and line.

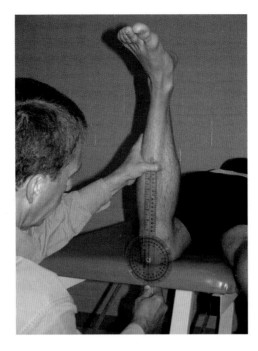

Moving arm	Anterior midline of tibia, along tibial crest.
	Read scale of goniometer.
Patient/Examiner action	Perform passive, or have patient perform active, hip lateral rotation. Patient should be instructed not to allow the hips to come off the support surface (Fig. 11.54).
Confirmation of alignment	Repalpate landmarks and confirm proper goniometric alignment at end of ROM, correcting alignment as necessary (see Fig. 11.54). Read scale of goniometer.
Documentation	Record patient's ROM.
Precaution	Do not allow patient to raise hips from support surface during measurement, as doing so will result in a falsely increased ROM.

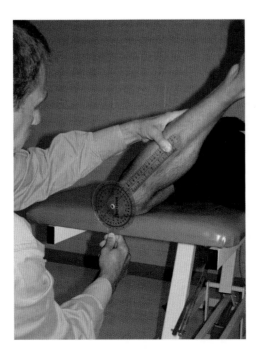

Hip Medial Rotation With Hip Extended—Goniometer (Video 11.10)

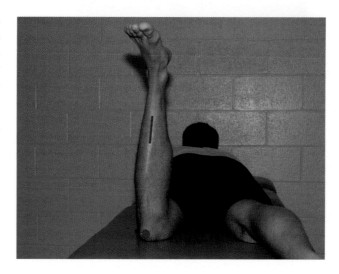

Fig. 11.55 Starting position for measurement of hip medial rotation in prone position. Bony landmarks for goniometer alignment (midpoint of patella, tibial crest) indicated by red dot and line.

Patient position	Prone, with knees at end of table, knee of lower extremity being measured is flexed to 90 degrees; contralateral lower extremity is slightly abducted (Fig. 11.55).
Stabilization	None needed; pelvis and thigh are stabilized by patient's weight.
Examiner action	After instructing patient in motion desired, medially rotate patient's hip through available ROM by keeping the thigh stationary and moving the leg, foot, and ankle laterally. Return limb to starting position. Performing passive movement provides an estimate of the ROM and demonstrates to patient exact motion desired (Fig. 11.56).
Goniometer alignment	Palpate following bony landmarks as shown in Fig. 11.55 and align goniometer accordingly (Fig. 11.57).
Stationary arm	Perpendicular to floor.
Axis	Midpoint of patella.
Moving arm	Anterior midline of tibia, along tibial crest.
	Read scale of goniometer.

Fig. 11.56 End of hip medial rotation ROM. Bony landmarks for goniometer alignment (midpoint of patella, tibial crest) indicated by red dot and line.

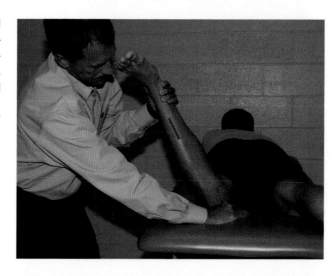

Fig. 11.57 Starting position for measurement of hip medial rotation ROM in prone position, demonstrating proper initial alignment of goniometer.

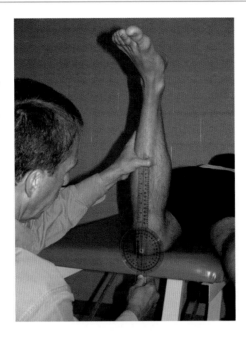

Patient/Examiner action	Perform passive, or have patient perform active, hip medial rotation. Patient should be instructed not to allow hips to come off the support surface (Fig. 11.58).
Confirmation of alignment	Repalpate landmarks and confirm proper goniometric alignment at end of ROM, correcting alignment as necessary (see Fig. 11.58). Read scale of goniometer.
Documentation	Record patient's ROM.
Precaution	Do not allow patient to raise hips from support surface during measurement, as doing so will result in a falsely increased ROM.

Fig. 11.58 End of hip medial rotation ROM, demonstrating proper alignment of goniometer at end range.

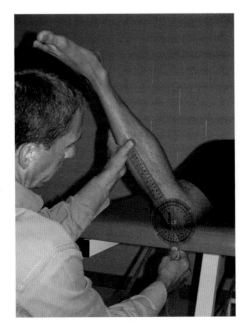

Hip Lateral Rotation With Hip Extended—Inclinometer (Video 11.11)

Fig. 11.59 Starting position for measurement of hip lateral rotation in prone position.

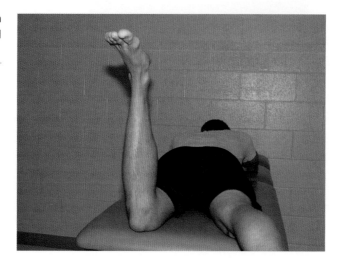

Patient position	Prone, knees at end of table, knee of lower extremity being measured is flexed to 90 degrees, contralateral lower extremity is slightly abducted (Fig. 11.59).
Stabilization	None needed; pelvis and thigh are stabilized by patient's weight.
Examiner action	After instructing patient in motion desired, laterally rotate patient's hip through available ROM by keeping the thigh stationary and moving the leg, foot, and ankle medially. Return limb to starting position. Performing passive movement provides an estimate of the ROM and demonstrates to patient exact motion desired (Fig. 11.60).
Inclinometer alignment	On lateral aspect of lower leg, proximal to the lateral malleolus. Ensure that the inclinometer is set to 0 degrees once it is positioned on patient (Fig. 11.61).

Fig. 11.60 End of hip lateral rotation ROM.

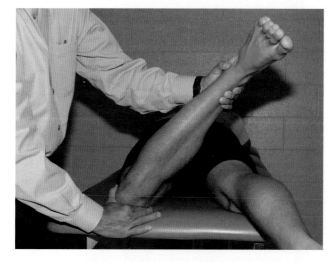

Fig. 11.61 Starting position for measurement of hip lateral rotation ROM in prone position, demonstrating proper initial alignment of inclinometer.

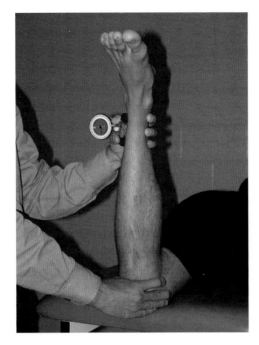

Patient/Examiner action   Perform passive, or have patient perform active, hip lateral rotation. Patient should be instructed not to allow the hips to come off the support surface (Fig. 11.62).

Documentation   Record patient's ROM.

Precaution   Do not allow patient to raise hips from support surface during measurement, as doing so will result in a falsely increased ROM.

Fig. 11.62 End of hip lateral rotation ROM, demonstrating proper alignment of inclinometer at end of range.

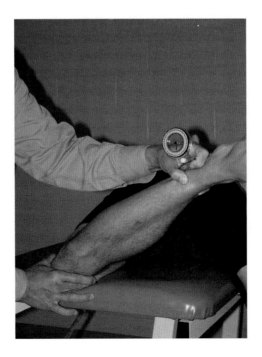

Hip Medial Rotation With Hip Extended—Inclinometer (Video 11.12)

Fig. 11.63 Starting position for measurement of hip medial rotation in prone position.

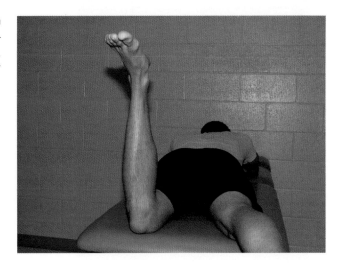

Patient position	Prone, knees at end of table, knee of lower extremity being measured is flexed to 90 degrees; contralateral lower extremity shows slight abduction (Fig. 11.63).
Examiner action	After instructing patient in motion desired, medially rotate patient's hip through available ROM by keeping the thigh stationary and moving the leg, foot, and ankle laterally. Return limb to starting position. Performing passive movement provides an estimate of the ROM and demonstrates to patient exact motion desired (Fig. 11.64).
Stabilization	None needed; pelvis and thigh are stabilized by patient's weight.
Inclinometer alignment	On medial aspect of lower leg, proximal to the medial malleolus. Ensure that the inclinometer is set to 0 degrees once it is positioned on patient (Fig. 11.65).

Fig. 11.64 End of hip medial rotation ROM.

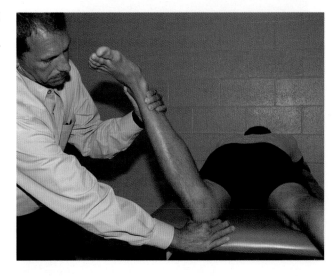

Fig. 11.65 Starting position for measurement of hip medial rotation ROM in prone position, demonstrating proper initial alignment of inclinometer.

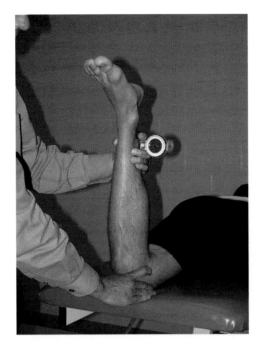

Patient/Examiner action	Perform passive, or have patient perform active, hip medial rotation. Patient should be instructed not to allow the hips to come off the support surface (Fig. 11.66).
Confirmation of alignment	Ensure that feet of inclinometer remain in firm contact with medial aspect of lower leg. Read scale of inclinometer (see Fig. 11.66).
Documentation	Record patient's ROM.
Precaution	Do not allow patient to raise hips from support surface during measurement, as doing so will result in a falsely increased ROM.

Fig. 11.66 End of hip medial rotation ROM, demonstrating proper alignment of inclinometer at end of range.

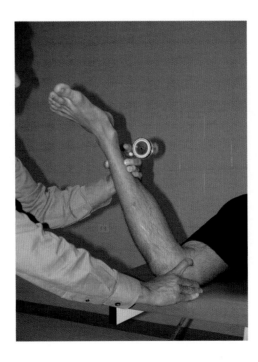

Hip Lateral Rotation With Hip Extended— Smartphone Method

Fig. 11.67 Starting position for measurement of hip lateral rotation in prone position.

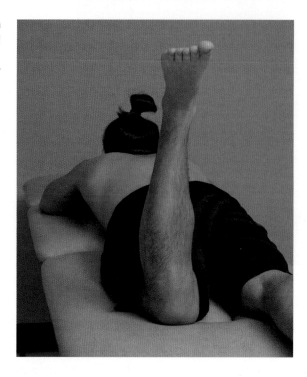

Patient position	Prone, knees at end of table, knee of lower extremity being measured is flexed to 90 degrees, contralateral lower extremity is slightly abducted (Fig. 11.67).
Stabilization	None needed; pelvis and thigh are stabilized by patient's weight.
Examiner action	After instructing patient in motion desired, laterally rotate patient's hip through available ROM by keeping the thigh stationary and moving the leg, foot, and ankle medially. Return limb to starting position. Performing passive movement provides an estimate of the ROM and demonstrates to patient exact motion desired (Fig. 11.68).

Fig. 11.68 End of hip lateral rotation ROM.

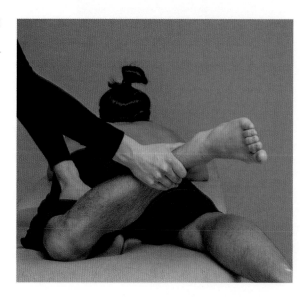

Fig. 11.69 Starting position for measurement of hip lateral rotation ROM in prone position, demonstrating proper initial alignment of smartphone.

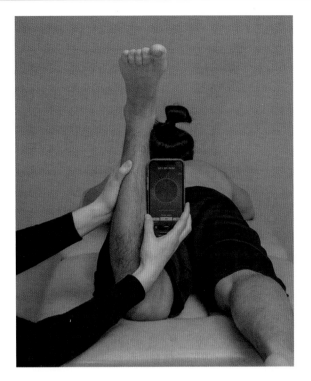

Smartphone alignment	On medial aspect of lower leg, proximal to the medial malleolus. Ensure that measurement app on Smartphone reads 0 degrees once it is positioned on patient (Fig. 11.69).
Patient/Examiner action	Perform passive, or have patient perform active, hip lateral rotation. Patient should be instructed not to allow the hips to come off the support surface (Fig. 11.70). Read angle on Smartphone at end of ROM.
Documentation	Record patient's ROM.
Precaution	Do not allow patient to raise hips from support surface during measurement, as doing so will result in a falsely increased ROM.

Fig. 11.70 End of hip lateral rotation ROM, demonstrating proper alignment of smartphone at end of range.

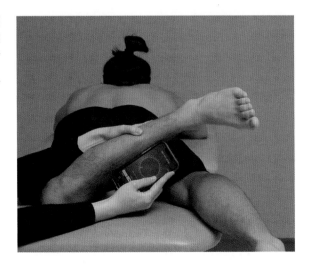

Hip Medial Rotation With Hip Flexed—Smartphone Method

Fig. 11.71 Starting position for measurement of hip medial rotation in prone position.

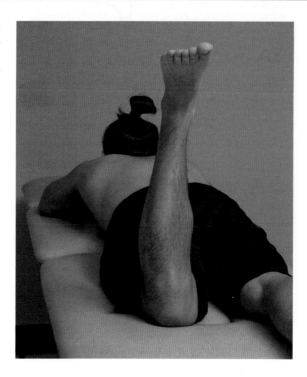

Patient position	Prone, knees at end of table, knee of lower extremity being measured is flexed to 90 degrees; contralateral lower extremity shows slight abduction (Fig. 11.71).
Examiner action	After instructing patient in motion desired, medially rotate patient's hip through available ROM by keeping the thigh stationary and moving the leg, foot, and ankle laterally. Return limb to starting position. Performing passive movement provides an estimate of the ROM and demonstrates to patient exact motion desired (Fig. 11.72).
Stabilization	None needed; pelvis and thigh are stabilized by patient's weight.

Fig. 11.72 End of hip medial rotation ROM.

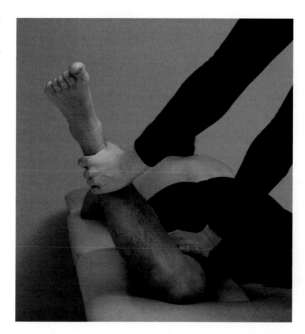

Fig. 11.73 Starting position for measurement of hip medial rotation ROM in prone position, demonstrating proper initial alignment of smartphone.

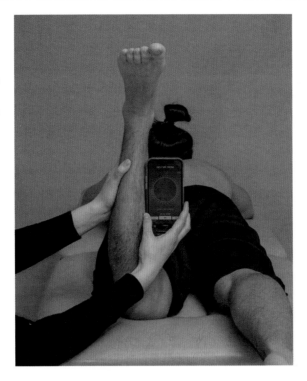

Smartphone alignment

On medial aspect of lower leg, proximal to the medial malleolus. Ensure that measurement app on Smartphone reads 0 degrees once it is positioned on patient (Fig. 11.73).

Patient/Examiner action

Perform passive, or have patient perform active, hip medial rotation. Patient should be instructed not to allow the hips to come off the support surface (Fig. 11.74). Read angle on Smartphone at end of ROM.

Documentation

Record patient's ROM.

Precaution

Do not allow patient to raise hips from support surface during measurement, as doing so will result in a falsely increased ROM.

Fig. 11.74 End of hip medial rotation ROM, demonstrating proper alignment of smartphone at end of range.

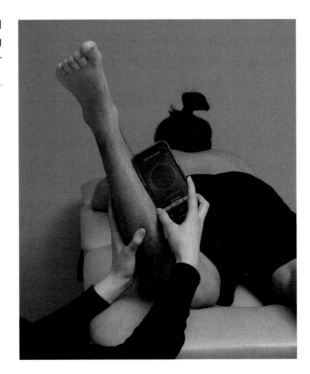

References

1. Clemente C. *Gray's Anatomy of the Human Body.* 13th ed. Philadelphia: Lea & Febiger; 1985.
2. Moore KL, Dalley AF, Agur AMR. *Clinically Oriented Anatomy.* 7th ed. Philadelphia: Wolters Kluwer Health/Lippincott Williams & Wilkins; 2013:1134.
3. Fuss FK, Bacher A. New aspects of the morphology and function of the human hip joint ligaments. *Am J Anat.* 1991;192(1):1–13.
4. Martin HD, et al. The function of the hip capsular ligaments: a quantitative report. *Arthroscopy.* 2008;24(2):188–195.
5. Levangie PK, Norkin CC. *Joint Structure and Function: A Comprehensive Analysis.* Philadelphia: F.A. Davis Co; 2011:588.
6. Neumann D. *Kinesiology of the Musculoskeletal System: Foundations for Rehabilitation.* 2nd ed. St. Louis, MO: Mosby/Elsevier; 2010.
7. Crowninshield RD, et al. A biomechanical investigation of the human hip. *J Biomech.* 1978;11(1–2):75–85.
8. Cyriax JH, Coldham M. *Textbook of Orthopaedic Medicine.* London: Baillière Tindall; 1982.
9. Kaltenborn F. *Mobilization of the Extremity Joints.* 3rd ed. Oslo: Olaf Norlis Bokhandel; 1980.
10. Johnston RC, Smidt GL. Measurement of hip-joint motion during walking. Evaluation of an electrogoniometric method. *J Bone Joint Surg Am.* 1969;51(6):1082–1094.
11. Oberg T, Karsznia A, Oberg K. Joint angle parameters in gait: reference data for normal subjects, 10–79 years of age. *J Rehabil Res Dev.* 1994;31(3):199–213.
12. Ostrosky KM, et al. A comparison of gait characteristics in young and old subjects. *Phys Ther.* 1994;74(7):637–646.
13. Steultjens MP, et al. Range of joint motion and disability in patients with osteoarthritis of the knee or hip. *Rheumatology (Oxford).* 2000;39(9):955–961.
14. Amigos RL. *Observational Gait Analysis.* Downey, CA: LAREI; 2001.
15. Jacobsen JS, et al. Changes in walking and running in patients with hip dysplasia. *Acta Orthop.* 2013;84(3):265–270.
16. Eitzen I, et al. Sagittal plane gait characteristics in hip osteoarthritis patients with mild to moderate symptoms compared to healthy controls: a cross-sectional study. *BMC Musculoskelet Disord.* 2012;13:258.
17. Diamond LE, et al. Hip joint biomechanics during gait in people with and without symptomatic femoroacetabular impingement. *Gait Posture.* 2016;43(1):198–203.
18. Han S, Cheng G, Xu P. Three-dimensional lower extremity kinematics of Chinese during activities of daily living. *J Back Musculoskelet Rehabil.* 2015;28:327–334.
19. Livingston LA, Stevenson JM, Olney SJ. Stairclimbing kinematics on stairs of differing dimensions. *Arch Phys Med Rehabil.* 1991;72(6):398–402.
20. Protopapadaki A, et al. Hip, knee, ankle kinematics and kinetics during stair ascent and descent in healthy young individuals. *Clin Biomech (Bristol, Avon).* 2007;22(2):203–210.
21. Ikeda ER, et al. Influence of age on dynamics of rising from a chair. *Phys Ther.* 1991;71(6):473–481.
22. Tully EA, Fotoohabadi MR, Galea MP. Sagittal spine and lower limb movement during sit-to-stand in healthy young subjects. *Gait Posture.* 2005;22(4):338–345.
23. Hyodo K, Masuda T, Aizawa J, Jinno T, Morita S. Hip, knee and ankle kinematics during activities of daily living: a cross-sectional study. *Braz J Phys Ther.* 2017;21:159–166.
24. Vander Linden DW, Wilhelm IJ. Electromyographic and cinematographic analysis of movement from a kneeling to a standing position in healthy 5- to 7-year-old children. *Phys Ther.* 1991;71(1):3–15.
25. Hemmerich A, et al. Hip, knee, and ankle kinematics of high range of motion activities of daily living. *J Orthop Res.* 2006;24(4):770–781.
26. Kapoor A, et al. Range of movements of lower limb joints in cross-legged sitting posture. *J Arthroplasty.* 2008;23(3):451–453.
27. Mulholland SJ, Wyss UP. Activities of daily living in non-Western cultures: range of motion requirements for hip and knee joint implants. *Int J Rehabil Res.* 2001;24(3):191–198.
28. American Medical Association. *Guides to the Evaluation of Permanent Impairment.* 4th ed. Chicago: American Medical Association; 1993:339.
29. Greene WB, Heckman JD. *The Clinical Measurement of Joint Motion.* Rosemont, IL: American Academy of Orthopaedic Surgeons; 1994.
30. Mundale MO, et al. Evaluation of extension of the hip. *Arch Phys Med Rehabil.* 1956;37(2):75–80.
31. Milch H. The pelvifemoral angle. *J Bone Joint Surg.* 1942;24:148–153.
32. Steindler A. *Mechanics of Normal and Pathological Locomotion in Man.* Springfield, IL: Thomas; 1935:424.
33. Kendall F, McCreary E, Provance P. *Muscles: Testing and Function.* 4th ed. Baltimore: Williams & Wilkins; 1993.
34. Milch H. The measurement of hip motion in the sagittal and coronal planes. *J Bone Joint Surg Am.* 1959;41(A(4)):731–736.
35. Moore M. Clinical assessment of joint motion. In: Basmajian JV, ed. *Therapeutic Exercise.* Baltimore: Williams & Wilkins; 1978.
36. Bartlett MD, et al. Hip flexion contractures: a comparison of measurement methods. *Arch Phys Med Rehabil.* 1985;66(9):620–625.
37. Drews JE, Vraciu JK, Pellino G. Range of motion of the joints of the lower extremities of newborns. *Phys Occup Ther Pediatr.* 1984;4:49–62.
38. Reese NB, Bandy WD. Use of an inclinometer to measure flexibility of the iliotibial band using the Ober test and the modified Ober test: differences in magnitude and reliability of measurements. *J Orthop Sports Phys Ther.* 2003;33(6):326–330.
39. Haley ET. Range of hip rotation and torque of hip rotator muscle groups. *Am J Phys Med.* 1953;32(5):261–270.
40. Simoneau GG, et al. Influence of hip position and gender on active hip internal and external rotation. *J Orthop Sports Phys Ther.* 1998;28(3):158–164.
41. Bierma-Zeinstra SM, et al. Comparison between two devices for measuring hip joint motions. *Clin Rehabil.* 1998;12(6):497–505.
42. Ellison JB, Rose SJ, Sahrmann SA. Patterns of hip rotation range of motion: a comparison between healthy subjects and patients with low back pain. *Phys Ther.* 1990;70(9):537–541.
43. Ahlback S, Lindahl O. Sagittal mobility of the hip joint. *Acta Orthop Scand.* 1964;34:310–322.
44. Ahlberg A, Moussa M, Al-Nahdi M. On geographical variations in the normal range of joint motion. *Clin Orthop Relat Res.* 1988;234:229–231.
45. Boone DC, et al. Reliability of goniometric measurements. *Phys Ther.* 1978;58(11):1355–1360.
46. Macedo LG, Magee DJ. Effects of age on passive range of motion of selected peripheral joints in healthy adult females. *Physiother Theory Pract.* 2009;25(2):145–164.
47. Roaas A, Andersson GB. Normal range of motion of the hip, knee and ankle joints in male subjects, 30-40 years of age. *Acta Orthop Scand.* 1982;53(2):205–208.
48. Roach KE, Miles TP. Normal hip and knee active range of motion: the relationship to age. *Phys Ther.* 1991;71(9):656–665.
49. Soucie JM, et al. Range of motion measurements: reference values and a database for comparison studies. *Haemophilia.* 2011;17(3):500–507.
50. Nussbaumer S, et al. Validity and test-retest reliability of manual goniometers for measuring passive hip range of motion in femoroacetabular impingement patients. *BMC Musculoskelet Disord .* 2010;11:194.
51. Pua YH, et al. Intrarater test-retest reliability of hip range of motion and hip muscle strength measurements in persons with hip osteoarthritis. *Arch Phys Med Rehabil.* 2008;89(6):1146–1154.
52. Hoaglund FT, Yau AC, Wong WL. Osteoarthritis of the hip and other joints in southern Chinese in Hong Kong. *J Bone Joint Surg Am.* 1973;55(3):545–557.
53. Svenningsen S, et al. Hip motion related to age and sex. *Acta Orthop Scand.* 1989;60(1):97–100.
54. Walker JM, et al. Active mobility of the extremities in older subjects. *Phys Ther.* 1984;64(6):919–923.
55. Gradoz MC, Bauer LE, Grindstaff TL, Bagwell JJ. Reliability of hip rotation range of motion in supine and seated positions. *J Sport Rehabil.* 2018. https://doi.org/10.1123/jsr.2017-0243.
56. Krause DA, Hollman JH, Krych AJ, Kalisvaart MM, Levy BA. Reliability of hip internal rotation range of motion measurement using a digital inclinometer. *Knee Surg Sports Traumatol Arthrosc.* 2015;23:2562–2567.

12

MEASUREMENT of RANGE of MOTION of the KNEE

Nancy Berryman Reese

ANATOMY

The knee joint consists of three separate articulations within a single joint capsule—one articulation between each convex femoral condyle and the corresponding tibial condyle and intervening meniscus and a third articulation between the patella and the anterior aspect of the distal femur (Fig. 12.1). The two tibial condyles are very slightly concave and are deepened somewhat by the fibrocartilaginous medial and lateral menisci, which are attached to the periphery of the tibial condyles.[1-3] Because there is significant bony incongruency at the knee joint (large convex femoral condyles articulating with relatively flat tibial condyles), stability of this joint occurs primarily via soft-tissue structures (capsule, ligaments, and particularly muscles) around and within the joint.[2,4-6] The articular capsule surrounding the knee joint is large, thin, and incomplete in some areas where muscle tendons replace fibers of the capsule.[2,4] Tendons of the quadriceps femoris, tensor fasciae latae, gastrocnemius, sartorius, and semimembranosus muscles all contribute fibers to and strengthen the articular capsule of the knee joint (Figs. 12.2 and 12.3).[2,3,7] Ligamentous reinforcement of the knee joint occurs via five extracapsular ligaments (patellar, oblique popliteal, arcuate popliteal, tibial collateral, and fibular collateral) (see Figs. 12.2 and 12.3) and two intraarticular ligaments (anterior and posterior cruciate) (Fig. 12.4).[2,4] Other ligaments that have been described as significant stabilizers of the knee joint include the fabellofibular ligament, the medial patellofemoral ligament, and the short lateral ligament.[3,8,9]

Each of the two articulations between the femoral and tibial condyles and the menisci can be described as separate joints,[2,10] but each is treated as a single joint, the tibiofemoral joint, during range of motion (ROM) measurements. Motion at the articulation between the patella and the anterior femur, the patellofemoral joint, typically is not measured clinically using a goniometer. Therefore only tibiofemoral motion is considered in the following discussion of the knee joint.

OSTEOKINEMATICS

Classic explanations of movements occurring at the knee joint describe active motion as including flexion and extension, which occur around a transverse axis passing through the femoral condyles, and rotation of the tibia, which occurs around a longitudinal axis passing through the medial intercondylar tubercle.[11-13] According to this description of knee motion, the axis for flexion and extension of the knee is not fixed but moves as the knee flexes.[13,14] Other investigators have challenged this classic description, asserting that flexion and extension of the knee occur around a fixed, oblique axis that extends from the lateral, posterior, inferior aspect of the knee to its medial, anterior, superior aspect.[15] This axis is described as passing through the lateral and medial femoral epicondyles (at the point of attachment of the collateral ligaments) and superior to the decussation of the cruciate ligaments. Thus the axis for knee flexion and extension lies not in the transverse plane but at an angle to all three cardinal planes, producing combined motions of flexion, adduction, and medial rotation, as well as extension, abduction, and lateral rotation.

Rotation at the knee, which occurs passively during flexion and extension motions and is associated with the locking mechanism of the knee, also may be produced actively but only when the knee is flexed.[12,16-18] Active rotation is impossible when the knee is extended fully because of the tightness of the collateral and cruciate ligaments.[2,12,17] Typically, only flexion and extension of the knee and not rotation are measured clinically.

ARTHROKINEMATICS

During the movements of knee flexion and extension, motion occurs as a result of rolling, spinning, and gliding of the femoral condyles upon the tibial plateaus.[5] Because motion occurs between the convex femoral condyles and the relatively flat tibial condyles, femoral roll and glide occur in opposite directions. As flexion is initiated with the tibia fixed, the femur rotates laterally, producing a spin of the femoral condyles. Continued knee flexion occurs as a result of posterior rolling and anterior gliding of the femoral condyles on the tibial plateaus. Most of the gliding motion appears to occur between the lateral femoral condyle and the lateral tibial plateau, with the medial

LATERAL VIEW

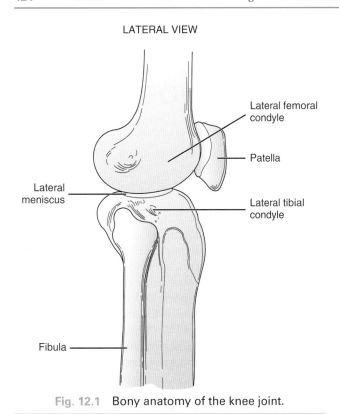

Fig. 12.1   Bony anatomy of the knee joint.

femoral condyle demonstrating only a small amount of anterior–posterior translation.[11,19] Motion in the opposite direction—anterior roll and posterior glide of the femoral condyles on the tibia—occurs during weight-bearing knee extension.[18]

LIMITATIONS OF MOTION: KNEE JOINT

Knee flexion is limited by soft-tissue approximation between the structures of the posterior thigh and calf, provided that the hip also is in some degree of flexion.[12,20] Flexion of the knee may be limited prematurely if the hip is extended because of tension in the rectus femoris muscle, which crosses the anterior aspect of both hip and knee joints.[21] The preferred position for measurement of knee flexion is with the patient supine and the hip flexed in order to avoid such premature stoppage of motion. Capsular and ligamentous structures provide the primary limitation of knee extension, provided the hip is extended as well.[12,14] When the hip is flexed, extension of the knee may be limited by tension in the hamstring muscle group.[18,21] Information regarding normal ranges of motion for the knee is found in Appendix B.

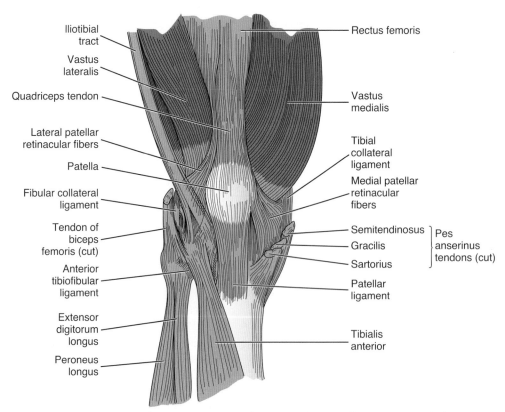

Fig. 12.2   Anterior view of knee joint illustrating muscular and ligamentous reinforcement.

POSTERIOR VIEW

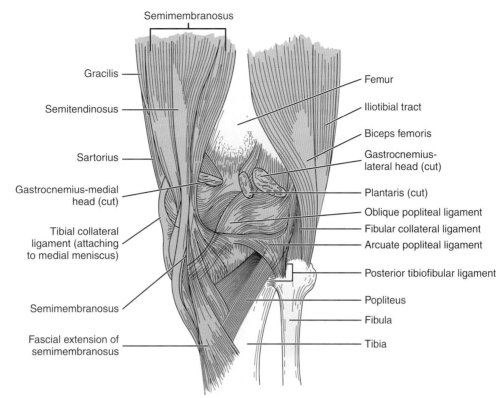

Fig. 12.3   Posterior view of knee joint illustrating muscular and ligamentous reinforcement.

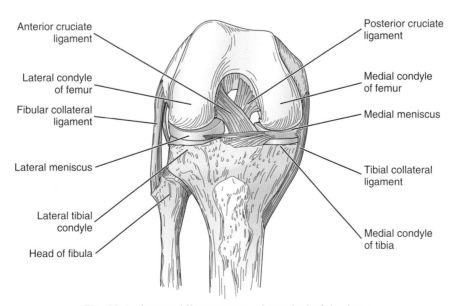

Fig. 12.4   Internal ligaments and menisci of the knee.

END-FEEL

Normal end-feels for knee flexion are soft (soft-tissue approximation) with the hip flexed and firm (muscular) and with the hip extended. Normal end-feels for knee extension are firm (capsular/ligamentous) with the hip extended and firm (muscular) with the hip flexed.

CAPSULAR PATTERN

The capsular pattern of the knee joint means that flexion is more limited than extension. Rotation of the tibia is not restricted if the capsule is involved.[22,23]

RANGE OF MOTION AND FUNCTIONAL ACTIVITY

Numerous authors have investigated the motion of the knee joint during functional activities. Much of this research has been related to knee motion during ambulatory activities such as walking on level ground,[24–31] walking up and down slopes,[27,31] and ascending (Fig. 12.5) and descending stairs.[24,26,27,31–34] Additional investigations have examined knee motion during other daily activities such as sitting onto and rising from a chair,[24,26,27,31,32,35] driving a car,[36] entering and exiting a bath,[27,31,37] lifting an object from the floor[32] (Fig. 12.6), dressing,[32,37] and transitioning from a kneeling to a standing position.[38] A few authors also have examined knee motion in so-called high range of motion activities such as kneeling (Fig. 12.7), squatting, and sitting cross-legged.[24,25,38–40]

A summary of knee ROM related to various functional activities is shown in Table 12.1. Most of the studies from which data were derived were performed in healthy adults, although some investigations included elderly and pediatric subjects. Essentials of the study populations and instrumentation used are included in the table. Caution should be used in extrapolating these data to the general population because the sample sizes for almost all of the studies were quite small. For more in-depth information on each study, the reader is referred to the reference list at the end of this chapter.

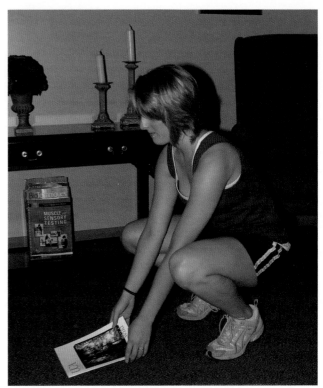

Fig. 12.6 Flexion of the knee while lifting an object from the floor.

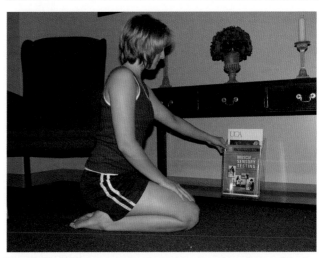

Fig. 12.7 Flexion of the knee during kneeling with the ankle plantarflexed.

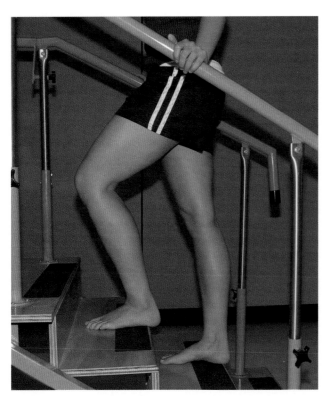

Fig. 12.5 Flexion of the knee during stair ascent.

Table 12.1   KNEE ROM DURING FUNCTIONAL ACTIVITIES

FUNCTIONAL ACTIVITY	MAXIMUM KNEE FLEXION REQUIRED	MAXIMUM KNEE EXTENSION REQUIRED	COMMENTS
Ambulation–Level Ground			
Desloovere et al.[24]	$64° \pm 5°$	$-3° \pm 4°$	Measured ROM using optical data capturing system (Vicon Motion Systems) in 10 healthy adults (1 F, 9 M; mean age 29 ± 9 years)
Han et al.[25]	$66° \pm 5°$		Measured 40 healthy Chinese adults; mean age 21 years (20 F, 20 M) using Optotrak system
Jevsevar et al.[26]	$65° \pm 7°$ (young group) $62° \pm 9°$ (old group)		Measured ROM using Selspot data acquisition system in 11 subjects divided into 2 groups according to age. Young group ($n=5$) aged <40 years; old group ($n=6$) aged >60 years
Myles et al.[27]	$67° \pm 6°$ (control group) $59° \pm 10°$ (subjects 18–24 months post TKA)	$-2° \pm 7°$ (control group) $-4° \pm 7°$ (subjects 18–14 months post TKA)	Measured ROM using an electrogoniometer in 50 patients following TKA (mean age$=70 \pm 9.2$ years) and in 20 age-matched controls (mean age$=67 \pm 8.2$ years)
Öberg et al.[28]	$57° - 73°$		Measured 116 M, 117 F aged 10–79 years at 3 different gait speeds, knee flexion ↑ as gait speed ↑, ↓ as age ↑
Ostrosky et al.[29]	$66° \pm 4°$ (young group) $69° \pm 5°$ (old group)	$-3° \pm 4°$ (young group) $-7° \pm 4°$ (old group)	Measured peak ROM during free speed walking using Expert Vision motion analysis system in 60 subjects divided into 2 groups according to age. Young group ($n=30$; 15 F, 15 M) aged 20–40 years; old group (n$=30$; 15 F, 15 M) aged 60–80 years
Rancho Los Amigos[30]	$60°$	$-5°$	Undefined subject group and methodology
Rowe et al.[31]	$67° \pm 6°$	$-2° \pm 7°$	Measured 20 healthy adults aged 49–80 years (16 F, 4 M) using Penny and Giles electrogoniometer
Ambulation–Ascending Slope			
Myles et al.[27]	$65° \pm 8°$ (control group) $58° \pm 10°$ (subjects 18 – 24 months post TKA)	$-2° \pm 7°$ (control group) $-7° \pm 7°$ (subjects 18–14 months post TKA)	Measured ROM using an electrogoniometer in 50 patients following TKA (mean age$=70 \pm 9.2$ years) and in 20 age-matched controls (mean age$=67 \pm 8.2$ years)
Rowe et al.[31]	$65° \pm 8°$	$-2° \pm 7°$	Measured 20 healthy adults aged 49–80 years (16 F, 4 M) using Penny and Giles electrogoniometer
Ambulation–Descending Slope			
Myles et al.[27]	$72° \pm 8°$ (control group) $62° \pm 10°$ (subjects 18–24 months post TKA)	$-3° \pm 8°$ (control group) $-4° \pm 7°$ (subjects 18–14 months post TKA)	Measured ROM using an electrogoniometer in 50 patients following TKA (mean age$=70 \pm 9.2$ years) and in 20 age-matched controls (mean age$=67 \pm 8.2$ years)
Rowe et al.[31]	$72° \pm 8°$	$-3° \pm 8°$	Measured 20 healthy adults aged 49–80 years (16 F, 4 M) using Penny and Giles electrogoniometer
Ambulation–Ascending Stairs			
Desloovere et al.[24]	$95° \pm 6°$	$-11° \pm 3°$	Measured ROM using optical data capturing system (Vicon Motion Systems) in 10 healthy adults (1 F, 9 M; mean age 29 ± 9 years)
Jevsevar et al.[26]	$99° \pm 7°$ (young group) $88° \pm 9°$ (old group)		Measured ROM using Selspot data acquisition system in 11 subjects divided into 2 groups according to age. Young group ($n=5$) aged <40 years; old group ($n=6$) aged >60 years; 18 cm stair rise height
Laubenthal et al.[32]	$83° \pm 8°$	$0°$	Measured 30 healthy males average age 25 years using electrogoniometer; no chair height cited
Livingston et al.[33] 20.3 cm stair rise height 20.3 cm stair rise height 12.7 cm stair rise height	$96° \pm 5° – 105° \pm 4°$ $96° \pm 4° – 102° \pm 5$ $83° \pm 3° – 92° \pm 3°$	$-5° \pm 1° – 15° \pm 1°$ $-6° \pm 4° – 11° \pm 1°$ $-2° \pm 4° – 8° \pm 3°$	Used cinematographic analysis to measure 15 healthy F aged 19–26 years divided into 3 groups according to height; taller subjects used ↓ knee flexion and ↑ knee extension compared with shorter subjects on identical steps

Continued

Table 12.1	KNEE ROM DURING FUNCTIONAL ACTIVITIES—cont'd		
FUNCTIONAL ACTIVITY	**MAXIMUM KNEE FLEXION REQUIRED**	**MAXIMUM KNEE EXTENSION REQUIRED**	**COMMENTS**
Myles et al.[27]	$99° \pm 10°$ (control group) $78° \pm 12°$ (subjects 18–24 months post TKA)	$-18° \pm 6°$ (control group) $-12° \pm 6°$ (subjects 18–14 months post TKA)	Measured ROM using an electrogoniometer in 50 patients following TKA (mean age = 70 ± 9.2 years) and in 20 age-matched controls (mean age = 67 ± 8.2 years)
Protopapadaki et al.[34]	$65° \pm 7°$		Measured 33 healthy adults aged 18–39 years (16 M, 17 F); stair rise height 18 cm
Rowe et al.[31]	$99° \pm 10°$	$18° \pm 6°$	Measured 20 healthy adults aged 49–80 years (16 F, 4 M) using Penny and Giles electrogoniometer; 16.5 stair rise height
Ambulation–Descending Stairs			
Desloovere et al.[24]	$66° \pm 56°$	$-5° \pm 3°$	Measured ROM using optical data capturing system (Vicon Motion Systems) in 10 healthy adults (1 F, 9 M; mean age 29 ± 9 years)
Jevsevar et al.[26]	$90° \pm 5°$ (young group) $84° \pm 5°$ (old group)		Measured ROM using Selspot data acquisition system in 11 subjects divided into 2 groups according to age. Young group ($n = 5$) aged <40 years; old group ($n = 6$) aged >60 years; 18 cm stair rise height
Laubenthal et al.[32]	$83° \pm 8°$	$0°$	Measured 30 healthy males average age 25 years using electrogoniometer; no chair height cited
Livingston et al.[33] 20.3 cm stair rise height 20.3 cm stair rise height 12.7 cm stair rise height	$93° \pm 2° - 102° \pm 2°$ $96° \pm 1° - 107° \pm 1°$ $86° \pm 1° - 96° \pm 3°$	$-7° \pm 2° - 15° \pm 4°$ $-1° \pm 4° - 18° \pm 2°$ $-3° \pm 2° - 13° \pm 3°$	Used cinematographic analysis to measure 15 healthy F aged 19–26 years divided into 3 groups according to height; taller subjects used ↓ knee flexion and ↑ knee extension compared with shorter subjects on identical steps
Myles et al.[27]	$97° \pm 9°$ (control group) $76° \pm 16°$ (subjects 18–24 months post TKA)	$-19° \pm 8°$ (control group) $-11° \pm 6°$ (subjects 18–14 months post TKA)	Measured ROM using an electrogoniometer in 50 patients following TKA (mean age = 70 ± 9.2 years) and in 20 age-matched controls (mean age = 67 ± 8.2 years)
Protopapadaki et al.[34]	$40° \pm 8°$		Measured 33 healthy adults aged 18–39 years (16 M, 17 F); stair rise height 18 cm
Rowe et al.[31]	$97° \pm 9°$	$19° \pm 8°$	Measured 20 healthy adults aged 49–80 years (16 F, 4 M); used Penny and Giles electrogoniometer; 16.5 stair rise height
Rising from a Chair			
Desloovere et al.[24]	$86° \pm 5°$	$-4° \pm 5°$	Measured ROM using optical data capturing system (Vicon Motion Systems) in 10 healthy adults (1 F, 9 M; mean age 29 ± 9 years)
Jevsevar et al.[26]	$97° \pm 9°$ (young group) $84° \pm 5°$ (old group)		Measured ROM using Selspot data acquisition system in 11 subjects divided into 2 groups according to age. Young group ($n = 5$) aged <40 years; old group ($n = 6$) aged >60 years; chair seat set at knee height for each subject
Myles et al.[27]	$105° \pm 10°$ (control group–low chair) $99° \pm 10°$ (control group–standard chair) $79° \pm 14°$ (subjects 18–24 months post TKA–low chair) $81° \pm 13°$ (subjects 18–24 months post TKA–standard chair)	$-8° \pm 7°$ (control group—low chair) $-8° \pm 9°$ (control group—standard chair) $-6° \pm 7°$ (subjects 18–14 months post TKA—low chair) $-6° \pm 5°$ (subjects 18–14 months post TKA–standard chair)	Measured ROM using an electrogoniometer in 50 patients following TKA (mean age = 70 ± 9.2 years) and in 20 age-matched controls (mean age = 67 ± 8.2 years)
Rowe et al.[31]	$105° \pm 10°$ (low chair; 38 cm high) $99° \pm 10°$ (standard chair; 46 cm high)	$-8° \pm 7°$ (low chair) $-8° \pm 9°$ (standard chair)	Measured 20 healthy adults aged 49–80 years (16 F, 4 M); used Penny and Giles electrogoniometer
Tully et al.[35]	$105° \pm 5°$	$0° \pm 6°$	Measured ROM using two-dimensional Peak Motus system in 47 healthy subjects (27 F, 20 M) aged 18–30 years

Table 12.1   KNEE ROM DURING FUNCTIONAL ACTIVITIES—cont'd

FUNCTIONAL ACTIVITY	MAXIMUM KNEE FLEXION REQUIRED	MAXIMUM KNEE EXTENSION REQUIRED	COMMENTS
Sitting onto Chair			
Laubenthal et al.[32]	93°±10° (45 cm seat height)	0°	Measured 30 healthy males average age 25 years using electrogoniometer
Myles et al.[27]	102°±12° (control group–low chair)	−8°±8° (control group–low chair)	Measured ROM using an electrogoniometer in 50 patients following TKA (mean age=70±9.2 years) and in 20 age-matched controls (mean age=67±8.2 years)
	99°±11° (control group–standard chair)	−6°±8° (control group–standard chair)	
	78°±17° (subjects 18–24 months post TKA–low chair)	−5°±4° (subjects 18–14 months post TKA–low chair)	
	79°±14° (subjects 18–24 months post TKA–standard chair)	−6°±6° (subjects 18–14 months post TKA–standard chair)	
Rowe et al.[31]	102°±12° (low chair; 38 cm high)	−8°±8° (low chair)	Measured 20 healthy adults aged 49–80 years (16 F, 4 M); used Penny and Giles electrogoniometer
	99°±11° (standard chair; 46 cm high)	−6°±8° (standard chair)	
Driving a Car			
Latz et al.[36]	80°–85°		Measured ROM using an electrogoniometer (Twin Axis type SG 65, Biometrics Ltd.) in 20 healthy adults (10F, 10M) with a mean age of 29.4±3.0 years
Entering Bath			
Myles et al.[27]	131°±13° (control group)	−1°±6° (control group)	Measured ROM using an electrogoniometer in 50 patients following TKA (mean age=70±9.2 years) and in 20 age-matched controls (mean age=67±8.2 years)
	78°±15° (subjects 18–24 months post TKA)	−4°±7° (subjects 18–14 months post TKA)	
Rowe et al.[31]	131°±13° (step in and sit down; 59 cm high)	−1°±6°	Measured 20 healthy adults aged 49–80 years (16 F, 4 M) using Penny and Giles electrogoniometer
Hyodo et al.[37]	124°±7° to 128°±7°	−1°±1° to −1°±2°	Measured 26 healthy adults aged 20±1 years (13F, 13M) using Fastrak system
Exiting Bath			
Myles et al.[27]	138°±14° (control group)	−3°±7° (control group)	Measured ROM using an electrogoniometer in 50 patients following TKA (mean age=70±9.2 years) and in 20 age-matched controls (mean age=67±8.2 years)
	78°±18° (subjects 18–24 months post TKA)	−5°±7° (subjects 18–14 months post TKA)	
Rowe et al.[31]	138°±14°	−3°±7°	Measured 20 healthy adults aged 49–80 years (16 F, 4 M) using Penny and Giles electrogoniometer
Hyodo et al.[37]	143°±8°	−31°±1°	Measured 26 healthy adults aged 20±1 years (13F, 13M) using Fastrak system
Putting on Pants (in sitting)			
Hyodo et al.[37]	119°±8°	−42°±11°	Measured 26 healthy adults aged 20±1 years (13F, 13M) using Fastrak system
Putting on Pants (in standing)			
Hyodo et al.[37]	115°±8°	−1°±2°	Measured 26 healthy adults aged 20±1 years (13F, 13M) using Fastrak system
Putting on Shoes (foot on ankle)			
Hyodo et al.[37]	103°±6°	−71°±9°	Measured 26 healthy adults aged 20±1 years (13F, 13M) using Fastrak system
Putting on Shoes (foot on knee)			
Hyodo et al.[37]	84°±10°	−55°±12°	Measured 26 healthy adults aged 20±1 years (13F, 13M) using Fastrak system
Tying Shoes			
Laubenthal et al.[32]	106°±9°	0°	Measured 30 healthy M average age 25 years using electrogoniometer
Hyodo et al.[37]	77°±9° to 78°±9°	−73°±11° to −75°±10°	Measured 26 healthy adults aged 20±1 years (13F, 13M) using Fastrak system
Lifting Object from Floor			
Laubenthal et al.[32]	117°±13°	0°	Measured 30 healthy M average age 25 years using electrogoniometer

Continued

	Table 12.1 KNEE ROM DURING FUNCTIONAL ACTIVITIES—cont'd		
FUNCTIONAL ACTIVITY	**MAXIMUM KNEE FLEXION REQUIRED**	**MAXIMUM KNEE EXTENSION REQUIRED**	**COMMENTS**
Kneeling			
Hemmerich et al.[38]	155° (ankle dorsiflexed) 144° (ankle plantarflexed)		Measured ROM in 30 Indian subjects average age 48 years (10 F, 20 M) using Fastrack system
Kneel-to-Stand			
Vander Linden and Wilhelm[39]	131° ± 3°	0° ± 9°	Measured ROM during kneel-to-stand movement in 10 healthy children aged 5–7 years (6 F, 4 M) using cinematography
Sitting Cross-Legged			
Hemmerich et al.[38]	150° ± 8°		Measured ROM in 30 Indian subjects average age 48 years (10 F, 20 M) using Fastrack system
Kapoor et al.[40]	135° ± 6°		Measured ROM in 44 Indian subjects (31 M, 13 F) aged 21–80 years using universal goniometer
Squatting			
Desloovere et al.[24]	79° ± 16° ("mild squat"– <90° knee flexion, mild exertion) 106° ± 22° ("deep squat"—as far and safely as possible)	−9° ± 6° (mild squat) −11° ± 5° (deep squat)	Measured ROM using optical data capturing system (Vicon Motion Systems) in 10 healthy adults (1 F, 9 M; mean age 29 ± 9 years)
Han et al.[25]	148° ± 11°		Measured 40 healthy Chinese adults; mean age 21 years (20 F, 20 M) using Optotrak system
Hemmerich et al.[38]	154° ± 10° (heels up) 157° ± 6° (heels down)		Measured ROM in 30 Indian subjects average age 48 years (10 F, 20 M) using Fastrack system

ROM, Range of motion; *TKA,* total knee arthroplasty.

Vicon Motion Analysis System by Vicon, MX, Oxford, UK. Optotrak System by NDI, Waterloo, Ontario, Canada. Expert Vision Motion Analysis System by Motion Analysis Corp, Santa Rosa, CA. Selspot Data Acquisition System by Selective Electronic Company (SELCOM), Molndal, Sweden. Peak Motus System by Vicon Peak, Centennial, CO. Fastrack System by Polhemus 3Space, Colchester, VT. Penny and Giles Twin Axis Goniometer by Biometrics Ltd., Newport, UK.

TECHNIQUES OF MEASUREMENT: KNEE FLEXION/EXTENSION

Motion of the knee may be measured with the subject in the supine or the prone position. The American Academy of Orthopaedic Surgeons[41] lists both supine and prone as optional starting positions for the measurement of knee motion. However, tightness in the rectus femoris muscle may limit knee flexion when the subject is positioned in prone. Therefore the supine position for measuring knee flexion, which is recommended by the American Medical Association,[42] is preferred.

Knee Flexion (Video 12.1)

Fig. 12.8 Starting position for measurement of knee flexion. Towel roll under ipsilateral ankle to promote full knee extension. Bony landmarks for goniometer alignment (greater trochanter, lateral femoral epicondyle, lateral malleolus) indicated by red dots.

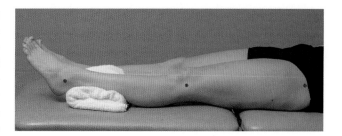

Normal ROM = 135–150 degrees.[43–50]

MDC for knee flexion goniometry measured by a single examiner = 7–8 degrees in normal and 5–23 degrees in pathological knees.[45,51–54]

Patient position

Supine, with lower extremities in anatomical position and towel roll under ipsilateral ankle (Fig. 12.8).

Stabilization

Over anterior aspect of thigh (Fig. 12.9).

Examiner action

After instructing patient in motion desired, flex patient's knee through available ROM by sliding patient's foot along table toward pelvis. Return to starting position. Performing passive movement provides an estimate of the ROM and demonstrates to patient the exact motion desired (see Fig. 12.9).

Goniometer alignment

Palpate following bony landmarks as shown in Fig. 12.8 and align goniometer accordingly (Fig. 12.10).

Fig. 12.9 End of knee flexion ROM, showing proper hand placement for stabilization of ipsilateral thigh. Bony landmarks for goniometer alignment (greater trochanter, lateral femoral epicondyle, lateral malleolus) indicated by red dots.

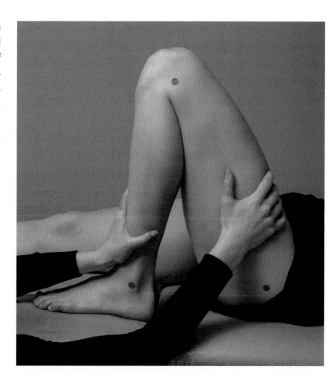

Fig. 12.10 Starting position for measurement of knee flexion demonstrating proper initial alignment of goniometer.

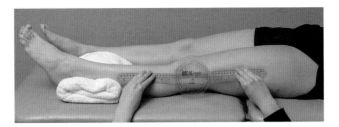

Stationary arm	Lateral midline of femur toward greater trochanter.
Axis	Lateral epicondyle of femur.
Moving arm	Lateral midline of fibula, in line with fibular head and lateral malleolus.
	Read scale of goniometer.
Patient/Examiner action	Perform passive, or have patient perform active, knee flexion by sliding foot toward pelvis (Fig. 12.11).
Confirmation of alignment	Repalpate landmarks and confirm proper goniometric alignment at end of ROM, correcting alignment as necessary (see Fig. 12.11).
	Read scale of goniometer.
Documentation	Record patient's ROM.
Note	Knee flexion may be measured with patient in prone position, but knee flexion ROM in prone may be limited owing to tightness of rectus femoris muscle.
Alternative patient position	Prone (see preceding Note) or side-lying; in either case, goniometer alignment remains the same.

Fig. 12.11 End of knee flexion ROM, demonstrating proper alignment of goniometer at end of range.

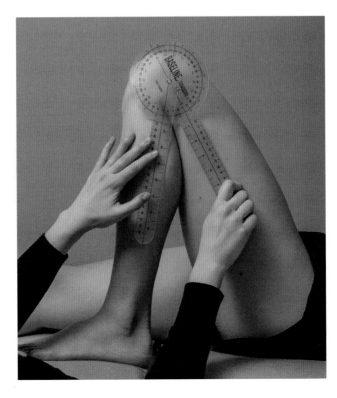

Knee Extension (Video 12.2)

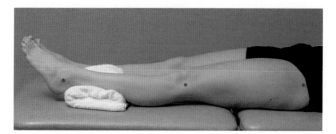

Fig. 12.12 Starting position for measurement of knee extension. Towel roll under ipsilateral ankle to promote full knee extension. Bony landmarks for goniometer alignment (greater trochanter, lateral femoral epicondyle, lateral malleolus) indicated by red dots.

Normal ROM = −2–5 degrees.[43,45,46,48–50]

MDC for knee extension goniometry measured by a single examiner = 5 degrees in normal and 4–10 degrees in pathological knees.[45,51–53]

Patient position	Supine, with knee extended as far as possible and towel roll under ipsilateral ankle (Fig. 12.12).
Stabilization	None needed.
Examiner action	Determine whether knee is extended as far as possible by (1) asking patient to straighten knee as far as possible (if measuring active ROM), or (2) providing passive pressure on the knee in the direction of extension (if measuring passive ROM) (Fig. 12.13).

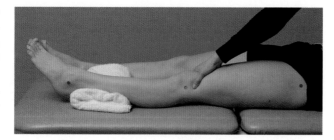

Fig. 12.13 End of knee extension ROM. Examiner is ensuring complete knee extension through posteriorly directed pressure on the distal thigh. Bony landmarks for goniometer alignment (greater trochanter, lateral femoral epicondyle, lateral malleolus) indicated by red dots.

Fig.   12.14   Measurement of knee extension demonstrating proper alignment of goniometer.

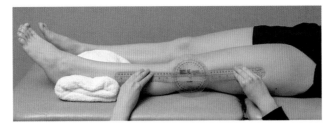

Goniometer alignment	Palpate following bony landmarks as shown in Fig. 12.12 and align goniometer accordingly (Fig. 12.14).
Stationary arm	Lateral midline of femur toward greater trochanter.
Axis	Lateral epicondyle of femur.
Moving arm	Lateral midline of fibula, in line with fibular head and lateral malleolus.
	Read scale of goniometer.
Documentation	Record patient's ROM.
Alternative patient position	Prone or side-lying. If prone position is used, it may be necessary to place a towel roll under the anterior aspect of the patient's thigh, and the patient's foot must be off the table in order to obtain full knee extension. With either position, goniometer alignment remains the same.

References

1. Messner K, Gao J. The menisci of the knee joint. Anatomical and functional characteristics, and a rationale for clinical treatment. *J Anat.* 1998;193(pt. 2):161–178.
2. Clemente C. *Gray's Anatomy of the Human Body.* 13th ed. Philadelphia: Lea & Febiger; 1985.
3. Goldblatt J, Richmond J. Anatomy and biomechanics of the knee. *Oper Tech Sports Med.* 2003;11:172–186.
4. Moore KL, Dalley AF, Agur AMR. *Clinically Oriented Anatomy.* 5th ed. Philadelphia: Lippincott Williams & Wilkins; 2006:1209.
5. Neumann D. *Kinesiology of the Musculoskeletal System.* St. Louis: Mosby; 2002.
6. Moore KL, Dalley AF, Agur AMR. *Clinically Oriented Anatomy.* 7th ed. Philadelphia: Wolters Kluwer Health/Lippincott Williams & Wilkins; 2014:1134.
7. Harner C, Giffin J, Vogrin T. Anatomy and biomechanics of the posterior cruciate ligament and posterolateral corner. *Oper Tech Sports Med.* 2001;9:39–46.
8. Kaplan EB. The fabellofibular and short lateral ligaments of the knee joint. *J Bone Joint Surg Am.* 1961;43-A:169–179.
9. Seebacher J, Inglis A, Marshall J. The structure of the posteriolateral aspect of the knee. *J Am Acad Orthop Surg.* 2000;8:97–110.
10. Greenfield B. Functional anatomy of the knee. In: *Rehabilitation of the Knee.* Philadelphia: FA Davis; 1993.
11. Freeman MA, Pinskerova V. The movement of the normal tibiofemoral joint. *J Biomech.* 2005;38(2):197–208.
12. Kapandji IA. *The Physiology of the Joints: Annotated Diagrams of the Mechanics of the Human Joints.* English ed. Edinburgh, New York: Churchill Livingstone; 1987.
13. Frankel V, Burstein A. *Orthopedic Biomechanics.* Philadelphia: Lea & Febiger; 1970.
14. Levangie PK, Norkin CC. *Joint Structure and Function: A Comprehensive Analysis.* 3rd ed. Philadelphia: Davis; 2001:495.
15. Hollister AM, et al. The axes of rotation of the knee. *Clin Orthop Relat Res.* 1993;290:259–268.
16. Barnett CH. Locking at the knee joint. *J Anat.* 1953;87(2):91–95.
17. Fuss FK, Bacher A. New aspects of the morphology and function of the human hip joint ligaments. *Am J Anat.* 1991;192(1):1–13.
18. Soderberg G. *Kinesiology: Application to Pathological Motion.* 2nd ed. Baltimore: Williams & Wilkins; 1997.
19. Johal P, et al. Tibio-femoral movement in the living knee. A study of weight bearing and non-weight bearing knee kinematics using 'interventional' MRI. *J Biomech.* 2005;38(2):269–276.
20. Smith L, Weiss E, Lehmkuhl L. *Brunnstrom's Clinical Kinesiology.* 5th ed. Philadelphia: Davis; 1996.
21. Kendall F, McCreary E, Provance P. *Muscles: Testing and Function.* 4th ed. Baltimore: Williams & Wilkins; 1993.
22. Cyriax JH, Coldham M. *Textbook of Orthopaedic Medicine.* London: Baillière Tindall; 1982.
23. Kaltenborn F. *Mobilization of the Extremity Joints.* 3rd ed. Oslo: Olaf Norlis Bokhandel; 1980.
24. Desloovere K, et al. Range of motion and repeatability of knee kinematics for 11 clinically relevant motor tasks. *Gait Posture.* 2010;32(4):597–602.
25. Han S, Cheng G, Xu P. Three-dimensional lower extremity kinematics of Chinese during activities of daily living. *J Back Musculoskelet Rehabil.* 2015;28:327–334.
26. Jevsevar DS, et al. Knee kinematics and kinetics during locomotor activities of daily living in subjects with knee arthroplasty and in healthy control subjects. *Phys Ther.* 1993;73(4):229–239 [discussion 240–242].
27. Myles CM, et al. Knee joint functional range of movement prior to and following total knee arthroplasty measured using flexible electrogoniometry. *Gait Posture.* 2002;16(1):46–54.
28. Oberg T, Karsznia A, Oberg K. Joint angle parameters in gait: reference data for normal subjects, 10–79 years of age. *J Rehabil Res Dev.* 1994;31(3):199–213.
29. Ostrosky KM, et al. A comparison of gait characteristics in young and old subjects. *Phys Ther.* 1994;74(7):637–644 [discussion 644–646].
30. Rancho Los Amigos. *Observational Gait Analysis.* Downey, CA: LAREI; 2001.
31. Rowe P, et al. Knee joint kinematics in gait and other functional activities measured using flexible electrogoniometry: how much knee motion is sufficient for normal daily life? *Gait Posture.* 2000;12(2):143–155.
32. Laubenthal KN, Smidt GL, Kettelkamp DB. A quantitative analysis of knee motion during activities of daily living. *Phys Ther.* 1972;52(1):34–43.
33. Livingston LA, Stevenson JM, Olney SJ. Stair climbing kinematics on stairs of differing dimensions. *Arch Phys Med Rehabil.* 1991;72(6):398–402.
34. Protopapadaki A, et al. Hip, knee, ankle kinematics and kinetics during stair ascent and descent in healthy young individuals. *Clin Biomech (Bristol, Avon).* 2007;22(2):203–210.
35. Tully EA, Fotoohabadi MR, Galea MP. Sagittal spine and lower limb movement during sit-to-stand in healthy young subjects. *Gait Posture.* 2005;22(4):338–345.
36. Latz D, Schiffner E, Schneppendahl J, et al. *Knee.* 2019;26(1):33–39.
37. Hyodo K, Masuda T, Aizawa J, Jinno T, Morita S. Hip, knee and ankle kinematics during activities of daily living: a cross-sectional study. *Braz J Phys Ther.* 2017;21:159–166.
38. Hemmerich A, et al. Hip, knee, and ankle kinematics of high range of motion activities of daily living. *J Orthop Res.* 2006;24(4):770–781.
39. Vander Linden DW, Wilhelm IJ. Electromyographic and cinematographic analysis of movement from a kneeling to a standing position in healthy 5- to 7-year-old children. *Phys Ther.* 1991;71(1):3–15.
40. Kapoor A, et al. Range of movements of lower limb joints in cross-legged sitting posture. *J Arthroplasty.* 2008;23(3):451–453.
41. Greene WB, Heckman JD. *The Clinical Measurement of Joint Motion.* Rosemont, IL: American Academy of Orthopaedic Surgeons; 1994.
42. American Medical Association. *Guides to the Evaluation of Permanent Impairment.* 4th ed. Chicago: American Medical Association; 1993:339.
43. Boone DC, et al. Reliability of goniometric measurements. *Phys Ther.* 1978;58(11):1355–1360.
44. Escalante A, Lichtenstein MJ, Hazuda HP. Determinants of shoulder and elbow flexion range: results from the San Antonio Longitudinal Study of Aging. *Arthritis Care Res.* 1999;12(4):277–286.
45. Macedo LG, Magee DJ. Effects of age on passive range of motion of selected peripheral joints in healthy adult females. *Physiother Theory Pract.* 2009;25(2):145–164.
46. Roaas A, Andersson GB. Normal range of motion of the hip, knee and ankle joints in male subjects, 30-40 years of age. *Acta Orthop Scand.* 1982;53(2):205–208.
47. Roach KE, Miles TP. Normal hip and knee active range of motion: the relationship to age. *Phys Ther.* 1991;71(9):656–665.
48. Soucie JM, et al. Range of motion measurements: reference values and a database for comparison studies. *Haemophilia.* 2011;17(3):500–507.
49. Smith J, Walker J. Knee and elbow range of motion in healthy older individuals. *Phys Occup Ther Geriatr.* 1983;2:31–38.
50. Walker JM, et al. Active mobility of the extremities in older subjects. *Phys Ther.* 1984;64(6):919–923.
51. Currier LL, et al. Development of a clinical prediction rule to identify patients with knee pain and clinical evidence of knee osteoarthritis who demonstrate a favorable short-term response to hip mobilization. *Phys Ther.* 2007;87(9):1106–1119.
52. Fritz JM, et al. An examination of the selective tissue tension scheme, with evidence for the concept of a capsular pattern of the knee. *Phys Ther.* 1998;78(10):1046–1056 [discussion 1057–1061].
53. Jakobsen TL, et al. Reliability of knee joint range of motion and circumference measurements after total knee arthroplasty: does tester experience matter? *Physiother Res Int.* 2010;15(3):126–134.
54. Hancock GE, Hepworth T, Wembridge K. Accuracy and reliability of knee goniometry methods. *J Exp Orthop.* 2018;5:46. https://doi.org/10.1186/s40634-018-0161-5.

13

MEASUREMENT of RANGE of MOTION
of the ANKLE and FOOT

Nancy Berryman Reese

ANATOMY

The ankle, or talocrural, joint consists of the articulation of a concave proximal, mortise-shaped joint surface formed by the distal tibia and fibular malleolus with the convex proximal surface of the talus (Fig. 13.1).[1–4] Ligamentous reinforcement of the talocrural joint is provided by collateral ligaments that span the medial and lateral aspects of the joint. The medial collateral ligament, also termed the *deltoid ligament,* originates from the medial malleolus and spreads in a fan-shaped manner over the medial aspect of the ankle to attach to the talus, calcaneus, and navicular bones (Fig. 13.2A).[3,4] This ligament consists of superficial and deep bands and provides strong reinforcement to the medial side of the joint.[5] The lateral collateral ligament of the ankle consists of three distinct components. From anterior to posterior, these include the anterior talofibular ligament, the calcaneofibular ligament, and the posterior talofibular ligament (Fig. 13.2B). All three of these ligaments have their origin on the lateral malleolus. The two talofibular ligaments attach to the anterior and posterior aspects of the talus, and the calcaneofibular ligament has its inferior attachment on the calcaneus.[1,4] The subtalar, or talocalcaneal, joint is formed by two articulations—a posterior and an anterior—between the talus and the calcaneus (Fig. 13.3). The posterior articulation occurs between the convex posterior talar facet of the calcaneus and the concave posterior calcaneal facet of the talus. The anterior articulation, formed by contact between the convex head of the talus and the concave middle and anterior talar facets of the calcaneus, is also part of the talocalcaneonavicular joint (an articulation between the anterior aspects of the talus and the calcaneus and the posterior aspect of the navicular).[2,6–8] A primary source of ligamentous stability for the subtalar joint comes from two ligaments located within the sinus tarsi: the cervical ligament and the interosseous talocalcaneal ligament. Each of these ligaments is broad and strong and interconnects the talus superiorly with the calcaneus inferiorly.[2,8,9] The subtalar joint receives additional reinforcement from the collateral ligaments of the ankle, as well as from anterior, posterior, and lateral talocalcaneal ligaments.[2,9,10]

The transverse tarsal joint is a collective term used for the combined talonavicular joint and the more laterally located calcaneocuboid joint (see Fig. 13.1). The talonavicular joint consists of the convex talar head articulating with a concave distal joint surface composed of the navicular bone and the spring ligament. Laterally, the joint surfaces of the transverse tarsal joint are irregular because the distal surface of the calcaneus and the proximal surface of the cuboid are both convex and concave. Reinforcement of the transverse tarsal joint is provided via several ligaments that span its joints (see Fig. 13.2A and B). The plantar calcaneonavicular, or spring, ligament supports the head of the talus by spanning the plantar surface of the talonavicular joint from the sustentaculum tali of the calcaneus to the navicular. More laterally, the plantar surface of the calcaneocuboid joint is supported by the long and short plantar ligaments, both of which originate from the plantar surface of the calcaneus and insert onto the metatarsal and cuboid bones. Dorsally, the transverse tarsal joint is reinforced by the dorsal talonavicular and calcaneocuboid ligaments and by the bifurcated ligament.[2,4,9,11]

OSTEOKINEMATICS

Traditional anatomical descriptions of motion at the ankle (talocrural), subtalar, and transverse tarsal joints depict motions that occur at these joints as dorsiflexion, plantarflexion, inversion, and eversion in their classical definitions[2] (see Chapter 1). More contemporary explanations describe motion at these joints as occurring around oblique axes that lie at angles to all three cardinal planes.[9,12–14] These axes allow motion in all three planes simultaneously. The motions thus produced have been termed *pronation* (a combination of dorsiflexion, abduction, and eversion) and *supination* (a combination of plantarflexion, adduction, and inversion).[9,10,12,14,15] Much confusion surrounds these terms in the literature, with some authors using supination and pronation instead of, or interchangeably with, inversion and eversion.[16–18] While acknowledging that

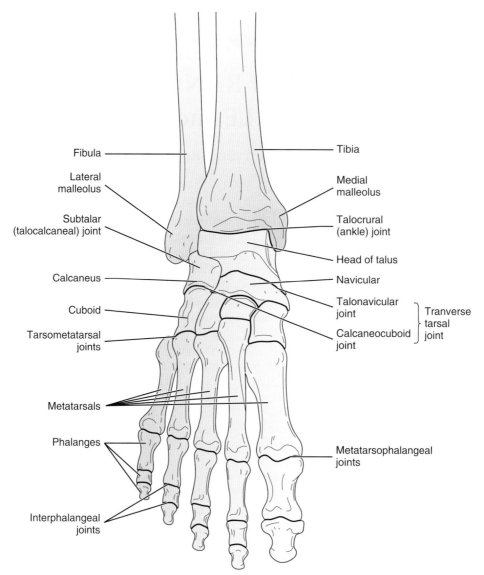

Fibula

Lateral
malleolus

Subtalar
(talocalcaneal) joint

Calcaneus

Cuboid

Tarsometatarsal
joints

Metatarsals

Phalanges

Interphalangeal
joints

Tibia

Medial
malleolus

Talocrural
(ankle) joint

Head of talus

Navicular

Talonavicular
joint

Calcaneocuboid
joint

⎫
⎬ Tranverse
⎭ tarsal
  joint

Metatarsophalangeal
joints

Fig. 13.1   Bony anatomy of the joints of the foot and ankle.

motions of the ankle, subtalar, and transverse tarsal joints are multi-planar, the terminology used for examination of range-of-motion in this text maintains the traditional terminology of dorsiflexion, plantarflexion, inversion, and eversion.

Motion at the ankle joint occurs around an oblique axis that is angled from lateral to medial anteriorly and dorsally and passes through the talus and the tips of the medial and lateral malleoli.[1,3,12] Movement around such an axis causes the major components of motion at the talocrural joint to be dorsiflexion and plantarflexion,[3,16] which are the motions measured clinically to examine this joint.

Motion at the subtalar joint occurs around an oblique axis that extends, from lateral to medial, in an anterior and dorsal direction, and passes through the head of the talus.[18,19] Because of the location and angulation of the subtalar joint axis, the principal components of motion at this joint are eversion and inversion and abduction and adduction.[13] Inversion and eversion are the

motions that are measured clinically to examine motion of this joint.[12]

Although the talonavicular and calcaneocuboid joints do not share a joint capsule, their joint lines traverse the foot from medial to lateral in a roughly S-shape, allowing motion to occur across the combined joints.[2] The primary components of motion that occur at this joint add to the component motions of dorsiflexion/plantarflexion at the ankle and eversion/inversion at the subtalar joint. Because no adequate means of measuring isolated transverse tarsal motion is commonly used clinically, motion at this joint is measured in this text in conjunction with subtalar motion as foot inversion and eversion.

ARTHROKINEMATICS

During dorsiflexion, the talus rolls anteriorly and slides posteriorly; the reverse movements occur during plantarflexion. Inversion and eversion at the subtalar joint

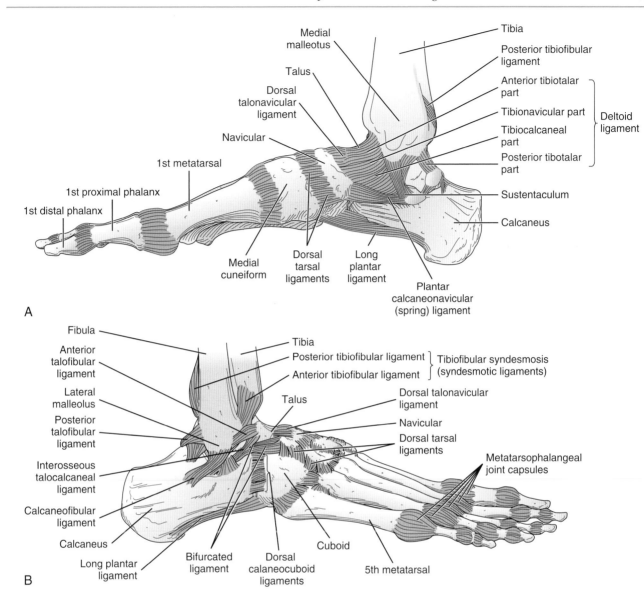

Fig. 13.2 Ligaments of the ankle, subtalar, and transverse tarsal joints. (A) Medial view. (B) Lateral view.

occur as a result of sliding of the calcaneus on the talus (open-chain motion) around an oblique axis. During motion at the transverse tarsal joint, spin occurs between the concave distal joint surface formed by the navicular and spring ligament and the convex talar head.[3]

LIMITATIONS OF MOTION

Dorsiflexion and plantarflexion of the ankle are limited by the joint capsule as well as by ligaments and muscles that cross the joint. Ankle plantarflexion is limited initially by tension in the muscles that dorsiflex the ankle and then by anterior capsular and ligamentous structures, including the anterior talofibular ligament and the tibionavicular fibers of the deltoid ligament.[3] Ankle dorsiflexion is limited by tension in the soleus and gastrocnemius muscles, particularly if the knee is extended when the movement occurs. Posterior capsular

and ligamentous structures, including the calcaneofibular ligament, the posterior talofibular ligament, and the tibiotalar fibers of the deltoid ligament, also limit ankle dorsiflexion, particularly with the knee flexed.[3] Inversion and eversion of the subtalar and transverse tarsal joints are limited by tension in the lateral and medial collateral ligaments of the ankle, respectively.[3,16] Information on normal ranges of motion for dorsiflexion, plantarflexion, inversion, and eversion is found in Appendix B.

END-FEEL

The normal end-feel for ankle plantarflexion is firm as the result of limitation first by muscular, then by ligamentous, structures. A firm end-feel also occurs at the limits of ankle dorsiflexion because of a muscular limitation to motion (when the knee is extended) or to

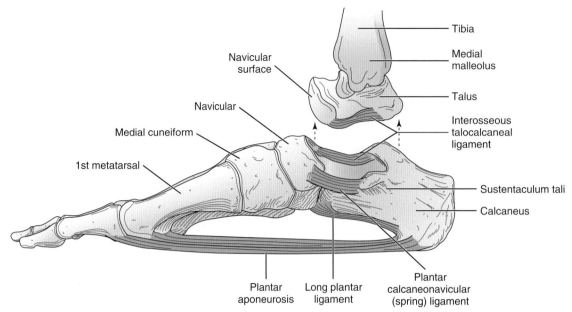

Fig. 13.3   Subtalar joint (disarticulated) and associated ligaments.

ligamentous and capsular limitations (when the knee is flexed). Ligamentous structures limit the range of inversion and eversion at the subtalar and transverse tarsal joints, producing a firm end-feel for motions at both joints.

CAPSULAR PATTERN

The capsular pattern for the ankle (talocrural) joint consists of more limitation of plantarflexion than dorsiflexion. For the subtalar joint, a capsular pattern is present when inversion is more limited than eversion.[20,21]

METATARSOPHALANGEAL AND INTERPHALANGEAL JOINTS

ANATOMY

The metatarsophalangeal (MTP) joints of the foot are similar in structure to the metacarpophalangeal joints of the hand.[12,16] Each of the five MTP joints is formed by the articulation of the convex metatarsal head with the concave base of the proximal phalanx of the corresponding digit[2] (see Fig. 13.1). A pair of collateral ligaments reinforces the sides of each MTP joint, and the plantar aspect of each joint is reinforced by the plantar plates (Fig. 13.4). These plantar plates, or ligaments, are composed of dense fibrous connective tissue, and all five are interconnected by the deep transverse metatarsal ligaments.[2,3]

The interphalangeal (IP) joints of the toes are classified as hinge joints, and each interphalangeal joint is composed of an articulation between the convex head of the more proximal phalanx and the concave

base of the more distal phalanx (see Fig. 13.1). Nine such interphalangeal joints are found in the toes—two (one proximal and one distal) in each of the lateral four toes and one interphalangeal joint in the great (first) toe. Ligamentous reinforcement of the interphalangeal joints is similar to that of the metatarsophalangeal joints, although the ligaments are smaller and the plantar plates are not interconnected[2,3,16] (see Fig. 13.4).

OSTEOKINEMATICS

Motions at the metatarsophalangeal joints, as at the metacarpophalangeal joints, consist of flexion, extension, abduction, and adduction, although the range of abduction and adduction available in the toes is much less than that seen in the fingers, with active abduction and adduction of the first MTP joint being impossible for some individuals. Only the movements of flexion and extension are available at the interphalangeal joints of the toes. More motion is possible at the proximal interphalangeal joints than at the distal, and flexion is generally greater than extension at all joints.[2,3,16]

ARTHROKINEMATICS

During flexion and extension at both the metatarsophalangeal and interphalangeal joints, the concave distal joint surface (base of the phalanx) rolls and slides on the convex proximal joint surface in the same direction as the external motion. For example, during MTP flexion, the base of the proximal phalanx rolls and slides in a plantar direction. The reverse motion occurs during MTP extension.[3]

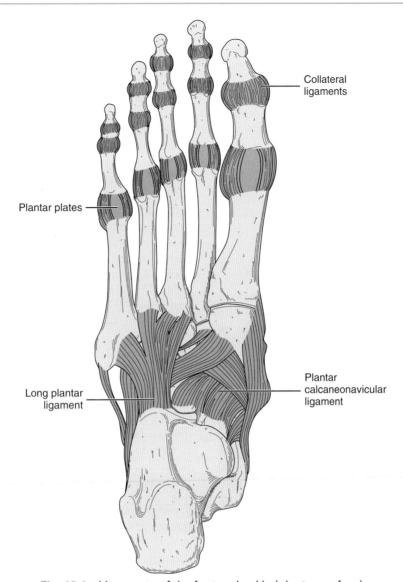

Fig. 13.4   Ligaments of the foot and ankle (plantar surface).

LIMITATIONS OF MOTION

MTP and IP joint flexion is limited by tension in the toe extensor muscles and tendons, whereas extension is limited by tension in the toe flexor muscles and tendons and the plantar ligaments. Abduction and adduction at the MTP joints are limited by the collateral ligaments of the joints or by approximation with adjacent toes.[2,3] Information regarding the normal ranges of motion for the MTP joints is located in Appendix B.

END-FEEL

The normal end-feel for flexion and extension at the metatarsophalangeal and interphalangeal joints is firm because of limitation by muscular, or muscular and ligamentous, structures. Normally the end-feel for MTP abduction and adduction is firm (ligamentous) unless movement is impeded by an adjacent toe, in which case the end-feel will be soft.

CAPSULAR PATTERN

The capsular pattern varies in the metatarsophalangeal and proximal and distal interphalangeal (PIP and DIP) joints depending on which joints are involved. For the first (great) toe, the capsular pattern is one of extension that is more limited than flexion. For the second through fifth toes, capsular involvement is suspected when flexion is more limited than extension.[20,21]

RANGE OF MOTION AND FUNCTIONAL ACTIVITY

Several investigators have examined the motion of the ankle joint during functional activities, particularly those related to ambulatory activities such as walking on level ground [22–26] and ascending and descending stairs[27,28] (Fig. 13.5). Additional investigations have examined ankle motion during other daily

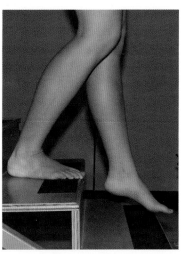

Fig. 13.5   Ankle ROM needed to descend stairs.

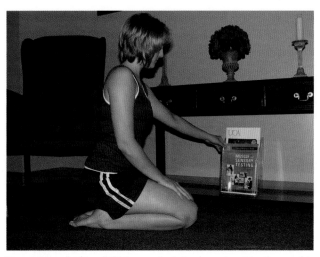

Fig. 13.6   Ankle ROM needed to kneel with the ankle plantarflexed.

activities such as dressing and bathing,[29] rising from a chair[30] and transitioning from a kneeling to a standing position.[31] A few authors also have examined ankle motion in so-called high range of motion (ROM) activities such as kneeling (Fig. 13.6), squatting, and sitting cross-legged.[32,33]

A summary of ankle range of motion related to various functional activities is shown in Table 13.1. Most of the studies from which data were derived were performed in healthy adults, although some investigations included elderly and pediatric subjects. Characteristics of the study populations and instrumentation used are included in the table. Caution should be used in extrapolating these data to the general population because the sample sizes for almost all of the studies were small. For more in-depth information on each study, the reader is referred to the reference list at the end of this chapter.

TECHNIQUES OF MEASUREMENT

ANKLE DORSIFLEXION/PLANTARFLEXION

Ankle dorsiflexion and plantarflexion may be measured using a variety of techniques and landmarks. The most common proximal landmark used for these measurements is the fibular shaft,[32] with the axis of the goniometer generally placed over, or distal to but aligned with, the lateral malleolus. Several distal landmarks have been used to measure ankle dorsiflexion and plantarflexion, including the shaft of the fifth metatarsal[34,35] and the plantar surface of the foot.[34,36] Although each of these distal landmarks appears to be reliable for measuring ankle dorsiflexion, techniques employing the heel as a distal landmark are less reliable than those in which the fifth metatarsal or the plantar surface of the foot is used.[34] Values obtained during the measurement of ankle dorsiflexion ROM have been shown to vary significantly according to the landmarks used during the measurement and according to the type of motion (active or passive) measured,[34] reinforcing the need for standardized positioning and technique during the measurement of range of motion. The position of the patient's knee during measurement also may influence the values obtained during dorsiflexion measurement, as tension in the calcaneal tendon may limit dorsiflexion with the knee extended.[37]

Many examiners recommend measuring ankle motion, and in particular dorsiflexion, while maintaining the subtalar joint in a neutral position.[38–42] The rationale behind such positioning is an attempt to minimize motion of the transverse tarsal joint while isolating talocrural motion.[42] Although the use of neutral positioning of the subtalar joint during ankle dorsiflexion does not completely eliminate forefoot motion,[40] a significant difference has been demonstrated in the amount of ankle dorsiflexion obtained when measurement is performed with the subtalar joint in the neutral compared with the pronated position.[41] Because of issues surrounding the reliability of determining and maintaining the neutral position of the subtalar joint,[41–44] techniques for measuring ankle dorsiflexion in subtalar neutral have been eliminated from this edition.

SUBTALAR INVERSION/EVERSION

The literature describes a variety of methods of measuring range of motion of inversion and eversion at the subtalar joint. Many individuals advocate measuring subtalar joint motion from a reference point of a neutral position of the subtalar joint;[18,43] others use anatomical zero as a reference.[45,46] Because of the time required and questionable reliability of these techniques, they have been eliminated from this edition.

Table 13.1 ANKLE ROM REQUIREMENTS FOR FUNCTIONAL ACTIVITIES			
FUNCTIONAL ACTIVITY	**ANKLE DORSIFLEXION**	**ANKLE PLANTARFLEXION**	**COMMENTS**
Ambulation—Level Ground			
Arndt et al.[23]	1° to 9°	7° to 10°	Measured peak ROM in 3 M subjects aged 36–45 years in whom intracortical pins were inserted. Data collected using MacReflex system
Begg and Sparrow[24]	17° (elderly group) 22° (young group)	17° (elderly group) 31° (young group)	Measured joint angles during gait in 24 healthy subjects, 12 young (mean age 28 years; 6 F, 6 M) and 12 elderly (mean age 69 years; 6 F, 6 M) using PEAK Motus motion analysis system
Han et al.[25]	32°	17°	Measured 40 healthy Chinese adults; mean age 21 years (20 F, 20 M) using Optotrak system
Ostrosky et al.[26]	12° ± 5° (young group) 14° ± 3° (older group)	28° ± 8° (young group) 24° ± 6° (older group)	Measured peak ROM during free speed walking using Expert Vision motion analysis system in 60 subjects divided into 2 groups according to age. Young group ($n = 30$; 15 F, 15 M) aged 20–40 years; old group ($n = 30$; 15 F, 15 M) aged 60–80 years
Rancho Los Amigos[22]	10°	15°	Undefined subject group and study method
Ambulation—Ascending Stairs			
Livingston et al.[27] 20.3 cm stair rise height 20.3 cm stair rise height 12.7 cm stair rise height	22° ± 1° to 27° ± 3° 20° ± 1° to 24° ± 2° 14° ± 1° to 19° ± 2°	24° ± 6° to 24° ± 1° 30° ± 7° to 24° ± 1° 28° ± 12° to 24° ± 1°	Used cinematographic analysis to measure 15 healthy F aged 19–26 years divided into 3 groups according to height
Protopapadaki et al.[28]	11° ± 4°	31° ± 5°	Measured 33 healthy adults aged 18–39 years (16 M, 17 F); stair rise height 18 cm
Ambulation—Descending Stairs			
Livingston et al.[27] 20.3 cm stair rise height 20.3 cm stair rise height 12.7 cm stair rise height	21° ± 7° to 32° ± 3° 26° ± 2° to 36° ± 2° 29° ± 3° to 32° ± 1°	28° ± 1° to 30° ± 2° 26° ± 2° to 31° ± 3° 24° ± 4° to 28° ± 4°	Used cinematographic analysis to measure 15 healthy F aged 19–26 years divided into 3 groups according to height
Protopapadaki et al.[28]	21° ± 4°	40° ± 6°	Measured 33 healthy adults aged 18–39 years (17 F, 16 M); stair rise height 18 cm
Entering Bath			
Hyodo et al.[29]	14° ± 4° to 17° ± 6°	13° ± 6° to 25° ± 10°	Measured 26 healthy adults aged 20 ± 1 years (13F, 13 M) using Fastrak system
Exiting Bath			
Hyodo et al.[29]	28° ± 7°	32° ± 10°	Measured 26 healthy adults aged 20 ± 1 years (13F, 13 M) using Fastrak system
Putting on Pants (in sitting)			
Hyodo et al.[29]	11° ± 7°	37° ± 8°	Measured 26 healthy adults aged 20 ± 1 years (13F, 13 M) using Fastrak system
Putting on Pants (in standing)			
Hyodo et al.[29]	7° ± 5° to 13° ± 6°	4° ± 4° to 37° ± 7°	Measured 26 healthy adults aged 20 ± 1 years (13F, 13 M) using Fastrak system
Putting on Shoes (Foot on ankle)			
Hyodo et al.[29]	5° ± 6°	21° ± 12°	Measured 26 healthy adults aged 20 ± 1 years (13F, 13 M) using Fastrak system
Putting on Shoes (Foot on knee)			
Hyodo et al.[29]	5° ± 5°	19° ± 12°	Measured 26 healthy adults aged 20 ± 1 years (13F, 13 M) using Fastrak system
Tying shoes			
Hyodo et al.[29]	3° ± 5°	1° ± 5° to 2° ± 7°	Measured 26 healthy adults aged 20 ± 1 years (13F, 13 M) using Fastrak system

Continued

Table 13.1	ANKLE ROM REQUIREMENTS FOR FUNCTIONAL ACTIVITIES—cont'd		
FUNCTIONAL ACTIVITY	**ANKLE DORSIFLEXION**	**ANKLE PLANTARFLEXION**	**COMMENTS**
Rising from a Chair Ikeda et al.[30]	27°±4° (young group) 29°±9° (older group)		Measured ROM using Selspot data acquisition system in 9 older subjects aged 61–74 years (6 M, 3 F) and compared with previous data on 9 healthy F aged 25–36 years; chair ht 80% of each subject's knee ht
Kneeling Hemmerich et al.[32] Ankle dorsiflexed Ankle plantarflexed	40°±5° 33°±7°	−3°±3° 24°±16°	Measured ROM in 44 Indian subjects (31 M, 13 F) aged 21–80 years using universal goniometer
Kneel-to-Stand Vander Linden and Wilhelm[31]	29°±4°	31°±11°	Measured ROM during kneel-to-stand movement in 10 healthy children aged 5–7 years (6 F, 4 M) using cinematography
Sitting Cross-Legged Hemmerich et al.[32]	32°±7°	26°±11°	Measured ROM in 30 Indian subjects, average age 48 years (10 F, 20 M) using Fastrack system
Kapoor et al.[33]	29°±3°		Measured ROM in 44 Indian subjects (31 M, 13 F) aged 21–80 years using universal goniometer
Squatting Han et al.[25]	34°±4° to 36°±5°		Measured 40 healthy Chinese adults; mean age 21 years (20 F, 20 M) using Optotrak system
Hemmerich et al.[32] Heels down Heels up	39°±6° 38°±5°	−3°±3° −4°±3°	Measured ROM in 44 Indian subjects (31 M, 13 F) aged 21–80 years using universal goniometer

Expert Vision Motion Analysis System by Motion Analysis Corp, Santa Rosa, CA.
Selspot Data Acquisition System by Selective Electronic Company (SELCOM), Molndal, Sweden.
Peak Motus System by Vicon Peak, Centennial, CO.
Optotrak System by NDI, Waterloo, Ontario Canada.
Fastrack System by Polhemus 3Space, Colchester, VT.
MacReflex system by Qualisys AB, Gothenbug, Sweden.

Measurement of inversion and eversion are most commonly measured clinically across the joints of the entire foot, resulting in the measurement of motion that occurs at several joints, including the talocrural, subtalar, and transverse tarsal joints. Although measurement of foot inversion and eversion does not include measurement of isolated motion at a single joint, such measurements are commonly used and easily performed, and they are useful as screening techniques.

METATARSOPHALANGEAL AND INTERPHALANGEAL FLEXION/ EXTENSION

Clinically, extension of the first MTP joint is the motion of the toes of most common concern, because limitation of that motion can cause significant impairment of foot function during gait. In fact, only articles examining MTP extension[47,48] and none examining MTP flexion or IP flexion or extension were found in the literature. The focus in the literature on measuring MTP extension is probably due to the need for sufficient MTP extension more than for other motions of the toes in normal functioning of the foot.

No fewer than four different methods of measuring extension of the first MTP joint have been described in the literature.[47,48] These methods vary according to the technique used by the examiner and according to the position in which the patient is placed during the measurement. Two basic measuring techniques and a variety of patient positions are described in the four methods. The measuring technique described in this text uses an approach in which motion is measured from the medial aspect of the joint with the goniometer aligned so that the axis is at the medial joint line, the moving arm is positioned along the medial midline of the proximal phalanx of the great toe, and the stationary arm is positioned along the medial midline of the first metatarsal. However, dorsal alignment of the goniometer also can be used. Subjects may be placed in a variety of positions when these measuring techniques are used, including non–weight-bearing and partial weight-bearing with the subject seated, and weight-bearing with the subject standing.[48]

Ankle Plantarflexion (Video 13.1)

Fig. 13.7 Starting position for measurement of ankle plantarflexion. Bony landmarks for goniometer alignment (fibular head, lateral malleolus, lateral midline of fifth metatarsal) indicated by red line and dots.

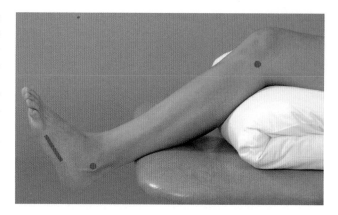

Normal ROM = 40–65 degrees.[47–53]

MDC for ankle plantarflexion goniometry measured by a single examiner = 13 degrees in normal ankles.[48]

Patient position	Supine or sitting (see Note), with knee flexed (as shown) or extended, and ankle in anatomical position (Fig. 13.7).
Stabilization	Over posterior aspect of distal leg (Fig. 13.8).
Examiner action	After instructing patient in motion desired, plantarflex patient's ankle through available ROM. Return to starting position. Performing passive movement provides an estimate of the ROM and demonstrates to patient exact motion desired (see Fig. 13.8).
Goniometer alignment	Palpate following bony landmarks as shown in Fig. 13.7 and align goniometer accordingly (Fig. 13.9).
Stationary arm	Lateral midline of fibula, in line with fibular head.
Axis	Distal to, but in line with, lateral malleolus at intersection of lines through lateral midline of fibula and lateral midline of fifth metatarsal.

Fig. 13.8 End of ankle plantarflexion ROM, showing proper hand placement for stabilizing leg. Bony landmarks for goniometer alignment (fibular head, lateral malleolus, lateral midline of fifth metatarsal) indicated by red line and dots.

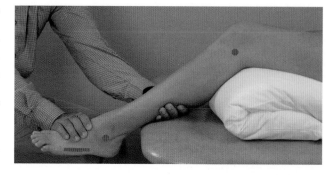

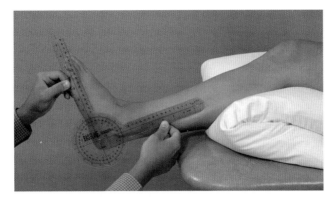

Fig. 13.9 Starting position for measurement of ankle plantarflexion, demonstrating proper initial alignment of goniometer. Note that axis of goniometer is positioned at the intersection point of lines through the lateral midline of the fibula and the fifth metatarsal.

Moving arm	Lateral midline of fifth metatarsal.
	Read scale of goniometer.
Patient/Examiner action	Perform passive, or have patient perform active, ankle plantarflexion (Fig. 13.10).
Confirmation of alignment	Repalpate landmarks and confirm proper goniometric alignment at end of ROM, correcting alignment as necessary.
	Read scale of goniometer (see Fig. 13.10).
Documentation	Record patient's ROM.
Note	Supine position is preferred over sitting position for measurements of ankle motion because bony landmarks are placed more easily at the examiner's eye level when the patient is supine.
Alternative patient position	Prone or side-lying. In either case, goniometer alignment remains the same.

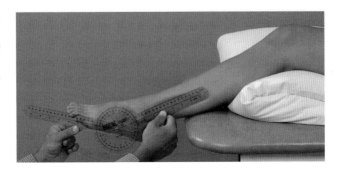

Fig. 13.10 End of ankle plantarflexion ROM, demonstrating proper alignment of goniometer at end of range.

Ankle Dorsiflexion (Video 13.2)

Fig. 13.11 Starting position for measurement of ankle dorsiflexion. Bony landmarks for goniometer alignment (fibular head, lateral malleolus, lateral midline of fifth metatarsal) indicated by red line and dots.

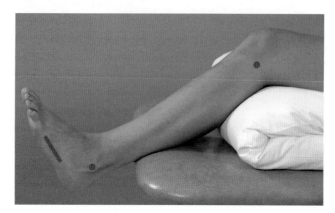

Normal ROM = 10–25 degrees.[49–55]

MDC for ankle dorsiflexion goniometry measured by a single examiner = 3–7 degrees in normal[50,56,57] and 3–8 degrees in pathological[40,56,58] ankles.

Patient position	Supine or sitting (see Note), with knee flexed at least 30 degrees, ankle in anatomical position (Fig. 13.11).
Stabilization	Over anterior aspect of distal leg (Fig. 13.12).
Examiner action	After instructing patient in motion desired, dorsiflex patient's ankle through available ROM. Return to starting position. Performing passive movement provides an estimate of the ROM and demonstrates to patient exact motion desired (see Fig. 13.12).
Goniometer alignment	Palpate following bony landmarks (shown in Fig. 13.11) and align goniometer accordingly (Fig. 13.13).

Fig. 13.12 End of ankle dorsiflexion ROM, showing proper hand placement for stabilizing leg and dorsiflexing joint. Note that motion is achieved through upward pressure on the plantar surfaces of metatarsals 4 and 5. Bony landmarks for goniometer alignment (fibular head, lateral malleolus, lateral midline of fifth metatarsal) indicated by red line and dots.

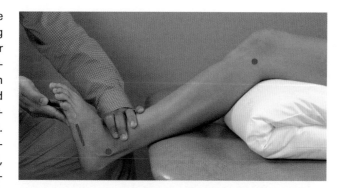

Fig. 13.13 Starting position for measurement of ankle dorsiflexion, demonstrating proper initial alignment of goniometer. Note that axis of goniometer is positioned at the intersection point of lines through the lateral midline of the fibula and the fifth metatarsal.

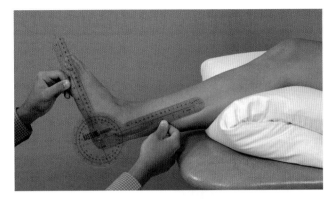

Stationary arm	Lateral midline of fibula, in line with fibular head.
Axis	Distal to but in line with lateral malleolus at intersection of lines through lateral midline of fibula and lateral midline of fifth metatarsal.
Moving arm	Lateral midline of fifth metatarsal.
	Read scale of goniometer.
Patient/Examiner action	Perform passive, or have patient perform active, ankle dorsiflexion (Fig. 13.14).
Confirmation of alignment	Repalpate landmarks and confirm proper goniometric alignment at end of ROM, correcting alignment as necessary. Read scale of goniometer (see Fig. 13.14).
Documentation	Record patient's ROM.
Note	Supine position is preferred over sitting position for measurements of ankle motion because bony landmarks are aligned more easily with the examiner's eye level when the patient is supine.
Alternative patient position	Prone or side-lying. In either case, goniometer alignment remains the same. Motion also can be measured with knee extended, providing an estimation of gastrocnemius tightness (see Figs. 14-35 to 14-37).

Fig. 13.14 End of ankle dorsiflexion ROM, demonstrating proper alignment of goniometer at end of range.

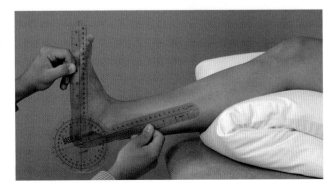

Ankle Dorsiflexion—Standing (Inclinometer)

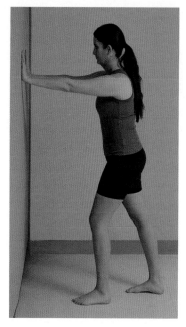

Fig. 13.15 Starting position for measurement of ankle dorsiflexion. Tested leg placed slightly anterior to stance leg, hands lightly touching wall for balance.

Normal ROM = 40–50 degrees using standing test with knee flexed.[49–55]

MDC for ankle dorsiflexion in standing with knee flexed measured by a single examiner using an inclinometer = 2–5 degrees in normal ankles.[49–55,59]

Patient position

Standing facing a wall with the foot to be tested slightly anterior to the contralateral foot. The patient may place the hands lightly on the wall for support (Fig. 13.15).

Stabilization

None required. Patients with balance issues should be either guarded by a second examiner during the test or tested in a non–weight-bearing position.

Examiner action

Ask the patient to keep the foot of the lower extremity to be tested flat on the floor while bending the knee of that extremity toward the wall. The knee should remain in line with the second toe. The contralateral leg is positioned as needed for balance. Correct errors in the patient's motion as needed and have the patient return to the staring position. Performing a trial movement provides an estimate of the ROM and demonstrates to patient exact motion desired (Fig. 13.16).

Fig. 13.16 End of ankle dorsiflexion ROM. Heel of tested leg remains in contact with floor with knee of tested leg in flexion. Hands lightly touching wall for balance.

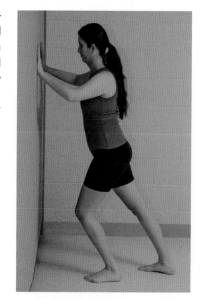

Fig. 13.17 Starting position for measurement of ankle dorsiflexion demonstrating proper initial alignment of inclinometer.

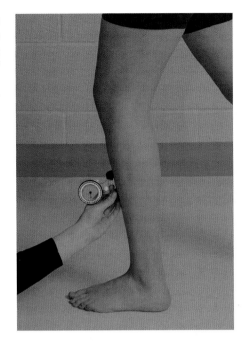

Inclinometer alignment	Along tibial crest midway between tibial tuberosity and ankle joint. Ensure the inclinometer is set to 0 degrees once it is positioned on the patient (Fig. 13.17).
Patient/Examiner action	Ask patient to repeat the lunge movement as previously instructed (Fig. 13.18).
Confirmation of alignment	Ensure that feet of inclinometer remain in firm contact with tibial crest. Read scale of inclinometer (see Fig. 13.18).
Documentation	Record patient's ROM.
Precaution	Ensure patient's heel remains in contact with the floor during the test. Lifting of the heel will result in a falsely increased ROM.

Fig. 13.18 End of ankle dorsiflexion ROM, demonstrating proper alignment of inclinometer at end of range. Heel of tested leg remains in full contact with floor.

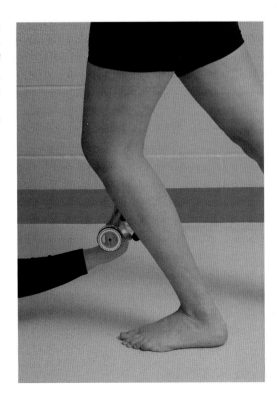

Ankle Dorsiflexion—Standing (Smartphone Method)

Fig. 13.19 Starting position for measurement of ankle dorsiflexion. Tested leg placed slightly anterior to stance leg, hands lightly touching wall for balance.

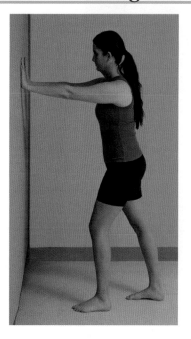

Normal ROM = 40–50 degrees using standing test with knee flexed.[49–55]

MDC for ankle dorsiflexion in standing with knee flexed measured by a single examiner using a Smartphone* = 3 degrees in normal ankles.[59]

Patient position	Standing facing a wall with the foot to be tested slightly anterior to the contralateral foot. The patient may place the hands lightly on the wall for support (Fig. 13.19).
Stabilization	None required. Patients with balance issues should be either guarded by a second examiner during the test or tested in a non–weight-bearing position.
Examiner action	Ask the patient to keep the foot of the lower extremity to be tested flat on the floor while bending the knee of that extremity toward the wall. The knee should remain in line with the second toe. The contralateral leg is positioned as needed for balance. Correct errors in the patient's motion as needed and have the patient return to the starting position. Performing a trial movement provides an estimate of the ROM and demonstrates to patient exact motion desired (Fig. 13.20).

*Using iPhone level app.

Fig. 13.20 End of ankle dorsiflexion ROM. Heel of tested leg remains in contact with floor with knee of tested leg in flexion. Hands lightly touching wall for balance.

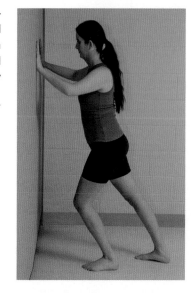

Fig. 13.21 Starting position for measurement of ankle dorsiflexion demonstrating alignment of Smartphone.

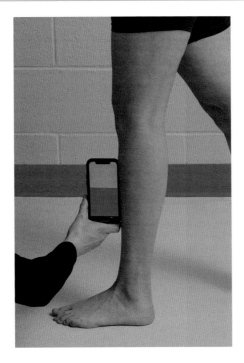

Smartphone alignment	Along tibial crest midway between tibial tuberosity and ankle joint. Ensure the smartphone app reads 0 degrees once it is positioned on the patient (Fig. 13.21).
Patient/Examiner action	Ask patient to repeat the movement as previously instructed (Fig. 13.22).
Confirmation of alignment	Ensure that smartphone remains in firm contact with tibial crest. Read scale of smartphone app (see Fig. 13.22).
Documentation	Record patient's ROM.
Precaution	Ensure patient's heel remains in contact with the floor during the test. Lifting of the heel will result in a falsely increased ROM.

Fig. 13.22 End of ankle dorsiflexion ROM, demonstrating alignment of Smartphone at end of range. Heel of tested leg remains in full contact with floor.

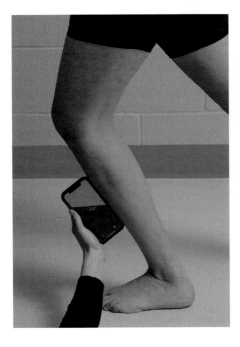

Ankle/Foot Inversion (Video 13.3)

Fig. 13.23 Starting position for measurement of combined ankle/foot inversion. Bony landmarks for goniometer alignment (tibial crest, anterior midline of talocrural joint, anterior midline of second metatarsal) indicated by red lines and dot.

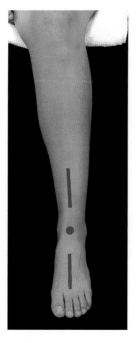

Normal ROM = 30–50 degrees.[5,49–51,53,60,61]

MDC for ankle/foot supination–inversion component goniometry measured by a single examiner in nonpathological ankles = 5–7 degrees with patient seated,[60] 3–4 degrees with patient in prone,[60] and 11 degrees with patient in supine.[50]

Patient position   Seated, with ankle in anatomical position (Fig. 13.23).

Stabilization   Over posterior aspect of distal leg (Fig. 13.24).

Examiner action   After instructing patient in motion desired, invert patient's foot/ankle through available ROM. Return to starting position. Performing passive movement provides an estimate of the ROM and demonstrates to patient exact motion desired (see Fig. 13.24).

Fig. 13.24 End of combined ankle/foot inversion ROM, showing proper hand placement for stabilizing tibia and inverting ankle/foot. Bony landmarks for goniometer alignment (tibial crest, anterior midline of talocrural joint, anterior midline of second metatarsal) indicated by red lines and dot.

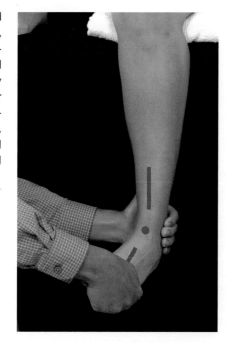

Fig. 13.25 Starting position for measurement of ankle/ foot inversion demonstrating proper initial alignment of goniometer.

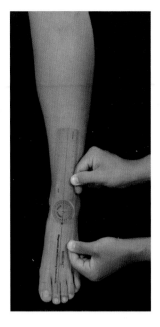

Goniometer alignment	Palpate following bony landmarks as shown in Fig. 13.23 and align goniometer accordingly (Fig. 13.25).
Stationary arm	Anterior midline of tibia, in line with tibial crest.
Axis	Anterior aspect of talocrural joint, midway between medial and lateral malleoli.
Moving arm	Anterior midline of second metatarsal.
	Read scale of goniometer.
Patient/Examiner action	Perform passive, or have patient perform active, ankle/foot inversion (Fig. 13.26).
Confirmation of alignment	Repalpate landmarks and confirm proper goniometric alignment at end of ROM, correcting alignment as necessary. Read scale of goniometer (see Fig. 13.26).
Documentation	Record patient's ROM.
Alternative patient position	Supine, with ankle in anatomical position; goniometer alignment remains the same.

Fig. 13.26 End of ankle/foot inversion ROM, demonstrating proper alignment of goniometer at end of range.

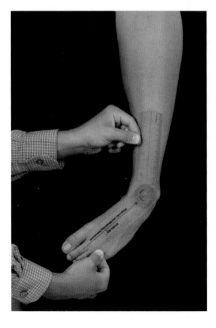

Ankle/Foot Eversion (Video 13.4)

Fig. 13.27 Starting position for measurement of combined ankle/foot eversion. Bony landmarks for goniometer alignment (tibial crest, anterior midline of talocrural joint, anterior midline of second metatarsal) indicated by red lines and dot.

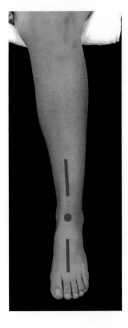

Normal ROM = 5–30 degrees.[49–53,55,59–61]

MDC for ankle/foot supination–eversion component goniometry measured by a single examiner in nonpathological ankles = 6–8 degrees with patient seated,[56] 3–4 degrees with patient in prone,[56] and 17 degrees with patient in supine.[48]

Patient position	Seated, with ankle in anatomical position (Fig. 13.27).
Stabilization	Over posterior aspect of distal leg (Fig. 13.28).
Examiner action	After instructing patient in motion desired, evert patient's foot/ankle through available ROM. Return to starting position. Performing passive movement provides an estimate of the ROM and demonstrates to patient exact motion desired (see Fig. 13.28).

Fig. 13.28 End of combined ankle/foot eversion ROM, showing proper hand placement for stabilizing tibia and inverting ankle/foot. Bony landmarks for goniometer alignment (tibial crest, anterior midline of talocrural joint, anterior midline of second metatarsal) indicated by red lines and dot.

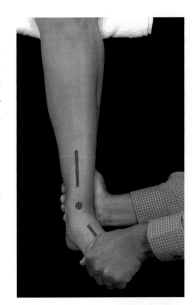

Fig. 13.29 Starting position for measurement of ankle/foot eversion, demonstrating proper initial alignment of goniometer.

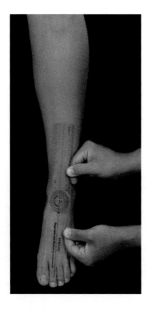

Goniometer alignment	Palpate following bony landmarks (shown in Fig. 13.27) and align goniometer accordingly (Fig. 13.29).
Stationary arm	Anterior midline of tibia, in line with tibial crest.
Axis	Anterior aspect of talocrural joint, midway between medial and lateral malleoli.
Moving arm	Anterior midline of second metatarsal.
	Read scale of goniometer.
Patient/Examiner action	Perform passive, or have patient perform active, ankle/foot eversion (Fig. 13.30).
Confirmation of alignment	Repalpate landmarks and confirm proper goniometric alignment at end of ROM, correcting alignment as necessary. Read scale of goniometer (see Fig. 13.30).
Documentation	Record patient's ROM.
Alternative patient position	Supine, with ankle in anatomical position; goniometer alignment remains the same.

Fig. 13.30 End of ankle/foot eversion ROM, demonstrating proper alignment of goniometer at end of range.

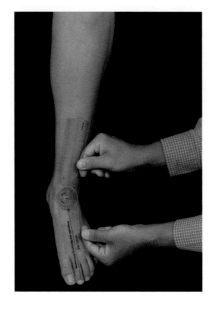

First Metatarsophalangeal (MTP) Joint Flexion (Plantarflexion) (Video 13.5)

Fig. 13.31 Starting position for measurement of first MTP joint flexion. Bony landmarks for goniometer alignment (medial midline of first metatarsal, medial aspect of first MTP joint, medial midline of proximal phalanx) indicated by red lines and dot.

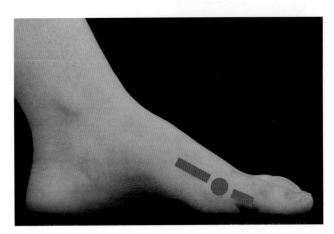

Patient position	Supine or seated with ankle in neutral position (Fig. 13.31).
Stabilization	Over first metatarsal (Fig. 13.32).
Examiner action	After instructing patient in motion desired, flex patient's first MTP joint through available ROM. Return limb to starting position. Performing passive movement provides an estimate of the ROM and demonstrates to patient exact motion desired (see Fig. 13.32).
Goniometer alignment	Palpate following bony landmarks as shown in Fig. 13.31 and align goniometer accordingly (Fig. 13.33).
Stationary arm	Medial midline of first metatarsal.
Axis	Medial aspect of first MTP joint.

Fig. 13.32 End of first MTP joint flexion ROM, showing proper hand placement for stabilizing first metatarsal and flexing MTP joint. Bony landmarks for goniometer alignment (medial midline of first metatarsal, medial aspect of first MTP joint, medial midline of proximal phalanx) indicated by red lines and dot.

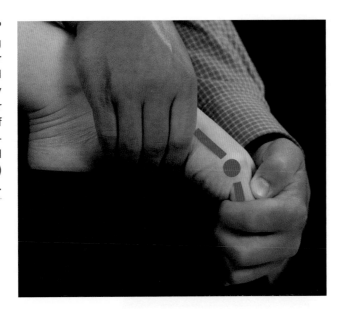

Fig. 13.33 Starting position for measurement of first MTP joint flexion, demonstrating proper initial alignment of goniometer.

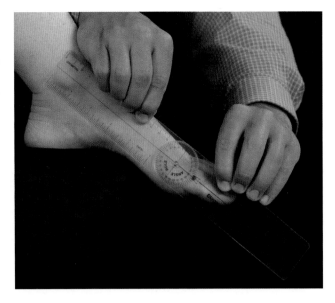

Moving arm	Medial midline of proximal phalanx of great toe.
	Read scale of goniometer.
Patient/Examiner action	Perform passive, or have patient perform active, MTP flexion (Fig. 13.34).
Confirmation of alignment	Repalpate landmarks and confirm proper goniometric alignment at end of ROM, correcting alignment as necessary. Read scale of goniometer (see Fig. 13.34).
Documentation	Record patient's ROM.
Note	Alternative alignment is with goniometer positioned over dorsum of the joint, similar to MTP flexion of lateral four toes (see Metatarsophalangeal [MTP] or Interphalangeal [PIP, DIP, IP] Flexion).

Fig. 13.34 End of first MTP joint flexion ROM, demonstrating proper alignment of goniometer at end of range.

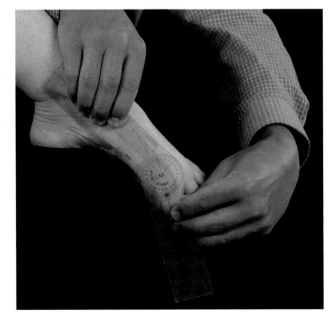

First Metatarsophalangeal (MTP) Joint Extension (Dorsiflexion) (Video 13.6)

Fig. 13.35 Starting position for measurement of first MTP joint extension. Bony landmarks for goniometer alignment (medial midline of first metatarsal, medial aspect of first MTP joint, medial midline of proximal phalanx) indicated by red lines and dot.

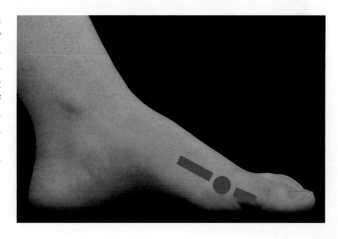

Normal ROM = 80–95 degrees.[48,49]

MDC for first MTP extension goniometry measured by a single examiner in non-pathological great toe = 3–4 degrees with patient in a non–weight-bearing position.[49]

Patient position	Supine or seated, with ankle in neutral position (Fig. 13.35).
Stabilization	Over first metatarsal (Fig. 13.36).
Examiner action	After instructing patient in motion desired, extend patient's first MTP joint through available ROM. Return limb to starting position. Performing passive movement provides an estimate of the ROM and demonstrates to patient exact motion desired (see Fig. 13.36).
Goniometer alignment	Palpate following bony landmarks as shown in Fig. 13.35 and align goniometer accordingly (Fig. 13.37).

Fig. 13.36 End of first MTP joint extension ROM, showing proper hand placement for stabilizing first metatarsal and extending MTP joint. Bony landmarks for goniometer alignment (medial midline of first metatarsal, medial aspect of first MTP joint, medial midline of proximal phalanx) indicated by red lines and dot.

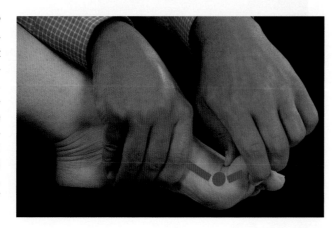

Fig. 13.37 Starting position for measurement of first MTP joint extension, demonstrating proper initial alignment of goniometer.

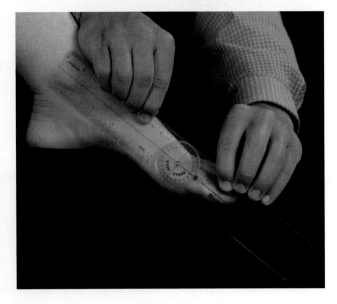

Stationary arm	Medial midline of first metatarsal.
Axis	Medial aspect of first MTP joint.
Moving arm	Medial midline of proximal phalanx of great toe.
	Read scale of goniometer.
Patient/Examiner action	Perform passive, or have patient perform active, MTP extension (Fig. 13.38).
Confirmation of alignment	Repalpate landmarks and confirm proper goniometric alignment at end of ROM, correcting alignment as necessary. Read scale of goniometer (see Fig. 13.38).
Documentation	Record patient's ROM.
Note	Alternative alignment is with goniometer positioned over dorsum of the joint, similar to MTP flexion of lateral four toes (see Metatarsophalangeal [MTP] or Interphalangeal [PIP, DIP, IP] Flexion).

Fig. 13.38 End of first MTP joint extension ROM, demonstrating proper alignment of goniometer at end of range.

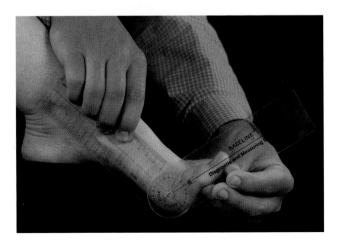

First Metatarsophalangeal (MTP) Joint Abduction (Video 13.7)

Fig. 13.39 Starting position for measurement of first MTP joint abduction. Bony landmarks for goniometer alignment (dorsal midline of first metatarsal, dorsal aspect of first MTP joint, dorsal midline of proximal phalanx) indicated by red lines and dot.

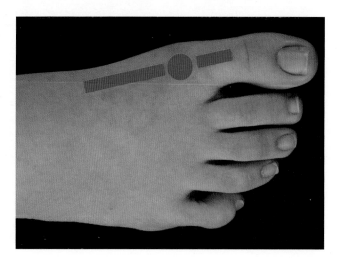

Patient position	Supine or seated, with ankle in neutral position (Fig. 13.39).
Stabilization	Over first metatarsal (Fig. 13.40).
Examiner action	After instructing patient in motion desired, abduct patient's first MTP joint through available ROM. Return limb to starting position. Performing passive movement provides an estimate of the ROM and demonstrates to patient exact motion desired (see Fig. 13.40).
Goniometer alignment	Palpate following bony landmarks as shown in Fig. 13.39 and align goniometer accordingly (Fig. 13.41).
Stationary arm	Dorsal midline of first metatarsal.

Fig. 13.40 End of first MTP joint abduction ROM, showing proper hand placement for stabilizing first metatarsal and abducting MTP joint. Bony landmarks for goniometer alignment (dorsal midline of first metatarsal, dorsal aspect of first MTP joint, dorsal midline of proximal phalanx) indicated by red lines and dot.

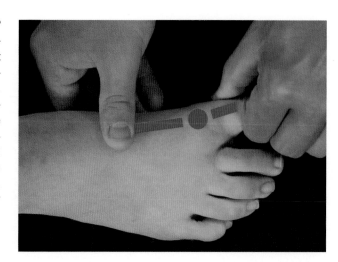

Fig. 13.41 Starting position for measurement of first MTP joint abduction, demonstrating proper initial alignment of goniometer.

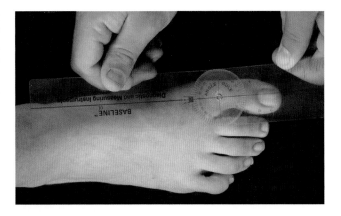

Axis	Dorsal midline of first MTP joint.
Moving arm	Dorsal midline of proximal phalanx of great toe.
	Read scale of goniometer.
Patient/Examiner action	Perform passive MTP abduction (Fig. 13.42; see Note).
Confirmation of alignment	Repalpate landmarks and confirm proper goniometric alignment at end of ROM, correcting alignment as necessary. Read scale of goniometer (see Fig. 13.42).
Documentation	Record patient's ROM.
Note	Active abduction of the first MTP joint may be difficult or impossible for many individuals.

Fig. 13.42 End of first MTP joint abduction ROM, demonstrating proper alignment of goniometer at end of range.

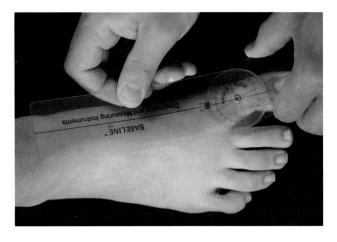

First Metatarsophalangeal (MTP) Joint Adduction (Video 13.8)

Fig. 13.43 Starting position for measurement of first MTP joint adduction. Bony landmarks for goniometer alignment (dorsal midline of first metatarsal, dorsal aspect of first MTP joint, dorsal midline of proximal phalanx) indicated by red lines and dot.

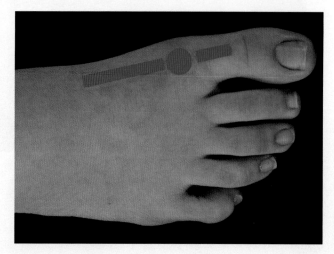

Patient position	Supine or seated, with ankle in neutral position (Fig. 13.43).
Stabilization	Over first metatarsal (Fig. 13.44).
Examiner action	After instructing patient in motion desired, adduct patient's first MTP joint through available ROM. Return limb to starting position. Performing passive movement provides an estimate of the ROM and demonstrates to patient exact motion desired (see Fig. 13.44).
Goniometer alignment	Palpate following bony landmarks as shown in Fig. 13.43 and align goniometer accordingly (Fig. 13.45).
Stationary arm	Dorsal midline of first metatarsal.
Axis	Dorsal midline of first MTP joint.

Fig. 13.44 End of first MTP joint adduction ROM, showing proper hand placement for stabilizing first metatarsal and adducting MTP joint. Bony landmarks for goniometer alignment (dorsal midline of first metatarsal, dorsal aspect of first MTP joint, dorsal midline of proximal phalanx) indicated by red lines and dot.

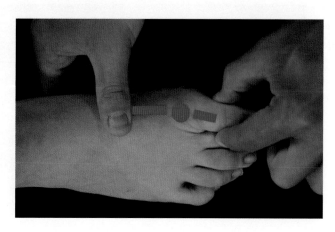

Fig. 13.45 Starting position for measurement of first MTP joint adduction, demonstrating proper initial alignment of goniometer.

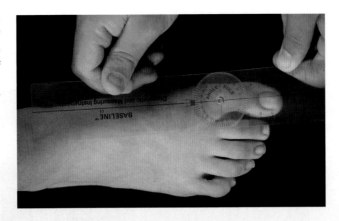

Moving arm	Dorsal midline of proximal phalanx of great toe.
	Read scale of goniometer.
Patient/Examiner action	Perform passive MTP adduction (Fig. 13.46; see Note).
Confirmation of alignment	Repalpate landmarks and confirm proper goniometric alignment at end of ROM, correcting alignment as necessary. Read scale of goniometer (see Fig. 13.46).
Documentation	Record patient's ROM.
Note	Active adduction of the first MTP joint may be difficult or impossible for many individuals.

Fig. 13.46 End of first MTP joint adduction ROM, demonstrating proper alignment of goniometer at end of range.

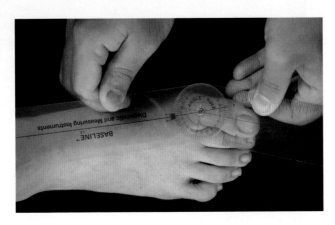

Metatarsophalangeal (MTP) or Interphalangeal (PIP, DIP, IP) Flexion (Video 13.9)

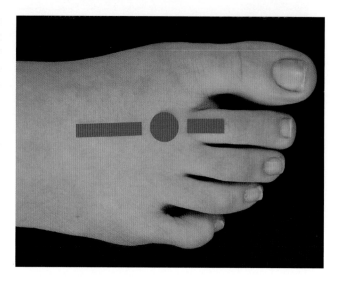

Fig. 13.47 Starting position for measurement of MTP joint flexion. Bony landmarks for goniometer alignment (dorsal midline of metatarsal, dorsal aspect of MTP joint, dorsal midline of proximal phalanx) indicated by red lines and dot.

Measurement of second MTP joint shown

Patient position	Supine or seated, with ankle in neutral position (Fig. 13.47).
Stabilization	Over more proximal bone of joint to be measured (in this case, stabilization of metatarsals is shown) (Fig. 13.48).
Examiner action	After instructing patient in motion desired, flex joint to be measured through available ROM. Return toe to starting position. Performing passive movement provides an estimate of the ROM and demonstrates to patient exact motion desired (see Fig. 13.48).
Goniometer alignment	Palpate following bony landmarks as shown in Fig. 13.47 and align goniometer accordingly (Fig. 13.49).
Stationary arm	Dorsal midline of more proximal bone of joint to be measured (in this case, the metatarsal).
Axis	Dorsal midline of joint to be measured (in this case, the MTP joint).

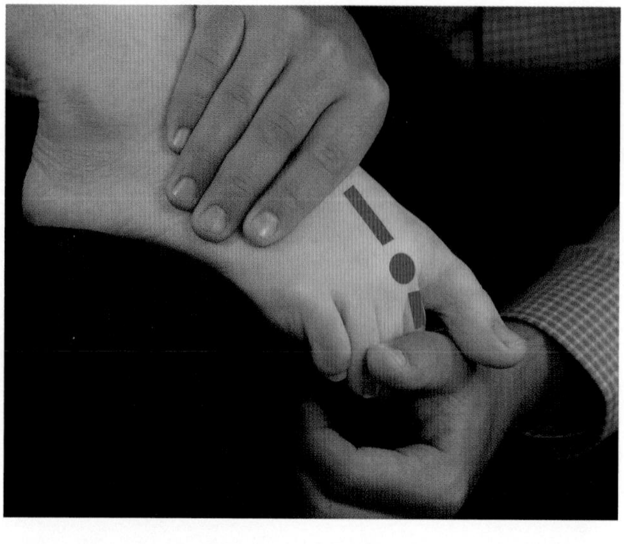

Fig. 13.48 End of MTP joint flexion ROM, showing proper hand placement for stabilizing metatarsal and flexing MTP joint. Bony landmarks for goniometer alignment (dorsal midline of metatarsal, dorsal aspect of MTP joint) indicated by red lines and dot.

Fig. 13.49 Starting position for measurement of MTP joint flexion, demonstrating proper initial alignment of goniometer.

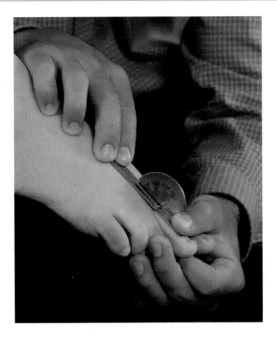

Moving arm	Dorsal midline of more distal bone of joint to be measured (in this case, the proximal phalanx).
	Read scale of goniometer.
Patient/Examiner action	Perform passive, or have patient perform active, flexion of joint to be measured (Fig. 13.50).
Confirmation of alignment	Repalpate landmarks and confirm proper goniometric alignment at end of ROM, correcting alignment as necessary. Read scale of goniometer (see Fig. 13.50).
Documentation	Record patient's ROM.
Alternative patient position	Side-lying; goniometer alignment remains same.
Note	This technique may be used to measure flexion of the MTP, DIP, or PIP joints of the lateral four toes, or flexion of the MTP or IP joint of the great toe. The figures shown here depict the measurement of MTP flexion of the second toe.

Fig. 13.50 End of MTP joint flexion ROM, demonstrating proper alignment of goniometer at end of range.

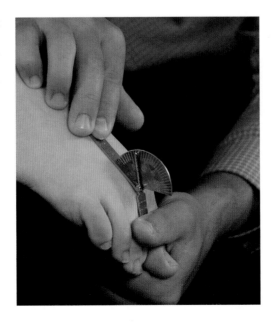

Metatarsophalangeal (MTP) or Interphalangeal (PIP, DIP, IP) Extension (Video 13.10)

Fig. 13.51 Starting position for measurement of MTP joint extension. Bony landmarks for goniometer alignment (dorsal midline of metatarsal, dorsal aspect of MTP joint, dorsal midline of proximal phalanx) indicated by red lines and dot.

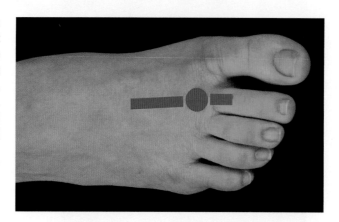

Measurement of second MTP joint shown

Patient position	Supine or seated, with ankle in neutral position (Fig. 13.51).
Stabilization	Over more proximal bone of joint to be measured (in this case, stabilization of metatarsals is shown) (Fig. 13.52).
Examiner action	After instructing patient in motion desired, extend joint to be measured through available ROM. Return limb to starting position. Performing passive movement provides an estimate of the ROM and demonstrates to patient exact motion desired (see Fig. 13.52).
Goniometer alignment	Palpate following bony landmarks as shown in Fig. 13.51 and align goniometer accordingly (Fig. 13.53).
Stationary arm	Dorsal midline of more proximal bone of joint to be measured (in this case, the metatarsal).
Axis	Dorsal midline of joint to be measured (in this case, MTP joint).

Fig. 13.52 End of MTP joint extension ROM, showing proper hand placement for stabilizing metatarsal and extending MTP joint. Bony landmarks for goniometer alignment (dorsal aspect of MTP joint, dorsal midline of proximal phalanx) indicated by red lines and dot.

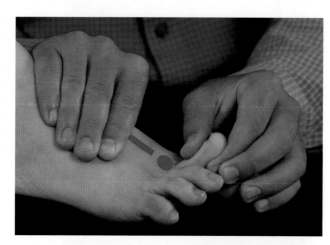

Fig. 13.53 Starting position for measurement of MTP joint extension, demonstrating proper initial alignment of goniometer.

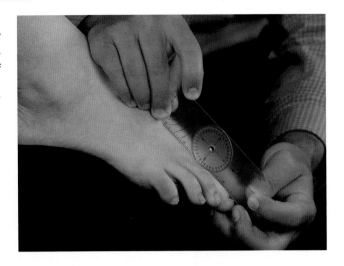

Moving arm	Dorsal midline of more distal bone of joint to be measured (in this case, the proximal phalanx).
	Read scale of goniometer.
Patient/Examiner action	Perform passive, or have patient perform active, extension of joint to be measured (Fig. 13.54).
Confirmation of alignment	Repalpate landmarks and confirm proper goniometric alignment at end of ROM, correcting alignment as necessary. Read scale of goniometer (see Fig. 13.54).
Documentation	Record patient's ROM.
Alternative patient position	Side-lying; goniometer alignment remains same.
Note	This technique may be used to measure extension of the MTP, DIP, or PIP joints of the lateral four toes, or extension of the MTP or IP joint of the great toe. The figures shown here depict the measurement of MTP extension of the second toe.

Fig. 13.54 End of MTP joint extension ROM, demonstrating proper alignment of goniometer at end of range.

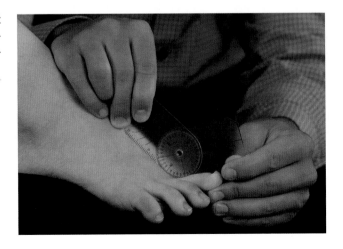

References

1. Bozkurt M, Doral MN. Anatomic factors and biomechanics in ankle instability. *Foot Ankle Clin.* 2006;11:451–463.
2. Clemente C. *Gray's Anatomy of the Human Body.* Philadelphia: Lea & Febiger; 1985.
3. Leardini A, O'Connor JJ, Catani F, Giannini S. The role of the passive structures in the mobility and stability of the human ankle joint: a literature review. *Foot Ankle Int.* 2000;21:602–615.
4. Moore KL, Dalley AF, Agur AMR. *Clinically Oriented Anatomy.* Philadelphia: Wolters Kluwer Health/Lippincott Williams & Wilkins; 2013:1134.
5. Pankovich AM, Shivaram MS. Anatomical basis of variability in injuries of the medial malleolus and the deltoid ligament. I. Anatomical studies. *Acta Orthop Scand.* 1979;50:217–223.
6. Keener BJ, Sizensky JA. The anatomy of the calcaneus and surrounding structures. *Foot Ankle Clin.* 2005;10:413–424.
7. Rockar PA. The subtalar joint: anatomy and joint motion. *J Orthop Sports Phys Ther.* 1995;21:361–372.
8. Stagni R, Leardini A, O'Connor JJ, Giannini S. Role of passive structures in the mobility and stability of the human subtalar joint: a literature review. *Foot Ankle Int.* 2003;24:402–409.
9. Neumann D. *Kinesiology of the Musculoskeletal System: Foundations for Rehabilitation.* St. Louis, MO: Mosby/Elsevier; 2010.
10. Lang LM. The anatomy of the foot. *Baillieres Clin Rheumatol.* 1987;1:215–240.
11. Donatelli R, Wolf SL. *The Biomechanics of the Foot and Ankle: Contemporary Perspectives in Rehabilitation.* Philadelphia: Davis; 1996:391.
12. Levangie PK, Norkin CC. *Joint Structure and Function a Comprehensive Analysis.* Philadelphia: F.A. Davis Co; 2011:588.
13. Root ML, Orien WP, Weed JH. *Normal and Abnormal Function of the Foot: Clinical Biomechanics.* Los Angeles: Clinical Biomechanics Corp; 1977:478.
14. Towers JD, Deible CT, Golla SK. Foot and ankle biomechanics. *Semin Musculoskelet Radiol.* 2003;7:67–74.
15. Kapandji IA. *The Physiology of the Joints: Annotated Diagrams of the Mechanics of the Human Joints.* Edinburgh, New York: Churchill Livingstone; 1987.
16. Lundberg A, Svensson OK, Bylund C, Goldie I, Selvik G. Kinematics of the ankle/foot complex—part 2: pronation and supination. *Foot Ankle.* 1989;9:248–253.
17. Smith-Oricchio K, Harris BA. Interrater reliability of subtalar neutral, calcaneal inversion and eversion. *J Orthop Sports Phys Ther.* 1990;12:10–15.
18. Manter J. Movements of the subtalar and transverse tarsal joints. *Anat Rec.* 1941;80:397–410.
19. Piazza SJ. Mechanics of the subtalar joint and its function during walking. *Foot Ankle Clin.* 2005;10:425–442.
20. Cyriax JH, Coldham M. *Textbook of Orthopaedic Medicine.* London: Baillière Tindall; 1982.
21. Kaltenborn F. *Mobilization of the Extremity Joints.* Oslo: Olaf Norlis Bokhandel; 1980.
22. Rancho Los Amigos. *Observational Gait Analysis.* Downey, CA: LAREI; 2001.
23. Arndt A, Westblad P, Winson I, Hashimoto T, Lundberg A. Ankle and subtalar kinematics measured with intracortical pins during the stance phase of walking. *Foot Ankle Int.* 2004;25:357–364.
24. Begg RK, Sparrow WA. Ageing effects on knee and ankle joint angles at key events and phases of the gait cycle. *J Med Eng Technol.* 2006;30:382–389.
25. Han S, Cheng G, Xu P. Three-dimensional lower extremity kinematics of Chinese during activities of daily living. *J Back Musculoskelet Rehabil.* 2015;28:327–334.
26. Ostrosky KM, VanSwearingen JM, Burdett RG, Gee Z. A comparison of gait characteristics in young and old subjects. *Phys Ther.* 1994;74:637–644. discussion 644–646.
27. Livingston LA, Stevenson JM, Olney SJ. Stairclimbing kinematics on stairs of differing dimensions. *Arch Phys Med Rehabil.* 1991;72:398–402.
28. Protopapadaki A, Drechsler WI, Cramp MC, Coutts FJ, Scott OM. Hip, knee, ankle kinematics and kinetics during stair ascent and descent in healthy young individuals. *Clin Biomech (Bristol, Avon).* 2007;22:203–210.
29. Hyodo K, Masuda T, Aizawa J, Jinno T, Morita S. Hip, knee and ankle kinematics during activities of daily living: a cross-sectional study. *Braz J Phys Ther.* 2017;21:159–166.
30. Ikeda ER, Schenkman ML, Riley PO, Hodge WA. Influence of age on dynamics of rising from a chair. *Phys Ther.* 1991;71:473–481.
31. Vander Linden DW, Wilhelm IJ. Electromyographic and cinematographic analysis of movement from a kneeling to a standing position in healthy 5- to 7-year-old children. *Phys Ther.* 1991;71:3–15.
32. Hemmerich A, Brown H, Smith S, Marthandam SS, Wyss UP. Hip, knee, and ankle kinematics of high range of motion activities of daily living. *J Orthop Res.* 2006;24:770–781.
33. Kapoor A, Mishra SK, Dewangan SK, Mody BS. Range of movements of lower limb joints in cross-legged sitting posture. *J Arthroplasty.* 2008;23:451–453.
34. Bohannon RW, Tiberio D, Zito M. Selected measures of ankle dorsiflexion range of motion: differences and intercorrelations. *Foot Ankle.* 1989;10:99–103.
35. Pandya S, Florence JM, King WM, Robison JD, Oxman M, Province MA. Reliability of goniometric measurements in patients with Duchenne muscular dystrophy. *Phys Ther.* 1985;65:1339–1342.
36. Ekstrand J, Wiktorsson M, Oberg B, Gillquist J. Lower extremity goniometric measurements: a study to determine their reliability. *Arch Phys Med Rehabil.* 1982;63:171–175.
37. Hornsby TM, Nicholson GG, Gossman MR, Culpepper M. Effect of inherent muscle length on isometric plantar flexion torque in healthy women. *Phys Ther.* 1987;67:1191–1197.
38. Bohannon RW, Tiberio D, Waters G. Motion measured from forefoot and hindfoot landmarks during passive ankle dorsiflexion range of motion. *J Orthop Sports Phys Ther.* 1991;13:20–22.
39. Diamond JE, Mueller MJ, Delitto A, Sinacore DR. Reliability of a diabetic foot evaluation. *Phys Ther.* 1989;69:797–802.
40. Tiberio D. Evaluation of functional ankle dorsiflexion using subtalar neutral position. A clinical report. *Phys Ther.* 1987;67:955–957.
41. Tiberio D, Bohannon RW, Zito MA. Effect of subtalar joint position on the measurement of maximum ankle dorsiflexic. *Clin Biomech (Bristol, Avon).* 1989;4:189–191.
42. Elveru RA, Rothstein JM, Lamb RL. Goniometric reliability in a clinical setting. Subtalar and ankle joint measurements. *Phys Ther.* 1988;68:672–677.
43. Picciano AM, Rowlands MS, Worrell T. Reliability of open and closed kinetic chain subtalar joint neutral positions and navicular drop test. *J Orthop Sports Phys Ther.* 1993;18:553–558.
44. Lattanza L, Gray GW, Kantner RM. Closed versus open kinematic chain measurements of subtalar joint eversion: implications for clinical practice. *J Orthop Sports Phys Ther.* 1988;9:310–314.
45. Greene WB, Heckman JD. *The Clinical Measurement of Joint Motion.* Rosemont, IL: American Academy of Orthopaedic Surgeons; 1994.
46. McPoil T, Brocato R. *The foot and ankle: Biomechanical evaluation and treatment, Orthopaedic and Sports Physical Therapy.* St. Louis: Mosby; 1985:313–325.
47. Buell T, Green DR, Risser J. Measurement of the first metatarsophalangeal joint range of motion. *J Am Podiatr Med Assoc.* 1988;78:439–448.
48. Hopson MM, McPoil TG, Cornwall MW. Motion of the first metatarsophalangeal joint. Reliability and validity of four measurement techniques. *J Am Podiatr Med Assoc.* 1995;85:198–204.
49. Boone DC, Azen SP. Normal range of motion of joints in male subjects. *J Bone Joint Surg Am.* 1979;61:756–759.
50. Macedo LG, Magee DJ. Effects of age on passive range of motion of selected peripheral joints in healthy adult females. *Physiother Theory Pract.* 2009;25:145–164.
51. Mecagni C, Smith JP, Roberts KE, O'Sullivan SB. Balance and ankle range of motion in community-dwelling women aged 64 to 87 years: a correlational study. *Phys Ther.* 2000;80:1004–1011.
52. Nigg BM, Fisher V, Allinger TL, Ronsky JR, Engsberg JR. Range of motion of the foot as a function of age. *Foot Ankle.* 1992;13:336–343.
53. Roaas A, Andersson GB. Normal range of motion of the hip, knee and ankle joints in male subjects, 30-40 years of age. *Acta Orthop Scand.* 1982;53:205–208.
54. Soucie JM, Wang C, Forsyth A, et al. Range of motion measurements: reference values and a database for comparison studies. *Haemophilia.* 2011;17:500–507.
55. Walker JM, Sue D, Miles-Elkousy N, Ford G, Trevelyan H. Active mobility of the extremities in older subjects. *Phys Ther.* 1984;64:919–923.
56. Denegar CR, Hertel J, Fonseca J. The effect of lateral ankle sprain on dorsiflexion range of motion, posterior talar glide, and joint laxity. *J Orthop Sports Phys Ther.* 2002;32:166–173.

57. Krause DA, Cloud BA, Forster LA, Schrank JA, Hollman JH. Measurement of ankle dorsiflexion: a comparison of active and passive techniques in multiple positions. *J Sport Rehabil.* 2011;20:333–344.

58. Kim D-H, An D-H, Yoo W-G. Validity and reliability of ankle dorsiflexion measures in children with cerebral palsy. *J Back Musculoskelet Rehabil.* 2018;31:465–468.

59. Banwell HA, Uden H, Marshall N, Altmann C, Williams CM. The iPhone Measure app level function as a measuring device for the weight bearing lunge test in adults: a reliability study. *J Foot Ankle Res.* 2019;12:37. https://doi.org/10.1186/s13047-019-0347-9.

60. Menadue C, Raymond J, Kilbreath SL, Refshauge KM, Adams R. Reliability of two goniometric methods of measuring active inversion and eversion range of motion at the ankle. *BMC Musculoskelet Disord.* 2006;7:60.

61. Milgrom C, Giladi M, Simkin A, et al. The normal range of subtalar inversion and eversion in young males as measured by three different techniques. *Foot Ankle.* 1985;6:143–145.

14

MUSCLE LENGTH TESTING
of the LOWER EXTREMITY

William D. Bandy

TESTS FOR MUSCLE LENGTH: ILIOPSOAS

Developed in 1876 as a method of measuring hip flexion contractures in children with tuberculosis, the Thomas test for determining iliopsoas muscle length has become "probably the most widely known and performed test for detecting decreased hip extension."[1] The original Thomas test was defined by Kendall et al.[2] as follows:

"The Thomas flexion test is founded upon our inability to extend a diseased hip without producing a lordosis. If there is flexion deformity, the patient is unable to extend the thigh on the diseased side, and it remains at an angle."

The original Thomas test has undergone modifications over the years. Today, the most frequent variation in the original technique is to use a goniometer to measure the amount of hip flexion while the subject holds the contralateral knee toward the chest.[3-5]

A second technique that can be used to measure iliopsoas muscle length is a modification of the technique used by the American Academy of Orthopaedic Surgeons (AAOS) to measure hip extension.[6] This technique is performed with the patient in the prone position with the knee flexed to 90 degrees.

TESTS FOR MUSCLE LENGTH: RECTUS FEMORIS

The Thomas test position also can be used to measure the length of the rectus femoris muscle. Kendall et al.[3] suggested that the Thomas test technique could be used not only to examine the iliopsoas muscle by taking measurements at the hip but also to examine the length of the rectus femoris muscle (a two-joint muscle) by taking measurements at the knee.

The length of the rectus femoris muscle also can be examined in the prone position. The knee is fully flexed through the full available range of motion (ROM), ensuring that the ipsilateral hip is not allowed to flex.

TESTS FOR MUSCLE LENGTH: HAMSTRINGS

According to Gajdosik et al.[7] the straight leg raise is the most common clinical test for measuring hamstring muscle length. A second type of test used for measuring hamstring muscle length is the knee extension test, which is described in the literature as performed in two ways, active[8] and passive.[9,10] Magee[4] refers to these tests as the "90/90 test." Measurements similar to the 90/90 knee extension test have been described in the pediatric medical literature for examination of infants; these tests are referred to as measurement of the "popliteal angle."[11,12]

Sit-and-Reach Test

The sit-and-reach test, a field test used to measure hamstring flexibility, is a part of most health-related physical fitness test batteries.[13] The test is performed by having the subject assume the long sitting posture and reach forward with both hands as far as possible, not allowing the knees to flex. A score is given based on the most distant point on a standardized box reached by both hands (Fig. 14.1).[14,15]

Although the sit-and-reach test has been shown to be reliable,[16,17] some authors suggest that the ability to reach is influenced by hamstring flexibility, range of motion of the lumbar and thoracic spine, anthropometric factors such as legs short or arms long relative to the length of the trunk, and the amount of scapular abduction, allowing a greater reach with the arms.[15,16] Jackson and Langford[13] suggest that "the sit and reach test does not possess criterion-related validity as a field test for hamstring and low back flexibility."

Chapter 1 includes information defining composite tests (tests that measure more than one motion or muscle), along with a rationale for avoiding these types of tests when examining muscle length. Given that the sit-and-reach test is influenced by so many factors, including muscle length of the upper and lower extremities and range of motion of the spine, a detailed description of this technique is not included in this chapter.

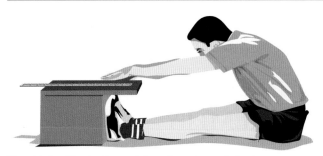

Fig. 14.1   Illustration of the sit-and-reach test, a composite test that measures multiple motions and muscles that is not included in this chapter.

TESTS FOR MUSCLE LENGTH: ILIOTIBIAL BAND AND TENSOR FASCIAE LATAE

Description of Tests

In 1935, Ober[18] described a test to examine the relationship between tightness in the tensor fasciae latae and the iliotibial band and low back pain and sciatica. This test, known today as the Ober test, was used originally to examine the length of the iliotibial band and of the tensor fasciae latae in individuals with low back pain, but now it is used to examine muscle length in anyone. In addition, use of the Ober test in patients with anterior knee pain and iliotibial band friction syndrome has been documented.[19,20]

In 1952, Kendall et al.[21] presented a modification of the original Ober test, suggesting that the examiner should keep the knee extended in the extremity to be tested (as opposed to flexing the knee to 90 degrees, as originally described by Ober) while performing the examination. The test is referred to as the modified Ober test. The following reasons have been offered for modifying the original Ober test: less stress to the medial knee joint, less tension on the patella, less potential interference by a tight rectus femoris muscle,[3] and a more functional test position.[22] Based on a review of the literature, the Ober test and the modified Ober test appear to be used with equal frequency; neither test has been shown to be more popular, more accurate, or easier to perform than the other.

Expressing concern that the Ober test was too difficult to be used "satisfactorily," Gautam and Anand[23] suggested the use of an alternative test for examining iliotibial band and tensor fasciae latae muscle length. These authors suggested that the problem with the Ober test arose from difficulty in maintaining the hip in 0-degree extension while at the same time attempting to examine the amount of hip adduction. They suggested that the Ober test is, therefore, a "two-plane" test (i.e., extension, abduction). Gautam and Anand[23] proposed an alternate test for estimating iliotibial band

contracture to be performed with the patient prone, thus eliminating the need to control hip extension. In this way, the two-plane Ober test is converted into a one-plane test of abduction. This "new test" for iliotibial band and tensor fasciae latae length is referred to in this text as the *prone technique.*

Quantification

Methods of quantifying the results of the Ober test and of modifications of the Ober test range from observation[16,18,23] to use of the goniometer,[12,24,25] the tape measure,[26] and the inclinometer.[22,27] Ober[18] relied on observation to quantify the results, stating that "if there is no contracture present, the thigh will adduct beyond the median line." Hoppenfeld[16] suggested that when the Ober test is performed, if the iliotibial tract is "normal" the thigh should drop to the adducted position, and if "contracture" is present in the tensor fasciae latae or the iliotibial band, the thigh remains abducted. Gose and Schweizer[28] presented a slightly more sophisticated classification system, which describes the position of the lower extremity relative to the horizontal body plane:

"If the leg can be passively stretched to a position horizontal but not completely adducted to the table, it constitutes 'minimal' tightness, especially in the proximal fascia. If the leg can be passively adducted to horizontal at best, it constitutes 'moderate' tightness of the iliotibial band and proximal fascia. If the leg cannot passively be adducted to horizontal, this constitutes a maximal contracture of the iliotibial band throughout its expanse."

Gajdosik et al.[24] suggested the use of a goniometer to quantify length of the iliotibial band and tensor fasciae latae muscles during performance of the Ober test. The stationary arm of the goniometer was aligned with both anterior superior iliac spines and the movable arm aligned with a line drawn on the midline of the thigh. (The location of the axis of the goniometer was not provided.) A value of 0 degrees was documented when the thigh was horizontal, positive values were recorded if the thigh was adducted past horizontal, and negative values were recorded if the thigh did not adduct to horizontal.

The use of a tape measure to quantify muscle length was described by Doucette and Goble.[26] Subjects were placed in the Ober test position, and the distance between the medial border of the patella and the support surface was measured. Melchione and Sullivan[22] and Reese and Bandy[27] described use of an inclinometer placed at the distal lateral thigh of the extremity on which the modified Ober test was performed.

TESTS FOR MUSCLE LENGTH: GASTROCNEMIUS AND SOLEUS

The key to differentiating between muscle length testing of the gastrocnemius and soleus muscles is realizing that because of its origin on the femur and insertion on the calcaneus, the gastrocnemius crosses two joints (the knee and the ankle joints). The soleus originates from the posterior surface of the fibula and tibia and crosses only the ankle joint as it inserts into the posterior surface of the calcaneus.

Therefore, flexing the knee during muscle length testing causes the gastrocnemius to become slack across the knee, and the amount of dorsiflexion is limited only by the soleus muscle. In testing the muscle length of the gastrocnemius, the knee is extended, which elongates the muscle across the knee and the ankle.[3,29]

Iliopsoas Muscle Length: Thomas Test (Video 14.1)

Fig. 14.2 Starting position for measuring iliopsoas muscle length using the Thomas test. Bony landmarks for goniometer alignment (lateral midline of trunk, greater trochanter, lateral femoral epicondyle) indicated by red line and dots.

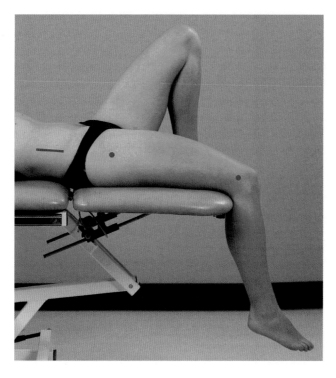

Patient position

Patient is supine, with hip of lower extremity to be measured extended. Buttock should be toward edge of support surface so knees extend just past the edge (Fig. 14.2).

Examiner action

After instructing patient in motion desired, flex contralateral hip, bringing knee toward chest. Knee is allowed to flex fully. The contralateral hip should be flexed only enough to flatten lumbar spine against support surface (Fig. 14.3). (Note: Extremity not being flexed is extremity to be measured with goniometer and is referred to as the "tested" extremity.)

Patient action

Patient is instructed to grasp knee to chest, only enough to flatten lumbar spine against support surface (Fig. 14.4).

Fig. 14.3 End of ROM for the Thomas test. Bony landmarks for goniometer alignment (lateral midline of trunk, greater trochanter, lateral femoral epicondyle) indicated by red line and dots.

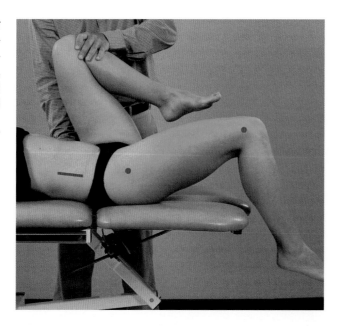

Fig. 14.4 Patient position for measuring iliopsoas muscle length using the Thomas test. Bony landmarks for goniometer alignment (lateral midline of trunk, greater trochanter, lateral femoral epicondyle) indicated by red line and dots.

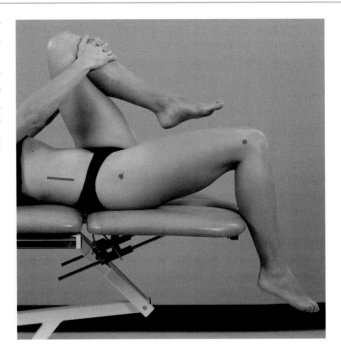

Goniometer alignment   Palpate following bony landmarks on tested lower extremity (shown in Fig. 14.2) and align goniometer accordingly (Fig. 14.5).

Stationary arm   Lateral midline of trunk.

Axis   Greater trochanter of femur.

Moving arm   Lateral epicondyle of femur.

If muscle length of iliopsoas is within normal limits, thigh of lower extremity being measured remains on examining table. No measurement is needed. If decreased muscle length of iliopsoas is present, patient's thigh being measured will rise off examining table. Maintaining proper goniometer alignment, read scale of goniometer for amount of hip flexion (see Fig. 14.5). (Note: If flexion of contralateral lower extremity to chest causes tested extremity to abduct rather than lift off support surface, patient may have a tight iliotibial band.)

Documentation   Record amount of hip flexion in tested extremity.

Precaution   Contralateral hip should be flexed by patient only enough to flatten lumbar spine against support surface. Pulling hip to chest and allowing inappropriate rotation of pelvis causes inaccurate measurement and should be avoided.

Fig. 14.5 Goniometer alignment at hip to examine iliopsoas muscle length using the Thomas test.

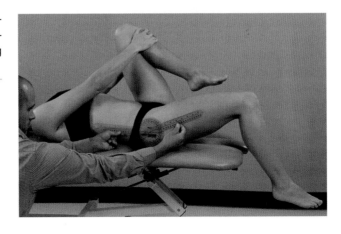

Iliopsoas Muscle Length: Prone Hip Extension Test (Video 14.2)

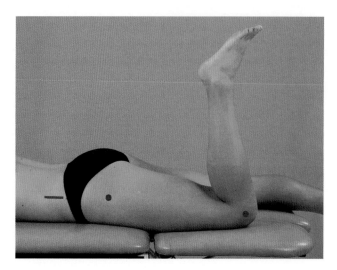

Fig. 14.6 Starting position for measuring iliopsoas muscle length using the prone extension test. Bony landmarks for goniometer alignment (lateral midline of trunk, greater trochanter, lateral femoral epicondyle) indicated by red line and dots.

An assistant is needed to perform this measurement correctly.

Patient position   Patient is prone, knee flexed to 90 degrees (Fig. 14.6).

Examiner action   After instructing the patient in motion desired, stabilize pelvis by placing one hand
(Examiner #1)   on ipsilateral side; with other hand, extend patient's hip maximally (indicated by pelvis beginning to rise), keeping knee flexed to 90 degrees (Fig. 14.7).

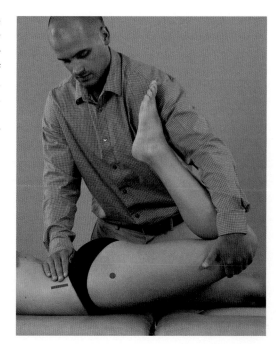

Fig. 14.7 End of ROM for the prone extension test. Bony landmarks for goniometer alignment (lateral midline of trunk, greater trochanter, lateral femoral epicondyle) indicated by red line and dot.

Fig. 14.8 Goniometer alignment to examine iliopsoas muscle length using the prone extension test.

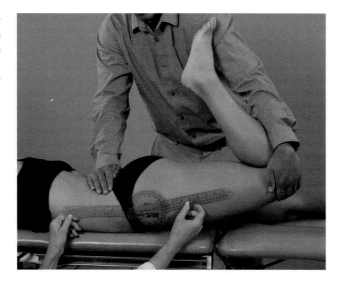

Goniometer alignment (Examiner #2)	Examiner #2 palpates following bony landmarks (shown in Fig. 14.6) and aligns goniometer accordingly (Fig. 14.8).
Stationary arm	Lateral midline of trunk.
Axis	Greater trochanter of femur.
Moving arm	Lateral epicondyle of femur. Maintaining goniometer alignment, examiner #2 reads scale of goniometer (see Fig. 14.8).
Documentation	Record patient's hip extension measurement.

Rectus Femoris Muscle Length: Thomas Test (Video 14.3)

Fig. 14.9 Starting position for measuring rectus femoris muscle length using the Thomas test. Bony landmarks for goniometer alignment (greater trochanter, lateral femoral epicondyle, lateral malleolus) indicated by red dots.

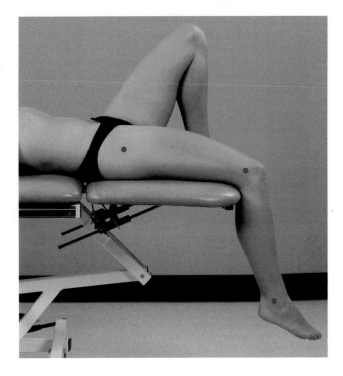

Patient position	Patient is supine, with hip of lower extremity to be measured extended. Buttock should be toward edge of support surface so knees extend just past the edge (Fig. 14.9).
Examiner action	After instructing patient in motion desired, flex contralateral hip, bringing knee toward chest. Knee is allowed to flex fully. The contralateral hip should be flexed only enough to flatten lumbar spine against support surface (Fig. 14.10). (Note: Extremity not being flexed is extremity to be measured with the goniometer and is referred to as the "tested" extremity.)
Patient action	Patient is instructed to grasp knee to chest, only enough to flatten lumbar spine against support surface (Fig. 14.11).

Fig. 14.10 End of ROM for the Thomas test. Bony landmarks for goniometer alignment (lateral midline of trunk, greater trochanter, lateral femoral epicondyle) indicated by red dots.

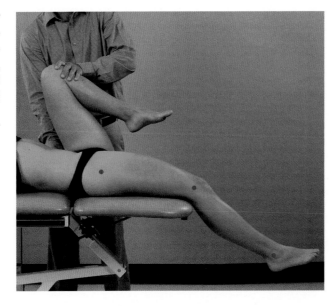

Fig. 14.11 Patient position for measuring rectus femoris muscle length using the Thomas test. Bony landmarks for goniometer alignment (lateral midline of trunk, greater trochanter, lateral femoral epicondyle) indicated by red dots.

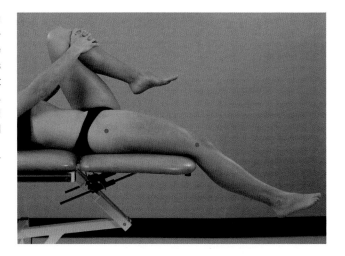

Goniometer alignment	Palpate following bony landmarks on tested lower extremity (shown in Fig. 14.9) and align goniometer accordingly (Fig. 14.12).
Stationary arm	Greater trochanter of femur.
Axis	Lateral epicondyle of femur.
Moving arm	Lateral malleolus. If muscle length of rectus femoris is within normal limits, knee being measured remains at 90 degrees of flexion. No measurement is needed. If decreased muscle length of rectus femoris is present, patient's knee being measured will extend slightly.
	Maintaining proper goniometer alignment, read scale of goniometer for amount of knee flexion (see Fig. 14.12).
Documentation	Record knee flexion in tested extremity.
Precaution	Contralateral hip should be flexed by patient only enough to flatten lumbar spine against support surface. Pulling hip to chest and allowing inappropriate rotation of pelvis causes inaccurate measurement and should be avoided.

Fig. 14.12 Goniometer alignment at knee to examine rectus femoris muscle length using the Thomas test.

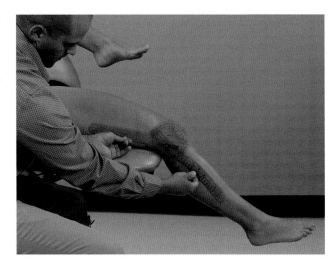

Rectus Femoris Muscle Length: Prone Technique (Ely Test) (Video 14.4)

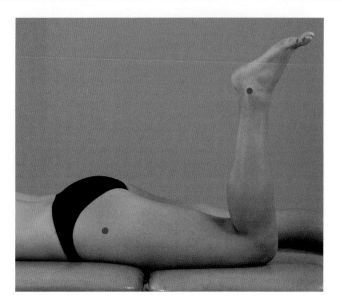

Fig. 14.13 Starting position for measuring rectus femoris muscle length using the prone technique. Bony landmarks for goniometer alignment (greater trochanter, lateral femoral epicondyle, lateral malleolus) indicated by red dots.

Patient position	Patient is prone, knee flexed to 90 degrees (Fig. 14.13).
Examiner action	After instructing patient in motion desired, flex patient's knee through full available ROM while maintaining the ipsilateral hip in full extension (Fig. 14.14).
Goniometer alignment	Palpate following bony landmarks (shown in Fig. 14.13) and align goniometer accordingly (Fig. 14.15).

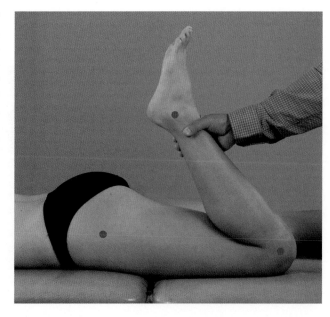

Fig. 14.14 End of ROM for rectus femoris muscle length test using the prone technique. Bony landmarks for goniometer alignment (greater trochanter, lateral femoral epicondyle, lateral malleolus) indicated by red dots.

Fig. 14.15 Patient position and goniometer alignment to examine rectus femoris muscle length using the prone technique.

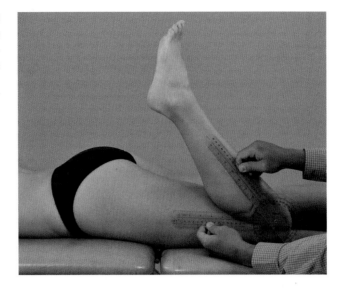

Stationary arm	Greater trochanter of femur.
Axis	Lateral epicondyle of femur.
Moving arm	Lateral malleolus.
	Maintaining proper goniometer alignment, read scale of goniometer (see Fig. 14.15).
Documentation	Record patient's maximum amount of knee flexion.
Note	The point at which the ipsilateral hip begins to flex during knee flexion marks the limit of rectus femoris muscle length. No further knee flexion should be attempted, and goniometric measurement of knee flexion should occur at that point. Fig. 14.16 illustrates inaccurate positioning for measurement caused by hip flexion of ipsilateral limb.

Fig. 14.16 Inaccurate positioning during the prone technique, allowing flexion of ipsilateral hip.

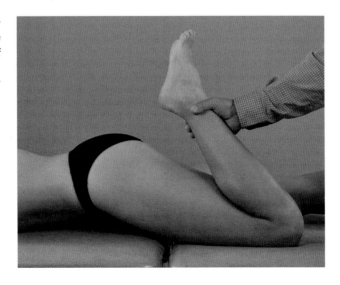

Hamstring Muscle Length: Straight Leg Raise Test (Video 14.5)

Fig. 14.17 Starting position for measuring hamstring muscle length using the straight leg raise. Bony landmarks for goniometer alignment (lateral midline of trunk, greater trochanter, lateral femoral epicondyle) indicated by red line and dot.

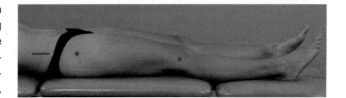

An assistant is needed to perform this measurement correctly.

Patient position	Patient is supine, with hip and knee extended (Fig. 14.17).
Examiner action (Examiner #1)	After instructing patient in motion desired, flex patient's hip through full available ROM while maintaining knee in full extension. One hand is placed over anterior thigh to ensure knee is maintained in full extension during movement, and hip is flexed until firm muscular resistance to further motion is felt (Fig. 14.18).
Goniometer alignment (Examiner 2)	Examiner #2 palpates following bony landmarks (shown in Fig. 14.17) and aligns goniometer accordingly (Fig. 14.19).
Stationary arm	Lateral midline of trunk.
Axis	Greater trochanter of femur.

Fig. 14.18 End of ROM for the straight leg raise test. Bony landmarks for goniometer alignment (lateral midline of trunk, greater trochanter, lateral femoral epicondyle) indicated by red line and dots.

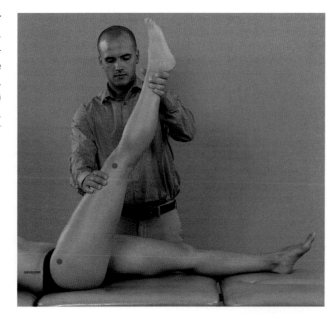

Fig. **14.19** Patient position and goniometer alignment at the end of the straight leg raise test.

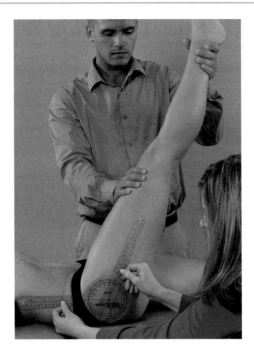

Moving arm	Lateral epicondyle of femur.
	Maintaining proper goniometer alignment, examiner #2 reads scale of goniometer (see Fig. 14.19).
Documentation	Record patient's maximum amount of hip flexion.
Precaution	Contralateral lower extremity should be maintained on support surface with knee fully extended to avoid inaccurate measurement caused by pelvic motion. Fig. 14.20 illustrates inaccurate positioning for measurement caused by hip flexion of contralateral limb.

Fig. **14.20** Incorrect positioning during the straight leg raise test, allowing hip and knee flexion of contralateral extremity.

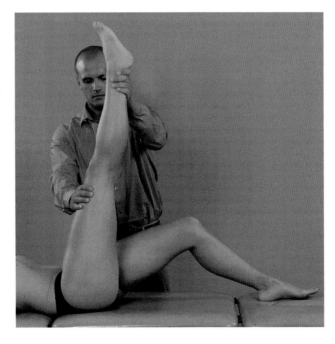

Hamstring Muscle Length: Knee Extension Test (Video 14.6)

Fig. 14.21 Starting position for measuring hamstring muscle length using the knee extension test. Bony landmarks for goniometer alignment (greater trochanter, lateral femoral epicondyle, lateral malleolus) indicated by red dots.

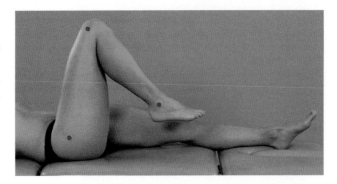

An assistant is needed to perform Option #2 of this measurement correctly.

Patient position	Patient is supine with hip flexed to 90 degrees. Contralateral lower extremity should be placed on support surface with knee fully extended. It is imperative that contralateral lower extremity be maintained in this position throughout testing (Fig. 14.21).
Examiner action	After instructing patient in motion desired, extend patient's knee through full available ROM while maintaining hip in 90 degrees of flexion. This passive movement allows an estimate of ROM available and demonstrates to patient exact movement desired (Fig. 14.22).
Patient/Examiner action	**Option #1** (Fig. 14.23)—Have patient perform active extension of knee until myoclonus is observed in hamstring muscles. **Option #2** (Fig. 14.24)—Examiner #1 passively extends knee until firm muscular resistance to further motion is felt.
Goniometer alignment	Palpate following bony landmarks (shown in Fig. 14.21) and align goniometer accordingly (see Figs. 14.23 and 14.24).

Fig. 14.22 End of ROM for the knee extension test. Bony landmarks for goniometer alignment (greater trochanter, lateral femoral epicondyle, lateral malleolus) indicated by red dots.

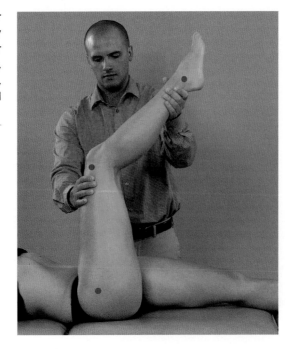

Fig. 14.23 Patient position and goniometer alignment at the end of the active knee extension test.

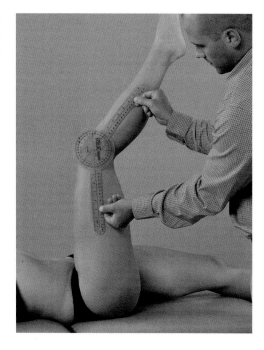

Stationary arm	Greater trochanter of femur.
Axis	Lateral epicondyle of femur.
Moving arm	Lateral malleolus.
	Maintaining proper goniometer alignment, read scale of goniometer (see Figs. 14.23 and 14.24). For Option #2, a second examiner is needed to align goniometer and read scale.
Documentation	Record patient's maximum amount of knee extension and which option was used.
Precaution	Contralateral lower extremity should be maintained on support surface with knee fully extended to avoid inaccurate measurement due to pelvic motion.

Fig. 14.24 Patient position and goniometer alignment at the end of the passive knee extension test.

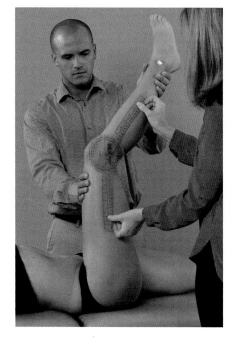

Iliotibial Band and Tensor Fasciae Latae Muscle Length: Ober Test and Modified Ober Test

Fig. 14.25 Starting position for measuring iliotibial band and tensor fasciae latae muscle length using the Ober test.

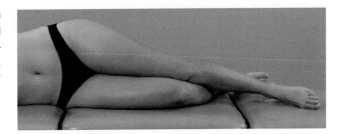

Patient position	Side-lying, with hip and knee of lowermost extremity flexed to 45 degrees to stabilize pelvis (Fig. 14.25).
Examiner action	After instructing patient in movement required, examiner places one hand on ipsilateral pelvis to stabilize it and maintain neutral pelvic alignment. Examiner uses other hand first to passively abduct hip and second to extend patient's hip on upper side in line with trunk, thereby bringing tensor fasciae latae over greater trochanter (Figs. 14.26 and 14.27).
Patient/Examiner action	Examiner asks patient to relax muscles of lower extremity while allowing uppermost limb to drop into adduction toward table through available ROM. As limb drops toward table, examiner prevents flexion and internal rotation of hip. If hip is allowed to internally rotate and flex, tensor fasciae latae and iliotibial band are no longer in lengthened position and are not accurately tested (see Figs. 14.26 and 14.27).
Ober test (Video 14.7)	During performance of test, examiner maintains patient's knee in 90 degrees of flexion (see Fig. 14.26).

Fig. 14.26 Position for performing the Ober test.

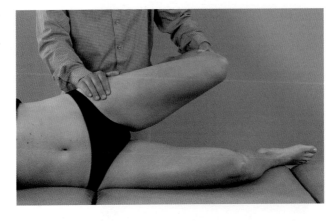

Fig. 14.27 Patient position when performing the modified Ober test.

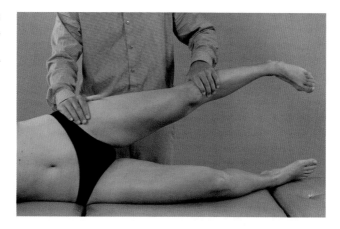

Modified Ober test (Video 14.8)

During performance of test, examiner maintains patient's knee in full extension (see Fig. 14.27).

Measurement

Review of literature yields very few reports of using goniometers, tape measures, or any other device for measurement when Ober and modified Ober tests are performed. Traditionally, this test is performed in an "all or none" fashion. Either test is positive and patient has tight tensor fasciae latae and iliotibial band, or test is negative and patient has ideal muscle length.

Positive test

For both Ober and modified Ober, the test is considered positive for tight tensor fasciae latae and iliotibial band if relaxed hip remains abducted and does not fall below horizontal. Test is considered negative for tight tensor fasciae latae and iliotibial band if relaxed and extended hip falls below horizontal.

Precaution

Extremity being measured should not be allowed to flex and internally rotate at the hip. Fig. 14.28 illustrates incorrect positioning for Ober test.

Fig. 14.28 Incorrect patient positioning for performing the Ober test, allowing flexion and internal rotation of the hip being tested.

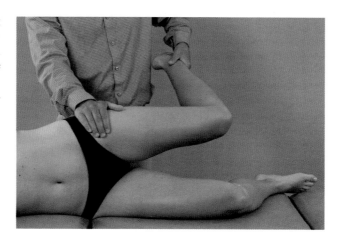

Iliotibial Band and Tensor Fasciae Latae Muscle Length: Ober Test and Modified Ober Test—Inclinometer

Fig. 14.29 Starting position for measurement of iliotibial band and tensor fasciae latae muscle length using the Ober test and modified Ober test.

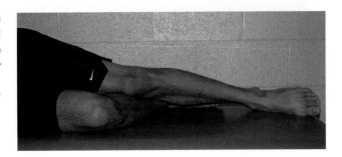

An assistant is needed to perform this measurement correctly.

Patient position   Side-lying, with hip and knee of lowermost extremity flexed to 45 degrees to stabilize pelvis (Fig. 14.29).

Examiner action (Examiner #1)   After instructing patient in movement required, examiner places one hand on ipsilateral pelvis to stabilize it and maintain neutral pelvic alignment. Examiner uses other hand first to passively abduct hip and second to extend patient's hip on upper side in line with trunk, thereby bringing tensor fasciae latae over greater trochanter (Figs. 14.30 and 14.31).

Patient/Examiner action   Examiner asks patient to relax muscles of lower extremity while allowing uppermost limb to drop into adduction toward table through available ROM. As limb drops toward table, examiner prevents flexion and internal rotation of hip. If hip is allowed to internally rotate and flex, tensor fasciae latae and iliotibial band are no longer in lengthened position and are not tested accurately (see Figs. 14.30 and 14.31).

Fig. 14.30 Position for performing the Ober test with inclinometer.

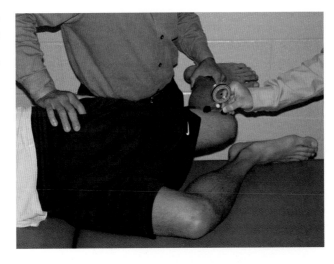

Fig. 14.31 Patient position when the modified Ober test and inclinometer are used.

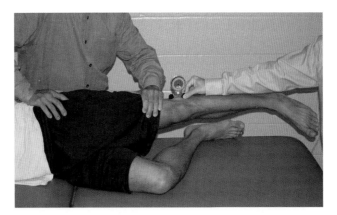

Ober test

During performance of test, examiner #1 maintains patient's knee in 90 degrees of flexion while examiner #2 places the inclinometer on the lateral epicondyle of the femur (see Fig. 14.30).

Modified ober test

During performance of test, examiner #1 maintains patient's knee in full extension while examiner #2 places the inclinometer on the lateral epicondyle of the femur (see Fig. 14.31).

Documentation

Read the inclinometer and record the amount of hip abduction. If during the test the limb remains horizontal, 0 degrees is recorded; if the limb falls below the horizontal (adducted), a positive number is recorded; and if the limb remains above the horizontal (abducted), a negative number is recorded.

Precaution

Extremity being measured should not be allowed to flex and internally rotate at the hip. Fig. 14.28 illustrates incorrect positioning for the Ober test.

Iliotibial Band (ITB) and Tensor Fasciae Latae (TFL) Muscle Length: Ober Test and Modified Ober Test—Smartphone

Fig. 14.32 Starting position for measurement of iliotibial band and tensor fasciae latae muscle length using the Ober test and modified Ober test.

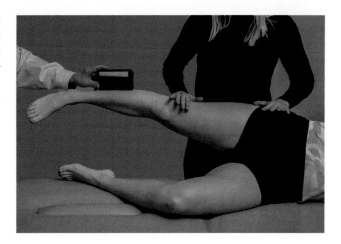

An assistant is needed to perform this measurement correctly.

Patient position

Side-lying, with hip and knee of lowermost extremity flexed to 45 degrees to stabilize pelvis (Fig. 14.32).

Examiner action (Examiner #1)

After instructing patient in movement required, examiner places one hand on ipsilateral pelvis to stabilize it and maintain neutral pelvic alignment. Examiner uses other hand first to passively abduct hip and second to extend patient's hip on upper side in line with trunk, thereby bringing tensor fasciae latae over greater trochanter (Figs. 14.33 and 14.34).

Fig. 14.33 Position for performing the Ober test with Smartphone.

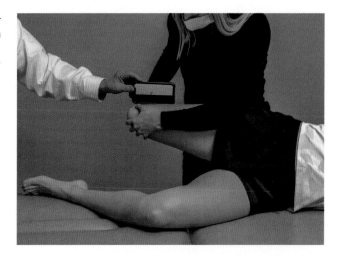

Fig. 14.34 Patient position when the modified Ober test and Smartphone are used.

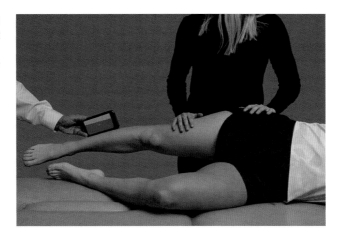

Patient/Examiner action

Examiner asks patient to relax muscles of lower extremity while allowing upper-most thigh to drop into adduction toward table through available muscle length. As limb drops toward table, examiner prevents flexion and internal rotation of hip (see Figs. 14.33 and 14.34).

Ober test

During performance of test, examiner #1 maintains patient's knee in 90 degrees of flexion, while examiner #2 places the Smartphone on the lateral epicondyle of the femur (see Fig. 14.33) with Smartphone screen facing toward therapist.

Modified ober test

During performance of test, examiner #1 maintains patient's knee in full extension while examiner #2 places the Smartphone on the lateral epicondyle of the femur (see Fig. 14.34) with Smartphone screen facing toward therapist. Ensure the Smartphone application starts at 0 degrees, move the patient's leg as needed.

Documentation

Read the Smartphone and record the amount of hip abduction. If during the test the limb remains horizontal, 0 degrees is recorded; if the limb falls below the horizontal (adducted), a positive number is recorded; and if the limb remains above the horizontal (abducted), a negative number is recorded.

Precaution

Extremity being measured should not be allowed to flex and internally rotate at the hip. If hip is allowed to internally rotate and flex, the tensor fasciae latae and iliotibial band are no longer in lengthened position and are not accurately tested. Fig. 14.28 illustrates incorrect positioning for the Ober test.

Iliotibial Band and Tensor Fasciae Latae Muscle Length: Prone Technique (Video 14.9)

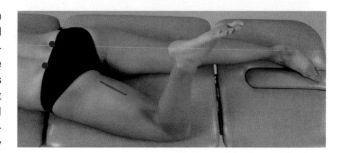

Fig. 14.35 Starting position for measuring iliotibial band and tensor fasciae latae muscle length using the prone technique. Bony landmarks for goniometer alignment (contralateral PSIS, ipsilateral PSIS, posterior midline of ipsilateral femur) indicated by red line and dots.

Patient position   Patient is prone, hip abducted and knee flexed to 90 degrees (Fig. 14.35).

Examiner action   After instructing patient in movement required, examiner stabilizes pelvis with one hand and adducts hip (maintaining 90-degree knee flexion) until movement of the pelvis is palpated. End point is defined as point at which initial pelvic movement is detected (Fig. 14.36).

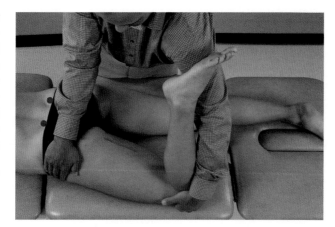

Fig. 14.36 End of ROM for the prone technique for measuring iliotibial band and tensor fasciae latae muscle length. Bony landmarks for goniometer alignment (contralateral PSIS, ipsilateral PSIS, posterior midline of ipsilateral femur) indicated by red line and dots.

Fig.   14.37 Goniometer alignment to examine iliotibial band and tensor fasciae latae muscle length using the prone technique.

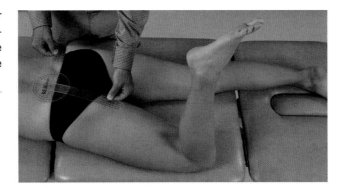

Goniometer alignment	Palpate following bony landmarks (shown in Fig. 14.35), and align goniometer accordingly (Fig. 14.37).
Stationary arm	Contralateral posterior superior iliac spine (PSIS).
Axis	Ipsilateral PSIS.
Moving arm	Posterior midline of ipsilateral femur.
	Maintaining goniometer alignment, read scale of goniometer (see Fig. 14.37).
Documentation	Record patient's hip abduction/adduction measurement.

Gastrocnemius Muscle Length Test (Video 14.10)

Fig. 14.38 Starting position for measuring gastrocnemius muscle length. Bony landmarks for goniometer alignment (fibular head, lateral malleolus, parallel to fifth metatarsal) indicated by red line and dots.

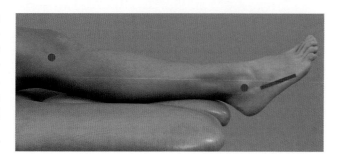

Patient position	Patient is supine with hip and knee extended (Fig. 14.38).
Examiner action	After instructing patient in motion desired, dorsiflex patient's ankle through full available ROM while maintaining knee in full extension. This passive movement allows an estimate of ROM available and demonstrates to patient exact movement desired (Fig. 14.39).
Patient/Examiner action	Maintaining full knee extension, perform passive, or have patient perform active, dorsiflexion of ankle (see Fig. 14.39).
Goniometer alignment	Palpate following bony landmarks (shown in Fig. 14.39) and align goniometer accordingly (Fig. 14.40).
Stationary arm	Head of fibula.
Axis	Lateral malleolus.

Fig. 14.39 End of ROM for the gastrocnemius muscle length test. Bony landmarks for goniometer alignment (fibular head, lateral malleolus, parallel to fifth metatarsal) indicated by red line and dots.

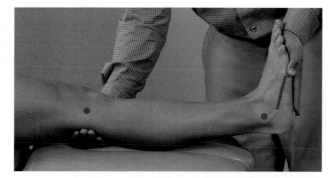

Fig. 14.40 Patient position and goniometer alignment at the end of the gastrocnemius muscle length test.

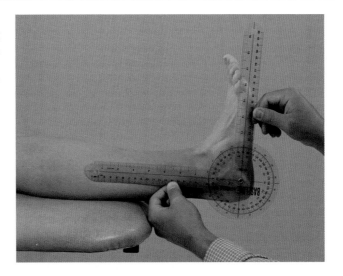

Moving arm

Parallel to fifth metatarsal.

Maintaining proper goniometer alignment, read scale of goniometer (see Fig. 14.40).

Documentation

Record patient's maximum amount of dorsiflexion.

Precaution

Examiner must ensure that knee remains in full extension during dorsiflexion movement.

Note

A suggested procedure for measuring dorsiflexion involves maintaining the subtalar joint in neutral position while dorsiflexing the patient's ankle. It is thought that in this way pronation and supination are avoided and pure dorsiflexion is measured. The procedure for maintaining neutral position of the subtalar joint is described in Chapter 13 (see Fig. 13.16).

Soleus Muscle Length Test: Supine (Video 14.11)

Fig. 14.41 Starting position for measuring soleus muscle length with patient supine. Bony landmarks for goniometer alignment (fibular head, lateral malleolus, parallel to fifth metatarsal) indicated by red line and dots.

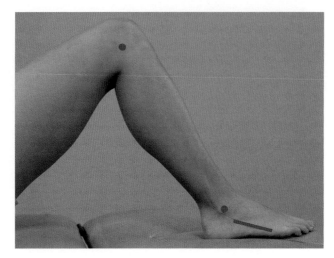

Patient position	Patient is supine with hip and knee flexed to 45 degrees. Placing knee in flexion relaxes gastrocnemius muscle and allows measurement of soleus muscle. Opposite lower extremity should be placed on support surface with knee fully extended (Fig. 14.41).
Examiner action	After instructing patient in motion desired, dorsiflex patient's ankle through full available ROM while maintaining hip and knee in 45 degrees of flexion. This passive movement allows an estimate of available ROM and demonstrates to patient exact movement desired (Fig. 14.42).
Patient/Examiner action	Maintaining hip and knee in 45 degrees of flexion, perform passive, or have patient perform active, dorsiflexion of ankle (see Fig. 14.42).
Goniometer alignment	Palpate following bony landmarks (shown in Fig. 14.41) and align goniometer accordingly (Fig. 14.43).
Stationary arm	Head of fibula.

Fig. 14.42 End of ROM for the soleus muscle length test—supine. Bony landmarks for goniometer alignment (fibular head, lateral malleolus, parallel to fifth metatarsal) indicated by red line and dots.

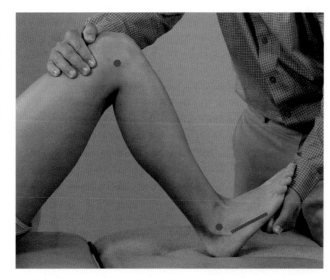

Fig. 14.43 Patient position and goniometer alignment at the end of the soleus muscle length test—supine.

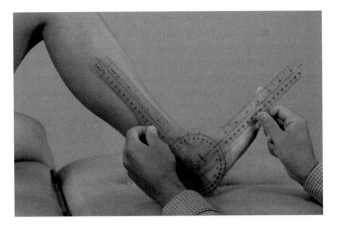

Axis	Lateral malleolus.
Moving arm	Parallel to fifth metatarsal.
	Maintaining proper goniometer alignment, read scale of goniometer (see Fig. 14.43).
Documentation	Record patient's maximum amount of dorsiflexion.
Note	A suggested procedure for measuring dorsiflexion involves maintaining the subtalar joint in neutral position while dorsiflexing the patient's ankle. It is thought that in this way pronation and supination are avoided and pure dorsiflexion is measured. The procedure for maintaining neutral position of the subtalar joint is described in Chapter 13 (see Fig. 13.16).

Soleus Muscle Length Test: Prone (Video 14.12)

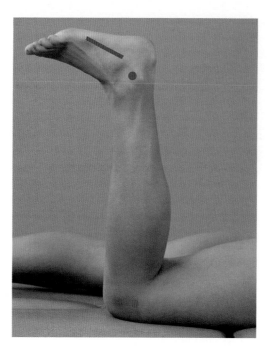

Fig. 14.44 Starting position for measuring soleus muscle length with patient prone. Bony landmarks for goniometer alignment (fibular head, lateral malleolus, parallel to fifth metatarsal) indicated by red line and dots.

Patient position

Patient is prone with knee flexed to 90 degrees. Placing knee in flexion relaxes gastrocnemius muscle and allows measurement of soleus muscle. Opposite lower extremity should be placed on support surface with knee fully extended (Fig. 14.44).

Examiner action

After instructing patient in motion desired, dorsiflex patient's ankle through full available ROM while maintaining knee in 90 degrees of flexion. This passive movement allows an estimate of available ROM and demonstrates to patient exact movement desired (Fig. 14.45).

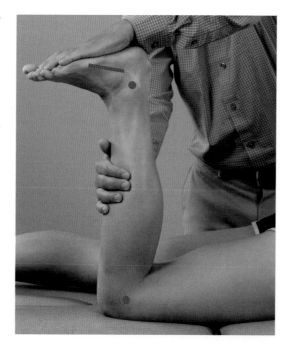

Fig. 14.45 End of ROM for soleus muscle length—prone. Bony landmarks for goniometer alignment (fibular head, lateral malleolus, parallel to fifth metatarsal) indicated by red line and dots.

Fig. 14.46 Patient position and goniometer alignment at the end of soleus muscle length test—prone.

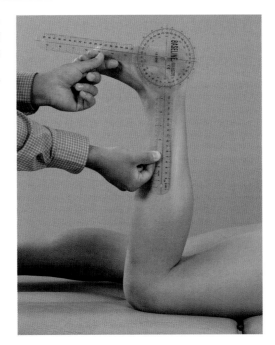

Patient/Examiner action	Maintaining hip and knee in 90 degrees of flexion, perform passive, or have patient perform active, dorsiflexion of ankle (see Fig. 14.45).
Goniometer alignment	Palpate following bony landmarks (shown in Fig. 14.44) and align goniometer accordingly (Fig. 14.46).
Stationary arm	Head of fibula.
Axis	Lateral malleolus.
Moving arm	Parallel to fifth metatarsal.
	Maintaining proper goniometer alignment, read scale of goniometer (see Fig. 14.46).
Documentation	Record patient's maximum amount of dorsiflexion.

Soleus (Gastrocnemius) Muscle Length: Standing Lunge Test—Tape Measure

Fig. 14.47 Starting position for measurement of dorsiflexion using the weight bearing lunge. Subject places hands against the wall. Toes of the tested leg (right) placed behind the tape 27 in. from the wall. Toes of the leg not being tested (left) placed behind the tape placed 12 in. from the wall.

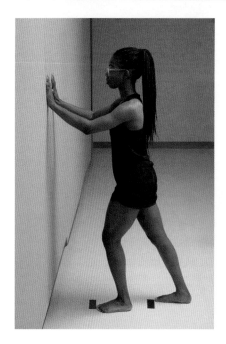

Patient position	Standing facing a wall with hands lightly against the wall for balance. Toes of the tested leg (right) placed behind the tape 27 in. from the wall. Toes of the leg not being tested (left) placed behind the tape placed 12 in. from the wall (Fig.14.47).
Examiner action	Ask the subject to place the forearms against the wall and perform a lunge on the extremity to be tested (right), keeping the foot of the tested extremity flat on the floor while flexing the knee of that extremity toward the wall. *(Note: To test the gastrocnemius muscle length, the knee of the extremity to be tested should be held in extension.)* The knee should remain in the line with the second toe. The opposite leg (left) acts as balance. Ensure that the subject does not move the knee and foot medial; return the subject to the starting position. Ensure the subject's heel remains in firm contact with the floor during movement. Performing a trial movement provides an estimate of muscle length and demonstrates to the subject the exact movement desired (Fig. 14.48).

Fig. 14.48 End range of ankle dorsiflexion. Subject moves hips forward toward the wall and lean against their forearms, as needed, for balance.

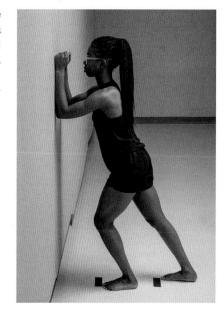

Fig. 14.49   End of ankle dorsiflexion demonstrating proper alignment of tape measure perpendicular between the base of the patella and the wall. Heel of both legs remain in full contact of the floor.

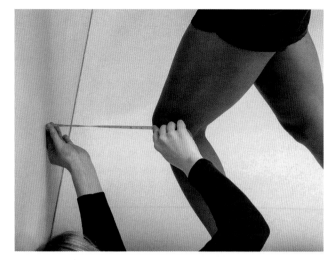

Tape measure alignment

Examiner places the "zero" end of the tape measure on the mid patella on the extremity to be measured (right).

Patient/Examiner action

Ask the subject to repeat the lunge movement as previously instructed (Fig. 14.48). Once the participant has reached end range, the other end of the tape measure is placed on the wall directly in front of and perpendicular to the mid patella. Read the tape measure (Fig. 14.49).

Documentation

The distance, in inches, is recorded.

Soleus (Gastrocnemius) Muscle Length: Standing Lunge Test—Inclinometer

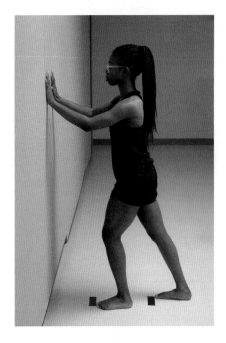

Fig. 14.50 Starting position for measurement of dorsiflexion using the weight bearing lunge. Subject places hands against the wall. Toes of the tested leg (right) placed behind the tape 27 in. from the wall. Toes of the leg not being tested (left) placed behind the tape placed 12 in. from the wall.

Patient position

Standing facing a wall with hands lightly against the wall for balance. Toes of the tested leg (right) placed behind the tape 27 in. from the wall. Toes of the leg not being tested (left) placed behind the tape placed 12 in. from the wall (Fig.14.50).

Examiner action

Ask the subject to place the forearms against the wall and perform a lunge on the extremity to be tested (right), keeping the foot of the tested extremity flat on the floor while flexing the knee of that extremity toward the wall. (Note: To test the gastrocnemius muscle length, the knee of the extremity to be tested should be held in extension.) The knee should remain in the line with the second toe. The opposite leg (left) acts as balance. Ensure that the subject does not move the knee and foot medial; return the subject to the starting position. Ensure the subject's heel remains in firm contact with the floor during movement. Performing a trial movement provides an estimate of muscle length and demonstrates to the subject the exact movement desired (Fig. 14.51).

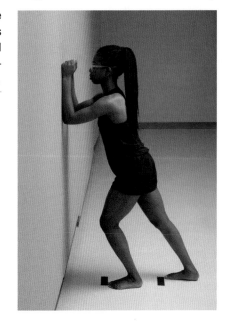

Fig. 14.51 End range of ankle dorsiflexion. Subject moves hips forward toward the wall and lean against their forearms, as needed, for balance.

Fig. 14.52 Starting position for measurement of dorsiflexion demonstrating proper initial alignment of inclinometer on the anterior tibia.

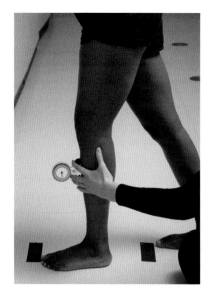

Inclinometer alignment	Along anterior tibial crest midway between the tibial tuberosity and ankle joint. Ensure the inclinometer is set at 0 degrees once positioned on the subject (Fig. 14.52).
Patient/Examiner action	Ask the subject to repeat the lunge movement as previously instructed. Ensure that the feet of the inclinometer remain in firm contact with the tibial crest (Fig. 14.51). Read scale of inclinometer (Fig. 14.53).
Documentation	Record subject's ROM.

Fig. 14.53 End of ankle dorsiflexion demonstrating proper alignment of inclinometer on the anterior tibia. Heel of both legs remain in full contact of the floor.

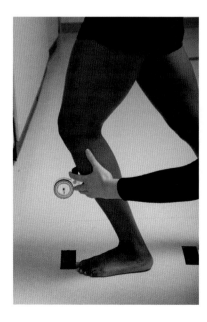

Soleus (Gastrocnemius) Muscle Length: Standing Lunge Test—Smartphone

Fig. 14.54 Starting position for measurement of dorsiflexion using the weight bearing lunge. Subject places hands against the wall. Toes of the tested leg (right) placed behind the tape 27 in. from the wall. Toes of the leg not being tested (left) placed behind the tape placed 12 in. from the wall.

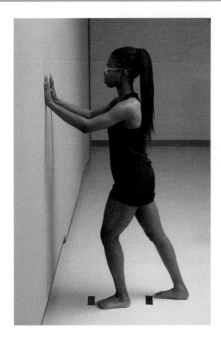

Patient position	Standing facing a wall with hands lightly against the wall for balance. Toes of the tested leg (right) placed behind the tape 27 in. from the wall. Toes of the leg not being tested (left) placed behind the tape placed 12 in. from the wall (Fig. 14.54).
Examiner action	Ask the subject to place the forearms against the wall and perform a lunge on the extremity to be tested (right), keeping the foot of the tested extremity flat on the floor while flexing the knee of that extremity toward the wall. *(Note: To test the gastrocnemius muscle length, the knee of the extremity to be tested should be held in extension.)* The knee should remain in the line with the second toe. The opposite leg (left) acts as balance. Ensure that the subject does not move the knee and foot medial; return the subject to the starting position. Ensure the subject's heel remains in firm contact with the floor during movement. Performing a trial movement provides an estimate of muscle length and demonstrates to the subject the exact movement desired (Fig. 14.55).

Fig. 14.55 End range of ankle dorsiflexion using the weight bearing lunge. Subject moves hips forward toward the wall and lean against their forearms, as needed, for balance.

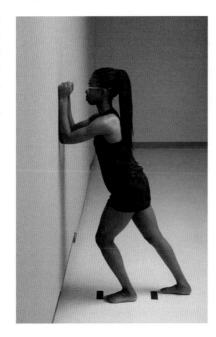

Fig. 14.56 Starting position for measurement of dorsiflexion demonstrating proper initial alignment of Smartphone on the anterior tibia.

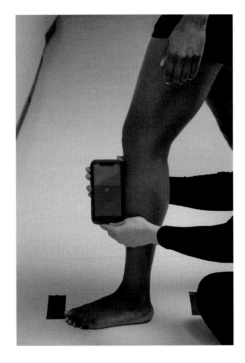

Smartphone alignment   Border of Smartphone along anterior tibial crest midway between the tibial tuberosity and ankle joint with screen facing therapist. Ensure the Smartphone is set at 0 degrees once positioned on the subject (Fig. 14.56).

Patient/Examiner action   Ask the subject to repeat the lunge movement as previously instructed (see Fig. 14.55). Ensure Smartphone remains in firm contact with the tibial crest. Read scale of Smartphone (Fig. 14.57).

Documentation   Record subject's ROM.

Fig. 14.57 End of ankle dorsiflexion demonstrating proper alignment of Smartphone on the anterior tibia. Heel of both legs remain in full contact of the floor.

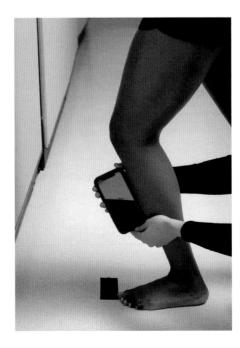

References

1. Lee LW, Kerrigan C, Croce LTD. Dynamic implications of hip flexion contractures. *Am J Phys Med Rehabil.* 1997;76:502–508.
2. Kendall FP. *Muscles: Testing and Function.* Baltimore: Williams & Wilkins; 1949.
3. Kendall FP, McCreary EK, Provance PG, et al. *Muscles: Testing and Function.* 5th ed. Baltimore: Williams & Wilkins; 2005.
4. Magee DJ. *Orthopedic Physical Assessment.* 5th ed. Philadelphia: WB Saunders; 2007.
5. Peeler J, Anderson JE. Reliability of the Thomas test for assessing range of motion about the hip. *Phys Ther Sport.* 2007;8:14–21.
6. Greene WB, Heckman JD. *The Clinical Measurement of Joint Motion.* 3rd ed. Rosemont, IL: American Academy of Orthopaedic Surgeons; 2003.
7. Gajdosik RL, Rieck MA, Sullivan DK, et al. Comparison of four clinical tests for assessing hamstring muscle length. *J Orthop Sports Phys Ther.* 1993;18:614–618.
8. Rakos DM, Shaw KA, Fedor RL, et al. Interrater reliability of the active-knee-extension test for hamstring length in school-aged children. *Pediatr Phys Ther.* 2001;13:37–41.
9. Fredriksen H, Dagfinrud H, V J, et al. Passive knee extension test to measure hamstring muscle tightness. *Scand J Med Sci Sports.* 1997;7:279–282.
10. Nelson RT, Bandy WD. Eccentric training and static stretching improve hamstring flexibility of high-school males. *J Athl Train.* 2004;39:31–35.
11. Katz K, Rosenthal A, Yosipovitch Z. Normal ranges of popliteal angle in children. *J Pediatr Orthop.* 1992;12:229–231.
12. Reade E, Horn L, A H, et al. Changes in popliteal angle measurement in infants up to one year of age. *Dev Med Child Neurol.* 1984;26:774–780.
13. Jackson A, Langford NJ. The criterion-related validity of the sit-and-reach test: replication and extension of previous findings. *Res Q Exerc Sport.* 1989;60:384–387.
14. Baltaci G, Un N, V T, et al. Comparison of three different sit and reach tests for measurement of hamstring flexibility in female university students. *Br J Sports Med.* 2003;37:59–61.
15. Cornbleet SL, Woolsey NB. Assessment of hamstring muscle length in school–aged children using the sit-and-reach test and the inclinometer measure of hip joint angle. *Phys Ther.* 1996;76:850–855.
16. Hoppenfeld S. *Physical Examination of the Spine and Extremities.* Norwalk: CT: Appleton & Lange; 1976.
17. Shephard RJ, Berridge M, Montelpare W. On the generality of the "sit and reach" test: an analysis of flexibility data for an aging population. *Res Q Exerc Sport.* 1990;61:326–330.
18. Ober FR. Back strain and sciatica. *JAMA.* 1935;104:1580–1581.
19. Ellis R, Hing W, Reid D. Iliotibial band friction syndrome–a systematic review. *Man Ther.* 2007;12:200–208.
20. Frederickson M, Weir A. Practical management of iliotibial band friction syndrome in runners. *Clin J Sport Med.* 2006;16:261–268.
21. Kendall HO, Kendall FP, Boynton DA. *Posture and Pain.* Baltimore: Williams & Wilkins; 1952.
22. Melchione WE, Sullivan MS. Reliability of measurements obtained by use of an instrument designed to indirectly measure iliotibial band length. *J Orthop Sports Phys Ther.* 1993;18:511–515.
23. Gautam VK, Anand S. A new test for estimating iliotibial band contracture. *J Bone Joint Surg Br.* 1998;80:474–475.
24. Gajdosik RL, Sandler MM, Marr HL. Influence of knee position and gender on the Ober test for length of the iliotibial band. *Clin Biomechan.* 2003;18:77–79.
25. Pandya S, Florence JM, King WM, et al. Reliability of goniometric measurements in patients with Duchenne muscular dystrophy. *Phys Ther.* 1985;65:1339–1342.
26. Doucette SA, Goble EM. The effect of exercise on patellar tracking in lateral patellar compression syndrome. *Am J Sports Med.* 1992;20:434–440.
27. Reese NB, Bandy WD. Use of inclinometer to measure flexibility of the iliotibial band using the Ober test and the modified Ober test: differences in magnitude and reliability of measurements. *J Orthop Sports Phys Ther.* 2003;33:326–330.
28. Gose JC, Schweizer P. Iliotibial band tightness. *J Orthop Sports Phys Ther.* 1989;10:399–407.
29. Wang SS, Whitney SL, Burdett RG, Janosky JE. Lower extremity muscular flexibility in long distance runners. *J Orthop Sports Phys Ther.* 1993;17:102–107.

15

RELIABILITY and VALIDITY of MEASUREMENTS of RANGE of MOTION and MUSCLE LENGTH TESTING of the LOWER EXTREMITY

Nancy Berryman Reese and William D. Bandy

RELIABILITY AND VALIDITY OF LOWER EXTREMITY GONIOMETRY

Chapters 11 through 14 presented techniques for measuring range of motion (ROM) of joints and length of muscles in the lower extremities. When selecting appropriate techniques for measuring ROM and muscle length, one must consider whether the technique selected has been shown to be reliable and valid.[1,2] This chapter presents information regarding the reliability and validity (when available) of techniques used for measuring lower extremity range of motion and muscle length. In accordance with the discussion of the preferred methods of analyzing reliability presented in Chapter 2, only those studies that examined reliability using the intraclass correlation coefficient (ICC) or Pearson product–moment correlation coefficient (Pearson's r) with a follow-up test are included.

As is apparent from the information and tables that follow, seldom has one method of goniometry or muscle length testing been shown to be clearly preferable in terms of reliability as demonstrated by more than one investigator. In fact, many studies are so vaguely described as to be unrepeatable by others, and studies that are repeated in some form often produce conflicting results. Therefore, unless obvious conclusions can be made regarding the efficacy of one technique over another, no interpretive comments are made regarding the information presented in this chapter. Rather, the chapter serves as a reference to the reader and, it is hoped, it will make obvious the areas of research in lower extremity ROM and muscle length testing that have yet to be addressed.

Hip Flexion/Extension

Several studies that examined the reliability of hip flexion and extension ROM have been published. Using a combination of the Thomas and Mundale techniques (see Chapters 11 and 14 for a description of the Mundale and Thomas techniques), Stuberg et al.[3] measured the reliability of measurements of passive hip flexion with the knee extended (straight leg raise) and passive hip extension in 20 individuals, aged 5 to 21 years, with moderate to severe hypertonicity. To examine interrater reliability, three pediatric physical therapists repeated each of the measurements three times on each subject in one testing session, using a blinded goniometer. Measurements were repeated 5 to 7 days later on five of the subjects to determine intrarater reliability. A two-way analysis of variance (ANOVA) for repeated measures was used to determine intrarater and interrater reliability for each motion. Analysis of intrarater reliability showed no significant differences among the three measures taken by a single examiner in one session, and intrarater error was calculated at less than or equal to 5 degrees for most measurements, based on the 95% confidence interval. Conversely, significant interrater variation was found in hip flexion and extension measurements.

Since Stuberg's study,[3] at least two additional studies have been published regarding the reliability of hip ROM in children with spastic cerebral palsy. As in the Stuberg[3] study, Kilgour et al.[4] measured hip extension using the Thomas test and measured hip flexion with the knee extended in a group of children with spastic diplegia (n = 25) and also in a group of age- and sex-matched controls (n = 25). However, unlike Stuberg et al.[3] the investigators in the Kilgour et al. study examined the reliability of "dynamic range of motion" measurements. A single experienced pediatric physical therapist performed all measurements in all 50 children using a goniometer and standardized techniques. Measurements were taken twice in the initial session and then repeated 7 days later. Intrarater reliability within the same session for measurements of hip flexion using the Thomas test was higher for the control group (0.09 to 0.91) than for the groups with spastic diplegia (0.17 to 0.66). Intrarater reliability for measurements of hip flexion with knee extended were higher for both groups of subjects within the same session (Controls: 0.79 to 0.87; Spastic diplegia: 0.97 to 0.99) than between the two sessions (Controls: 0.34 to 0.67; Spastic diplegia: 0.84 to 0.92).[4]

Mutlu et al.[5] also examined the reliability of goniometric measurements of passive hip ROM in children with spastic cerebral palsy (CP). In a group of 38 children with spastic CP, three different physical therapists with 3 to 16 years of experience measured passive hip flexion with the knee extended and passive hip extension using the Thomas test. All subjects were measured by each of the three examiners a second time, 1 week later. The authors calculated intrarater and interrater reliability of the measurements using ICCs. Intrarater reliability for measurements of hip flexion with the knee extended ranged from 0.60 to 0.86, while for hip extension, these values ranged from 0.61 to 0.99 (Table 15.1). Interrater reliability was higher, ranging from 0.77 to 0.83 for hip flexion with the knee extended, and from 0.92 to 0.95 for hip extension (Table 15.2).[5]

At least five groups of investigators have examined the reliability of hip ROM measurement in individuals

with musculoskeletal pathology involving the hip.[10,11,16–18] Nussbaumer et al.[10] examined the concurrent validity and intrarater reliability of the standard goniometer for measuring passive hip ROM in subjects with femoroacetabular impingement. Passive hip flexion (as well as abduction, adduction, and rotation) was simultaneously measured using a standard goniometer and an electromagnetic tracking system (ETS) (which served as the criterion device for concurrent validity). Two human movement scientists performed all goniometric assessments using a standardized protocol. The amount of force applied during passive ROM measurements was standardized and monitored using a hand-held dynamometer. Intrarater reliability for measurements of passive hip flexion was high, with an ICC of 0.92 and a standard error of measurement (SEM) of 4 degrees (see Table 15.1). However, concurrent validity between the standard goniometer and the ETS for

Table 15.1 INTRARATER RELIABILITY: HIP FLEXION/EXTENSION RANGE OF MOTION

HIP FLEXION

STUDY	TECHNIQUE	n	SAMPLE	r^*	ICC[†]
Aalto et al.[6]	PROM; supine; hip flexed with knee extended (SLR); goniometer; 2 examiners (PTs) measured ROM after 1 and 8, 1–2 s passive stretches	20 (40 hips)	Healthy adults (12 F, 8 M) (18–45 years; $\bar{x}$ = 23.3)		0.94–0.98
Clapper and Wolf[7]	AROM; supine standardized goniometer technique; 3 measures; 5 sessions; 1 examiner (MMSc)	20	Healthy adults 10 F, $\bar{x}$ = 28.3 years 10 M, $\bar{x}$ = 30.0 years	0.75	0.95
Kilgour et al.[4]	PROM; supine; hip flexed with knee extended (SLR); Intrasessional (Intra) and Intersessional (Inter) reliability; goniometer	50	25 Children with CP (CP); 25 age- and sex-matched controls (CTL) (28 F, 22 M) (6–17 years)		0.99 (CTL; Intra) 0.52–0.61 (CTL; Inter) 0.95–0.98 (CP; Intra) 0.62–0.63 (CP; Inter)
Macedo and Magee[8]	PROM; supine; hip neutral and knee extended; standardized goniometer technique; 1 examiner (PT)	12 (24 hips)	Healthy Caucasian women (18–59 years; $\bar{x}$ = 37.2)		0.85
Marques et al.[9]	PROM; supine; hip neutral and knee flexion; goniometer; 2 examiners	40	Healthy adults (32 F, 8 M) (18–28 years; $\bar{x}$ = 21.8 ± 4.2 years)		0.95
Mutlu et al.[5]	PROM; supine; hip flexed with knee extended (SLR); 3 examiners (PTs with 3–14 years experience); goniometer	38 (60 hips)	Children with spastic diplegia (CP) (18–108 months; $\bar{x}$ = 52.9 ± 19.6 months)		0.60–0.86
Nussbaumer et al.[10]	PROM; supine; hip flexed with knee flexion; 1 examiner (1 year experience in musculoskeletal examination)	30 (60 hips)	15 Patients with FAI (7 F, 8 M) (35 ± 11 years) 15 healthy subjects (7 F, 8 M) (34 ± 10 years)		0.92
Pua et al.[11]	PROM; supine; strap across contralateral distal thigh; hip flexed with knee flexion; 1 examiner (PT w/7 years experience); affected hip tested; digital inclinometer	22	Adults with hip OA (12 F, 10 M) (50–84 years; $\bar{x}$ = 62 ± 8.9)		0.97
Prather et al.[12]	PROM; supine; hip flexed with knee flexion; goniometer; 2 examiners (PT and MD)	28 (56 hips)	Healthy adults (18–51 years; $\bar{x}$ = 31 years)		0.95 (both hips) 0.94 (R hip) 0.96 (L hip)
Walker et al.[13]	AROM; AAOS standardized goniometer technique; 4 examiners	4	Healthy adults (60–84 years)	> 0.81	

Table 15.1	INTRARATER RELIABILITY: HIP FLEXION/EXTENSION RANGE OF MOTION—cont'd				

HIP EXTENSION

STUDY	TECHNIQUE	n	SAMPLE	r^*	ICC†
Bartlett et al.[14]	Four goniometer techniques utilized: AAOS; prone with contralateral hip flexed (AA); Mundale technique (MU); pelvifemoral angle technique (PA); and Thomas test technique (TT)	28	Children and young adults with Myelomeningocele (MM) ($n = 14$; 4–19 years) or spastic diplegia (SD) ($n = 14$; 6–20 years)	AA 0.93 (MM) 0.82 (SD) MU 0.91 (MM) 0.63 (SD) PA 0.92 (MM) 0.78 (SD) TT 0.93 (MM) 0.89 (SD)	
Clapper and Wolf[7]	AROM; supine standardized goniometer technique; 3 measures; 5 sessions; 1 examiner (MMSc)	20	Healthy adults 10 F, $\bar{x} = 28.3$ years 10 M, $\bar{x} = 30.0$ years		0.83
Macedo and Magee[8]	PROM; prone; hip neutral with knee extended; standardized goniometer technique; 1 examiner (PT)	12 (24 hips)	Healthy Caucasian women (18–59 years; $\bar{x} = 37.2$)		0.82
Prather et al.[12]	PROM; supine; hip flexed with knee flexion; goniometer; 2 examiners (PT and MD)	28 (56 hips)	Healthy adults (18–51 years; $\bar{x} = 31$ years)		0.83 (both hips) 0.80 (R hip) 0.85 (L hip)
Walker et al.[13]	AROM; AAOS standardized goniometer technique; 4 examiners	4	Healthy adults (60–84 years)	> 0.81	

AAOS, American Academy of Orthopedic Surgeons; *AROM*, active range of motion; *CP*, cerebral palsy; *CTL*, control; *F*, female; *FAI*, femoroacetabular impingement; *M*, male; *MM*, myelomeningocele; *MMSc*, Master of Medical Science; *OA*, osteoarthritis; *PROM*, passive range of motion; *SD*, spastic diplegia; *SLR*, straight leg raise.
*Pearson's *r*.
†Intraclass correlation coefficient.

Table 15.2	INTERRATER RELIABILITY: HIP FLEXION/EXTENSION RANGE OF MOTION				

HIP FLEXION

STUDY	TECHNIQUE	n	SAMPLE	r^*	ICC†
Aalto et al.[6]	PROM; supine; hip flexed with knee extended (SLR); 2 examiners (PTs) measured ROM after 1 and 8, 1–2 s passive stretches; goniometer	20 (40 hips)	Healthy adults (12 F, 8 M) (18–45 years; $\bar{x} = 23.3$)		0.90–0.94 (intraday) 0.66–0.99 (interday)
Marques et al.[9]	PROM; supine; hip neutral and knee flexion; goniometer; 2 examiners	40	Healthy adults (32 F, 8 M) (18–28 years; $\bar{x} = 21.8 \pm 4.2$ years)		0.92
Mutlu et al.[5]	PROM; supine; hip flexed with knee extended (SLR); 3 examiners (PTs with 3–14 years experience); goniometer	38 (60 hips)	Children with spastic diplegia (CP) (18–108 months; $\bar{x} = 52.9 \pm 19.6$ months)		0.77–0.83
Owen et al.[15]	AROM; AAOS technique; subjects at 4 separate sites; number of examiners not provided; goniometer	82 (164 hips)	Children 15–24 months postfemoral shaft fracture (4–10 years; $\bar{x} = 6$)		0.31–0.48
Poulsen et al.[16]	PROM; supine; hip flexed with knee flexed; 4 examiners (2 MDs, 2 chiropractors—DCs); goniometer	61 (122 hips)	Adults with hip OA (32 F, 29 M) ($\bar{x} = 65.6 \pm 8$ years)		0.73 (MDs) 0.79 (DCs)
Prather et al.[12]	PROM; supine; hip flexed with knee flexion; 2 examiners (PT and MD); goniometer	28 (56 hips)	Healthy adults (18–51 years; $\bar{x} = 31$ years);		0.87 (both hips) 0.82 (R hip) 0.89 (L hip)
Sutlive et al.[17]	AROM; supine, contralateral hip and knee flexed; examiners DPT students; goniometer	72 (first 30 used for reliability study)	Adults with pain in hip region (40 F, 32 M) ($\bar{x} = 58.6 \pm 11.2$ years)		0.85

Continued

Table 15.2	INTERRATER RELIABILITY: HIP FLEXION/EXTENSION RANGE OF MOTION—cont'd					
			HIP EXTENSION			
STUDY	TECHNIQUE	n	SAMPLE	r*		ICC†
Bartlett et al.[14]	Four goniometer techniques utilized: AAOS; prone with contralateral hip flexed (AA); Mundale technique (MU); Pelvifemoral angle technique (PA); and Thomas test technique (TT)	28	Children and young adults with Myelomeningocele (MM) (n = 14; 4–19 years) or spastic diplegia (SD) (n = 14; 6–20 years)	AA 0.92 (MM) 0.80 (SD) MU 0.79 (MM) 0.84 (SD) PA 0.73 (MM) 0.77 (SD) TT 0.90 (MM) 0.70 (SD)		
Poulsen et al.[16]	PROM; prone; 4 examiners (2 MDs, 2 chiropractors—DCs); goniometer	61 (122 hips)	Adults with hip OA (32 F, 29 M) ($\bar{x}$ = 65.6 ± 8 years)			0.68 (MDs) 0.33 (DCs)
Prather et al.[12]	PROM; prone; goniometer; 2 examiners (PT and MD)	28 (56 hips)	Healthy adults (18–51 years; $\bar{x}$ = 31 years)			0.44 (both hips) 0.44 (R hip) 0.46 (L hip)
Sutlive et al.[17]	AROM; prone with knee extended; examiners DPT students; goniometer	72 (1st 30 used for reliability study)	Adults with pain in hip region (40 F, 32 M) ($\bar{x}$ = 58.6 ± 11.2 years)			0.68

AAOS, American Academy of Orthopedic Surgeons; *AROM,* active range of motion; *CP,* cerebral palsy; *DPT,* Doctor of Physical Therapy; *F,* female; *M,* male; *OA,* osteoarthritis; *PROM,* passive range of motion; *SLR,* straight leg raise.
*Pearson's *r*.
†Intraclass correlation coefficient.

measurements of hip flexion was low (ICC = 0.44). The authors attributed this lack of concurrent validity to a variety of possibilities, including uncontrolled pelvic tilt, visual estimation of anatomical references, and the two-dimensional characteristics of hip ROM measurements using the goniometer.

Both Pua et al.[11] and Poulsen et al.[16] investigated the reliability of measurements of passive range of motion in subjects with hip osteoarthritis (OA). Pua et al. examined intrarater reliability of hip flexion, extension, abduction, and rotation in 22 adults with hip OA. A single examiner (physical therapist) with over 7 years of experience performed all measurements on two separate occasions at least 1 week apart. Standardized measurement and positioning techniques were used. Hip flexion and extension were measured using an inclinometer. During hip flexion measurements, the subject was supine with a strap across the contralateral thigh and the inclinometer positioned parallel to the femur. Hip extension was measured with the patient supine and the contralateral hip in sufficient flexion to flatten the lumbar spine. The angle between the ipsilateral femur and the table was then measured using the inclinometer, first with the knee in 80 degrees of flexion and then with the knee hanging freely. Intrarater reliability was reported using ICC, SEM, and minimal detectable change (MDC) values. Intrarater reliability for hip flexion was high, with an ICC value of 0.97, SEM of

3.5 degrees, and MDC of 8 degrees. Reliability of hip extension was lower and fairly similar with the knee flexed or hanging freely (ICC = 0.86 to 0.89; SEM = 4.5 to 4.7 degrees; MDC = 10.5 to 11 degrees).

Poulson et al.[16] focused on interrater reliability of passive hip ROM measurements in subjects with hip OA. Examiners consisted of two orthopedists and two chiropractors who measured hip flexion and extension ROM (along with four other hip motions) in 48 subjects with unilateral hip OA using a standard goniometer. Measurements were taken in both the affected and unaffected hip with all measurements recorded to the nearest 5 degrees. Standardized protocols were used for all ROM measurements. Reliability was reported using the ICC and SEM and was higher for the chiropractors for measurements of hip flexion (ICC = 0.79, SEM = 7 degrees) and higher for the orthopedists for measurements of hip extension (ICC = 0.68, SEM = 4 degrees).

In a study aimed at developing a clinical prediction rule for the diagnosis of OA in individuals with hip pain, Sutlive et al.[17] examined hip ROM limitations in 72 adults with unilateral hip pain. As part of the study, the investigators used the first 30 subjects to establish interrater reliability of goniometric measurements of active hip flexion, abduction, and adduction and interrater reliability of measurements of passive hip medial and lateral rotation using an inclinometer. Measurements were performed by DPT students following multiple training sessions to standardize procedures. A description of the specific positioning and technique used to measure ROM was not included. The authors reported reliability using the ICC and also reported values for SEM and MDC. For hip flexion, these values were 0.85 (ICC), 2 degrees (SEM), and 5.5 degrees (MDC).

Similarly, Currier et al.[18] undertook a study aimed at identifying a clinical prediction rule for identifying patients with knee pain and knee OA who would respond favorably to hip mobilizations. As part of that study, they examined the interrater reliability of goniometric measurements of hip abduction and adduction and knee flexion and extension, and the reliability of measurements of hip flexion, extension, medial rotation, and lateral rotation using an inclinometer. Sixty subjects with knee OA, aged 51 to 79 years, were administered a battery of examination procedures, including ROM measurements, by two physical therapist students. Although the examiners underwent seven training sessions in which the various examination procedures were practiced, the article included no details regarding the specific techniques used for ROM measurement, with the exception of hip medial rotation for which a detailed description of procedures was provided. The authors reported ICCs and SEM values for each measurement. Interrater reliability for ROM measurements using an inclinometer was higher for hip flexion than for hip extension (hip flexion: ICC = 0.56, SEM = 6 degrees; hip extension: ICC = 0.20, SEM = 4 degrees).

Active hip flexion and extension, along with 26 other motions of the upper and lower extremities, were measured in 60 adults, aged 60 to 84 years, by Walker et al.[13] Techniques recommended by the American Academy of Orthopedic Surgeons[19] (AAOS) were used for all measurements. Before data were collected, intrarater reliability was determined using four subjects. Although the exact number of motions measured to determine reliability is unclear from the procedure, the authors reported a Pearson's r for intrarater reliability greater than 0.81 for all hip motions (see Table 15.1). Mean error between measurements was calculated to be 5 degrees +1 degree.

Macedo and Magee[8] measured passive rather than active ROM of 30 extremity movements, including hip flexion and extension, in a study of the effects of aging on ROM in 90 healthy women. Reliability was tested in 12 subjects before initiation of the larger study. A single examiner measured passive hip flexion and extension ROM twice within a 6-h period using standardized measurement techniques. Hip flexion was measured with the subjects in a supine position with the contralateral hip and knee in the anatomical position. Hip extension was measured with the subjects in prone, again with the contralateral hip and knee in the anatomical

position. Intraclass correlation coefficients were 0.85 for hip flexion, with SEM and MDC values of 3 degrees and 8 degrees, respectively. For hip extension, the ICC was 0.82, SEM was 2 degrees, and MDC was 6 degrees (see Table 15.1).

Marques and colleagues[9] also examined the reliability of passive range of motion measurements of hip flexion, comparing the universal goniometer and computerized photogrammetry. Measurements of passive hip flexion in a group of healthy volunteers ($n = 40$, aged 18–28 years) were taken with the subject in a supine position without attempts at stabilizing the pelvis during the motion. Relative reliability (intra- and interrater) of measurements was reported using the ICC, and intrarater reliability (ICC = 0.95; see Table 15.1) was slightly higher than interrater reliability (ICC = 0.92; see Table 15.2).

In a study designed to compare reliability of the Orthoranger (an electronic, computerized goniometer) and the universal goniometer, Clapper and Wolf[7] examined intrarater reliability of active hip flexion and extension goniometry, in addition to eight other motions of the lower extremities. Twenty healthy adults were included in the examination of reliability. The specific technique for measuring hip flexion and extension was not delineated in the article, so comparison with other studies is difficult. Intraclass correlation coefficients reported for hip flexion and extension were 0.95 and 0.83, respectively (see Table 15.1).

Prather et al.[12] also examined the reliability of goniometric measurements of hip flexion and extension, along with other hip ROM measurements, in asymptomatic adults. As in the study by Clapper and Wolf, the specific technique for measuring hip flexion and extension was not delineated in the article, although the authors did indicate that hip flexion was measured with the subjects in supine and hip extension was measured in prone and that standardized techniques were used. Unlike Clapper and Wolf[7], Prather et al.[12] measured passive hip ROM and reported both intrarater and interrater reliability. Sixteen examiners (including physical therapists, physiatrists, and orthopedic surgeons) performed the measurements on both hips of each subject. Intrarater reliability was reported for all examiners and also was broken down by type of examiner (physical therapist or "clinician"). Reliability was reported for the right and left hips and for both hips combined (see Table 15.1). Interrater reliability was reported for all examiners (see Table 15.2) and for a subgroup of physical therapist versus "clinician." Intrarater reliability for hip flexion ranged from 0.92 to 0.94 for clinicians and from 0.95 to 0.97 for physical therapists. The intrarater reliability of hip extension measurements was lower, ranging from 0.80 to 0.85 for clinicians and from 0.80 to 0.86 for physical therapists. Interrater reliability for hip flexion ranged from 0.82 to 0.89 and from 0.44 to 0.46

for hip extension. The reliability of all measurements was slightly lower for the right hip than for the left.

Because of the variation in measuring techniques for hip flexion and extension, reliability of measurement of these two motions would be expected to vary, depending on the technique used. Two different groups of investigators compared reliability characteristics of different methods of measuring hip flexion or extension. Bartlett et al.[14] measured hip extension in healthy children and in children with meningomyelocele or spastic diplegia. All subjects were between the ages of 4 and 20 years. Four different positioning techniques were compared: AAOS (contralateral hip flexed), Mundale, pelvifemoral angle, and Thomas (see Chapters 11 and 14 for a description of techniques). Intrarater and interrater reliability was reported using Pearson's r. Values for intrarater reliability ranged from 0.63 for the Mundale test in the group with spastic diplegia to 0.93 for the AAOS test in the group with meningomyelocele (see Table 15.1). Single-rater error in the group of healthy children was reported as 5 degrees when the AAOS and Thomas techniques were used, and 10 degrees when the Mundale and pelvifemoral angle techniques were used. Interrater reliability was generally lower than intrarater reliability, and correlation values ranged from 0.70 for the Thomas test in patients with spastic diplegia to 0.92 for the AAOS technique in patients with meningomyelocele (see Table 15.2). Rater error was calculated based on the 95% confidence interval for the mean difference between raters, and was reported as 10 degrees for all techniques except the Mundale (14 degrees) in children with meningomyelocele, 10 degrees for the Mundale and pelvifemoral angle techniques in healthy children, 3 degrees for the AAOS and Thomas techniques in healthy children, and 11.5 degrees and 12.2 degrees, respectively, for the AAOS and Thomas techniques in patients with spastic diplegia.

A second group of investigators measured hip extension (along with four additional motions) in both lower extremities of 25 children (50 hips) with cerebral palsy using the Staheli and Thomas tests.[20] The examiner was a pediatric physical therapist with over 10 years of experience. For 37 lower extremities, the examiner visually estimated the subject's ROM before measuring it with a goniometer. Each of the five motions was measured four times, twice using an assistant to stabilize the subject and twice with the examiner stabilizing the subject without assistance. The assistant, who was a doctor of physical therapy student, read and recorded all measurements. The authors compared the intrarater reliability of one-person versus two-person goniometry and of the Staheli and Thomas tests for measuring hip extension. There was no significant difference in the reliability of one-person (ICC=0.98) versus two-person (ICC=0.98) goniometry for measures of hip extension, nor for any of the other motions measured. The Staheli and Thomas tests both yielded excellent reliability with

ICCs of 0.98 for both methods, regardless of whether one or two people were used during the measurement. Visual estimations were compared with one-person goniometry using the Pearson product–moment correlation, and r values ranged from 0.89 when comparing visual estimation to the Thomas test method to 0.92 when comparing visual estimation to the Staheli method.

A group of investigators[21] measured hip flexion in 20 healthy adults of unstated age using both the AAOS technique (but with the contralateral hip extended) and the pelvifemoral angle technique, as well as hip extension in the same 20 healthy adults using the pelvifemoral angle technique. Two examiners performed the same measurements in each subject to examine variability between raters (intrarater reliability was not considered). Although the investigators did not use inferential statistics to report interrater reliability, raw data were reported, allowing the reader to calculate the ICCs for interrater reliability for each test. Intraclass correlation coefficients and the SEM were calculated by the author of this text for each set of data (hip flexion, AAOS technique with contralateral hip extended; hip flexion, pelvifemoral angle technique; hip extension, pelvifemoral angle technique). Intraclass correlation coefficients were calculated using a two-way random effects model with absolute agreement. The ICCs, which are reported in Table 15.2, indicate higher interrater reliability for measuring hip flexion when the AAOS technique rather than the pelvifemoral angle technique was used in this group of examiners. Reliabilities for measuring hip extension using the pelvifemoral angle technique were similar to those obtained in measuring hip flexion using the same technique. The SEM for hip flexion was 4.2 degrees using the pelvifemoral angle technique and 5.2 degrees using the AAOS technique with the contralateral hip extended. When hip extension was performed using the pelvifemoral angle technique, the SEM was 1.9 degrees.

Hip Abduction/Adduction

As was true in hip flexion and extension, several studies have examined the reliability of hip abduction and adduction ROM measurements. Intrarater and interrater reliability of active hip abduction measurement, along with five other motions of the upper and lower extremities, was examined in a group of 12 healthy adult males aged 26 to 54 years.[22] All motions were measured in each subject three times per session by each of four different physical therapists. Values were reported as 0.75 for intrarater reliability and 0.55 for interrater reliability (ICC) (Tables 15.3 and 15.4). Repeated measures ANOVA revealed significant intrarater variation for two of the four examiners, and significant interrater variation among all four examiners, for measurements of hip abduction.

Table 15.3   INTRARATER RELIABILITY: HIP ABDUCTION/ADDUCTION RANGE OF MOTION

HIP ABDUCTION

STUDY	TECHNIQUE	n	SAMPLE	r^*	ICC[†]
Boone et al.[22]	AROM; supine; knee extended, hip neutral; 4 examiners (PTs)	12	Healthy males (26–54 years)		0.75
Clapper and Wolf[7]	AROM; standing position; goniometer technique; 3 measures; 5 sessions; 1 examiner (MMSc)	20	Healthy adults 10 F, $\bar{x} = 28.3$ years 10 M, $\bar{x} = 30.0$ years		0.86
Fosang et al.[23]	PROM; supine; standardized technique; 6 examiners; two measures per examiner	18	Children with spastic CP (2–10 years)		0.58–0.83
Glanzman et al.[20]	PROM; supine; hip neutral; compared goniometry with 1 examiner (1E) to goniometry with 1 examiner and 1 assistant (2E)	25 (50 hips)	Children with CP (6–18 years)		0.97 (1E) 0.98 (2E)
Herrero et al.[24]	PROM; compared goniometry (G) to inclinometry (I); goniometric measurements taken in supine; hip neutral; contralateral leg stabilized by assistant; inclinometric measurements taken in supine with hip flexed to 90°, contralateral hip stabilized in maximum extension; 5 examiners (PTs; 1–8 years experience)	7 (14 hips)	Children with spastic CP (2 F, 5 M) (7.0–15.2 years)	0.71–0.92 (G) 0.74–0.98 (I)	0.83–0.95 (G) 0.85–0.98 (I)
Macedo and Magee[8]	PROM; supine, hip and knee extended; standardized goniometer technique; 1 examiner (PT)	12 (24 hips)	Healthy Caucasian women (18–59 years; $\bar{x} = 37.2$)		0.90
Marques et al.[9]	AROM; standing with lateral support; goniometer; 2 examiners	40	Healthy adults (32 F, 8 M) (18–28 years; $\bar{x} = 21.8 \pm 4.2$ years)		0.92
Mutlu et al.[5]	PROM; supine; hip neutral; 3 examiners (PTs with 3–14 years experience); goniometer	38 (60 hips)	Children with spastic diplegia (CP) (18–108 months; $\bar{x} = 52.9 \pm 19.6$ months)		0.48–0.70
Nussbaumer et al.[10]	PROM; supine; hip neutral; contralateral leg hanging off edge of examining table; 1 examiner (1 year experience in musculoskeletal examination)	30 (60 hips)	15 patients with FAI (7 F, 8 M) (35 ± 11 years) 15 healthy subjects (7 F, 8 M) (34 ± 10 years)		0.92
Prather et al.[12]	PROM; supine; goniometer; 2 examiners (PT and MD)	28 (56 hips)	Healthy adults (18–51 years; $\bar{x} = 31$ years)		0.85 (both hips) 0.86 (R hip) 0.85 (L hip)
Pua et al.[11]	PROM; supine; contralateral hip in 10° abduction; 1 examiner (PT w/7 years experience); affected hip tested; digital inclinometer	22	Older adults with hip OA (12 F, 10 M) (50–84 years; $\bar{x} = 62 \pm 8.9$ years)		0.94
Walker et al.[13]	AROM; AAOS standardized goniometer technique; 4 examiners	4	Healthy adults (60–84 years)	> 0.81	

HIP ADDUCTION

STUDY	TECHNIQUE	n	SAMPLE	r^*	ICC[†]
Clapper and Wolf[7]	AROM; standing position; goniometer technique; 3 measures; 5 sessions; 1 examiner (MMSc)	20	Healthy adults 10 F, $\bar{x} = 28.3$ years 10 M, $\bar{x} = 30.0$ years		0.80
Macedo and Magee[8]	PROM; supine, hip neutral; standardized goniometer technique; 1 examiner (PT)	12 (24 hips)	Healthy Caucasian women (18–59 years; $\bar{x} = 37.2$ years)		0.90
Nussbaumer et al.[10]	PROM; supine; hip neutral; contralateral leg hanging off edge of examining table; 1 examiner (1 year experience in musculoskeletal examination)	30 (60 hips)	15 Patients with FAI (7 F, 8 M) (35 ± 11 years) 15 healthy subjects (7 F, 8 M) (34 ± 10 years)		0.84
Prather et al.[12]	PROM; supine; goniometer; 2 examiners (PT and MD)	28 (56 hips)	Healthy adults (18–51 years; $\bar{x} = 31$ years)		0.88 (both hips) 0.86 (R hip) 0.89 (L hip)
Walker et al.[13]	AROM; AAOS standardized goniometer technique; 4 examiners	4	Healthy adults (60–84 years)	> 0.81	

AAOS, American Acadamy of Orthopedic Surgeons; *AROM,* active range of motion; *CP,* cerebral palsy; *F,* female; *FAI,* femoroacetabular impingement; *M,* male; *MMSc,* Master of Medical Science; *OA,* osteoarthritis; *PROM,* passive range of motion.

*Pearson's *r*.

[†]Intraclass correlation coefficient.

Table 15.4   INTERRATER RELIABILITY: HIP ABDUCTION/ADDUCTION RANGE OF MOTION

HIP ABDUCTION

STUDY	TECHNIQUE	n	SAMPLE	r*	ICC†
Boone et al.[22]	AROM; supine; knee extended, hip neutral; 4 examiners (PTs)	12	Healthy males (26–54 years)		0.55
Currier et al.[18]	Technique not described; 2 examiners (DPT students)	60 (120 hips) subset of 25 (50 hips) used for reliability study	Adults with knee OA (27 F, 33 M) (51–79 years; $\bar{x}$ = 65.8 years)		0.54
Drews et al.[25]	PROM; comparison of two techniques: supine with maximal hip and knee extension (HE), and supine with hip and knee 90° flexion (HF); goniometer placed on a protractor; 2 PT examiners	9	Infants (12 h–6 days)	HE 0.87 (R) 0.97 (L) HF 0.59 (R) 0.57 (L)	
Fosang et al.[23]	PROM; supine; standardized technique; 6 examiners; two measures per examiner	18	Children with spastic CP (2–10 years)		0.62–0.73
Marques et al.[9]	AROM; standing with lateral support; goniometer; 2 examiners	40	Healthy adults (32 F, 8 M) (18–28 years; $\bar{x}$ = 21.8 ± 4.2 years)		0.91
McWhirk and Glanzman[26]	PROM; supine, hip neutral; standardized goniometer technique; 2 PT examiners (1 and 10 years experience)	25 (46 LEs)	Children with spastic CP (2–18 years)		0.91
Mutlu et al.[5]	PROM; supine; hip neutral; contralateral leg stabilized; 3 examiners (PTs with 3–14 years experience); goniometer	38 (60 hips)	Children with spastic diplegia (CP) (18–108 months; $\bar{x}$ = 52.9 ± 19.6 months)		0.61–0.77
Owen et al.[15]	PROM; supine; hips neutral, knees extended; subjects at 4 separate sites; number of examiners not provided; goniometer	82 (164 hips)	Children 15–24 months post femoral shaft fracture (4–10 years; $\bar{x}$ = 6)		0.28–0.43
Poulsen et al.[16]	PROM; supine; hip neutral; goniometer axis midway between ASIS and symphysis pubis, stationary arm parallel to midline; 4 examiners (2 MDs, 2 chiropractors—DCs); goniometer	61 (122 hips)	Adults with hip OA (32 F, 29 M) ($\bar{x}$ = 65.6 ± 8 years)		0.63 (MDs) 0.45 (DCs)
Prather et al.[12]	PROM; supine; goniometer; 2 examiners (PT and MD)	28 (56 hips)	Healthy adults (18–51 years; $\bar{x}$ = 31 years)		0.34 (both hips) 0.48 (R hip) 0.20 (L hip)
Sutlive et al.[17]	AROM; supine; hip neutral; examiners DPT students; goniometer	72 (1st 30 used for reliability study)	Adults with pain in hip region (40 F, 32 M) ($\bar{x}$ = 58.6 ± 11.2 years)		0.85

HIP ADDUCTION

STUDY	TECHNIQUE	n	SAMPLE	r*	ICC†
Currier et al.[18]	Technique not described; 2 examiners (DPT students)	60 (120 hips) subset of 25 (50 hips) used for reliability study	Adults with knee OA (27 F, 33 M) (51–79 years; $\bar{x}$ = 65.8 years)		0.37
Drews et al.[25]	PROM; supine; standardized technique; goniometer placed on a protractor; 2 PT examiners	9	Infants (12 h–6 days)	0.62 (R) 0.70 (L)	
Owen et al.[15]	PROM; supine; hips neutral, knees extended; subjects at 4 separate sites; number of examiners not provided; goniometer	82 (164 hips)	Children 15–24 months postfemoral shaft fracture (4–10 years; $\bar{x}$ = 6)		0.19–0.20
Poulsen et al.[16]	PROM; supine; hip neutral; goniometer axis midway between ASIS and symphysis pubis, stationary arm parallel to midline; 4 examiners (2 MDs, 2 chiropractors, DCs); goniometer	61 (122 hips)	Adults with hip OA (32 F, 29 M) ($\bar{x}$ = 65.6 ± 8 years)		0.65 (MDs) 0.14 (DCs)
Prather et al.[12]	PROM; supine; goniometer; 2 examiners (PT and MD)	28 (56 hips)	Healthy adults (18–51 years; $\bar{x}$ = 31 years)		0.54 (both hips) 0.42 (R hip) 0.65 (L hip)
Sutlive et al.[17]	AROM; supine; hip neutral; examiners DPT students; goniometer	72 (1st 30 used for reliability study)	Adults with pain in hip region (40 F, 32 M) ($\bar{x}$ = 58.6 ± 11.2 years)		0.54

AROM, Active range of motion; *ASIS*, anterior superior iliac spine; *CP*, cerebral palsy; *DPT*, Doctor of Physical Therapy; *F*, female; *Fx*, fracture; *L*, left; *LE*, lower extremity; *M*, male; *OA*, osteoarthritis; *PROM*, passive range of motion; *R*, right.

*Pearson's r.
†Intraclass correlation coefficient.

Other investigators who have examined the reliability of active hip abduction and adduction include Clapper and Wolf[7] and Walker et al.[13] although these investigators examined only intrarater reliability. Both studies have been described previously, and each used a different statistical method for reporting reliability. Clapper and Wolf[7] reported ICC levels of 0.86 and 0.80 for hip abduction and adduction, respectively, whereas Walker et al.[13] used Pearson's r and reported values "greater than 0.81" for both hip abduction and hip adduction (see Table 15.3) and a mean error between repeated measures of 5 degrees.

The reliability of passive hip abduction and adduction ROM has also been studied in healthy adults. In studies described previously, Macedo and Magee[8] reported intrarater reliability of hip abduction and adduction in healthy adult females, Prather et al.[12] examined both intrarater and interrater reliability of the same motions in young adults of both sexes, and Marques et al.[9] examined intrarater and interrater reliability of hip abduction, but not adduction range of motion in healthy young adults. Intraclass correlation coefficients for intrarater reliability were fairly similar in the studies, with Macedo and Magee[8] reporting an ICC of 0.9 for both abduction and adduction, Prather et al.[12] reporting ICC levels ranging from 0.80 to 0.91 for hip abduction and from 0.78 to 0.92 for hip adduction, depending on the examiner and the side being tested (see Table 15.3), and Marques et al.[9] reporting ICCs of 0.92 and 0.91 for intrarater and interrater reliability, respectively (see Tables 15.3 and 15.4). Macedo and Magee[8] also reported values for SEM and MDC, which were higher for hip abduction (SEM = 3 degrees, MDC = 9 degrees) than for adduction (SEM = 1 degree, MDC = 4 degrees).

At least five groups of investigators have examined the reliability of hip ROM measurements in adults with musculoskeletal disorders. All studies have been described previously. Four of these studies examined passive ROM[10,11,16,18] and the fifth[17] examined active ROM measurements. Most investigators measured ROM using a standard goniometer, although some use an inclinometer. Two groups limited their studies to examination of intrarater reliability. Nussbaumer et al.[10] reported intrarater reliability of hip abduction and adduction measurements using a standard goniometer and found higher reliability for hip abduction (ICC = 0.92, SEM = 2 degrees) than adduction (ICC = 0.84, SEM = 2 degrees). Pua et al.[11] used a digital inclinometer to measure hip adduction and reported an ICC of 0.84 with an SEM of 12 degrees. The other three groups all reported interrater reliability of hip abduction and adduction ROM measurements using a goniometer in subjects with hip or knee osteoarthritis (OA). Both Currier et al.[18] and Poulsen et al.[16] examined passive hip motion. Intraclass correlation coefficients reported by the two studies were fairly low, ranging from 0.14 to 0.65 in the Poulsen study and from 0.37 to 0.54 in the

Currier study. Both groups reported values for SEM, and these ranged from 6 to 8 degrees for measurements of hip abduction and from 4 to 6 degrees for measurements of hip adduction. The interrater reliability of active hip measurements was examined by Sutlive et al.[17] They reported higher reliability for the measurement of both motions (hip abduction: ICC = 0.85, SEM = 2 degrees, MDC = 4 degrees; hip adduction: ICC = 0.54, SEM = 1 degree, MDC = 3 degrees).

Several studies involving the reliability of passive hip abduction and adduction ROM in children have been published. Interrater reliability was examined for hip abduction and adduction measurements in a subgroup of 54 healthy infants aged 12h to 6 days old.[25] The subgroup consisted of nine infants in whom passive hip abduction and adduction were measured. Abduction was measured twice, once with the hip in 0 degrees of extension, and once with the hip flexed to 90 degrees. Adduction was measured with the hip in 0 degrees of extension. Seven other motions of the lower extremities also were examined in this study (see the remainder of this chapter for other motions of the lower extremity). Specific goniometric alignment and techniques were difficult to discern from the description of the study. Interrater reliabilities (Pearson's r) ranged from a high of 0.97 for hip abduction with the hip extended in the left lower extremity, to a low of 0.57 for hip abduction with the hip flexed in the same extremity (see Table 15.4). The SEM from the Drews et al.[25] study (calculated by the author of this text from data provided) ranged from 1.7 degrees for left hip abduction with the hip extended to 6.4 degrees for left hip abduction with the hip flexed.

Much lower reliability for the measurements of hip abduction and adduction was reported by Owen et al.[15] who examined the reliability of goniometric measurements of all motions of the hip in a group of 82 children (aged 4 to 10 years) at 15 and 24 months postfemoral shaft fracture. Subjects from four separate clinical sites were included in the study. Measurements were taken of both hips of each subject by an undefined number of examiners with undefined levels of experience, using AAOS measurement techniques and the examiner's choice of goniometer. Reliability was calculated using ICCs and 95% confidence intervals. Interrater reliability for hip abduction ranged from 0.28 to 0.43 with 95% confidence intervals of 24 to 32 degrees. For hip adduction, ICCs ranged from 0.19 to 0.20, with 95% confidence intervals ranging from 15 to 20 degrees (see Table 15.4).

At least five groups of investigators have examined the reliability of ROM measurements of the hip and other joints in children with spastic cerebral palsy. Stuberg et al.[3] examined intrarater and interrater reliability for hip abduction and adduction using a two-way ANOVA for repeated measures (see "Hip Flexion/Extension" section of this chapter). No significant difference was found between the three measures of hip abduction or adduction taken by a single examiner, and intrarater error was calculated at less than or equal to 5 degrees for most measurements, based on the 95% confidence interval. Significant within-session interrater variation was noted for hip adduction but not for abduction, although across-session interrater variation was significant for both measures.

Fosang et al.[23] investigated the reliability of selected ROM measurements, including hip abduction, as part of a larger study of reliability of various lower extremity clinical measures. Eighteen children (aged 2 to 10 years) participated in the study, in which six experienced physical therapists measured the spastic hip of each of the subjects twice over 6 days. All examiners received a day of training in measurement techniques before the time of data collection. Intrarater and interrater reliability was calculated using ICCs. Standard errors of the measurements and 95% confidence intervals also were calculated. Intraclass correlation coefficients ranged from 0.58 to 0.83 for intrarater reliability (see Table 15.3), and from 0.62 to 0.73 for interrater reliability (see Table 15.4). Standard errors of measurements for individual raters ranged from 3.7 to 6.9 degrees, and between examiners, ranges were from 5.3 to 5.6 degrees.

McWhirk and Glanzman[26] investigated the ability of an experienced and an inexperienced examiner to achieve similar ROM measurements of five lower extremity motions in children with spastic cerebral palsy. Forty-six lower extremities were measured in 25 children by two physical therapists, one with 10 years and one with a single year of experience. Standardized measurement techniques were reviewed and used during the data collection process. In addition, each examiner served as an assistant for the other by stabilizing the extremities as needed during the measuring process. Interrater reliability for hip abduction measurements was high with an ICC of 0.91 (see Table 15.4) and a 95% confidence interval of 3.57 ± 1.35 degrees.

In a study designed to compare the intrarater and interrater reliability of measurements of hip abduction using a universal goniometer versus an electronic inclinometer, Herrero et al.[24] measured both lower extremities of a group of children with spastic cerebral palsy. Five physical therapists, with anywhere from 1 to 8 years of experience in pediatric physical therapy, served as the examiners for the study. A standardized protocol was used to perform all measurements. Goniometric measurements were performed with the subjects in a supine position and the hips in 0 degrees of extension, while measurements made with the inclinometer were performed with the subjects in supine and the hip to be measured in 90 degrees of flexion (the contralateral hip was positioned in 0 degrees of hip extension). An assistant stabilized the contralateral lower extremity during all measurements, regardless of the instrument used. Subjects were measured once by each examiner

in two separate sessions. Subjects were measured using only one instrument; those measured with the goniometer were not measured with the inclinometer, and vice versa. The authors reported ICCs for intrarater reliability for the goniometer ranging from 0.83 to 0.95 and for the inclinometer from 0.85 to 0.98. Interrater reliability was lower for the goniometer (ICC = 0.38 to 0.48) than for the inclinometer (ICC = 0.97 to 0.98).

Glanzman et al.[20] conducted a study to compare the reliability of using one versus two people to perform ROM measurements in children with cerebral palsy. In addition, they examined the correlation of visual estimation to goniometric measurements of motion in this population. Measurements were made of hip abduction with subjects in supine, and intrarater reliability was calculated. Additional details of this study have been described previously (see "Hip Flexion/Extension" section of this chapter). Results showed no difference in intrarater reliability regardless of whether one (ICC = 0.97) or two (ICC = 0.98) persons were used to perform the measurements (see Table 15.3). Visual estimations of hip abduction correlated highly with goniometric measurements (Pearson's correlation coefficient = 0.96).

Hip Medial-Lateral Rotation

Intrarater reliability of hip rotation measurements has been reported by at least six groups of investigators, whose studies have been described previously (see "Hip Flexion/Extension" and "Hip Abduction/Adduction" sections of this chapter).[7,13] One of the studies indicated that goniometric measurements were performed as described by the AAOS[13] while another study did not describe the goniometric techniques used.[7] However, in neither of these two studies can the relative flexed or extended position of the hip be determined, as the AAOS guidelines describe techniques for measuring hip rotation with the hip flexed or extended.[19,27] Intrarater reliability of hip medial and lateral rotation measurements was reported as "greater than 0.81" by Walker et al.,[13] with a mean error between repeated measures of 5 degrees. The study by Clapper and Wolf[7] demonstrated lower reliability for hip lateral rotation measurements (0.80) than for measurements of hip medial rotation (0.92) (Table 15.5).

The remaining four previously described studies each provided descriptions of subject positioning during measurements of hip rotation range of motion. Macedo and Magee[8] and Pua et al.[11] measured hip rotation with the subjects in a seated position with the hip and knee flexed to 90 degrees using a goniometer and digital inclinometer, respectively. Intrarater reliability reported in the two studies was similar, with Macedo and Magee reporting slightly higher reliability using the goniometer in healthy women (Medial rotation: ICC = 0.91, SEM = 2 degrees, MDC = 6 degrees; Lateral rotation: ICC = 0.90, SEM = 2 degrees, MDC = 6 degrees) than Pua et al. did

Table 15.5   INTRARATER RELIABILITY: HIP MEDIAL/LATERAL ROTATION RANGE OF MOTION

HIP MEDIAL ROTATION

STUDY	TECHNIQUE	n	SAMPLE	r^*	ICC[†]
Aalto et al.[6]	PROM; seated; hip and knee flexed to 90°; 2 examiners (PTs) measured ROM after 1 and 8, 1–2 s passive stretches; goniometer	20 (40 hips)	Healthy adults (12 F, 8 M) (18–45 years; $\bar{x}=23.3$)		0.93–0.97
Clapper and Wolf[7]	AROM; supine standardized goniometer technique; 3 measures; 5 sessions; 1 examiner (MMSc)	20	Healthy adults 10 F, $\bar{x}=28.3$ years 10 M, $\bar{x}=30.0$ years		0.92
Ellison et al.[28]	PROM; prone with hip in 0° abduction, knee flexed to 90°; contralateral hip in 30° abduction; pelvis manually stabilized; 3 examiners; gravity inclinometer	150	Healthy adults (HA) ($n=100$; 75 F, 25 M) (20–41 years; $\bar{x}=26\pm5$ years) Subjects with LBP ($n=50$; 29 F, 21 M) (23–61 years; $\bar{x}=37.4\pm10.9$ years)		0.98–0.99 (HA) 0.96–0.97 (LBP)
Gradoz et al.[29]	PROM; seated (S) and supine (SU); hip and knee flexed to 90°; goniometer; 3 examiners (1 PT w/10 years experience, 2 first year PT students)	19	Healthy adults (11 F, 8 M) ($\bar{x}=23.5\pm1.2$ years)		0.69–0.71 (S) 0.78–0.91 (SU)
Krause et al.[30]	PROM and AROM; AROM performed unilaterally and bilaterally; seated; hip and knee flexed to 90°; digital inclinometer; 2 examiners (PTs w/15–25 years experience)	25	Healthy Adults (17 F, 8 M) (22–42 years; $\bar{x}=24.2\pm3.8$ years)		0.84 (PROM) 0.92 (AROM, unilateral) 0.86 (AROM, bilateral)
Macedo and Magee[8]	PROM; seated; hip and knee flexed to 90°; 1 examiner (PT)	12 (24 hips)	Healthy Caucasian women 18–59 years; $\bar{x}=37.2$ years		0.91
Nussbaumer et al.[10]	PROM; supine; hip and knee flexed to 90°; 1 examiner (1 year experience in musculoskeletal examination)	30 (60 hips)	15 patients with FAI (7 F, 8 M) (35 ± 11 years) 15 healthy subjects (7 F, 8 M) (34 ± 10 years)		0.95
Prather et al.[12]	PROM; tested in supine (SU) with hip and knee flexed to 90° and in prone (PR) with hip neutral and knee flexed to 90°; goniometer; 2 examiners (PT and MD)	28 (56 hips)	Healthy adults (18–51 years; $\bar{x}=31$ years)		0.88 (SU; both hips) 0.94 (PR; both hips) 0.86 (SU; R hip) 0.94 (PR; R hip) 0.91 (SU; L hip) 0.94 (PR; L hip)
Pua et al.[11]	PROM; Seated with hip and knee flexed to 90°; 1 examiner (PT w/7 years experience); affected hip tested; digital inclinometer	22	Older adults with hip OA (12 F, 10 M) (50–84 years; $\bar{x}=62\pm8.9$ years)		0.93
Walker et al.[13]	AROM; AAOS standardized goniometer technique; 4 examiners	4	Healthy adults (60–84 years)	>0.81	

HIP LATERAL ROTATION

STUDY	TECHNIQUE	n	SAMPLE	r^*	ICC[†]
Clapper and Wolf[7]	AROM; supine standardized goniometer technique; 3 measures; 5 sessions; 1 examiner (MMSc)	20	Healthy adults 10 F, $\bar{x}=28.3$ years 10 M, $\bar{x}=30.0$ years		0.80
Ellison et al.[28]	PROM; prone with hip in 0° abduction, knee flexed to 90°; contralateral hip in 30° abduction; pelvis manually stabilized; 3 examiners; gravity inclinometer	150	Healthy adults (HA) ($n=100$; 75 F, 25 M) (20–41 years; $\bar{x}=26\pm5$ years) Subjects with LBP ($n=50$; 29 F, 21 M) (23–61 years; $\bar{x}=37.4\pm10.9$ years)		0.96 (HA) 0.95–0.96 (LBP)
Gradoz et al.[29]	PROM; seated (S) and supine (SU); hip and knee flexed to 90°; goniometer; 3 examiners (1 PT w/10 years experience, 2 first year PT students)	19	Healthy adults (11 F, 8 M) ($\bar{x}=23.5\pm1.2$ years)		0.65–0.82 (S) 0.86–0.91 (SU)
Macedo and Magee[8]	PROM; seated; hip and knee flexed to 90°; 1 examiner (PT)	12 (24 hips)	Healthy Caucasian women (18–59 years; $\bar{x}=37.2$ years)		0.91
Mutlu et al.[5]	PROM; seated; hip and knee flexed to 90°; contralateral leg stabilized; 3 examiners (PTs with 3–14 years experience); goniometer	38 (60 hips)	Children with spastic diplegia (CP) (18–108 months; $\bar{x}=52.9\pm19.6$ months)		0.80–0.85
Nussbaumer et al.[10]	PROM; supine; hip and knee flexed to 90°; 1 examiner (1 year experience in musculoskeletal examination)	30 (60 hips)	15 patients with FAI (7 F, 8 M) (35 ± 11 years) 15 healthy subjects (7 F, 8 M) (34 ± 10 years)		0.91

Continued

Table 15.5	INTRARATER RELIABILITY: HIP MEDIAL/LATERAL ROTATION RANGE OF MOTION—cont'd				
	HIP LATERAL ROTATION				
STUDY	TECHNIQUE	n	SAMPLE	r^*	ICC[†]
Prather et al.[12]	PROM; tested in supine (SU) with hip and knee flexed to 90°and in prone (PR) with hip neutral and knee flexed to 90°; goniometer; 2 examiners (PT and MD)	28 (56 hips)	Healthy adults (18–51 years; $\bar{x}$=31 years)		0.95 (SU; both hips) 0.85 (PR; both hips) 0.95 (SU; R hip) 0.86 (PR; R hip) 0.95 (SU; L hip) 0.84 (PR; L hip)
Pua et al.[11]	PROM; seated with hip and knee flexed to 90°; 1 examiner (PT w/7 years experience); affected hip tested; digital inclinometer	22	Older adults with hip OA (12 F, 10 M) (50–84 years; $\bar{x}$=62±8.9 years)		0.96
Walker et al.[13]	AROM; AAOS standardized goniometer technique; 4 examiners	4	Healthy adults (60–84 years)	>0.81	

AAOS, American Academy of Orthopedic Surgeons; *AROM*, active range of motion; *CP*, cerebral palsy; *F*, female; *FAI*, femoroacetabular impingement; *LBP*, low back pain; *M*, male; *MMSc*, Master of Medical Science; *OA*, osteoarthritis; *PROM*, passive range of motion; *PSIS*, posterior superior iliac spine.
*Pearson's *r*.
[†]Intraclass correlation coefficient.

using the digital inclinometer in adults with hip OA (Medial rotation: ICC=0.93, SEM=3 degrees, MDC=8 degrees; Lateral rotation: ICC=0.96, SEM=3 degrees, MDC=7 degrees). Hip rotation was measured with subjects positioned in supine with the hip and knee flexed to 90 degrees in studies carried out by Nussbaumer et al.[10] and Prather et al.[12] Prather et al.[12] also measured hip rotation with subjects in prone with the knee flexed to 90 degrees. Subjects in the Prather et al.[12] study were healthy adults, while those in the study by Nussbaumer et al.[10] had a diagnosis of femoroacetabular impingement. In general, higher reliability was reported from measurements taken with the subject in a supine rather than a prone position. Reliability ranged from 0.88 to 0.95 for measurements of internal rotation taken with the subject supine[10,12] and from 0.86 to 0.94 for the same measurements taken with the subject prone.[12] Reliability of lateral rotation measurements ranged from 0.90 to 0.95 when taken in a supine position[10,12] and from 0.84 to 0.86 when taken in a prone position.[12]

Aalto et al.[6] investigated the reliability of passive hip internal rotation ROM goniometry as part of a larger study designed to examine the effects of passive stretch on the reliability of hip ROM measurements. Measurements were taken in 20 healthy adults (aged 18 to 45 years) by two experienced physical therapists. Subjects were seated with the hip and knee flexed to 90 degrees. During the initial measurement session, each examiner measured hip internal rotation ROM twice following a single passive stretch of the internal rotators, and twice again following eight passive stretches of the internal rotators. During the second measurement session, each examiner repeated the prior measurements a single time per stretching session. Measurements were taken with subjects placed in a sitting position. Reliability was determined through

the calculation of ICCs. Intrarater reliability ranged from 0.93 to 0.97 within session and from 0.72 to 0.97 between sessions (see Table 15.5). Interrater reliability ranged from 0.83 to 0.91 within session and from 0.75 to 0.82 between sessions (Table 15.6).

Gradoz and colleagues[29] compared the reliability of measuring passive hip rotation with subjects in seated, as compared to supine, positions. Measurements were taken using a universal goniometer by one experienced and two novice examiners in healthy young adult subjects (n=19) with the hip and knee flexed to 90 degrees. Relative reliability was reported using the ICC, and absolute reliability was reported using minimal detectable change (MDC). Intrarater reliability for measurements taken in the supine position ranged from 0.78 to 0.9, while those in the seated position were lower, ranging from 0.65 to 0.82 (see Table 15.5). Interrater reliability ranged from 0.64 to 0.79 (see Table 15.6) and were lower for measurements taken in the seated position. Minimal detectable change values ranged from a low of 6.1 degrees for external rotation measured in the seated position to a high of 7.9 degrees for internal rotation measured in the supine position (see Tables 15.5 and 15.6).

Studies that investigated the interrater reliability of hip rotation have been described previously[15,25] (see "Hip Flexion/Extension" and "Hip Abduction/Adduction" sections of this chapter). Drews et al.[25] and Poulsen et al.[16] measured passive hip rotation with the hip and knee flexed to 90 degrees and the subject in the supine position. Owen et al.[15] measured hip rotation with the subject supine, the hip in neutral, and the knee flexed to 90 degrees. Currier et al.[18] and Sutlive et al.[17] measured passive hip rotation with the subject in the prone position and the knee flexed to 90 degrees. Two of these five studies measured hip rotation ROM in children using a goniometer,[15,25] while the other three measured

Table 15.6 INTERRATER RELIABILITY: HIP MEDIAL/LATERAL ROTATION MEASUREMENT

HIP MEDIAL ROTATION

STUDY	TECHNIQUE	n	SAMPLE	r*	ICC†
Aalto et al.[6]	PROM; seated; hip and knee flexed to 90°; 2 examiners (PTs) measured ROM after 1 and 8, 1–2 s passive stretches; goniometer	20 (40 hips)	Healthy adults (12 F, 8 M) (18–45 years; x̄ = 23.3)		0.83–0.91 (intraday) 0.72–0.97 (interday)
Currier et al.[18]	PROM; prone; hip neutral, knee flexed to 90°; contralateral hip in 15° abduction; 2 examiners (DPT students); inclinometer	60 (120 hips) subset of 25 (50 hips) used for reliability study	Adults with knee OA (27 F, 33 M) (51–79 years; x̄ = 65.8 years)		0.76
Drews et al.[25]	PROM; supine; hip and knee flexed 90°; goniometer placed on protractor; 2 PT examiners	9	Infants (12 h–6 days)	0.78 (R) 0.91 (L)	
Ellison et al.[28]	PROM; prone with hip in 0° abduction, knee flexed to 90°; contralateral hip in 30° abduction; pelvis manually stabilized; 3 examiners; gravity inclinometer	150	Healthy adults (HA) (n = 100; 75 F, 25 M) (20–41 years; x̄ = 26 ± 5 years) Subjects with LBP (n = 50; 29 F, 21 M) (23–61 years; x̄ = 37.4 ± 10.9 years)		0.98–0.99 (HA) 0.96–0.97 (LBP)
Gradoz et al.[29]	PROM; seated (S) and supine (SU); hip and knee flexed to 90°; goniometer; 3 examiners (1 PT w/10 years experience, 2 first year PT students)	19	Healthy adults (11 F, 8 M) (x̄ = 23.5 ± 1.2 years)		0.64 (S) 0.79 (SU)
Krause et al.[30]	PROM and AROM; AROM performed unilaterally and bilaterally; seated; hip and knee flexed to 90°; digital inclinometer; 2 examiners (PTs w/15–25 years. experience)	25	Healthy Adults (17 F, 8 M) (22–42 years; x̄ = 24.2 ± 3.8 years)		0.93 (PROM) 0.89 (AROM, unilateral) 0.89 (AROM, bilateral)
Owen et al.[15]	PROM; prone; hips neutral, knees flexed to 90°; subjects at 4 separate sites; number of examiners not provided; goniometer	82	Children 15 and 24 months postfemoral shaft Fx		0.41 (R) 0.30 (L)
Poulsen et al.[16]	PROM; supine; hip and knee flexed to 90°; stationary arm parallel to midline of body; 4 examiners (2 MDs, 2 chiropractors—DCs); goniometer	61 (122 hips)	Adults with hip OA (32 F, 29 M) (x̄ = 65.6 ± 8 years)		0.63 (MDs) 0.44 (DCs)
Prather et al.[12]	PROM; tested in supine (SU) with hip and knee flexed to 90°and in prone (PR) with hip neutral and knee flexed to 90°; goniometer; 2 examiners (PT and MD)	28 (56 hips)	Healthy adults (18–51 years; x̄ = 31 years)		0.75 (SU; both hips) 0.79 (PR; both hips) 0.72 (SU; R hip) 0.80 (PR; R hip) 0.78 (SU; L hip) 0.77 (PR; L hip)
Simoneau et al.[31]	AROM; compared two techniques: prone with hip extended (P), and seated with hip flexed (S); 3 teams of 2 examiners	60	Healthy adults (18–27 years)		0.94 (P) 0.91 (S)
Sutlive et al.[17]	AROM; prone with hip neutral, knee flexed to 90°; examiners DPT students; inclinometer	72 (1st 30 used for reliability study)	Adults with pain in hip region (40 F, 32 M) (x̄ = 58.6 ± 11.2 years)		0.88

HIP LATERAL ROTATION

STUDY	TECHNIQUE	n	SAMPLE	r*	ICC†
Currier et al.[18]	Technique not described; 2 examiners (DPT students); inclinometer	60 (120 hips) subset of 25 (50 hips) used for reliability study	Adults with knee OA (27 F, 33 M) (51–79 years; x̄ = 65.8 years)		0.29
Drews et al.[25]	PROM; supine; hip and knee flexed 90°; goniometer placed on protractor; 2 PT examiners	9	Infants (12 h–6 days)	0.63 (R) 0.79 (L)	
Ellison et al.[28]	PROM; prone with hip in 0° abduction, knee flexed to 90°; contralateral hip in 30° abduction; pelvis manually stabilized; 3 examiners; gravity inclinometer	150	Healthy adults (HA) (n = 100; 75 F, 25 M) (20–41 years; x̄ = 26 ± 5 years) Subjects with LBP (n = 50; 29 F, 21 M) (23–61 years; x̄ = 37.4 ± 10.9 years)		0.96–0.97 (HA) 0.95 (LBP)

Continued

Table 15.6 INTERRATER RELIABILITY: HIP MEDIAL/LATERAL ROTATION MEASUREMENT—cont'd

HIP LATERAL ROTATION

STUDY	TECHNIQUE	n	SAMPLE	r*	ICC†
Gradoz et al.[29]	PROM; seated (S) and supine (SU); hip and knee flexed to 90°; goniometer; 3 examiners (1 PT w/10 years experience, 2 first year PT students)	19	Healthy adults (11 F, 8 M) ($\bar{x}$ = 23.5 ± 1.2 years)		0.65 (S) 0.75 (SU)
Mutlu et al.[5]	PROM; seated; hip and knee flexed to 90°; contralateral leg stabilized; 3 examiners (PTs with 3–14 years experience); goniometer	38 (60 hips)	Children with spastic diplegia (CP) (18–108 months; $\bar{x}$ = 52.9 ± 19.6 months)		0.69–0.87
Owen et al.[15]	PROM; prone; hips neutral, knees flexed to 90°; subjects at 4 separate sites; number of examiners not provided; goniometer	82	Children 15 and 24 months post femoral shaft Fx		0.06 (R) 0.33 (L)
Poulsen et al.[16]	PROM; supine; hip and knee flexed to 90°; stationary arm parallel to midline of body; 4 examiners (2 MDs, 2 chiropractors—DCs); goniometer	61 (122 hips)	Adults with hip OA (32 F, 29 M) ($\bar{x}$ = 65.6 ± 8 years)		0.53 (MDs) 0.48 (DCs)
Prather et al.[12]	PROM; tested in supine (SU) with hip and knee flexed to 90° and in prone (PR) with hip neutral and knee flexed to 90°; goniometer; 2 examiners (PT and MD)	28 (56 hips)	Healthy adults (18–51 years; $\bar{x}$ = 31 years)		0.63 (SU; both hips) 0.18 (PR; both hips) 0.48 (SU; R hip) 0.24 (PR; R hip) 0.77 (SU; L hip) 0.12 (PR; L hip)
Simoneau et al.[31]	AROM; compared two techniques: prone with hip extended (P), and seated with hip flexed (S); 3 teams of 2 examiners	60	Healthy adults (18–27 years)		0.94 (P) 0.90 (S)
Sutlive et al.[17]	AROM; prone with hip neutral, knee flexed to 90°; examiners DPT students; inclinometer	72 (1st 30 used for reliability study)	Adults with pain in hip region (40 F, 32 M) ($\bar{x}$ = 58.6 ± 11.2 years)		0.77

AROM, Active range of motion; *CP*, cerebral palsy; *DPT*, Doctor of Physical Therapy; *F*, female; *Fx*, fracture; *L*, left; *LBP*, low back pain; *M*, male; *OA*, osteoarthritis; *PROM*, passive range of motion; *R*, right.
*Pearson's *r*.
†Intraclass correlation coefficient.

hip rotation in adults with OA using either a goniometer[16] or an inclinometer.[10,11,16–18] In the pediatric studies, interrater reliability appeared to be higher when measurements were taken with the hip flexed rather than in neutral. Drews et al.[25] measured rotation with the hip flexed and reported correlation values (Pearson's *r*) for interrater reliability of hip medial rotation as 0.78 on the right and 0.91 on the left, and for hip lateral rotation as 0.63 on the right and 0.79 on the left (see Table 15.6). The SEM from the Drews et al.[25] study (calculated by the author of this text from data provided) ranged from 2.8 degrees for medial rotation of the left hip to 7.0 degrees for lateral rotation of the right hip. Interrater reliability in the study by Owen et al.[15] who measured hip rotation with the hip in neutral, ranged from 0.06 for measurements of lateral rotation of the right hip to 0.41 for measurements of medial rotation of the right hip (see Table 15.6). In adult subjects with OA, interrater reliability was highest in the study by Sutlive et al.[17] with measurements of medial rotation using an inclinometer

(ICC = 0.88, SEM = 2 degrees, MDC = 5 degrees) slightly more reliable than lateral rotation (ICC = 0.77, SEM = 2 degrees, MDC = 5 degrees). Currier et al.[18] also used an inclinometer and techniques similar to those by Sutlive et al., but found lower interrater reliability for both medial (ICC = 0.76, SEM = 6 degrees) and lateral (ICC = 0.29, SEM = 10 degrees) rotation. The interrater reliability reported by Poulsen et al.[16] also was fairly low. These researchers used a goniometer for measurement and reported reliability for medial rotation ranging from 0.44 to 0.63 with SEM of 9 and 10 degrees, respectively. The reliability for measurements of lateral rotation was similar, ranging from 0.48 to 0.53 with SEM of 8 and 6 degrees, respectively (see Table 15.6).

Simoneau et al.[31] compared the influence of hip position and sex on active hip rotation in 60 college-age individuals. Hip medial and lateral rotation was measured in each individual by two examiners with the subject in the seated and the prone position. Interrater reliabilities were calculated using ICCs and were reported to range from 0.90 to 0.94 for all measurements of hip rotation (see Table 15.6), regardless of whether the hip was flexed or extended when the measurement was taken. Calculation of the SEM from the data provided in the Simoneau et al.[31] study revealed SEM values between 2.1 and 2.6 degrees for all measurements of hip rotation, again regardless of whether the hip was flexed or extended during the measurement.

The reliability of the inclinometer in measuring hip rotation ROM was investigated by Ellison et al.[28] in healthy subjects and subjects with low back pain. Reliability information was calculated as part of a larger study that compared hip rotation ROM in the two groups. During the reliability segment of the study, 22 healthy subjects and 15 patients with low back pain, all of unstated age, had their hip ROM measured in a prone position with both a gravity inclinometer and a standard goniometer. Healthy patients also were measured with the goniometer in a seated position for purposes of comparing ROM measurements between the two positions. No significant difference was found between ROM measured in the two positions or between measurements obtained with the inclinometer versus the goniometer in the prone position. Intraclass correlation coefficients were calculated to determine intrarater and interrater reliability for both instruments, although only ICCs for the inclinometer were reported by the authors. Intrarater reliability for the inclinometer ranged from 0.95 for lateral rotation measurements of the left hip in patients with low back pain to 0.99 for medial rotation measurements of the right hip in healthy subjects (see Table 15.5). Similar levels of interrater reliability were reported, ranging from 0.95 for measurements of lateral rotation of the right hip in patients with low back pain to 0.99 for measurements of medial rotation of the right hip in healthy subjects (see Table 15.6).

Krause and colleagues[30] also reported high intrarater and interrater reliability for measurements of hip internal rotation range of motion using the inclinometer. Measurements of both active and passive range of motion in a seated position were taken in 25 adults aged 22–42 without known hip pathology. The authors reported intrarater reliability (ICC) ranging from.84 to 0.92, interrater reliability from 0.89 to 0.93, and MDC from 5.4 to 8.6 degrees (see Tables 15.5 and 15.6).

Knee Flexion/Extension

Various investigators have examined the reliability of goniometric measurement of knee flexion and extension. A few of these investigators included only knee flexion[22,32–36] or knee extension[4,25,37–39] measurements as their focus of study. Those studies focusing only on knee flexion measurements reported generally good to excellent reliability, both within and between raters.

Brosseau et al.[32] compared the reliability of the universal goniometer with that of the parallelogram goniometer for measuring active knee flexion in 60 healthy college-age adults. Measurements were made with the universal goniometer, using standard landmarks, with subjects positioned supine and with the knee in two separate positions, slightly flexed and flexed at a larger angle. Intraclass correlation coefficients for intrarater reliability for the two positions of knee flexion ranged from a low of 0.86 to a high of 0.97 (Table 15.7); interrater reliability ranged from a low of 0.62 to a high of 0.94 (Table 15.8). Intrarater error ranged from 3.8 to 5.5 degrees, and interrater error ranged from 7.3 to 18.1 degrees. The actual level of reliability and the measurement error obtained depended on the examiner performing the measurement, which measurement was used for the analysis, and the position of the knee (less or more flexed). Intrarater and interrater reliability levels were higher with the knee more flexed and were lower with the knee in the less flexed position.

Similarly, Hancock and colleagues[36] compared the intrarater and interrater reliability (ICC), as well as minimum significant difference, of different measurement methods (Halo digital goniometer, long arm goniometer, short arm goniometer, Smartphone app, and visual estimation) in measuring three set positions of knee flexion as well as full knee flexion and extension. Two experienced examiners measured six knees free of known pathology. Reliability for all methods was high, with intrarater and interrater reliability higher than 0.98 and 0.99, respectively for each method. The values reported for minimal detectable change were more variable and ranged from a low of 5.83 degrees for the Halo digital goniometer to a high of 14.31 degrees for visual estimation (see Tables 15.7 and 15.8).

Gogia et al.[33] examined interrater reliability and validity of measurements of the knee joint in 30 healthy adults between the ages of 20 and 60 years. Subjects were positioned passively in some arbitrarily determined degree of knee flexion, then goniometric measurement of the knee position was taken separately by two examiners. An X-ray was taken of each subject's knee before the subject was allowed to move. Interrater reliability and validity of goniometric measurements were calculated using both the ICC and Pearson's r. Reliabilities ranged from 0.98 (Pearson's r) to 0.99 (ICC) for interrater reliability, and from 0.97 (Pearson's r) to 0.99 (ICC) for validity. This study, as did the study by Brosseau et al.[32] as described previously, provided support for the reliability and validity of goniometric measurements of knee flexion (see Table 15.8).

High interrater reliability of knee flexion measurements taken with a universal goniometer also was

Table 15.7 INTRARATER RELIABILITY: KNEE RANGE OF MOTION

KNEE FLEXION

STUDY	TECHNIQUE	n	SAMPLE	r*	ICC†
Boone et al.[22]	AROM; supine; foot maintained on table; goniometer aligned with tibia, rather than fibula; 4 examiners (PTs)	12	Healthy males (25–54 years)		0.87
Brosseau et al.[40]	AROM; supine; knee placed in maximal flexion and held in place with Velcro strap; standardized goniometer technique; 2 PT examiners	60	Adults with knee ROM restrictions ($\bar{x}=52$ years)		0.99
Brosseau et al.[32]	AROM; supine; standardized goniometer techniques; quad roll placed under the knee in two different positions with resulting different flexion angles; 4 examiners (4th year PT students)	60	Healthy adults ($\bar{x}=20.6$ years)	0.86–0.97‡	
Clapper and Wolf[7]	AROM; supine standardized goniometer technique; 3 measures; 5 sessions; 1 examiner (MMSc)	20	10M, $\bar{x}=28.3$ years 10F, $\bar{x}\geq30.0$ years		0.95
Hancock et al.[36]	AROM; supine; foot bolster placed on anterior leg to maintain position; measured with short arm goniometer (SG), long arm goniometer (LG), Goniometer Pro smartphone application (SP), Halo digital inclinometer (DI) and visual estimation (VE); 3 examiners (2 orthopedic surgeons, 1 PT)	3 (6 knees)	Healthy adults		0.986 (SG) 0.993 (LG) 0.991 (SP) 0.994 (DI) 0.989 (VE)
Jakobsen et al.[41]	AROM and PROM; supine with foot flat on table, knee pointed to ceiling; subject asked to bend knee maximally for AROM; examiner flexed knee to end of ROM or point of pain for PROM; 2 examiners, PT student (IE) and experienced PT (EE); standardized technique	19 (23 knees)	Adults within 2.5 months posttotal knee arthroplasty (10F, 9M) (50–76 years; $\bar{x}=63.7\pm9.1$ years)		0.96 (AROM, IE) 0.98 (PROM, IE) 0.97 (AROM, EE) 0.97 (PROM, EE)
Peters et al.[42]	PROM; supine; compared goniometry (G) to visual estimation (VE) and radiographic goniometry (RG); 5 examiners (3 MDs, 2 PTs); standardized procedures	21 (subset of 13 used to measure intrarater reliability)	Healthy adult males (22–42 years, $\bar{x}=29.6\pm4.9$ years)		0.97 (G) 0.94 (RG) 0.96 (VE)
Rothstein et al.[43]	PROM; 3 goniometers (metal, plastic, and small plastic); 12 examiners (PTs with 1–4 years of experience); each examiner chose their preferred technique	12	Patients; no ages or diagnoses supplied	0.97–0.99§	0.97–0.99§
Walker et al.[13]	AROM; AAOS standardized goniometer technique; 4 examiners	4	Healthy adults (60–84 years)	>0.81	
Watkins et al.[44]	PROM; position not specified; blinded goniometer; 14 examiners (PTs with 7.2±4 years of experience); examiners randomly paired per subject; 2 measures per examiner	43	Patients (18–80 years; $\bar{x}=39.5$)		0.99
Macedo and Magee[8]	PROM; supine; standardized technique; 1 examiner	12 (24 hips)	Healthy Caucasian women (18–59 years; $\bar{x}=37.2$)		0.72
Verhaegen et al.[45]	AROM; supine; four examiners; compared goniometry of knee motion (G) to computerized measurement of digital photographs (DP); standardized techniques	49	Adults presenting for orthopedic consultation (unaffected knee measured) (no ages supplied)		0.94–0.97 (G) 0.99 (DP)

KNEE EXTENSION

STUDY	TECHNIQUE	n	SAMPLE	r*	ICC†
Brosseau et al.[40]	AROM; supine; roll under the knee for standardization when not able to achieve full extension; standardized goniometer technique; 2 PT examiners	60	Adults with knee ROM restrictions ($\bar{x}=52$ years)		0.97–0.98
Clapper and Wolf[7]	AROM; supine standardized goniometer technique; 3 measures; 5 sessions; 1 examiner (MMSc)	20	Healthy adults 10M, $\bar{x}=28.3$ years 10F, $\bar{x}=30.0$ years		0.85
Hancock et al.[36]	AROM; supine; bolster under ankle; measured with short arm goniometer (SG), long arm goniometer (LG), Goniometer Pro smartphone application (SP), Halo digital inclinometer (DI) and visual estimation (VE); 3 examiners (2 orthopedic surgeons, 1 PT)	3 (6 knees)	Healthy adults		0.986 (SG) 0.993 (LG) 0.991 (SP) 0.994 (DI) 0.989 (VE)

Table 15.7   INTRARATER RELIABILITY: KNEE RANGE OF MOTION—cont'd

KNEE EXTENSION

STUDY	TECHNIQUE	n	SAMPLE	r^*	ICC[†]
Jakobsen et al.[41]	AROM and PROM; supine with roll under heel; subject asked to extend knee maximally for AROM; examiner moved knee to end of ROM or point of pain for PROM; 2 examiners—PT student (IE) and experienced PT (EE); standardized technique	19 (23 knees)	Adults within 2.5 months posttotal knee arthroplasty (10 F, 9 M) (50–76 years; $\bar{x} = 63.7 \pm 9.1$ years)		0.91 (AROM, IE) 0.78 (PROM, IE) 0.94 (AROM, EE) 0.89 (PROM, EE)
Kilgour et al.[4]	PROM; supine; intrasessional (Intra) and intersessional (Inter) reliability; goniometer	50	25 children with CP; 25 age and sex-matched controls (CTL) (28 F, 22 M) (6–17 years)		0.79–0.87 (CTL; Intra) 0.34–0.67 (CTL; Inter) 0.97–0.99 (CP; Intra) 0.89–0.92 (CP; Inter)
Mollinger and Steffan[37]	PROM; supine; standardized technique; 2 examiners (PTs); goniometer	112 (subset of 10 used for reliability study)	Nursing home residents with range of ambulatory or cognitive dysfunction (87% F) (45–100 years, $\bar{x} = 83 \pm 8$ years)		0.99
Pandya et al.[38]	PROM; supine; standardized goniometer technique; 5 examiners (experienced PTs)	150	Duchenne muscular dystrophy (<1–20 years)		0.93
Peters et al.[42]	PROM; supine; compared goniometry (G) to visual estimation (VE) and radiographic goniometry (RG); 5 examiners (3 MDs, 2 PTs); standardized procedures	21 (subset of 13 used to measure intrarater reliability)	Healthy adult males (22–42 years, $\bar{x} = 29.6 \pm 4.9$ years)		0.85 (G) 0.87 (RG) 0.95 (VE)
Rothstein et al.[43]	PROM; 3 goniometers (metal, plastic, and small plastic); 12 examiners (PTs with 1–4 years experience); each examiner chose their preferred technique	12	Patients; no ages or diagnoses supplied	0.91–0.96[§]	0.91–0.97[§]
Shamsi et al.[39]	AROM; supine; hip at 90° flexion; measured with universal goniometer (G) and electrogoniometer (EG); 1 examiner (PT)	45	Adults with chronic low back pain and hamstring shortness (14 F, 31 M) (19–59 years, $\bar{x} = 38.8 \pm 11.14$ years)		0.96 (G) 0.99 (EG)
Walker et al.[13]	AROM; AAOS standardized goniometer technique; 4 examiners	4	Healthy adults (60–84 years)	>0.81	
Watkins et al.[44]	PROM; position not specified; blinded goniometer; 14 examiners (PTs with 7.2 ± 4 years experience); examiners randomly paired per subject; 2 measures per examiner	43	Patients (18–80 years; $\bar{x} = 39.5$ years)		0.98
Macedo and Magee[8]	PROM; supine; standardized technique; 1 examiner	12 (24 hips)	Healthy Caucasian women (18–59 years; $\bar{x} = 37.2$ years)		0.76
Verhaegen et al.[45]	AROM; supine; 4 examiners; compared goniometry of knee motion (G) to computerized measurement of digital photographs (DP); standardized techniques	49	Adults presenting for orthopedic consultation (unaffected knee measured) (no ages supplied)		0.78–0.86 (G) 0.78–0.94 (DP)

AAOS, American Academy of Orthopedic Surgeons; *AROM*, active range of motion; *CP*, cerebral palsy; *F*, female; *M*, male; *MMSc*, Master of Medical Science; *PROM*, passive range of motion; *ROM*, range of motion.

*Pearson's *r*.

[†]Intraclass correlation coefficient.

[‡]Dependent on patient position and tester performing the measurement.

[§]Dependent on type of goniometer used.

Table 15.8 INTERRATER RELIABILITY: KNEE RANGE OF MOTION

KNEE FLEXION

STUDY	TECHNIQUE	n	SAMPLE	r^*	ICC[†]
Boone et al.[22]	AROM; supine; foot maintained on table; goniometer aligned with tibia, rather than fibula; 4 examiners (PTs)	12	Healthy M (25–54 years)		0.50
Brosseau et al.[32]	AROM; supine; standardized goniometer techniques; quad roll placed under the knee in 2 different positions with resulting different flexion angles; 4 examiners (4th year PT students)	60	Healthy adults ($\bar{x}$=20.6 years)		0.62–0.94[‡]
Brosseau et al.[40]	AROM; supine; knee placed in maximal flexion and held in place with Velcro strap; standardized goniometer technique; 2 PT examiners	60	Adults with knee ROM restrictions ($\bar{x}$=52 years)		0.98
Currier et al.[18]	PROM; supine; 2 examiners (DPT students); goniometer	60 (120 hips) subset of 25 (50 hips) used for reliability study	Adults with knee OA (27 F, 33 M) (51–79 years; $\bar{x}$=65.8 years)		0.87
Fritz et al.[46]	PROM; supine; affected (A) and nonaffected (NA) knees tested; standardized instructions provided; 8 examiners (PTs) at 2 centers; goniometer	152 (subset of 35 used for reliability study)	Subjects with unilateral knee dysfunction (13–82 years; $\bar{x}$=40 ± 15.9 years)		0.97 A 0.80 NA
Gogia et al.[33]	PROM; side-lying position; standardized goniometer; 2 PT examiners	30	Healthy adults (20–60 years; $\bar{x}$=35 years)	0.98	0.99
Hancock et al.[36]	AROM; supine; foot bolster placed on anterior leg to maintain position; measured with short arm goniometer (SG), long arm goniometer (LG), Goniometer Pro smartphone application (SP), Halo digital inclinometer (DI) and visual estimation (VE); 3 examiners (2 orthopedic surgeons, 1 PT)	3 (6 knees)	Healthy adults		0.991 (SG) 0.996 (LG) 0.994 (SP) 0.999 (DI) 0.991 (VE)
Jakobsen et al.[41]	AROM and PROM; supine with foot flat on table, knee pointed to ceiling; subject asked to bend knee maximally for AROM; examiner flexed knee to end of ROM or point of pain for PROM; 2 examiners—PT student (IE) and experienced PT (EE); standardized technique	19 (23 knees)	Adults within 2.5 months posttotal knee arthroplasty (10 F, 9 M) (50–76 years; $\bar{x}$=63.7 ± 9.1 years)		0.81–0.87 (AROM) 0.96 (PROM)
Lenssen et al.[47]	AROM; comparison of 4 measurements: AROM sitting position (AST), AROM supine position (ASU), PROM sitting position (PST), and PROM supine position (PSU); standardized technique; 2 PT examiners	30	Patients 3 days posttotal knee arthroplasty (51–77 years)		0.86 AST 0.89 ASU 0.88 PST 0.88 PSU
McWhirk and Glanzman[26]	PROM; standardized goniometer technique; 2 PT examiners (1 and 10 years experience)	25 (46 LEs)	Children with spastic CP (2–18 years)		0.78
Mitchell et al.[34]	AROM; goniometer aligned parallel to anterior aspects of thigh and tibia; 2 novice examiners	20	Healthy adults and adults with arthritis (ages not provided)	0.96	
Peters et al.[42]	PROM; supine; compared goniometry (G) to visual estimation (VE) and radiographic goniometry (RG); 5 examiners (3 MDs, 2 PTs); standardized procedures	21	Healthy adult M (22–42 years; $\bar{x}$=29.6 ± 4.9 years)		0.88 (G) 0.99 (RG) 0.80 (VE)

Table 15.8   INTERRATER RELIABILITY: KNEE RANGE OF MOTION—cont'd

KNEE FLEXION

STUDY	TECHNIQUE	n	SAMPLE	r^*	ICC[†]
Phillips et al.[48]	AROM; supine with foot flat on examining table, knee flexed and pointed toward ceiling; multiple examiners; compared direct goniometry of knee (G) to goniometry of radiographic images (RI) using 4 different sets of landmarks for the latter	43 (50 knees)	Adults posttotal knee arthroplasty (22 F, 21 M) (45–92 years; $\bar{x}=73$ years)		0.85 (G) 0.95–0.99 (RI)
Rheault et al.[35]	AROM; prone with towel roll under anterior distal femur; compared universal goniometer (G) with "fluid-based goniometer" (gravity inclinometer, GI); 2 examiners; standardized technique	20	Healthy adults (15 F, 5 M) ($\bar{x}=24.8$ years)	0.87 (G) 0.83 (GI)	
Rothstein et al.[43]	PROM; 3 goniometers (metal, plastic, and small plastic); 12 examiners (PTs with 1–4 years experience); each examiner chose their preferred technique	12	Patients; no ages or diagnoses supplied	0.88–0.91[§]	0.91–0.99[§]
Verhaegen et al.[45]	AROM; supine; 4 examiners; compared goniometry of knee motion (G) to computerized measurement of digital photographs (DP); standardized techniques	49	Adults presenting for orthopedic consultation (unaffected knee measured) (no ages supplied)		0.93 (G) 0.97 (DP)
Watkins et al.[44]	PROM; position not specified; blinded goniometer; 14 examiners (PTs with 7.2 ± 4 years experience); examiners randomly paired per subject; 2 measures per examiner	43	Patients (18–80 years; $\bar{x}=39.5$ years)		0.90

KNEE EXTENSION

STUDY	TECHNIQUE	n	SAMPLE	r^*	ICC[†]
Brosseau et al.[40]	AROM; supine; roll under the knee for standardization when not able to achieve full extension; standardized goniometer technique; 2 PT examiners	60	Adults with knee ROM restrictions ($\bar{x}=52$ years)		0.89–0.93
Currier et al.[18]	PROM; supine; 2 examiners (DPT students); goniometer	60 (120 hips) subset of 25 (50 hips) used for reliability study	Adults with knee OA (27 F, 33 M) (51–79 years; $\bar{x}=65.8$ years)		0.69
Drews et al.[25]	PROM; supine; standardized technique; goniometer placed on protractor; 2 PT examiners	9	Healthy infants (12 h–6 days)	0.69 (L) 0.89 (R)	
Fritz et al.[46]	PROM; supine; affected (A) and nonaffected (NA) knees tested; standardized instructions provided; 8 examiners (PTs) at 2 centers; goniometer	152 (subset of 35 used for reliability study)	Subjects with unilateral knee dysfunction (13–82 years; $\bar{x}=40\pm15.9$ years)		0.94 A 0.72 NA
Hancock et al.[36]	AROM; supine; bolster under ankle; measured with short arm goniometer (SG), long arm goniometer (LG), Goniometer Pro smartphone application (SP), Halo digital inclinometer (DI) and visual estimation (VE); 3 examiners (2 orthopedic surgeons, 1 PT)	3 (6 knees)	Healthy adults		0.991 (SG) 0.996 (LG) 0.994 (SP) 0.999 (DI) 0.991 (VE)

Continued

Table 15.8 INTERRATER RELIABILITY: KNEE RANGE OF MOTION—cont'd

KNEE EXTENSION

STUDY	TECHNIQUE	n	SAMPLE	r[*]	ICC[†]
Jakobsen et al.[41]	AROM and PROM; supine with roll under heel; subject asked to extend knee maximally for AROM; examiner moved knee to end of ROM or point of pain for PROM; 2 examiners—PT student (IE) and experienced PT (EE); standardized technique	19 (23 knees)	Adults within 2.5 months posttotal knee arthroplasty (10 F, 9 M) (50–76 years; $\bar{x}=63.7\pm9.1$ years)		0.86–0.87 (AROM) 0.70–0.72 (PROM)
Lenssen et al.[47]	AROM and PROM; supine position; standardized goniometer technique; 2 PT examiners (3 and 5 years experience)	30	Patients 3 days posttotal knee arthroplasty		0.64 AROM 0.62 PROM
McWhirk and Glanzman[26]	PROM; standardized goniometer technique; 2 PT examiners (1 and 10 years experience)	25 (46 LEs)	Children with spastic CP (2–18 years)		0.78
Mollinger and Steffan[37]	PROM; supine; standardized technique; 2 examiners (PTs); goniometer	112 (subset of 10 used for reliability study)	Nursing home residents with range of ambulatory or cognitive dysfunction (87% F) (45–100 years; $\bar{x}=83\pm8$ years)		0.97
Pandya et al.[38]	PROM; supine; standardized goniometer technique; 5 examiners (experienced PTs)	21	Duchenne muscular dystrophy (4–20 years)		0.58
Peters et al.[42]	PROM; supine; compared goniometry (G) to visual estimation (VE) and radiographic goniometry (RG); 5 examiners (3 MDs, 2 PTs); standardized procedures	21	Healthy adult M (22–42 years; $\bar{x}=29.6\pm4.9$ years)		0.21 (G) 0.84 (RG) 0.80 (VE)
Phillips et al.[48]	AROM; supine with roll under Achilles tendon, subject asked to push knee toward table; multiple examiners; compared direct goniometry of knee (G) to goniometry of radiographic images (RI) using 4 different sets of landmarks for the latter	43 (50 knees)	Adults posttotal knee arthroplasty (22 F, 21 M) (45–92 years; $\bar{x}=73$ years)		0.91 (G) 0.90–0.98 (RI)
Rothstein et al.[43]	PROM; 3 goniometers (metal, plastic, and small plastic); 12 examiners (PTs with 1–4 years of experience); each examiner chose their preferred technique	12	Patients; no ages or diagnoses supplied	0.63–0.70[§]	0.64–0.71[§]
Verhaegen et al.[45]	AROM; supine; 4 examiners; compared goniometry of knee motion (G) to computerized measurement of digital photographs (DP); standardized techniques	49	Adults presenting for orthopedic consultation (unaffected knee measured) (no ages supplied)		0.64 (G) 0.65 (DP)
Watkins et al.[44]	PROM; position not specified; blinded goniometer; 14 examiners (PTs with 7.2±4 years experience); examiners randomly paired per subject; 2 measures per examiner	43	Patients (18–80 years; $\bar{x}=39.5$ years)		0.86

AROM, Active range of motion; *CP,* cerebral palsy; *DPT,* Doctor of Physical Therapy; *F,* female; *L,* left; *LE,* lower extremity; *M,* male; *OA,* osteoarthritis; *PROM,* passive range of motion; *R,* right; *ROM,* range of motion.

[*]Pearson's *r.*

[†]Intraclass correlation coefficient.

[‡]Dependent on patient position and tester performing the measurement.

[§]Dependent on type of goniometer used.

reported by Mitchell et al.[34] This group of investigators measured active knee flexion in a group of 20 adults who were healthy or who had a diagnosis of rheumatoid arthritis. A standardized technique was used for aligning the goniometer that involved positioning the proximal and distal arms of the instrument parallel to the anterior aspect of the thigh and the tibia and the axis parallel to the lateral knee joint line. Despite the fact that neither examiner had previous clinical experience in using a goniometer, interrater reliabilities (Pearson's *r*) were high (0.96), with a standard error reported of 0.16 degree (see Table 15.8).

Another study involved examination of interrater reliability of knee flexion ROM using a universal goniometer, and the reliability and concurrent validity of knee flexion measurements using a gravity inclinometer, in a group of 20 healthy adults.[35] Data were analyzed using Pearson's *r* to determine correlation and paired *t*-tests to determine whether a significant difference could be discerned between data obtained by the two examiners. Pearson's *r* values of 0.87 and 0.83 were obtained for the universal goniometer and the gravity inclinometer, respectively. However, paired *t*-tests revealed a significant difference between examiners for measurements obtained using both instruments. Concurrent validity between the two instruments was 0.82 and 0.83 for the two examiners.[35]

Finally, Boone et al.[22] examined both the intrarater and interrater reliability of measurements of active knee flexion in a group of 12 healthy adult males aged 25 to 54 years. Subjects in this study were positioned supine for knee measurement, but the distal arm of the goniometer was aligned with the tibia rather than with the fibula. Standardized patient positioning and landmarks for goniometry were used. Other details of the study have been described previously (see "Hip Abduction/Adduction" section of this chapter). Reliability was calculated using ICCs, and intrarater reliability equaled 0.87 while interrater reliability equaled 0.50. Repeated measures of ANOVA revealed significant intrarater variation for one of the four examiners and significant interrater variation among all four examiners.

As with knee flexion, generally good to excellent reliability has been reported for knee extension among those investigators whose studies have focused on measurement of this parameter of range of motion. Three of these studies, all of which have been described previously (see "Hip Abduction/Adduction" section of this chapter), involved measurements taken in children. One group measured passive knee extension in a sample of 150 children with Duchenne's muscular dystrophy and reported intrarater reliability of 0.93 (ICC)[38] (see Table 15.7). Measurements of knee extension in a group of 25 children with spastic cerebral palsy and a group of 25 age- and sex-matched controls yielded intrarater reliability values ranging from 0.89 to 0.99 for subjects with CP and from 0.34 to 0.87 for controls, depending on whether measures were taken on the same

or different days[4] (see Table 15.7). In a study of healthy infants aged 12h to 6days old, Drews et al.[25] used Pearson's *r* to analyze the data and reported interrater reliability for knee extension goniometry as 0.69 for the left knee and 0.89 for the right knee. The SEM from this study (calculated by the author of this text from data provided) was 2.2 degrees for the right knee and 3.7 degrees for the left knee.

Mollinger and Steffan[37] measured knee extension ROM in a group of 112 nursing home residents with a range of ambulatory or cognitive dysfunction. A subset of 10 subjects was used to examine the both intrarater and interrater reliability of the measurements. Two examiners participated in the study using standardized goniometric techniques. Reliability of knee extension measurements was high, both within examiners (ICC = 0.99) and between examiners (ICC = 0.97) (see Tables 15.7 and 15.8). An additional study of knee extension in adults, this time in 45 patients with chronic low back pain, reported high levels of intrarater reliability when measuring knee extension with both a universal goniometer and an electrogoniometer.[39] Investigators reported ICCs and standard error of the measurement (SEM) for measurements using each of the two instruments. For the universal goniometer, intrarater reliability was 0.96 with SEM of 1.04 degrees while reliability for the electrogoniometer was 0.99 with SEM of 2.16 degrees (see Table 15.7).

The vast majority of studies that have included measurements of both knee flexion and extension ROM have reported higher reliability for measurements of knee flexion than for knee extension.[7,13,22,30,40] At least three of these studies were conducted in groups of healthy subjects. In an investigation of 21 young, healthy, male subjects, Peters et al.[42] compared the reliability and agreement of measurements of passive knee flexion and extension using universal goniometry, radiographic goniometry, and visual estimation techniques. Five examiners (three physicians and two physical therapists) participated in the study. Universal goniometry was performed by the physical therapists, using standardized techniques. The remaining measurements (radiographic goniometry and visual estimation) were performed by the physician examiners. Intrarater and interrater reliability were assessed using the ICC. Intrarater reliability was higher for measurements of knee flexion (ICCs ranging from 0.94 to 0.97) than for knee extension (ICCs ranging from 0.85 to 0.87) when using universal or radiographic goniometry but was virtually identical when using visual estimation (flexion = 0.96, extension = 0.95) (see Table 15.7). Visual estimation techniques also yielded identical interrater reliability for knee flexion and extension (ICC = 0.80). Interrater reliability using the goniometric techniques was much higher for knee flexion (ICCs = 0.88 to 0.99) than knee extension (ICCs = 0.21 to 0.84) (see Table 15.8).

Verhaegen et al.[45] compared ROM measurements of the knee from digital photographs to measurements made using standard goniometry in the unaffected knee of 49 subjects. Goniometric measurements were made using a standardized protocol. ROM from digital photographs was assessed using a computer software program. All assessments of digital photographs and goniometric measurements were performed twice by each of four examiners who were blinded to the results. The authors reported ICCs and SEM values for intrarater and interrater reliability for measurements of active knee flexion and extension using the two techniques. Intrarater reliability for knee flexion was slightly higher when using digital photography (ICC = 0.99, SEM = 2 degrees) than when using goniometry (ICC = 0.96, SEM = 3 degrees), although both methods demonstrated high reliability. Results were similar for measurements of knee extension (Digital photography: ICC = 0.84, SEM = 2 degrees; Goniometry: ICC = 0.82, SEM = 2 degrees), although ICC levels were lower for extension than for flexion (see Table 15.7). Interrater reliability for measurements of knee flexion was high, regardless of whether digital photography (ICC = 0.97) or goniometry (ICC = 0.93) was used. Extension measurements demonstrated much lower interrater reliability, ranging from 0.65 when using digital photography to 0.64 when using goniometry (see Table 15.8).

In a study described previously (see "Hip" section of this chapter), Clapper and Wolf[7] examined the intrarater reliability of active knee flexion and extension goniometry in a group of healthy subjects. Exact positioning of subjects in the study was not described in sufficient detail to determine whether subjects were positioned prone or supine, nor were the landmarks that were listed. The investigators used ICCs for determining intrarater reliability and obtained values of 0.85 for knee extension and 0.95 for knee flexion (see Table 15.7).[7,22]

Several groups of investigators have found higher reliability of knee flexion than knee extension measurements when studying subjects with knee pathology. In a follow up to their 1997 investigation, Brosseau et al.[40] repeated their study of active knee ROM with slight modifications in a group of 60 subjects (average age, 52 years) with knee restrictions. Reliability of the universal goniometer versus that of the parallelogram goniometer again was compared, but in this study, measurements and radiographs were taken in each subject's maximally flexed and maximally extended positions. Standard positioning and measurement techniques were used by both examiners, and the ROM of the knee also was measured on radiographs for the purpose of establishing validity. Reliability of the goniometric measurements was calculated using ICC values, and intrarater reliability was 0.99 for knee flexion and 0.97 to 0.98 for knee extension (see Table 15.7). Interrater reliability was 0.98 for knee flexion measurements

and 0.89 to 0.93 for knee extension measurements (see Table 15.8). Criterion validity was examined through the calculation of Pearson's product–moment correlation coefficients, which between the radiograph and the universal goniometer were 0.98 for knee flexion and between 0.39 and 0.44 for knee extension.

Rothstein et al.[43] and Watkins et al.[44] examined the reliability of passive knee flexion and extension measurements in groups of 12 and 43 patients, respectively, who had been given a variety of diagnoses. No standardization of subject positioning or landmarks was used in either study. Subjects in the study conducted by Rothstein et al.[43] had measurements of knee motion taken with three different goniometers, and reliability using each instrument was compared. Data were analyzed using both Pearson's r[43] and ICCs.[43,44] Intrarater reliability for all measurements was high (see Table 15.7), regardless of the type of goniometer used.[43] Interrater reliability was lower for knee extension than for knee flexion goniometry in both of the studies, although the difference was more dramatic in the study by Rothstein et al.[43] (see Table 15.8).

In a study described previously (see "Hip" section of this chapter), Currier et al.[18] examined the interrater reliability of goniometric measurements of passive knee flexion and extension as part of a study aimed at developing a clinical prediction rule for identifying patients with knee pain and knee OA who would respond favorably to hip mobilizations. Reliability was investigated in a subset of 25 of the 60 subjects involved in the study. Interrater reliability of knee flexion was higher (ICC = 0.87, SEM = 8 degrees) than knee extension (ICC = 0.69, SEM = 3 degrees).

Fritz et al.[46] also reported higher interrater reliability for measurements of passive knee flexion than for knee extension. These investigators examined reliability of goniometric measurements in a subgroup of 35 subjects as part of a study to determine the presence of evidence of a capsular pattern of motion restriction in patients with knee pathology. Eight examiners at two different centers were involved in the reliability study. Examiners were provided with instructions for performing the ROM measurements but no training on the procedures. Interrater reliability was highest for measurements of knee flexion on the involved side (ICC = 0.97, SEM = 4 degrees) and lowest for measurements of knee extension on the uninvolved side (ICC = 0.72, SEM = 2 degrees) (see Table 15.8).

Lenssen et al.[47] looked at reliability of measurements of active and passive knee ROM in patients in the first few days following total knee arthroplasty. Thirty patients (aged 51 to 77) had both active and passive knee motions measured by two experienced examiners, who used standardized techniques. Interrater reliability was calculated using ICCs and ranged from a low of 0.62 for passive knee flexion to a high of 0.89 for active knee flexion (see Table 15.8).

One group of investigators examined the reliability of measurements of both active and passive knee ROM and found the lowest reliability levels for measurements of passive knee extension. Jakobsen et al.[41] investigated the influence of examiner experience on intrarater and interrater reliability of goniometric measurements of active and passive knee flexion and extension in a group of 19 subjects who were within 2.5 months of total knee arthroplasty. All motions were measured using standardized techniques with the subjects in the supine position. Two examiners, one physical therapist with 10 years of experience in orthopedic physical therapy and one physical therapist student, performed measurements on each subject twice in the same day. The authors reported intrarater reliability for each examiner and interrater reliability between the two examiners for each of the four motions measured (active and passive knee flexion, active and passive knee extension). Reliability was reported using ICC, SEM, and what the authors referred to as the smallest real difference (SRD), which is equivalent to, and will be referred to henceforward as the MDC. Few differences were revealed in the reliability of the experienced versus inexperienced examiner in this study. Measurements of active and passive knee flexion and active knee extension demonstrated intrarater reliability levels above 0.9 (ICC = 0.91 to 0.98, SEM = 2 degrees, MDC = 4 to 7 degrees), regardless of experience level of the examiner (see Table 15.7). The lowest intrarater reliability was seen for measurements of passive knee extension, with the experienced examiner demonstrating slightly higher reliability (ICC = 0.89, SEM = 2 degrees, MDC = 7 degrees) than the inexperienced examiner (ICC = 0.78, SEM = 2 degrees, MDC = 7 degrees). Interrater reliability was highest for measurements of passive knee flexion (ICC = 0.96, SEM = 2 to 3 degrees, MDC = 6 to 7 degrees) and lowest for measurements of passive knee extension (ICC = 0.70 to 0.72, SEM = 3 degrees, MDC = 9 to 10 degrees) (see Table 15.8).

Only four studies were located in which reliability for measurements of knee extension were reported to be the same or slightly higher than for knee flexion. Macedo and Magee[8] used the ICC to analyze intrarater reliability in a group of healthy women and reported higher reliability for measures of knee extension (ICC = 0.76, SEM = 2 degrees, MDC = 5 degrees) than for knee flexion (ICC = 0.72, SEM = 3 degrees, MDC = 7 degrees) (see Table 15.7). In a study described previously (see "Hip" section of this chapter) Walker et al.[13] also examined the intrarater reliability of knee goniometry in healthy adults. These investigators calculated reliability using Pearson's r and obtained values for intrarater reliability of greater than 0.81 (see Table 15.7) and a mean error between repeated measures of 5 degrees for each motion.

The remaining two studies reported the same or higher interrater reliability of knee extension compared with knee flexion in subjects with pathology. McWhirk and Glanzman[26] measured passive knee motion in children with spastic cerebral palsy and reported the same ICC values for the interrater reliability of knee extension as for knee flexion (ICC = 0.78) (see Table 15.8). Phillips et al.[48] measured active flexion and extension of the knee from radiographs of the knees of subjects following knee arthroplasty and compared those measurements with goniometric measurements of the subjects' actual knee joint motion. Measurements were made of 50 knees at least 6 months following total knee replacement using standardized measurement techniques and anatomical landmarks. A universal goniometer with extended arms was used to measure ROM in the subjects and on their radiographs. Intraclass correlation coefficients were used to examine interrater reliability of goniometric measurements, intrarater and interrater reliability of radiographic measurements, and agreement between goniometric and radiographic measurements. Interrater reliability for goniometric measurements was higher for knee extension (ICC = 0.91) than for knee flexion (ICC = 0.85). Interrater reliability for radiographic measurements ranged from 0.95 to 0.99 for knee flexion and from 0.90 to 0.98 for knee extension, depending on which of four different sets of anatomical landmarks was used. Intrarater reliability of radiographic measurements was 0.99 for both motions, regardless of which landmarks were used. Agreement between goniometric and radiographic measurements ranged from 0.81 to 0.95 for knee flexion and from 0.70 to 0.86 for knee extension, again depending on which set of landmarks was used for the measurements.

Ankle Dorsiflexion/Plantar Flexion

Most reliability studies of active ankle dorsiflexion and plantar flexion ROM measurements have been performed on healthy adult subjects. Two of these studies were described previously (see the "Hip" and "Knee" sections of this chapter); these investigators obtained intrarater reliability of 0.92 (ICC)[7] and greater than 0.81 (Pearson's r)[13] for ankle dorsiflexion, and 0.96 (ICC)[7] and greater than 0.81 (Pearson's r)[13] for ankle plantar flexion (Table 15.9). The mean error between repeated measures in the Walker et al.[13] study was 5 degrees.

Both intrarater and interrater reliability were investigated by Krause et al.[61] in their study examining the reliability of five different techniques of measuring ankle dorsiflexion. Two novice examiners (DPT students) measured both active and passive ankle dorsiflexion ROM with the knee extended and flexed to 90 degrees using a blinded universal goniometer. Ankle dorsiflexion also was measured with the subject in a modified lunge position using a digital inclinometer. A third examiner recorded the measurements and positioned the subject's foot during measurements of passive dorsiflexion.

Table 15.9   INTRARATER RELIABILITY: ANKLE RANGE OF MOTION

ANKLE DORSIFLEXION

STUDY	TECHNIQUE	n	SAMPLE	r*	ICC†
Allington et al.[49]	PROM; supine; compared visual estimation with knee flexed (VEKF) and extended (VEKE) to goniometry with knee flexed (GKF) and extended (GKE); 2 examiners "junior" PTs	24 (46 ankles)	Children with spastic CP (3–14 years)	0.91–0.94 (VEKF) 0.92–0.93 (VEKE) 0.93–0.95 (GKF) 0.94–0.95 (GKE)	
Bennell et al.[50]	PROM; standing, weight-bearing lunge position; compared tape measure (TM) and gravity inclinometer (GI); 4 examiners—3 PTs and 1 PT student	13	Healthy adults (5 F, 8 M) ($\bar{x}$ = 18.8 ± 2 years)		0.97–0.98 (TM) 0.98 (GI)
Bohannon et al.[51]	PROM and AAROM; 3 different distal landmarks used; 1 examiner; reliability of each separate technique not provided	36	Healthy females		0.80–0.93‡
Cipriani et al.[52]	PROM; standing; weight-bearing lunge test (WBLT) and modified weight bearing lunge test (mWBLT) with foot place 35 cm from wall; tape measure; DPT student examiners	41	Healthy adults 20F ($\bar{x}$ = 27.25 years), 21 M ($\bar{x}$ = 28.19 years)		0.95 (WBLT) 0.95 (mWBLT)
Clapper and Wolf[7]	AROM; supine standardized goniometer technique; 3 measures; 5 sessions; 1 examiner (MMSc)	20	Healthy adults (20–36 years) 10 F, $\bar{x}$ = 30.0 years 10 M, $\bar{x}$ = 28.3 years		0.92
Custer and Cosby[53]	PROM; standing; weight bearing lunge; knee straight stance (KS) or knee bent stance (KB); inclinometer placed at tibial tuberosity (TT), distal tibia (DT), and fibula (F); bubble inclinometer; 2 examiners (AT w/10 years experience, AT student)	18	Healthy adults (12 F, 6 M) ($\bar{x}$ = 22.1 ± 3.4 years)		0.847–0.917 (KS, DT) 0.878–0.824 (KS, F) 0.776–0.884 (KS, TT) 0.944–0.975 (KB, DT) 0.842–0.938 (KB, F) 0.903–0.911 (KB, TT)
Denegar et al.[54]	PROM; 5 different measurement techniques: (1) sitting, knee extended (SKE), (2) prone, knee flexed (PKF), (3) standing, knee extended (STKE), (4) standing, knee flexed (STKF); 2 examiners; injured (I) and uninjured (UI) ankles measured	12 (24 ankles)	Healthy college athletes with history of unilateral ankle sprain (18–22 years) 7 F, $\bar{x}$ = 19.3 ± 1.4 years 5 M, $\bar{x}$ = 19.8 ± 1.3 years		0.96 (SKE, I) 0.97 (SKE, UI) 0.97 (PKF, I) 0.97 (PKF, UI) 0.98 (STKE, I) 0.99 (STKE, UI) 0.99 (STKF, I) 0.99 (STKF, UI)
Diamond et al.[55]	PROM, measurements taken in STJN	25	Diabetes (34–77 years)		0.89 (R) 0.96 (L)
Dobija & Jankowski[56]	PROM; supine; knee extended; bubble inclinometer; 4 examiners	16	Older Adults with orthopedic problems (11 F, 5 M) 79 ± 7 years		0.91–0.95
Dobija & Jankowski[56]	PROM; supine; knee flexed; bubble inclinometer; 4 examiners	16	Older Adults with orthopedic problems (11 F, 5 M) 79 ± 7 years		0.92–0.97
Elveru et al.[57]	PROM; position chosen by examiner; 14 PT examiners (6.5 ± 3 years experience)	43 (50 ankles)	Neurologic or orthopedic disorders (12–81 years)		0.90
Glanzman et al.[20]	PROM; supine; hip and knee extended; compared goniometry with 1 examiner (1E) to goniometry with 1 examiner and 1 assistant (2E)	25 (50 ankles)	Children with CP (6–18 years)		0.97 (1 E) 0.98 (2 E)

Table 15.9 INTRARATER RELIABILITY: ANKLE RANGE OF MOTION—cont'd					
ANKLE DORSIFLEXION					
STUDY	**TECHNIQUE**	**n**	**SAMPLE**	**r***	**ICC†**
Jonson and Gross[58]	AAROM; prone with knee extended; 2 examiners, both orthopedic PTs	63 (subgroup of 18 used for reliability study)	Healthy Naval midshipmen (18–30 years) 6 F, $\bar{x}$ = 20.2 ± 1.7 years 57 M, $\bar{x}$ = 21.2 ± 2.9 years		0.74
Kilgour et al.[4]	PROM; supine; hip flexed with knee extended (SLR); Intrasessional (Intra) and Intersessional (Inter) reliability; goniometer	50	25 children with CP (CP); 25 age and sex-matched controls (CTL) (28 F, 22 M) (6–17 years)		0.97–0.98 (CTL; Intra) 0.70–0.75 (CTL; Inter) 0.98–0.99 (CP; Intra) 0.75–0.90 (CP; Inter)
Kim et al.[59]	AAROM; supine; measurements of right (R) and left (L) ankles taken in STJN with knee extended (KE) and knee flexed (KF); AAROM involved asking subject to assist with passive motion supplied by examiner; 5 examiners (podiatric physicians and student) with 0–26 years experience	14	Healthy adults (6 F, 8 M) (23–52 years; $\bar{x}$ = 28.2 years)		0.74 (RKE) 0.81 (RKF) 0.84 (LKE) 0.86 (LKF)
Konor et al.[60]	PROM; standing, weight-bearing lunge; compared goniometer (G), digital inclinometer (DI), and tape measure (TM); 1 examiner (4th year exercise science student)	20	Healthy adults (13 F, 7 M) $\bar{x}$ = 24 ± 3 years		0.85 (G) 0.96 (DI) 0.98 (TM)
Krause et al.[61]	AROM and PROM; 5 different measurement techniques: (1) AROM knee extended (AKE), (2) AROM knee flexed (AKF), (3) PROM knee extended (PKE), (4) PROM knee flexed (PKF), and (5) modified lunge (ML); PROM measurements taken in STJN; lunge measured with inclinometer; 2 examiners (2nd year DPT students)	39	Healthy adults (26 F, 13 M) (22–33 years; $\bar{x}$ = 24.2 ± 2.72 years)		0.81–0.82 (AKE) 0.68–0.81 (AKF) 0.70–0.76 (PKE) 0.78–0.83 (PKF) 0.88–0.89 (ML)
Macedo and Magee[8]	PROM; sitting, knee flexed to 90°; 1 examiner (PT)	12 (24 ankles)	Healthy Caucasian women (18–59 years; $\bar{x}$ = 37.2 years)		0.77
Munteanu et al.[62]	PROM; standing, weight-bearing lunge; compared digital inclinometer (DI) to acrylic plate apparatus (AP); 4 examiners (podiatrists) w/0, 3, 10, and 20 years experience	30	Healthy adults (20 F, 10 M) 19–42 years; $\bar{x}$ = 22.1 ± 5.6 years		. 0.77–0.91 (DI) 0.67–0.96 (AP)
Mutlu et al.[5]	PROM; supine; 3 examiners (PTs with 3–14 years experience); goniometer	38 (60 hips)	Children with spastic diplegia (CP) (18–108 months; $\bar{x}$ = 52.9 ± 19.6 months)		0.81–0.90
Pandya et al.[38]	PROM; supine; standardized goniometer technique; 5 examiners (experienced PTs)	150	Duchenne muscular dystrophy (4–20 years)		0.90
Searle et al.[63]	PROM; supine Modified Lindcombe with 80.4 N pressure; digital inclinometer; 2 examiners	30	Healthy individuals (14 F, 16 M) 28 ± 6.8 years		0.89
Searle et al.[63]	PROM; supine Modified Lindcombe with 80.4 N pressure; digital inclinometer; 2 examiners	30	People with Diabetes Mellitus (17 F, 13 M) 65.8 ± 16 years		0.90–0.94

Continued

Table 15.9   INTRARATER RELIABILITY: ANKLE RANGE OF MOTION—cont'd

ANKLE DORSIFLEXION

STUDY	TECHNIQUE	n	SAMPLE	r^*	ICC[†]
Searle et al.[63]	PROM; standing, weight-bearing lunge; digital protractor; 2 examiners	30	Healthy individuals (14 F, 16 M) 28 ± 6.8 years		0.85–0.89
Searle et al.[63]	PROM; standing, weight-bearing lunge; digital protractor; 2 examiners	30	People with Diabetes Mellitus (17 F, 13 M) 65.8 ± 16 years		0.83–0.85
Van der Worp et al.[64]	PROM; standing, weight-bearing lunge; digital inclinometer; 2 examiners (sports PTs)	42	Recreational runners (20 F, 22 M) ($\bar{x}$ = 38.2 ± 12.4 years)		0.86
Walker et al.[13]	AROM; AAOS standardized goniometer technique; 4 examiners	4	Healthy adults (60–84 years)	>0.81	
Youdas et al.[65]	AROM; position chosen by examiner; 2 measures; 10 PT examiners (5–13 years experience)	38 (45 ankles)	Orthopedic problems (13–71 years)		0.78–0.96[§]

ANKLE PLANTAR FLEXION

STUDY	TECHNIQUE	n	SAMPLE	r^*	ICC[†]
Allington et al.[49]	PROM; supine; compared visual estimation (VE) to goniometry (G); 2 examiners "junior" PTs	24 (46 ankles)	Children with spastic CP (3–14 years)	0.84–0.86 (VE) 0.85–0.86 (G)	
Clapper and Wolf[7]	AROM; supine standardized goniometer technique; 3 measures; 5 sessions; 1 examiner (MMSc)	20	Healthy adults 10 M, $\bar{x}$ = 28.3 years 20 F, $\bar{x}$ = 30.0 years		0.96
Dobija & Jankowski[56]	PROM; supine; knee extended; bubble inclinometer; 4 examiners	16	Older Adults with orthopedic problems (11 F, 5 M) 79 ± 7 years		0.66–0.96
Dobija & Jankowski[56]	PROM; supine; knee flexed; bubble inclinometer; 4 examiners	16	Older Adults with orthopedic problems (11 F, 5 M) 79 ± 7 years		0.84–0.93
Elveru et al.[57]	PROM; position chosen by examiner; 14 PT examiners (6.5 ± 3 years experience)	43 (50 ankles)	Neurologic or orthopedic disorders (12–81 years)		0.86
Macedo and Magee[8]	PROM; sitting, knee flexed to 90°; 1 examiner (PT)	12 (24 ankles)	Healthy Caucasian women (18–59 years; $\bar{x}$ = 37.2 years)		0.90
Walker et al.[13]	AROM; AAOS standardized goniometer technique; 4 examiners	4	Healthy adults (60–84 years)	>0.81	
Youdas et al.[65]	AROM; position chosen by examiner; 2 measures; 10 PT examiners (5–13 years experience)	38 (45 ankles)	Orthopedic disorders (13–71 years)		0.64–0.98[§]

AAOS, American Academy of Orthopedic Surgeons; *AAROM,* active assisted range of motion; *AROM,* active range of motion; *CP,* cerebral palsy; *DPT,* Doctor of Physical Therapy; *F,* female; *L,* left; *M,* male; *MMSc,* Master of Medical Science; *PROM,* passive range of motion; *R,* right; *STJN,* subtalar joint neutral.

*Pearson's *r*.

[†]Intraclass correlation coefficient.

[‡]Dependent on type of measurement and distal landmark used.

[§]10 testers performed measurement.

All goniometric measurements were taken with the subject lying prone. Passive dorsiflexion was performed by the third examiner by positioning the subject's subtalar joint in neutral and applying a standardized force of 6.4 kg using a hand-held dynamometer. The investigators calculated intrarater and interrater reliability using the ICC and also reported the MDC for each measurement. Intrarater reliability ranged from 0.68 with a MDC of 7 degrees for measurement of active dorsiflexion with the knee flexed to an ICC of 0.89 and a MDC of 6 degrees for measurement of dorsiflexion using the modified lunge

Table 15.10	INTERRATER RELIABILITY: ANKLE RANGE OF MOTION				
ANKLE DORSIFLEXION					
STUDY	**TECHNIQUE**	**n**	**SAMPLE**	**r***	**ICC†**
Allington et al.[49]	PROM; supine; compared visual estimation with knee flexed (VEKF) and extended (VEKE) to goniometry with knee flexed (GKF) and extended (GKE); 2 examiners "junior" PTs	24 (46 ankles)	Children with spastic CP (3–14 years)	0.94 (VEKF) 0.90 (VEKE) 0.95 (GKF) 0.94 (GKE)	
Bennell et al.[50]	PROM; standing, weight-bearing lunge position; compared tape measure (TM) and gravity inclinometer (GI); 4 examiners—3 PTs and 1 PT student	13	Healthy adults (5 F, 8 M) ($\bar{x}$ = 18.8 ± 2 years)		0.99 (TM) 0.97 (GI)
Custer and Cosby[53]	PROM; standing; weight bearing lunge; knee straight stance (KS) or knee bent stance (KB); inclinometer placed at tibial tuberosity (TT), distal tibia (DT), and fibula (F); bubble inclinometer; 2 examiners (AT w/10 years experience, AT student)	18	Healthy adults (12 F, 6 M) ($\bar{x}$ = 22.1 ± 3.4 years)		0.927 (KS, DT) 0.915 (KS, F) 0.877 (KS, TT) 0.964 (KB, DT) 0.924 (KB, F) 0.935 (KB, TT)
Diamond et al.[55]	PROM, measurements taken in STJN	31	Diabetes (34–77 years)		0.74 (R) 0.87 (L)
Dobija & Jankowski[56]	PROM; supine; knee extended; bubble inclinometer; 4 examiners	16	Older adults with orthopedic problems (11 F, 5 M) 79 ± 7 years		0.91
Dobija & Jankowski[56]	PROM; supine; knee flexed; bubble inclinometer; 4 examiners	16	Older adults with orthopedic problems (11 F, 5 M) 79 ± 7 years		0.90
Elveru et al.[57]	PROM; position chosen by examiner; 14 PT examiners (6.5 ± 3 years experience)	43 (50 ankles)	Orthopedic and neurologic disorders (12–81 years)		0.50
Jonson and Gross[58]	AAROM; prone with knee extended; 2 examiners, both orthopedic PTs	63 (subgroup of 18 used for reliability study)	Healthy Naval midshipmen (18–30 years) 6 F, $\bar{x}$ = 20.2 ± 1.7 years 57 M, $\bar{x}$ = 21.2 ± 2.9 years		0.65
Kim et al.[59]	AAROM; supine; measurements of right (R) and left (L) ankles taken in STJN with knee extended (KE) and knee flexed (KF); AAROM involved asking subject to assist with passive motion supplied by examiner; 5 examiners (podiatric physicians and student) with 0–26 years experience	14	Healthy adults (6 F, 8 M) (23–52 years; $\bar{x}$ = 28.2 years)		0.39 (RKE) 0.54 (RKF) 0.34 (LKE) 0.48 (LKF)
Krause et a[61]	AROM and PROM; 5 different measurement techniques: (1) AROM knee extended (AKE), (2) AROM knee flexed (AKF), (3) PROM knee extended (PKE), (4) PROM knee flexed (PKF), and (5) modified lunge (ML); PROM measurements taken in STJN; lunge measured with inclinometer; 2 examiners (2nd year DPT students)	39	Healthy adults (26 F, 13 M) (22–33 years; $\bar{x}$ = 24.2 ± 2.72 years)		0.62 (AKE) 0.55 (AKF) 0.67 (PKE) 0.79 (PKF) 0.82 (ML)
McWhirk and Glanzman[26]	PROM; standardized goniometer technique; 2 PT examiners (1 and 10 years experience)	25 (46 ankles)	Children with spastic CP (2–18 years)		0.87
Munteanu et al.[62]	PROM; standing, weight-bearing lunge; compared digital inclinometer (DI) to acrylic plate apparatus (AP); 4 examiners (podiatrists) with 0, 3, 10, and 20 years experience	30	Healthy adults (20 F, 10 M) (19–42 years; $\bar{x}$ = 22.1 ± 5.6 years)		0.92–0.95 (DI) 0.93–0.97 (AP)

Continued

Table 15.10 INTERRATER RELIABILITY: ANKLE RANGE OF MOTION—cont'd					
ANKLE DORSIFLEXION					
STUDY	**TECHNIQUE**	**n**	**SAMPLE**	**r***	**ICC†**
Mutlu et al.[5]	PROM; supine; 3 examiners (PTs with 3–14 years experience); goniometer	38 (60 hips)	Children with spastic diplegia (CP) (18–108 months; $\bar{x}=52.9\pm19.6$ months)		0.88
Pandya et al.[38]	PROM; supine; standardized goniometer technique; 5 examiners (experienced PTs)	21	Duchenne muscular dystrophy (<1–20 years)		0.73
Searle et al.[63]	PROM; supine Modified Lindcombe with 80.4N pressure; digital inclinometer; 2 examiners	30	Healthy individuals (14F, 16M) 28±6.8 years		0.91
Searle et al.[63]	PROM; supine Modified Lindcombe with 80.4N pressure; digital inclinometer; 2 examiners	30	People with Diabetes Mellitus (17F, 13M) 65.8±16 years		0.91
Searle et al.[63]	PROM; standing, weight-bearing lunge; digital protractor; 2 examiners	30	Healthy individuals (14F, 16M) 28±6.8 years		0.93
Searle et al.[63]	PROM; standing, weight-bearing lunge; digital protractor; 2 examiners	30	People with Diabetes Mellitus (17F, 13M) 65.8±16 years		0.88
Van der Worp et al.[64]	PROM; standing, weight-bearing lunge; digital inclinometer; 2 examiners (sports PTs)	42	Recreational runners (20F, 22M) $\bar{x}=38.2\pm12.4$ years		0.88
Youdas et al.[65]	AROM; position chosen by examiner; 2 measures; 10 PT examiners (5–13 years experience)	38 (45 ankles)	Orthopedic disorders (13–71 years)		0.28
ANKLE PLANTAR FLEXION					
STUDY	**TECHNIQUE**	**n**	**SAMPLE**	**r***	**ICC†**
Allington et al.[49]	PROM; supine; compared visual estimation (VE) to goniometry(G); 2 examiners "junior" PTs	24 (46 ankles)	Children with spastic CP (3–14 years)	0.83 (VE) 0.84 (G)	
Dobija & Jankowski[56]	PROM; supine; knee extended; bubble inclinometer; 4 examiners	16	Older Adults with orthopedic problems (11F, 5M) 79±7 years		0.72
Dobija & Jankowski[56]	PROM; supine; knee flexed; bubble inclinometer; 4 examiners	16	Older Adults with orthopedic problems (11F, 5M) 79±7 years		0.86
Drews et al.[25]	PROM; supine; hip and knee flexed 90°; goniometer placed on protractor; 2 PT examiners	9	Healthy infants (12h–6days)	0.84 (L) 0.89 (R)	
Elveru et al.[57]	PROM; position chosen by examiner; 14 PT examiners (6.5±3 years experience)	43 (50 ankles)	Orthopedic and neurologic disorders (12–81 years)		0.72
Youdas et al.[65]	AROM; position chosen by examiner; 2 measures; 10 PT examiners (5–13 years experience)	38 (45 ankles)	Orthopedic disorders (13–71 years)		0.25

AAOS, American Academy of Orthopedic Surgeons; *AAROM,* active assistive range of motion; *AROM,* active range of motion; *CP,* cerebral palsy; *DPT,* Doctor of Physical Therapy; *F,* female; *L,* left; *M,* male; *PROM,* passive range of motion; *R,* right; *STJN,* subtalar joint neutral.
Pearson's r.
†Intraclass correlation coefficient.

position (see Table 15.9). Interrater reliability was lowest for measurement of active dorsiflexion with the knee extended (ICC = 0.62, SEM = 3.7) and highest for measurement of active dorsiflexion using the modified lunge position (ICC = 0.82, SEM = 2.8) (Table 15.10).

Jonson and Gross[58] examined the reliability of ankle dorsiflexion measurement, along with eight other lower extremity skeletal measures, in a group of healthy naval midshipmen. A subgroup of 18 subjects was used to determine reliability. Two experienced examiners measured active assisted dorsiflexion in each subject. Measurements were taken with a standard goniometer with the subject positioned prone and the knee extended. Reliability was calculated using the ICC and was reported as 0.74 for intrarater and 0.65 for interrater reliability (see Tables 15.9 and 15.10).

One group of investigators compared visual estimation and goniometric measurements of active ankle dorsiflexion and plantar flexion ROM in 45 ankles of a group of 38 patients with orthopedic disorders, aged 13 to 71 years.[65] No standardized method was used for patient positioning or for goniometric measurement. Measurements were taken by 10 examiners, and intrarater reliability was determined for each examiner. Intrarater reliability was calculated using ICCs only for measurements of ankle motion made with the universal goniometer and ranged from 0.78 to 0.96 for ankle dorsiflexion and from 0.64 to 0.98 for ankle plantar flexion[65] (see Table 15.9). However, interrater reliability for ankle dorsiflexion and plantar flexion was poor, whether goniometric measurement or visual estimation was used (see Table 15.10). The lack of a standardized measurement procedure and standardized patient positioning probably contributed to these poor reliabilities. The authors of this study concluded that the same therapist should perform any repeated measurements of ankle ROM because of the poor interrater reliability found in this study.

Kim et al.[59] found similarly poor interrater reliability when measuring active assisted and passive ankle joint dorsiflexion. Five examiners with varying years of experience (0 to 26 years) measured bilateral ankle dorsiflexion in a group of 14 healthy adults during three sessions spaced at least 1 week apart. Four of the examiners measured active assisted ankle dorsiflexion using a modified Root technique in which the examiner places the subtalar joint in a neutral position, the midtarsal joint in maximal pronation, and then dorsiflexes the subject's ankle with assistance from the subject. The fifth examiner used an alternate technique that differed from the modified Root technique only in that the subject was not asked to assist in dorsiflexing the ankle. Measurements were made with the subjects in supine and the knee in both the extended and flexed positions. The investigators used the ICC to calculate intrarater and interrater reliability. Intrarater reliability ranged from 0.74 to 0.86 (see Table 15.9) and interrater reliability ranged from 0.34 to 0.54 (see Table 15.10). These authors reported no effects on reliability with years of experience or technique employed.

Several investigators who have examined the reliability of measurements of passive motion of the ankle joint have done so within the pediatric population. These studies included investigations in healthy infants and in children with a variety of diagnoses. Passive ankle plantarflexion was measured by two examiners in a group of 54 healthy infants between the ages of 12h and 6days.[25] A subgroup of nine of the infants was used to examine interrater reliability of passive ankle plantar flexion measurements using Pearson's r. Values for interrater reliability reported in this study were 0.84 for the left ankle and 0.89 for the right ankle (see Table 15.10). The SEM from this study (calculated by

the author of this text from data provided) was 2.6 degrees for right ankle plantar flexion and 3.1 degrees for the left ankle.

In a study designed to investigate the intrarater and interrater reliability of goniometry and visual estimations of passive ankle joint ROM in children with cerebral palsy, Allington et al.[49] measured ankle motion in both ankles of 24 children with spastic CP. Two examiners measured ankle dorsiflexion and plantar flexion, as well as subtalar inversion and eversion, in both lower extremities of each subject, using goniometry and visual estimation on three separate occasions over a 10-day period. All measurements were performed by two individuals—one who positioned the joint and the other who performed the measurement. Subjects were positioned supine for all measurements. Ankle dorsiflexion was performed with the knee extended and again with the knee flexed. Reliability was calculated using Pearson's correlation coefficient. Intrarater reliability ranged from 0.85 to 0.86 for ankle plantar flexion and from 0.93 to 0.95 for ankle dorsiflexion (see Table 15.9). Interrater reliability was 0.84 for ankle plantar flexion and 0.95 for ankle dorsiflexion (see Table 15.10).

Glanzman et al.[20] also compared goniometric measurements of passive ankle motion to visual estimation of that motion in a group of 25 children with cerebral palsy. Ankle dorsiflexion, but not plantar flexion, was measured with the subject's knee in extension using either one or two examiners. When a second examiner was employed, that person held the knee in extension while the first examiner positioned the ankle and performed the measurement. Additional details of this study have been described previously (see "Hip" section of this chapter). Intrarater reliability for goniometric measurements was high (ICC = 0.98), regardless of whether one or two examiners were used (see Table 15.9). Additionally, measurements using visual estimation were highly correlated with goniometric measurements made using a single examiner (Pearson's r = 0.96).

At least four other groups of investigators have examined the reliability of goniometric measurements of passive ankle dorsiflexion ROM in children with spastic cerebral palsy. Kilgour et al.[4] measured ankle dorsiflexion range of motion, along with nine other motions of the lower extremity, in 25 children with spastic cerebral palsy and 25 age- and sex-matched controls. (The reliability of measurements of the remaining nine motions is discussed in Section "Reliability of Muscle Length Testing" of this chapter.) A single physical therapist performed all measurements, assisted by two other physical therapists—one who maintained the ankle position, and the other who recorded the measurement. ROM was measured twice per motion in each of two sessions, spaced 7days apart. Intrarater reliability was calculated with the use of ICCs, both within session and between sessions, for controls and subjects with CP. Within-session reliability for controls was 0.97 to 0.98, and for subjects with CP, 0.98 to 0.99. Reliability between sessions was less, with ICC values for control subjects ranging from 0.70 to 0.75, and for subjects with CP from 0.75 to 0.90 (see Table 15.9).

In a study described previously (see "Hip Abduction/ Adduction" section of this chapter), McWhirk and Glanzman[26] investigated the within-session interrater reliability of goniometric measurements of passive ankle dorsiflexion in children with spastic cerebral palsy using an experienced and a novice examiner. Interrater reliability was good, with an ICC of 0.87 and a 95% confidence interval of 3.56 ± 1.23 (see Table 15.10).

Interrater reliability similar to that in the McWhirk and Glanzman study[26] was found by Mutlu et al.[5] The latter group of investigators measured passive ankle dorsiflexion in a group of 38 children with spastic cerebral palsy using three different examiners who performed the measurements in two separate sessions 1 week apart. An assistant was used during all measurements to maintain the position of the subjects and record the measurements. All measurements were taken with the subjects in supine and the knee extended. Intrarater and interrater reliability was calculated using the ICC. Intrarater reliability ranged from 0.81 to 0.90 (see Table 15.9) and interrater reliability was 0.88 (see Table 15.10), similar to the 0.87 value reported by McWhirk and Glanzman.[26]

Stuberg et al.[3] measured the reliability of passive ankle goniometry in a group of children with cerebral palsy; however, this group of investigators examined ankle dorsiflexion measurements. Specifics about the study's protocol have been described previously (see "Hip" section of this chapter). A two-way ANOVA for repeated measures was used to determine intrarater and interrater reliability of passive ankle dorsiflexion measurement. Analysis of intrarater reliability showed no significant difference between the three measures taken by a single examiner in one session, and intrarater error was calculated at less than or equal to 5 degrees. Conversely, significant interrater variation was found.

Reliability of passive ankle dorsiflexion measurement also was examined in a group of children with Duchenne's muscular dystrophy.[38] Goniometric measurements were performed using standardized procedures and positioning. Interrater and intrarater reliability was calculated for 21 and 150 patients, respectively, using ICCs. Reliabilities were 0.73 for interrater and 0.90 for intrarater reliability of passive ankle dorsiflexion measurement (see Tables 15.9 and 15.10).

Numerous investigators have examined the reliability of passive ankle dorsiflexion measurements in the adult population.[55,57] Several of these groups investigated the intrarater reliability of passive ankle dorsiflexion ROM measurements in healthy adults. Macedo and Magee[8] gathered their data from a group of 90 Caucasian women aged 18 to 59 years and reported good to excellent reliability (ankle dorsiflexion:

ICC = 0.77, SEM = 3 degrees, MDC = 7 degrees; ankle plantar flexion: ICC = 0.90, SEM = 5 degrees, MDC = 13 degrees; see Table 15.9). Additional details of this study have been described previously (see "Hip" section of this chapter).

Bohannon et al.[51] examined the reliability of measurements of ankle motion in healthy adults using various distal landmarks and various methods of dorsiflexing the ankle. Ankle dorsiflexion was measured in 36 female subjects. Dorsiflexion motion was accomplished in three different ways: (1) passively to the point of notable tension, (2) passively with maximal force, and (3) passively with maximal force and active assistance by the subject. Each motion was measured three times, and the distal landmark was altered each time by using the fifth metatarsal, the heel, or the plantar surface of the foot for alignment of the moving arm of the goniometer. ANOVA revealed a significant difference in ankle dorsiflexion measurements under the three conditions and when different landmarks were used. The amount of ankle dorsiflexion obtained was greatest when the examiner passively dorsiflexed the ankle with maximal force and was actively assisted by the subject. The least amount of dorsiflexion was obtained when the examiner performed passive ankle dorsiflexion to notable tension. Variations in the landmark used also influenced the amount of dorsiflexion obtained. Dorsiflexion measurements were highest when the heel was used as the distal landmark and lowest when the fifth metatarsal was used. Intrarater reliability of each measurement was calculated using ICCs, and all measurements were found to be reliable (range, 0.80 to 0.93). However, measurements of ankle dorsiflexion that involved using the heel as the distal landmark or passive dorsiflexion to notable tension were the least reliable[9,51] (see Table 15.9).

Of the remaining studies in healthy adults, all examined the reliability of ankle dorsiflexion measures taken with the subjects in a weight-bearing lunge position.[50,51,57,60,62,66] Ekstrand et al.[66] appear to have been the first to examine the reliability of this method of measuring ankle dorsiflexion, which they performed using a gravity inclinometer. When employing strict measuring protocols, this group of investigators reported an intrarater coefficient of variation of 2.6%. Ankle dorsiflexion measurements in most of the remaining studies were performed using some type of inclinometer, either digital[50,60,62,66] or gravity.[51,53] Some studies employed additional measurement techniques such as a tape measure,[51,66] an acrylic plate marked in 2-degree increments,[50] or a goniometer[52,66] as part of their measurement of ankle dorsiflexion in a weight-bearing lunge position. Intrarater reliability of ankle dorsiflexion measurement using an inclinometer ranged from 0.86 to 0.98 or higher in all studies using this instrument (see Table 15.9). Interrater reliability was equally high, ranging from 0.88 to 0.97 (see Table 15.10). The tape measure method also demonstrated high reliability, with ICCs reported from 0.97 to 0.99 for intrarater reliability (see Table 15.9) and at 0.99 for interrater reliability (see Table 15.10). Reliability of the goniometer in performing this measurement was slightly lower than the other two instruments, with ICC values ranging from 0.85 to 0.96 for intrarater reliability (see Table 15.9). Hall and Docherty[67] provided evidence of strong concurrent validity of measurements of dorsiflexion range of motion employing a tape measure or inclinometer as compared to a motion capture system with subjects in a weight-bearing lunge position.

The remaining studies involving passive ankle dorsiflexion were performed using adult patient populations. Denegar et al.[54] examined the reliability of passive ankle ROM measurements as part of a study of the effect of ankle sprains on dorsiflexion ROM and arthrokinematic movement. Measurements of ankle dorsiflexion were performed in a group of 12 college athletes with a history of unilateral ankle sprain. Both the injured and uninjured ankles were measured using a gravity inclinometer. Ankle dorsiflexion was measured with the subject in four different positions: (1) sitting with the knee extended, (2) prone with the knee flexed to 90 degrees, (3) standing with the knee extended (lunge position), and (4) standing with the knee flexed (unilateral squat). Intrarater reliability was calculated using the ICC and SEM, and was high for all measurements, with ICC values ranging from 0.91 to 0.99 (see Table 15.9) and SEM values all approximating 1 degree.

Elveru et al.[57] measured passive ankle dorsiflexion and plantar flexion in 50 ankles of 43 patients with neurological or orthopedic disorders. No standardized patient positioning or goniometric technique was used in the study. Two measurements of ankle plantar flexion and dorsiflexion were taken on each patient by two examiners using a blinded goniometer. The first of each pair of measurements was used to calculate intertester reliability. Intraclass correlation coefficients were used to determine intrarater and interrater reliability. Intrarater reliability for ankle motions equaled 0.90 for dorsiflexion and 0.86 for plantar flexion; interrater reliability was 0.50 for dorsiflexion and 0.72 for plantar flexion (see Tables 15.9 and 15.10).

Reliability of passive ankle dorsiflexion but not of plantar flexion was examined by Diamond et al.[55] in a group of 31 patients with diabetes mellitus. Two examiners measured passive ankle dorsiflexion ROM using a standardized procedure that involved maintaining the subtalar joint in a neutral position during measurement. Extensive training (20 training sessions over 18 months) was undertaken by each examiner before data were collected. Intrarater and interrater reliability was assessed using ICCs. Values reported for reliability of ankle dorsiflexion were 0.89 (right ankle) and 0.96 (left ankle) for intrarater, and 0.74 (right ankle) and 0.87 (left ankle) for interrater (see Tables 15.9 and 15.10). The SEM also

was reported for all goniometric data. Values for SEM were 1 degree (left ankle) and 3 degrees (right ankle) for repeated measurements taken by the same examiner, and 2 degrees (left ankle) and 3 degrees (right ankle) for measurements taken by different examiners.[55]

Reliability of passive ankle dorsiflexion in weight bearing and nonweight-bearing was examined by Searle et al.[63] in 30 individuals with diabetes mellitus and 30 adults without diabetes. Two examiners measured passive ankle dorsiflexion ROM with the knee extended using a modified Lindcombe template with a standard force of 80.4 N (nonweight-bearing) and a Lunge test (weight bearing). Intrartester and intertester reliability was assessed using ICCs and SEM was calculated using 95% confidence intervals. Values reported for reliability of ankle dorsiflexion when nonweight-bearing were 0.90 to 0.94 (diabetes group) and 0.89 (nondiabetes group) for intratester reliability, and 0.91 (diabetes group) and 0.91 (nondiabetes group) for intertester reliability. Values reported for reliability of ankle dorsiflexion when performing the lunge test were 0.83 to 0.85 (diabetes group) and 0.85 to 0.89 (nondiabetes group) for intratester reliability, and 0.88 (diabetes group) and 0.93 (nondiabetes group) for intertester reliability (see Tables 15.9 and 15.10). Values reported for SEM when nonweight-bearing were 1.9 degrees (diabetes group) and 1.7 degrees (nondiabetes group). Values reported for SEM during the lunge test (weight bearing) were 2.1 degrees for both the diabetes and nondiabetes groups.

Dobija and Jankowski[56] examined the reliability of passive ankle dorsiflexion and plantarflexion using a bubble inclinometer in 16 older adults with orthopedic problems. Four examiners measured passive ankle dorsiflexion and plantarflexion ROM with the knee extended and with the knee flexed with the subject in supine using standardized procedures. The SEM was calculated and intra and intertester reliability were assessed using ICCs. Values reported for reliability of ankle dorsiflexion were 0.91 to 0.95 (knee extended) and 0.92 to 0.97 (knee flexed) for intratester reliability, and 0.91 (knee extended) and 0.90 (knee flexed) for intertester reliability. Values reported for reliability of ankle plantarflexion were 0.66 to 0.96 (knee extended) and 0.84 to 0.93 (knee flexed) for intratester reliability, and 0.72 (knee extended) and 0.86 (knee flexed) for intertester rater reliability (see Tables 15.9 and 15.10). Values reported for SEM for dorsiflexion were 2.5 degrees (knee extended) and 2.8 degrees (knee flexed). Values reported for SEM for plantarflexion were 4.4 degrees (knee extended) and 3.5 degrees (knee flexed).

Subtalar Inversion/Eversion

Reliability of goniometric inversion and eversion measurements varies widely depending on the technique used to perform the measurement. Elveru et al.[57] measured passive inversion and eversion of the subtalar joint in 43 patients (50 ankles) with neurologic and orthopedic disorders. Examiners measured subtalar inversion and eversion motion and the neutral position of the subtalar joint using a universal goniometer, with the patient in a prone, nonweight-bearing position. The neutral subtalar position was determined through palpation. Measurements of inversion and eversion were taken without referencing them to the neutral position of the subtalar joint, but later, the measurements were recalculated based on the subtalar neutral position. Each examiner was provided with standardized written instructions detailing techniques used for determining the neutral position of the subtalar joint and for measuring passive inversion and eversion. ROM measurements were taken by placing the goniometer on the posterior aspect of the joint, with the proximal arm aligned along the midline of the calf and the distal arm aligned with the posterior midline of the calcaneus. Intrarater and interrater reliability was calculated using ICCs. In the case of both intrarater and interrater reliability, ICC levels were lower when the measurement was referenced to the neutral position of the subtalar joint compared with measurements taken with no reference used (Tables 15.11 and 15.12). The authors attributed this decreased reliability to the error associated with determining the subtalar neutral position.[57]

Low interrater reliability for subtalar inversion and eversion measurements also was found by a group of investigators who used a similar technique to that used by Elveru et al.[57] Smith-Oricchio and Harris[69] measured subtalar inversion and eversion in reference to the subtalar neutral position in 20 patients with recent ankle pathology. Patients were measured in the prone, nonweight-bearing position, as well as in a standing, weight-bearing position. Goniometric alignment, as described in the previous study,[57] was seen along the posterior aspect of the joint.[57] Interrater reliability was calculated using ICCs. Low interrater reliability was found for calcaneal inversion and eversion measurements taken in the prone, nonweight-bearing position (see Table 15.12). However, interrater reliability of subtalar eversion measurements taken with the patient standing on both feet was high (ICC = 0.91). The authors attributed this difference to the fact that the subtalar motion measured with the patient in the prone position was passive, whereas the motion measured with the patient in the standing position was active eversion; this eliminates a variable and a potential source of error for the examiner.[69]

Yet a third group of investigators examined the reliability of measurements of subtalar inversion and eversion by using goniometric techniques similar to those described in the studies by Elveru et al.[57] and Smith-Oricchio and Harris.[69] Subtalar inversion and eversion ROM was measured in a group of 31 patients with diabetes mellitus.[55] Measurements were taken with the goniometer placed along the posterior aspect of the joint and with the arms of the goniometer aligned as

described in the previous studies.[57] No attempt was made by these examiners to reference subtalar measurements to the subtalar neutral position. Instead, motion of the subtalar joint was referenced to "anatomical zero."[55] In contrast to the examiners in the previous two studies, the examiners in this study underwent a period of extensive training (18 months) before the time of data collection. Intrarater and interrater reliability was calculated using ICCs. For calcaneal inversion, intrarater reliability (calculated on data from 25 patients) was 0.96 for the left and 0.92 for the right, and for calcaneal eversion, it equaled 0.96 in both extremities (see Table 15.11). Interrater reliability (calculated on data from 31 patients) ranged from a low of 0.78 for calcaneal eversion on the left to a high of 0.89 for calcaneal inversion on the left (see Table 15.12). The SEM was reported as 2 degrees for measurements of calcaneal inversion taken by the same examiner and 3 degrees for measurements taken by two different examiners, regardless of the side (right or left) measured. For calcaneal eversion, the SEM for measurements taken by the same examiner was 1 degree, regardless of the side measured, and the SEM for measurements taken by two different examiners was 2 degrees on the right and 4 degrees on the left. The higher levels of reliability obtained in this study compared with other investigations were attributed by the authors to the extensive period of training undertaken by the examiners before the time of data collection.[55]

Other investigators have used different methods of measuring eversion and inversion ROM in their studies of reliability. Walker et al.[13] measured inversion and eversion in a group of four healthy adults, using the anterior approach described by the AAOS in its 1965 publication.[19] Only inversion motion was measured by Boone et al.[22] in a group of 12 healthy adult males, using the same technique used by investigators in the Walker et al.[13] study. Because both groups measured active range of motion, presumably the motion measured was combined forefoot and hindfoot motion, although this fact could not be clearly discerned from either study. Boone et al.[22] calculated reliability using the ICC and reported intrarater reliability for inversion measurements of 0.80 (see Table 15.11). Intrarater reliabilities for both inversion and eversion measurements were reported as greater than 0.81 (Pearson's r) by Walker et al.,[13] with a mean error between repeated measures of 5 degrees. Interrater reliability, which was calculated by only one group[11,22] and only for inversion, equaled 0.69 (ICC) (see Table 15.12).

The reliability of ankle inversion and eversion measurements taken in the prone and sitting positions was compared by Menadue et al.[68] Active ROM was measured in 60 ankles of 30 subjects (aged 21 to 59 years) by three examiners who had varying amounts of previous experience. Measurements of each motion were performed three times by each examiner in each testing position on two separate occasions. Standardized

Table 15.11 INTRARATER RELIABILITY: SUBTALAR JOINT RANGE OF MOTION					
SUBTALAR INVERSION					
STUDY	**TECHNIQUE**	**n**	**SAMPLE**	**r^***	**ICC†**
Allington et al.[49]	PROM; supine; compared visual estimation (VE) to goniometry (G); 2 examiners "junior" PTs	24 (46 ankles)	Children with spastic CP (3–14 years)	0.75–0.80 (VE) 0.76–0.78 (G)	
Boone et al.[22]	AROM; supine; knee extended; goniometer aligned with 2nd metatarsal and shaft of tibia; 4 examiners (PTs)	12	Healthy adult males (26–54 years)		0.80
Diamond et al.[55]	PROM, referenced from anatomical zero	25	Diabetes (34–77 years)		0.92 (R) 0.96 (L)
Elveru et al.[57]	PROM; prone; measurements taken with and without reference to subtalar joint neutral (STJN); 14 PT examiners (6.5 ± 3 years experience)	43 (50 ankles)	Orthopedic and neurological disorders (12–81 years)		0.62 referenced to STJN 0.74 not referenced to STJN
Macedo and Magee[8]	PROM; sitting, knee flexed to 90°; standardized goniometer technique; 1 PT examiner	12 (24 ankles)	Healthy Caucasian women (18–59 years; $\bar{x}$ = 37.2 years)		0.68
Menadue et al.[68]	AROM; measured in 2 positions: prone (P) and sitting (S); standardized technique; 3 examiners (exercise scientist, 4th-year PT student, and a manipulative PT with 25 years experience)	30 (60 ankles)	Healthy adults (21–59 years)		Within session: 0.94 P 0.91–0.96 S Between sessions: 0.53–0.76 P 0.62–0.80 S
Walker et al.[13]	AROM; AAOS standardized goniometer technique; 4 examiners	4	Healthy adults (60–84 years)	> 0.81	
SUBTALAR EVERSION					
STUDY	**TECHNIQUE**	**n**	**SAMPLE**	**r^***	**ICC†**
Allington et al.[49]	PROM; supine; compared visual estimation (VE) to goniometry (G); 2 examiners "junior" PTs	24 (46 ankles)	Children with spastic CP (3–14 years)	0.84–0.90 (VE) 0.84–0.90 (G)	
Diamond et al.[55]	PROM, referenced from anatomical zero	25	Diabetes (34–77 years)		0.96 (R) 0.96 (L)
Elveru et al.[57]	PROM; prone; measurements taken with and without reference to subtalar joint neutral (STJN); 14 PT examiners (6.5 ± 3 years experience)	43 (50 ankles)	Orthopedic and neurological disorders (12–81 years)		0.59 referenced to STJN; 0.75 not referenced to STJN
Macedo and Magee[8]	PROM; sitting, knee flexed to 90°; standardized goniometer technique; 1 PT examiner	12 (24 hips)	Healthy Caucasian women (18–59 years; $\bar{x}$ = 37.2 years)		0.69
Menadue et al.[68]	AROM; measured in 2 positions: prone (P) and sitting (S); standardized technique; 3 examiners (exercise scientist, 4th-year PT student, and a manipulative PT with 25 years experience)	30 (60 ankles)	Healthy adults (21–59 years)		Within session: 0.83–0.94 P 0.82–0.93 S Between sessions: 0.54–0.60 P 0.42–0.64 S
Walker et al.[13]	AROM; AAOS standardized goniometer technique; 4 examiners	4	Healthy adults (60–84 years)	> 0.81	

AAOS, American Academy of Orthopedic Surgeons; *AROM,* active range of motion; *CP,* cerebral palsy; *L,* left; *PROM,* passive range of motion; *R,* right; *STJN,* subtalar joint neutral.

*Pearson's r.
†Intraclass correlation coefficient.

techniques for measuring ROM were followed. As in the study by Diamond et al.,[55] no attempt was made by the examiners in this study to reference subtalar motions to subtalar neutral. Intrarater (both within session and between sessions) and interrater reliability was calculated using ICCs (version 2.1). Standard error of the measurement and 95% confidence intervals also were calculated. Within-session intra-rater reliability ranged from 0.82 for measurement of ankle eversion in a sitting position to 0.96 for measurement of ankle inversion in a sitting position (see Table 15.11). Between-session intrarater reliability was lower and ranged from 0.42 for measurement of ankle eversion in a sitting position to 0.80 for

Table 15.12   INTERRATER RELIABILITY: SUBTALAR JOINT RANGE OF MOTION

SUBTALAR INVERSION

STUDY	TECHNIQUE	n	SAMPLE	r*	ICC†
Allington et al.[49]	PROM; supine; compared visual estimation (VE) to goniometry (G); 2 examiners "junior" PTs	24 (46 ankles)	Children with spastic CP (3–14 years)	0.82 (VE) 0.80 (G)	
Boone et al.[22]	AROM; supine; knee extended; goniometer aligned with 2nd metatarsal and shaft of tibia; 4 examiners (PTs)	12	Healthy adult males (26–54 years)		0.69
Diamond et al.[55]	PROM, referenced from anatomical zero	31	Diabetes (34–77 years)		0.86 (R) 0.89 (L)
Drews et al.[25]	PROM; supine; standardized technique; goniometer placed on protractor; 2 PT examiners	9	Healthy infants (12h–6days)	0.56 (L) 0.71 (R)	
Elveru et al.[57]	PROM; prone; measurements taken with and without reference to subtalar joint neutral (STJN); 14 PT examiners (6.5±3 years experience)	43 (50 ankles)	Orthopedic and neurological disorders (12–81 years)		0.15 referenced to STJN 0.32 not referenced to STJN
Menadue et al.[68]	AROM; measured in 2 positions: prone (P) and sitting (S); standardized technique; 3 examiners (exercise scientist, 4th-year PT student, and a manipulative PT with 25 years experience)	30 (60 ankles)	Healthy adults (21–59 years)		0.54 P 0.73 S
Smith-Oricchio and Harris[69]	PROM, referenced to STJN	20	Ankle pathology (18–53 years)		0.42

SUBTALAR EVERSION

STUDY	TECHNIQUE	n	SAMPLE	r*	ICC†
Allington et al.[49]	PROM; supine; compared visual estimation (VE) to goniometry (G); 2 examiners "junior" PTs	24 (46 ankles)	Children with spastic CP (3–14 years)	0.93 (VE) 0.93 (G)	
Diamond et al.[55]	PROM, referenced from anatomical zero	31	Diabetes (34–77 years)		0.79 (R) 0.78 (L)
Drews et al.[25]	PROM; supine; standardized technique; goniometer placed on protractor; 2 PT examiners	9	Healthy infants (12h–6days)	0.33 (L) 0.62 (R)	
Elveru et al.[57]	PROM; prone; measurements taken with and without reference to subtalar joint neutral (STJN); 14 PT examiners (6.5±3 years experience)	43 (50 ankles)	Orthopedic and neurological disorders (12–81 years)		0.12 referenced to STJN 0.17 not referenced to STJN
Menadue et al.[68]	AROM; measured in 2 positions: prone (P) and sitting (S); standardized technique; 3 examiners (exercise scientist, 4th-year PT student, and a manipulative PT with 25 years experience)	30 (60 ankles)	Healthy adults (21–59 years)		0.41 P 0.62 S
Smith-Oricchio and Harris[69]	PROM, referenced to STJN	20	Ankle pathology (18–53 years)		0.60

AROM, Active range of motion; *CP,* cerebral palsy; *L,* left; *PROM,* passive range of motion; *R,* right; *STJN,* subtalar joint neutral.
*Pearson's *r.*
†Intraclass correlation coefficient.

measurement of ankle inversion in a sitting position (see Table 15.11). Standard error of measurement ranged from 1 degree for eversion in a prone position to 2.9 degrees for eversion in a sitting position; 95% confidence intervals ranged from 2 to 6 degrees. Interrater reliability ranged from 0.41 for measurement of ankle eversion in a prone position to 0.73 for measurement of ankle inversion in a sitting position (see Table 15.12). Standard error of the measurement between raters ranged from 2.8 degrees for eversion in prone to 4.6 degrees for inversion in sitting; 95% confidence intervals ranged from 6 to 9 degrees.

Macedo and Magee[8] measured "ankle inversion and eversion" of 90 healthy adult females who were positioned in supine for the measurements. No description was provided of the goniometer placement for these measurements. Intrarater reliability was calculated using the ICC, and SEM and MDC also were reported. Measurements of inversion (ICC = 0.68, SEM = 4 degrees, MDC = 11 degrees) were somewhat more reliable than eversion (ICC = 0.69, SEM = 6 degrees, MDC = 17 degrees) in this study.

Finally, two groups of investigators examined the reliability of passive inversion and eversion measurements of the foot in children.[25,49] In the Drews et al.[25] study, investigators used a unique and rather vaguely described technique for measuring inversion and eversion, in which measurements were taken by aligning the moving arm of the goniometer along the midline of the plantar surface of the foot. The alignment of the stationary arm was not provided in the published report, nor was an explanation of the reference position against which the measurement was taken provided. Interrater reliability was calculated using Pearson's r, and values ranged from a low of 0.33 for eversion of the left foot to a high of 0.71 for inversion of the right foot (see Table 15.12). The SEM for this study (calculated by the author of this text from data provided) ranged from 3.8 degrees for

measurements of inversion on the right foot to 7 degrees for measurements of eversion on the left foot.

Similarly, in their study of children with spastic cerebral palsy (described in the "Ankle Dorsiflexion/Plantar Flexion" section of this chapter), Allington et al.[49] provided a vague description of the methods used to measure inversion and eversion range of motion. Although the authors stated that a "strict protocol" was used, only the positioning of subjects in supine during the measurement was included in the description of measurement methods. These investigators calculated intrarater and interrater reliability using Pearson's r. Intrarater reliability ranged from 0.76 to 0.78 for inversion and from 0.84 to 0.90 for eversion (see Table 15.11). Results for interrater reliability were higher than for intrarater, with values of 0.80 for inversion and 0.93 for eversion (see Table 15.12).

Metatarsophalangeal Flexion/Extension

Very few studies were found that used inferential statistics to examine the reliability of goniometric measurements of extension of the first metatarsophalangeal (MTP) joint. Hopson et al.[70] calculated the intrarater reliability of four different methods of measuring extension of the first MTP joint in a group of 20 healthy adults aged 21 to 43 years. Methods compared included the following: (1) measuring from the medial side of the joint with the subject in a nonweight-bearing position, (2) measuring from the dorsal surface of the joint with the subject in a nonweight-bearing position; (3) measuring from the medial side of the joint with the subject seated in a partial weight-bearing position; and (4) measuring from the medial side of the joint with the subject standing in a full weight-bearing position. Intrarater reliability of each method was calculated using ICC. Reliabilities ranged from a low of 0.91 for method 2 to a high of 0.98 for method 4 (Table 15.13). The authors

Table 15.13 INTRARATER RELIABILITY: FIRST MTP JOINT EXTENSION				
STUDY	**TECHNIQUE**	**n**	**SAMPLE**	**ICC***
Hopson et al.[70]	PROM; long sitting (nonweight-bearing) position with axis on the medial side (medial side NWB) and with axis on dorsum (dorsum NWB); seated, knee 90° flexion and foot on floor (partial WB); and static weight bearing (full WB); 1 examiner	20	Healthy adults (21–43 years)	0.95, medial side NWB 0.91, dorsum NWB 0.95, partial WB 0.98, full WB
Otter et al.[71]	PROM; compared measurements made using universal goniometer (G) and smartphone goniometer (SG); goniometric alignment on medial side of joint; starting position in maximal plantar flexion; 8 examiners (final year podiatry students)	26	Healthy adults (11 F, 15 M) 18–51 years; x̄ = 27 ± 10.7 years	0.71–0.86 (G) 0.77–0.93 (SG)
Van der Worp et al.[64]	PROM; standing, knee extended, ankle plantarflexed, 1st metatarsal in maximum dorsiflexion; pocket goniometer; 2 examiners (sports PTs)	42	Recreational runners (20 F, 22 M) x̄ = 38.2 ± 12.4 years	0.62

F, Female; *M*, male; *NWB*, nonweight-bearing; *PROM*, passive range of motion; *WB*, weight-bearing.
*Intraclass correlation coefficient.

STUDY	TECHNIQUE	n	SAMPLE	ICC*
Otter et al.[71]	PROM; compared measurements made using universal goniometer (G) and smartphone goniometer (SG); goniometric alignment on medial side of joint; starting position in maximal plantar flexion; 8 examiners (final year podiatry students)	26	Healthy adults (11 F, 15 M) 18–51 years; $\bar{x}=27 \pm 10.7$ years	0.79 (G) 0.83 (SG)
Van der Worp et al.[64]	PROM; standing, knee extended, ankle plantarflexed, 1st metatarsal in maximum dorsiflexion; pocket goniometer; 2 examiners (sports PTs)	42	Recreational runners (20 F, 22 M) $\bar{x}=38.2 \pm 12.4$ years	0.42

Table 15.14   INTERRATER RELIABILITY: FIRST MTP JOINT EXTENSION

F, Female; *M*, male; *PROM*, passive range of motion.
*Intraclass correlation coefficient.

concluded that all four methods of measuring extension of the first MTP were reliable, but the measurements should not be considered interchangeable.[70]

Measurement of MTP extension in a standing position also was investigated by van der Worp et al.[64] This group of investigators used a protocol slightly modified from that used in the study by Hopson et al.[70] in that the size of the subjects' step length was not standardized. Two sports physical therapists used a pocket goniometer to perform measurements from the medial side of the joint in a group of 42 recreational runners. Reliability was calculated using the ICC. Intrarater reliability was lower for this study (ICC = 0.62, SEM = 10 degrees) than for the study by Hopson et al. (ICC = 0.98).[70] Interrater reliability was also calculated by van der Worp et al.[64] (Table 15.14) and was low (ICC = 0.42, SEM = 34 degrees).

A third group of investigators examined the reliability of measurements of MTP extension and MTP static position.[71] Two measuring instruments, a standard goniometer and a smartphone goniometer application (DrGoniometer), were used and compared for reliability. Measurement of static joint position was performed in 26 healthy adults by five podiatry students in their final year of the program. Each subject stood on an elevated platform, and the first MTP joint was positioned in dorsiflexion and maintained in that position with a prop under the hallux. Relevant anatomical landmarks were located and marked on each subject by a single researcher before the measurement session. Goniometric measurements were taken twice by each examiner, followed by two measurements with the smartphone application, all in the same session. The examiners were blinded to all measurements. Passive ROM of the first MTP joint was performed in 32 healthy adults by three podiatry students. For all measurements, subjects were seated with the first MTP joint in full flexion. Two measurements using the goniometer, followed by two measurements with the smartphone application, were made in a single session by each examiner. Intraclass correlations for intrarater reliability of static joint position measurements with the goniometer ranged from 0.71 to 0.86 with SEM ranging from 1 to 2 degrees. The smartphone application demonstrated slightly higher reliability with ICCs ranging from 0.77 to 0.93

and SEM ranging from 1 to 2 degrees. When measuring PROM of the first MTP joint, both instruments showed good to excellent reliability (goniometer: ICC = 0.77 to 0.87, SEM = 1 to 2 degrees; smartphone application: ICC = 0.87 to 0.89, SEM = 1 to 2 degrees). Interrater reliability was higher for measurements of static joint position (goniometer = 0.79, smartphone application = 0.83) than for PROM (goniometer = 0.69, smartphone application = 0.71).

Kwon et al.[72] investigated the validity of goniometric measurements of ROM measurements of the MTP joints of toes 2 to 4 by comparing such measurements to ROM measurements obtained from computed tomography (CT) images (gold standard). The feet of 29 healthy adult subjects (58 ft) were used in the study. Hammer toe deformity was present in 27 of the feet. ROM measurements were performed with the subjects in long sitting with the ankle in 30 degrees of plantar flexion and the goniometer placed over the dorsal surface of the joint. Goniometric measurements were compared with measurements obtained from CT images of the same foot using the Pearson correlation coefficient. Goniometric measurements were found to be highly correlated with CT measurements (Pearson's $r = 0.84$ to 0.90), demonstrating validity of the goniometric measures. However, the two measurement techniques demonstrated consistent differences, preventing the two techniques from being interchangeable.

RELIABILITY OF MUSCLE LENGTH TESTING

Tests for Iliopsoas Muscle Length

Adults

When the reliability of the Thomas test (described in Chapter 14) in measuring the flexibility of the iliopsoas muscle was explored, the vast majority of research used the goniometer. Therefore, the reader should assume that studies presented in this section used the goniometer unless it is specifically stated that another device was used.

Wang et al.[73] performed intrarater reliability measurements on 10 subjects using the Thomas test (described in Chapter 14) to examine the length of the iliopsoas muscle. Results indicated reliability correlations (ICC) for both the dominant and the nondominant iliopsoas muscle equal to 0.97. During the flexibility examination of 117 elite athletes, Harvey[74] included the Thomas test for examination of muscle length of both the iliopsoas and the rectus femoris muscle. Harvey[74] reported intratester reliability correlations (ICC) for all flexibility tests performed in the study as ranging from 0.91 to 0.94 and did not specify which test yielded which correlation. Similar high reliability with use of the Thomas test was reported by Aalto et al.,[6] who examined 20 healthy adults and reporting intratester reliability above 0.92 and intertester reliability greater than 0.74 in the right and left extremities (ICC). In a unique study that used the Thomas test to examine hip motion in 22 older individuals with a diagnosis of hip osteoarthritis, Pua et al.[11] reported intratester reliability of 0.86 (ICC).

Two studies established the reliability of the Thomas test for measurement of iliopsoas muscle length before investigating the effects of an exercise program for increasing flexibility of the muscle. Godges et al.[75] and Winters et al.[76] reported intratester reliability (ICC) greater than 0.80 for measurements using the Thomas test. In addition, Winters et al. reported intertester reliability (ICC) of 0.98.

Clapis et al.[77] examined intertester reliability of the goniometer and the inclinometer between two testers who measured 42 healthy adults. Results indicated high intertester reliability (ICC) for both the goniometer (ICC=0.92) and the inclinometer (ICC=0.89). In addition, the authors reported excellent reliability (ICC) between measurements performed with the two instruments for both testers. The inclinometer-goniometer reliability for tester one was 0.93 and 0.91 for tester two. The authors concluded that because of high reliability when the same instrument is used, as well as high reliability when both instruments are used to measure the same person, the goniometer and inclinometer "can be used interchangeably for measuring hip extensor flexibility."

Conversely, research by Peeler and Anderson[78] reported lower reliability for the Thomas test than was described in previous studies. The authors examined the reliability of the Thomas test in 54 subjects and reported intrarater reliability of 0.52 and interrater reliability of 0.60 (both were ICCs).

Additionally, examining 22 healthy adults, Wakefield et al.[79] found similar low reliability to Peeler and Anderson.[78] Intratester reliability among two testers was 0.51 and 0.54. The resulting intertester reliability was 0.65. The consensus among Peeler and Anderson[78] and Wakefield et al.[79] was that the goniometer has limitations when used to measure iliopsoas muscle length.

Children

Other researchers used the Thomas test to measure the length of the iliopsoas muscle as indicated by the amount of hip extension in children. When measuring intertester reliability in healthy children using the Thomas test, Pandya et al.[38] reported intratester and intertester reliability (ICC) of 0.85 and 0.74, respectively. Drews et al.[25] modified the Thomas test position by placing infants in the side-lying position for measurement and reporting intertester reliability of 0.56 for the left hip and 0.74 for the right. In contrast, after using the Thomas test on 25 healthy children, Kilgour et al.[4] reported intratester reliability (ICC) ranging from 0.09 to 0.91.

Kilgour et al.[4] also used the Thomas test to examine children in whom cerebral palsy had been diagnosed. Intratester reliability (ICC) was also low in this group, ranging from 0.17 to 0.66. Using the Thomas test, Pandya et al.[38] (measuring children with Duchenne muscular dystrophy) and Bartlett et al.[14] (measuring children with myelomeningocele and spastic dysplasia) reported on intrarater and interrater reliability. Both studies reported lower interrater than intrarater reliability, with Pandya et al.[38] (ICC) reporting interrater at 0.74 and intrarater at 0.85. Describing separate reliability correlations for children with myelomeningocele and spastic dysplasia, Bartlett et al.[14] reported intertester reliability (Pearson's r) at 0.90 and 0.70, respectively. (Note: This information from Bartlett et al.[14] is repeated from an earlier section of this chapter to provide here a complete analysis of information related to the Thomas test.) Examining only intertester reliability, McWhirk and Glanzman[26] also reported less than excellent reliability of the Thomas test. After measuring 25 children with spastic cerebral palsy, the authors reported interrater reliability of 0.58. A second study including Glanzman et al.[20] also measured intrarater reliability on 25 children with spastic diplegia using the Thomas test. The authors reported a high reliability of 0.98. Mutlu et al.[5] also examined children with spastic diplegia, determining the intertester reliability on 38 children. The authors reported reliability of the mean of three testers performed on two separate occasions as 0.95 and 0.92.

Children with an orthopedic medical condition were examined by Owen et al.[15] using the Thomas test. Measuring 101 children 2 years after a fracture to the shaft of the femur, the authors reported a poor interrater reliability (ICC) of below 0.25.

Kilgour et al.[4] used the prone hip extension test (described in Chapter 14) as a completely different test to measure flexibility of the iliopsoas muscle. After 25 healthy children and 25 children with cerebral palsy were examined, reported intratester reliability (ICC) ranged from 0.80 to 0.92 and from 0.78 to 0.91, respectively. In the study by Glanzman et al.,[20] the investigators also measured intrarater reliability using the prone hip extension test. Reliability was reported as 0.98 in a sample of 25 children with spastic diplegia.

Table 15.15 INTRATESTER RELIABILITY OF TESTS FOR ILIOPSOAS MUSCLE LENGTH

STUDY	TECHNIQUE	n	SAMPLE	ICC*
Aalto et al.[6]	Thomas	20	Healthy adults ($\bar{x}=23.3$)	0.96 (R) 0.92 (L)[†] 0.95 (R) 0.93 (L)
Bartlett et al.[14]	Thomas	14	Myelomeningocele (4–19 years)	0.93
Bartlett et al.[14]	Thomas	14	Spastic diplegia (6–20 years)	0.89
Clapis et al.[69]		42	Healthy adults ($\bar{x}=22.8$ years)	0.92
Glanzman et al.[20]	Thomas	25	Children with spastic diplegia (6–18 years)	0.98
Glanzman et al.[20]	Prone	25	Children with spastic diplegia (6–18 years)	0.98
Godges et al.[75]	Thomas	25	Healthy adults ($\bar{x}=21.0$ years)	0.80 (R) 0.88 (L)[†]
Harvey[74]	Thomas	117	Elite athletes	0.91–0.94[‡]
Kilgour et al.[4]	Thomas	25	Children with CP ($\bar{x}=10.0$ years)	0.17–0.66[§]
Kilgour et al.[4]	Thomas	25	Healthy children ($\bar{x}=10.0$ years)	0.09–0.91[§]
Kilgour et al.[4]	Prone	25	Children with CP ($\bar{x}=10.0$ years)	0.78–0.91[§]
Kilgour et al.[4]	Prone	25	Healthy children ($\bar{x}=10.0$ years)	0.80–0.92[§]
Pandya et al.[38]	Thomas	150	Duchenne muscular dystrophy (<1–20 years)	0.85
Peeler and Anderson[78]	Thomas	54	Healthy adults (18–45 years)	0.52
Pua et al.[11]	Thomas	22	Hip osteoarthritis ($\bar{x}=62.0$ years)	0.86
Wakefield et al.[79]	Thomas	22	Health adults (18–36 years)	0.51, 0.54
Wang et al.[73]	Thomas	10	Healthy adults (18–37 years)	0.97 (dominant) 0.97 (nondominant)
Winters et al.[76]	Thomas	20	Healthy adults (age not reported)	0.98

CP, Cerebral palsy; L, left; R, right.
*Intraclass correlation coefficient.
†Refer to text for explanation.
‡Two testers performed measurements.
§Three testers performed measurements.

Table 15.16 INTERTESTER RELIABILITY OF THE THOMAS TEST FOR ILIOPSOAS MUSCLE LENGTH

STUDY	n	SAMPLE	ICC*
Aalto et al.[6]	20	Healthy adults ($\bar{x}=23.3$ years)	0.83 (R), 0.74 (L)
Bartlett et al.[14]	14	Myelomeningocele (4–19 years)	0.90
Bartlett et al.[14]	14	Spastic diplegia (6–20 years)	0.70
Drews et al.[25]	9	Healthy infants (12h–6days)	0.56 (L), 0.74 (R)
McWhirk and Glanzman[26]	25	Children with spastic CP (2–18 years)	0.58
Mutlu et al.[5]	38	Children with spastic diplegia (18–108 months; $\bar{x}=52.9\pm19.6$ months)	0.95, 0.92[†]
Owen et al.[15]	101	Children s/p femoral shaft fracture (4–10 years)	0.19 (R), 0.22 (L)
Pandya et al.[38]	21	Duchenne muscular dystrophy (<1–20 years)	0.74
Peeler and Anderson[78]	54	Healthy adults (18–45 years)	0.60
Wakefield et al.[79]	22	Healthy adults (18–56 years)	0.65
Winters et al.[76]	20	Healthy adults (ages not reported)	0.98

CP, Cerebral palsy; L, left; R, right; s/p, status post.
*Intraclass correlation coefficient.
†Mean of three different testers performed on two occasions.

Summary of Tests for Iliopsoas Muscle Length

Table 15.15 provides a summary of studies related to intratester reliability of the measurement of iliopsoas muscle length. Information on intertester reliability is presented in Table 15.16.

Tests for Rectus Femoris Muscle Length

Among studies previously presented in which the Thomas test was used to measure test–retest reliability of iliopsoas muscle length measurement, three investigations also used the Thomas test to measure rectus femoris muscle length by taking measurements at the knee (the technique is described in Chapter 14). Wang et al.[73] reported intrarater reliability coefficients for the dominant rectus femoris muscle equal to 0.97 and for the nondominant rectus femoris muscle equal to 0.96 (ICC). As was indicated previously, Harvey[74] reported intrarater reliability correlations (ICC) for measurements of muscle length of the iliopsoas and rectus femoris muscles as ranging from 0.91 to 0.94, without specifying which test resulted in which correlation. Conversely, using the Thomas test to measure muscle length of the rectus femoris muscle on 20 healthy adults, Aalto et al.[6]

Table 15.17 INTRATESTER RELIABILITY FOR RECTUS FEMORIS MUSCLE LENGTH				
STUDY	TECHNIQUE	n	SAMPLE	ICC*
Aalto et al.[6]	Thomas	20	Healthy adults ($\bar{x} \geq 23.3$ years)	0.60 (R), 0.86 (L) 0.52 (R), 0.72 (L)
Harvey[74]	Thomas	117	Elite athletes (age not reported)	0.91–0.94[†]
Peeler and Anderson[78]	Thomas	57	Healthy adults (18–45 years; $\bar{x}$=29.0 years)	0.65, 0.65, 0.72[‡]
Peeler and Anderson[78]	Prone	57	Healthy adults (18–45 years; $\bar{x}$=29.0 years)	0.54, 0.77, 0.66[‡]
Piva et al.[81]	Prone	20	Subjects with patellofemoral pain syndrome ($\bar{x}$=29.0 years)	0.90, 0.93[§]
Wang et al.[73]	Thomas	10	Healthy adults (18–37 years)	0.97 (dominant), 0.96 (nondominant)

L, Left; *R*, right.
*Intraclass correlation coefficient.
[†]Refer to text for explanation.
[‡]Three testers.
[§]Two testers.

reported intrarater reliability (ICC) ranging from 0.52 to 0.86. These authors also investigated intertester reliability of the Thomas test for rectus femoris muscle length, reporting reliability correlations of 0.60 for the right hip and 0.50 for the left.

In a second study by Peeler and Anderson,[80] the authors examined intrarater and interrater reliability in 57 subjects across three testers. Results indicated intrarater reliability to range from 0.65 to 0.72, and interrater reliability to range from 0.44 to 0.59. Table 15.17 provides a summary of studies related to intrarater reliability of rectus femoris muscle length measurement with use of the Thomas test.

A second test to the Thomas test for measuring rectus femoris muscle length is performed by lying the subject prone and measuring the amount of knee flexion, sometimes referred to as Ely's test. Piva et al.[81] reported intrarater reliability of the prone test as 0.90 and 0.93 for two testers. Also using this prone measurement technique for measuring rectus femoris muscle length in their study, Peeler and Anderson[80] reported intratester reliability of 0.50 to 0.83 and intertester reliability ranging from 0.54 to 0.66 among three examiners.

Tests for Hamstring Muscle Length

Review of the literature indicates that of all research on muscle length tests for the extremities (upper and lower), most has been conducted on the reliability of hamstring muscle length testing. Three tests have been presented in the literature as a means to measure the length of the hamstring muscles: straight leg raise, knee extension test–active, and knee extension test–passive. These tests are described in detail in Chapter 14.

Straight Leg Raise

As part of a larger reliability study, Hsieh et al.[82] evaluated the reliability of the straight leg raise test on 10 subjects using a test–retest design. Results indicated

an intrarater correlation coefficient (Pearson's *r*) of 0.95 (SEM=1.8 degrees). Rose[83] investigated the reliability of the straight leg raise test as a part of a larger study that examined other clinical ROM measurements. Each lower extremity of 18 subjects was measured twice, resulting in intrarater reliability coefficients (Pearson's *r*) of 0.86 and 0.83 for the right and left lower extremity, respectively. The author reported the least significant difference as 17.4 degrees for the right lower extremity and 18.9 degrees for the left lower extremity.

Before examining the muscle flexibility of the lower extremity of long distance runners, Wang et al.[73] established the intrarater reliability of the straight leg raise in 10 subjects. Results indicated an ICC of 0.90 for the dominant limb and 0.91 for the nondominant limb. In a study intended to determine the appropriate method of increasing hamstring flexibility, Hanten and Chandler[84] measured the left leg of 75 females two times to establish the reliability of the straight leg raise test. The intrarater reliability ICC was reported to be 0.91.

Aalto et al.[6] used the straight leg raise test to measure motion in 20 adults and reported intratester reliability (ICC) ranging from 0.94 to 0.98 for the right and left extremities. In addition, in a rare study that examined the intertester reliability (ICC) of the straight leg raise, the authors reported reliability of 0.93 for the right extremity and 0.90 for the left. In a second study examining the interrater reliability of measurement of hamstring flexibility, Mutlu et al.[5] reported reliability of 0.83 as the mean of three testers performed on two separate occasions. Examining only the intrarater reliability (ICC) of 20 subjects with symptoms of patellofemoral syndrome, Piva et al.[81] reported intrarater reliability of 0.88 and 0.98 among two testers.

In addition to conducting previous studies that included healthy adults, Kilgour et al.[4] examined the reliability of two groups of children, one group of 25 healthy children and one group of 25 children with a diagnosis of cerebral palsy. Intratester reliability was reported to be above 0.95, irrespective of which group of children was tested.

Knee Extension Test–Active

The earliest reported study on the reliability of the active knee extension test was conducted by Gajdosik and Lusin.[85] These authors suggested that the straight leg raise was not a valid test for measuring hamstring muscle length because of difficulty in controlling movement at the pelvis, and because the straight leg raise was primarily a test to examine neurological tissue (sciatic nerve), not muscle length. Therefore Gajdosik and Lusin[85] introduced the active knee extension test (described in Chapter 14) and examined intratester reliability on 15 males using a test–retest design. Reported correlation coefficients (Pearson's r) were 0.99 for both the right and the left lower extremity. However, appropriate follow-up testing to analyze for random and systematic error was not included (refer to Chapter 2). This study is presented in this chapter because it is one of the first investigations to use the active 90/90 test.

In establishing the reliability of the active knee extension test for measurement of hamstring muscle length on 12 subjects as part of a study intended to determine the most efficient muscle stretching technique, Sullivan et al.[36] examined intratester reliability and intertester reliability between two testers. The authors reported the intratester reliability (ICC) on the active knee extension test as 0.99 for both testers and the intertester reliability (ICC) between the two testers as 0.93.

In a study undertaken to determine the effects of increasing the length of hamstring muscles on the strength of those muscles, Worrell et al.[86] examined intratester reliability of the active knee extension test in 10 subjects measured twice. The authors reported a correlation coefficient (ICC) of 0.93. In another study that compared two types of stretching techniques for increasing hamstring flexibility, Webright et al.[87] reported on intratester and intertester reliability of the active knee extension test between two examiners. Using a test–retest design on 12 subjects, both examiners achieved an intratester reliability coefficient of 0.98; intertester reliability between the examiners also was reported as 0.98. More recently, Shepard et al.[88] measured the intratester reliability of hamstring muscle length in 37 athletes and reported 0.92 for the right leg and 0.97 for the left. In a study that examined intertester reliability of the active knee extension test, Rakos et al.[89] had three different testers measure 101 children who ranged from 10 to 13 years of age. The authors reported an ICC of 0.79 across all three testers.

Knee Extension Test–Passive

Fredriksen et al.[90] agreed with Gajdosik et al.[91] that the straight leg raise was an inadequate measure of hamstring muscle length because of difficulty involved in controlling pelvic movement. However, these authors questioned the validity of the active knee extension test because the test depended on the strength of the quadriceps muscles, as well as on the ability of the subject to simultaneously contract the quadriceps muscles and relax the hamstring muscles. Therefore, Fredriksen et al.[90] suggested that the passive knee extension test (described in Chapter 14), in which the examiner moved the leg through the available range of motion, was the most appropriate test to measure hamstring muscle length. Two testers examined the reliability of the passive knee extension test on two subjects (one male, one female) measured across 8 days. A total of 28 measurements were taken by each tester, and these measurements were analyzed with a Pearson correlation and paired t-tests. The authors reported intertester correlation coefficients of 0.99 and no significant difference between testers, concluding that "the passive knee extension test is a simple and reliable method."

Bandy et al.[92,93] performed two studies to attempt to determine the optimal length of time that the hamstring muscles should be placed in a sustained stretch position. As part of these studies, the authors reported reliability of the passive knee extension test performed before and after 6 weeks on the control group. Correlation values reported for the control group's pretest and posttest measurements when the passive knee extension test was used were 0.91 (ICC) for the 15 control subjects in the first study[92] and 0.97 (ICC) for the 20 control subjects in the second study.[93]

Before a study was begun to determine whether a special eccentric exercise program could change the flexibility of the hamstring muscles, Nelson and Bandy[94] established the reliability of the passive knee extension test. The authors used a test–retest design in measuring passive knee extension in 15 subjects with a mean age of 29.8 years. Results indicated intratester reliability of 0.96.

Three studies used the passive knee extension test to examine children. In addition to measuring children by using the straight leg test, Kilgour et al.[4] measured the same two groups of children using the passive knee extension test. Authors reported high intratester reliability (ICC) for the children who were healthy (0.99) and for the children in whom cerebral palsy had been diagnosed (0.96 to 0.99). Fosang et al.[23] also measured 18 children with cerebral palsy; an extensive review of the literature revealed that this was one of the only studies to report low intratester reliability (ICC), which ranged from 0.55 to 0.97. In addition, Fosang et al.[23] reported intertester reliability of 0.72. In contrast to this finding, McWhirk and Glanzman[26] measured 25 children with cerebral palsy and reported an intertester reliability (ICC) of 0.93.

Comparison of Three Measurement Techniques

In a study intended to compare the reliability of the three previously described techniques of hamstring muscle length measurement, Gajdosik et al.[91] performed the straight leg raise test, the knee extension test–active, and the knee extension test–passive on 30 males, using a test–retest design. Reported intrarater reliability coefficients (ICC) were 0.83 for the straight leg raise test, 0.86 for the knee extension test–active, and 0.90 for the knee extension test–passive. The authors concluded that study results suggest that the tests "probably represent similar, yet indirect measurements of hamstring length."

Summary: Tests for Hamstring Muscle Length

Summary of studies that examined the reliability of tests to measure hamstring muscle length are presented in Tables 15.18 and 15.19. As is indicated in the tables, irrespective of the measurement test used, or whether

Table 15.18	INTRATESTER RELIABILITY OF TESTS FOR HAMSTRING MUSCLE LENGTH					
STUDY	**TECHNIQUE**	**n**	**SAMPLE**	**r***	**ICC†**
Aalto et al.[6]	SLR	20	Healthy adults ($\bar{x}$ = 23.3 years)		0.94 (R), 0.96 (L)
					0.96 (R), 0.98 (L)
Gajdosik et al.[91]	SLR	30	Healthy adults (18–40 years)		0.83
Hanten and Chandler[84]	SLR	75	Healthy females (18–29 years)		0.91
Hsieh et al.[82]	SLR	10	Healthy adults (26–30 years)	0.95	
Kilgour et al.[4]	SLR	25	Healthy children ($\bar{x}$ = 10.0 years)		0.99–0.99‡
Kilgour et al.[4]	SLR	25	Children with CP ($\bar{x}$ = 10 years)		0.95–0.98‡
Piva et al.[81]	SLR	20	Subjects with patellofemoral pain syndrome ($\bar{x}$ = 29.0 years)		0.88, 0.98§
Rose[83]	SLR	18	Healthy adults ($\bar{x}$ = 19.5 years)	0.86 (R)	
				0.83 (L)	
Wang et al.[73]	SLR	10	Healthy adults (18–37 years)		0.90‖
					0.91¶
Gajdosik and Lusin[85]	Active**	15	Healthy males (18–26 years)	0.99 (R)	
				0.99 (L)	
Gajdosik et al.[91]	Active		Healthy adults (18–40 years)		0.86
Shepard et al.[88]	Active	37	Athletes (18–40 years)		0.92 (R)
					0.97 (L)
Sullivan et al.[95]	Active	12	Healthy adults		0.99, 0.99§
Webright et al.[87]	Active	12	Healthy adults		0.98, 0.98§
Worrell et al.[86]	Active	10	Healthy adults		0.93
Bandy and Irion[92]	Passive††	15	Healthy adults (22–36 years)		0.91
Bandy et al.[93]	Passive	20	Healthy adults (20–40 years)		0.97
Fosang et al.[23]	Passive	18	Children with CP ($\bar{x}$ = 6.4 years)		0.55–0.97‡‡
Gajdosik et al.[91]	Passive	30	Healthy adults (18–40 years)		0.90
Nelson and Bandy[94]	Passive	15	Healthy adults ($\bar{x}$ = 29.8 years)		0.96
Kilgour et al.[4]	Passive	25	Healthy children ($\bar{x} \geq$ 10.0 years)		0.99–0.99‡
Kilgour et al.[4]	Passive	25	Children with CP ($\bar{x}$ = 10 years)		0.96–0.99‡

CP, Cerebral palsy; *L*, left; *R*, right; *SLR*, straight leg raise.
*Pearson's *r*.
†Intraclass correlation coefficient.
‡Three testers performed measurement.
§Two testers performed measurement.
‖Dominant.
¶Nondominant.
**Active knee extension test (90/90 active).
††Passive knee extension test (90/90 passive).
‡‡Six testers performed measurement.

Table 15.19	INTERTESTER RELIABILITY OF TESTS FOR HAMSTRING MUSCLE LENGTH				
STUDY	**TECHNIQUE**	**n**	**SAMPLE**	**r***	**ICC†**
Aalto et al.[6]	SLR	20	Healthy adults ($\bar{x}$ = 23.3)		0.93 (R), 0.90 (L)
Mutlu et al.[5]	SLR	38	Children with spastic cerebral palsy (18–108 months; $\bar{x}$ = 52.9 ± 19.6 months)		0.83‡
Rakos et al.[89]	Active	101	Healthy children (10–13 years)		0.79
Sullivan et al.[95]	Active§	12	Healthy adults		0.93
Webright et al.[87]	Active	12	Healthy adults		0.98
Fosang et al.[23]	Passive	18	Children with CP ($\bar{x}$ = 6.4 years)		0.72‖
Fredriksen et al.[90]	Passive¶	2	Healthy adults	0.99	
McWhirk and Glanzman[26]	Passive	25	Children with spastic CP (2–18 years)		0.93

CP, Cerebral palsy; *SLR*, straight leg raise; *L*, left; *R*, right.
*Pearson's *r*.
†Intraclass correlation coefficient.
‡Mean of three different testers performed on two occasions.
§Active knee extension test (90/90 active).
‖Six testers performed measurements.
¶Passive knee extension test (90/90 passive).

adults or children were tested, the vast majority of studies reported reliability above 0.90 for both intratester reliability (see Table 15.18) and intertester reliability (see Table 15.19).

Tests for Iliotibial Band and Tensor Fasciae Latae Muscle Length

Examination of the reliability of any of the measurement techniques (observation, tape measure, goniometer, inclinometer) used during the Ober test or during modification of the Ober test is very rare. Only three published studies that examined the reliability of the Ober or modified Ober test and only one published study that analyzed the reliability of the prone test could be found through an extensive review of the literature (Ober tests are described in Chapter 14).

As is indicated in Chapter 14, Melchione and Sullivan[96] described use of an inclinometer placed at the distal lateral thigh of the extremity on which the modified Ober test was being performed. Intrarater and interrater reliability of the technique was examined with the use of a test–retest design on 10 subjects with anterior knee pain. Results indicated intratester reliability coefficients (ICC) of 0.94 and intertester reliability coefficients (ICC) of 0.73. The authors concluded that the "repeated measurements obtained with the described method (inclinometer) demonstrated good reliability between testers and excellent reliability within testers."

A similar inclinometer technique was used by Reese and Bandy[97] to measure intrarater reliability of the Ober knee flexed and the modified Ober knee extended tests. Sixty-one healthy adults were measured on two occasions by the same researcher. Results indicated values of 0.90 and 0.91 for the Ober (knee extended) and modified Ober (knee flexed), respectively. Additional analysis revealed a significantly greater ROM when the modified Ober test compared with the Ober test was used, indicating that the two examination procedures should not be used interchangeably. In their study on individuals with patellofemoral syndrome, Piva et al.[81] reported intrarater reliability of 0.90 and 0.99 for two testers.

Gajdosik et al.[98] also reported that the modified Ober performed with the knee extended allowed greater adduction ROM than was seen with the original Ober test (knee flexed). During this investigation, the author established reliability of the Ober test on 23 women and 26 men using a goniometer and reported intratester reliability to range from 0.82 to 0.92. Details of the studies on reliability of the Ober and the modified Ober are presented in Table 15.20.

Pandya et al.[38] examined the reliability of using a goniometer to quantify the prone test (described in Chapter 14) for measurement of iliotibial band and tensor fasciae latae muscle length. Intrarater reliability testing was performed on 150 children, with a reported reliability ICC value of 0.81; intertester reliability testing was performed on 21 children, with ICC reported as 0.25.

Tests for Gastrocnemius and Soleus Muscle Length

In a study with the ultimate purpose of examining the lower extremity flexibility of long-distance runners, Wang et al.[73] reported intratester reliability of measurements of the length of the gastrocnemius muscle (measured supine) and of the soleus muscle (measured prone) in 10 subjects. (Their tests are described in Chapter 14.) Results indicated a reliability correlation (ICC) for gastrocnemius muscle length of 0.98 for both the dominant and the nondominant limb; soleus muscle reliability correlations (ICC) were 0.93 for the dominant limb and 0.94 for the nondominant limb. When examining the measurement of the gastrocnemius muscle length in healthy adults, Jonson and Gross[87] found lower reliability (ICC) than did Wang et al.,[73] who reported intratester reliability of 0.74 and intertester reliability of 0.65. Piva et al.[81] reported intrarater reliability of 0.78 and 0.97 for two examiners in their study. Kim et al.[59] and Krause et al.[61] measured intrarater reliability of the examination of gastrocnemius muscle flexibility in healthy adults and reported reliability coefficients greater than 0.74 for all measurements.

Using the supine measurement with the knee extended to measure gastrocnemius muscle length, Kilgour et al.[4] examined intratester reliability of three testers who measured children between the ages of 6 and 17 years. After investigating 25 healthy children and 25 children with cerebral palsy, the authors reported intratester reliability (ICC) greater than 0.95, irrespective of the group being measured. Also examining intrarater reliability of the gastrocnemius muscle in children with cerebral palsy were Glanzman et al.[20] and Mutlu et al.[5] Glanzman et al. reported intrarater reliability as 0.98 in 25 children with cerebral palsy while Mutlu et al. reported intrarater reliability that was slightly lower at 0.88.

Also after children with cerebral palsy were examined, Fosang et al.[23] and Allington et al.[49] determined intertester reliability and intratester reliability. When 18 children were examined, Fosang et al.[23] reported intrarater reliability (ICC) ranging from 0.74 to 0.91 and interrater reliability of 0.72 across six testers. Allington et al.[49] measured 24 children, yielding an intratester reliability of 0.94 and 0.95 for two testers (Pearson's correlation; mean measurement error of 4 degrees for both) and an interrater reliability of 0.94 across the two testers (Pearson's correlation; mean measurement error of 4 degrees). A summary of studies related to intratester reliability of measurement of gastrocnemius muscle length that included both healthy adults and children as well as children diagnosed with cerebral palsy is presented in Table 15.21.

Table 15.20 INTRATESTER RELIABILITY FOR OBER AND MODIFIED OBER TESTS OF THE ILIOTIBIAL BAND				
STUDY	**TECHNIQUE**	**n**	**SAMPLE**	**ICC[*]**
Melchione and Sullivan[96]	Inclinometer	10	Subjects with knee pain (16–43 years; x̄=23.8)	0.94 (modified)
Piva et al.[81]	Inclinometer	20	Subjects with patellofemoral pain syndrome (x̄=29.0 years)	0.90, 0.99[†]
Reese and Bandy[97]	Inclinometer	61	Healthy adults (21–30 years; x̄=24.2 years)	0.91 (modified)
				0.90 (Ober)
Gajdosik et al.[98]	Goniometer	26 (men)	Healthy adults (20–43 years; x̄=27.0)	0.92 (modified)[‡]
		23 (women)		0.87 (Ober) [‡]
				0.82 (modified) [‡]
				0.83 (Ober) [§]

[*]Intraclass correlation.
[†]Two testers performed measurement.
[‡]For women.
[§]For men.

Table 15.21 INTRARATER RELIABILITY OF MEASUREMENT FOR GASTROCNEMIUS MUSCLE LENGTH				
STUDY	**n**	**SAMPLE**	**r[*]**	**ICC[†]**
Jonson and Gross[58]	18	Healthy adults (18–30 years)		0.74
Kilgour et al.[4]	25	Healthy children (x̄=10.0 years)		0.95–0.98[‡]
Kim et al.[59]	14	Healthy adults (x̄=28.2 years)		0.74 (R); 0.84 (L)
Krause et al.[61]	39	Healthy adults (22–33 years)		0.83, 0.78[§]
Wang et al.[73]	10	Healthy adults (18–37 years)		0.98
Allington et al.[49]	24	Children with CP (3–14 years)	0.94, 0.95	
Fosang et al.[23]	18	Children with CP (x̄=6.4 years)		0.74–0.91[∣∣]
Glanzman et al.[20]	25	Children with CP (6–18 years)		0.98
Kilgour et al.[4]	25	Children with spastic CP (x̄=10.0 years)		0.96–0.99[‡]
Mutlu et al.[5]	38	Children with CP (18–108 months; x̄=52.9±19.6 months)		0.88 [¶]
Piva et al.[81]	20	Subjects with patellofemoral pain syndrome (x̄=29.0 years)		0.78, 0.97[§]

CP, Cerebral palsy; *L*, left; *R*, right.
[*]Intraclass correlation coefficient.
[†]Pearson's *r*.
[‡]Three testers performed measurement.
[§]Two testers performed measurement.
[∣∣]Six testers performed measurement.
[¶]Mean of three different testers performed on two different occasions.

Only two investigators examined the interrater reliability of the gastrocnemius muscle. Kim et al.[59] reported interrater reliability of 0.74 for the right limb and 0.84 for the left limb in 14 healthy adults. Lower interrater reliability was reported by Krause et al.,[61] who determined reliability to be 0.67 in 39 healthy adults.

Examining reliability of the measurement of soleus muscle flexibility, Piva et al.[81] measured 20 subjects with patellofemoral syndrome. The authors reported intrarater reliability of 0.85 and 0.92 among two examiners. Kim et al.[59] calculated intrarater and interrater reliability of measurement of the soleus muscle in 14 healthy adults. The authors reported intrarater reliability of 0.81 on the right limb and 0.86 on the left, but lower reliability when reporting interrater reliability of 0.54 on the right and 0.48 on the left. Intrarater and interrater reliability was also reported by Krause et al.[61] Soleus reliability was reported in 39 healthy adults as 0.83 and 0.78 for two testers performing intrarater reliability and 0.79 for interrater reliability. Data on reliability of the soleus muscle is presented in Table 15.22.

Tests for Gastrocnemius and Soleus Muscle Length—Lunge Test

Intratester Reliability

Two methods have been reported in the literature to examine muscle flexibility of the calf muscles using the lunge test. One method has the subject stand with the forearms against the wall for balance, the knee held against the wall, and the foot and toes slightly away from that same wall. This method of measurement then asks the subject to slowly move the foot away from the wall as far as able, while keeping the knee against the wall. At this end of muscle length, the distance from the toe to the wall is measured. A concern exists in using this method of the lunge test because the numerous repositioning of the foot to achieve a single measure may be more challenging for the subject and the examiner. Therefore, this lunge test method was not used in this book.

The method used in the book is placing the foot and toes a set distance away from the wall and have the subject lean into the wall on their elbows until the end of muscle length is achieved (described in Figs. 14.47

	Table 15.22	RELIABILITY OF MEASUREMENT FOR SOLEUS MUSCLE LENGTH			
STUDY	**TYPE OF RELIABILITY**	**n**	**SAMPLE**		**ICC***
Kim et al.[59]	Intrarater	14	Healthy adults ($\bar{x}$ = 28.2 years)		0.81 (R); 0.86 (L)
Kim et al.[59]	Interrater	14	Healthy adults ($\bar{x}$ = 28.2 years)		0.54 (R); 0.48 (L)
Krause et al.[61]	Intrarater	39	Healthy adults (22–33 years)		0.83, 0.78[†]
Krause et al.[61]	Interrater	39	Healthy adults (22–33 years)		0.79
Piva et al.[81]	Intrarater	20	Subjects with patellofemoral pain syndrome ($\bar{x}$ = 29.0 years)		0.85, 0.92[†]

L, Left; *R*, right.

*Intraclass correlation coefficient.

[†]Two testers performed measurements.

to 14.57). Several authors have used this lunge test as a method to examine the muscle length of the soleus muscle, with a few also looking at the gastrocnemius muscle.

Examining both the soleus and gastrocnemius muscles in 13 males and 9 females ($\bar{x}$ = 22.9 years) using the lunge, Banwell et al.[50] reported excellent intratester reliability (ICC above 0.91) using the inclinometer for both muscles, and lower reliability for using the Smartphone (0.85 to 0.95). (Of interest, the study by Banwell et al.[50] is the only study reporting on the intratester reliability using the Smartphone to measure the reliability of the gastrocnemius muscle.) Investigating only the gastrocnemius muscle, Searle et al.[63] used the inclinometer in 30 older subjects with diabetes (13 males, 17 females; $\bar{x}$ = 65.8 years) and 30 healthy younger subjects (16 males, 14 females; $\bar{x}$ = 28.0). The authors reported intratester reliability among two testers of 0.83 and 0.89 for the older subjects with diabetes; and 0.85 and 0.89 for the younger, healthy subjects.

Other studies have evaluated the tape measure, goniometer, and inclinometer in measuring the intratester reliability of the lunge with the knees flexed, thereby, measuring the soleus muscle length. In the only study using a tape measure, Cipriani et al.[52] had two examiners determine the intratester reliability of the lunge test in 41 subjects (21 males, 20 females; $\bar{x}$ = 27.9 years). The authors reported a reliability of 0.91 and 0.97 for the two examiners.

Konor et al.[60] used both the goniometer and inclinometer to assess the reliability of 20 subjects (7 males, 13 females; $\bar{x}$ = 24.0 years). The authors reported specific data on both the right and left leg. Similar reliability was found for both the right and left legs, as well as measurement using the goniometer and inclinometer with three out of four reliabilities being above 0.95. The measurement of the right soleus using the goniometer was the only measurement below 0.95, as the reliability was 0.85.

Three studies used only the inclinometer to examine the reliability of the lunge test for measuring soleus intratester reliability. An early study by Bennell et al.[99] examined soleus reliability using the lunge test in 13 teenagers (8 males, 5 females; $\bar{x}$ = 18.8 years). Using two examiners, the authors reporter reliability of 0.98 and 0.97. Results from studies by Krause et al.[61] and Langarika-Rocafort et al.,[100] although reporting good reliability, did not produce the same high reliability as

Bennell et al.[50] Krause et al.[61] reported intratester reliability of the soleus among two investigators of 0.88 and 0.89 in 39 individuals (13 males, 26 females; $\bar{x}$ = 24.2 years), while Langarika-Rocafort et al.[100] studied 25 female high school volleyball players ($\bar{x}$ = 15.5 years) and reported intratester reliability of 0.87.

All studies reported results that agree with Searle et al.[63] who indicated "the lunge test to be reliable tests to measure weight bearing ankle dorsiflexion in adults. Table 15.23 presents a summary of the intratester reliability studies just described.

Intertester Reliability

As an extension of their study on intratester reliability, four studies also examined the reliability between two testers (intertester reliability) using the lunge test and the same methods and subjects as described in the previous section on the intratester reliability. Studying the intertester reliability of the gastrocnemius muscle in patients with diabetes, as well as healthy adults, Searle et al.[63] reported reliability of 0.88 for the subjects with diabetes and 0.93 for the healthy adults.

Banwell et al.[50] examined the intertester reliability of both the gastrocnemius and soleus muscles using both the inclinometer and the Smartphone and reported reliability of greater than 0.85 for all tests. Studies by both Bennell et al.[99] and Krause et al.[61] examined the intertester reliability of using an inclinometer for examining soleus muscle length and reported reliability of 0.97 and 0.82, respectively.

Finally, two studies examined intertester reliability of the lunge test to measure soleus muscle length as the sole purpose of their investigation and reported reliability above 0.90. Using the inclinometer to measure the reliability of 43 subjects (14 males, 29 females; $\bar{x}$ = 25.5 years), Rabin and Kozol[101] found the reliability to be 0.93. In the only study examining the intertester reliability of the Smartphone, Awatani et al.[102] examined the soleus muscle in 18 subjects (9 males, 9 females; $\bar{x}$ = 25.3 years) and reported a reliability of 0.94.

The majority of the studies reviewed reported intertester reliability above 0.90 using the lunge test. A summary of intertester reliability of measuring the gastrocnemius and soleus muscle length using the lunge test is presented in Table 15.24.

Table 15.23	INTRATESTER RELIABILITY OF SOLEUS AND GASTROCNEMIUS (GASTROC) MUSCLE LENGTH—LUNGE TEST			
STUDY	TECHNIQUE	n	SAMPLE	ICC*
Banwell et al.[99]	Inclinometer, Smartphone	21	Healthy Subjects ($\bar{x}$=22.9 years)	Gastroc (Inclinometer)=0.91, 0.95 Gastroc (Smartphone)=0.85, 0.85 Soleus (Inclinometer)=0.97, 0.91 Soleus (Smartphone)=0.95, 0.95
Bennell et al.[50]	Inclinometer	13	Healthy Subjects ($\bar{x}$=18.8 years)	Soleus=0.98, 0.97
Konor et al.[60]	Inclinometer, Goniometer	20	Healthy Subjects ($\bar{x}$=24.0 years)	Soleus (Goniometer)=0.85 (Right) 0.96 (left) Soleus (Inclinometer)=0.96 (Right) 0.97 (Left)
Krause et al.[61]	Inclinometer	39	Healthy Subjects ($\bar{x}$=24.2 years)	Soleus=0.88, 0.89
Langarika – Rocafort et al.[100]	Inclinometer	25	Female Athletes ($\bar{x}$=15.5 years)	Soleus=0.87
Cipriani et al.[52]	Tape Measure	41	Healthy Subjects ($\bar{x}$=27.9 years)	Soleus=0.91, 0.97
Searle et al.[63]	Inclinometer	30	Subject with Diabetes ($\bar{x}$=65.8 years)	Gastrocnemius=0.83, 0.89
		30	Healthy Subjects ($\bar{x}$=28.0 years)	Gastrocnemius=0.85, 0.89

*ICC=Intraclass correlation coefficient.

Table 15.24	INTERTESTER RELIABILITY OF SOLEUS AND GASTROCNEMIUS (GASTROC) MUSCLE LENGTH—LUNGE TEST			
STUDY	TECHNIQUE	n	SAMPLE	ICC*
Awatani et al.[102]	Smartphone	18	Healthy Subjects ($\bar{x}$=25.3 years)	Soleus=0.94
Banwell et al.[99]	Inclinometer, Smartphone	21	Healthy Subjects ($\bar{x}$=22.9 years)	Gastroc (Inclinometer)=0.85 Gastroc (Smartphone)=0.94 Soleus (Inclinometer)=0.96 Soleus (Smartphone)=0.98
Bennell et al.[50]	Inclinometer	13	Healthy Subjects ($\bar{x}$=18.8 years)	Soleus=0.97
Krause et al.[61]	Inclinometer	39	Healthy Subject ($\bar{x}$=24.2 years)	Soleus=0.82
Rabin et al.[101]	Inclinometer	43	Healthy Subjects ($\bar{x}$=25.5 years)	Soleus=0.93
Searle et al.[63]	Inclinometer	30	Subject with Diabetes ($\bar{x}$=65.8 years)	Gastrocnemius=0.88
		30	Healthy Subject ($\bar{x}$=28.0 years)	Gastrocnemius=0.93

*ICC=Intraclass correlation coefficient.

Table 15.25	VALIDITY OF SOLEUS MUSCLE LENGTH—LUNGE TEST			
STUDY	TECHNIQUE	n	SAMPLE	ICC*
Awatani et al.[102]	Smartphone–X-Ray	18	Healthy Subjects ($\bar{x}$=25.3 years)	Soleus=0.94
Balsalobre-Fernandez et al.[103]	Smartphone, Inclinometer	12	Healthy Subjects ($\bar{x}$=28.6 years)	Soleus=0.97

*ICC=Intraclass correlation coefficient.

Validity

Only two studies examining the validity of the Smartphone to measure the soleus muscle length have been reported in the literature—one study using X-ray as the criterion measure, while the second study used the criterion measure as the inclinometer. Examining the validity of the Smartphone for measuring soleus muscle during the lunge test using the inclinometer as the criterion measure in 12 subjects (7 males, 5 females; $\bar{x}$=28.6 years), Balsalobre-Fernandez et al.[103] reported a validity reliability of 0.99. Similar results were found by a study by Awatani et el,[102] who used x ray as the criterion measure. Studying 18 subjects (9 males, 9 females; $\bar{x}$=25.3 years), the authors reported a reliability between the Smartphone and X-ray (validity) to be 0.94. The authors of both studies agreed that "the application measurements under appropriate conditions are precise and accurate for weight-bearing ankle dorsiflexion." Information on the two studies examining validity of the Smartphone for the measurement of the soleus muscle length in the weight bearing position (lunge) is presented in Table 15.25.

References

1. Domholdt E. *Physical Therapy Research: Principles and Applications.* 2nd ed. Philadelphia: Saunders; 2000.
2. Domholdt E. *Rehabilitation Research: Principles and Applications.* 3rd ed. Philadelphia: WB Saunders; 2004.
3. Stuberg WA, Fuchs RH, Miedaner JA. Reliability of goniometric measurements of children with cerebral palsy. *Dev Med Child Neurol.* 1988;30(5):657–666.
4. Kilgour G, McNair P, Stott NS. Intrarater reliability of lower limb sagittal range-of-motion measures in children with spastic diplegia. *Dev Med Child Neurol.* 2003;45(6):391–399.
5. Mutlu A, Livanelioglu A, Gunel MK. Reliability of goniometric measurements in children with spastic cerebral palsy. *Med Sci Monit.* 2007;13(7):CR323–CR329.
6. Aalto TJ, et al. Effect of passive stretch on reproducibility of hip range of motion measurements. *Arch Phys Med Rehabil.* 2005;86(3):549–557.
7. Clapper MP, Wolf SL. Comparison of the reliability of the Orthoranger and the standard goniometer for assessing active lower extremity range of motion. *Phys Ther.* 1988;68(2):214–218.
8. Macedo LG, Magee DJ. Effects of age on passive range of motion of selected peripheral joints in healthy adult females. *Physiother Theory Pract.* 2009;25(2):145–164.
9. Marques AP, et al. Inter- and intra-rater reliability of computerized photogrammetry and universal goniometer in the measurement of hip flexion and abduction. *Fisioter Pesqui.* 2017;24:22–28.
10. Nussbaumer S, et al. Validity and test-retest reliability of manual goniometers for measuring passive hip in femoroacetabular impingement patients. *BMC Musculoskelet Disord.* 2010;11:194.
11. Pua YH, et al. Intrarater test-retest reliability of hip range of motion and hip muscle strength measurements in persons with hip osteoarthritis. *Arch Phys Med Rehabil.* 2008;89(6):1146–1154.
12. Prather H, et al. Reliability and agreement of hip range of motion and provocative physical examination tests in asymptomatic volunteers. *PM R.* 2010;2(10):888–895.
13. Walker JM, et al. Active mobility of the extremities in older subjects. *Phys Ther.* 1984;64(6):919–923.
14. Bartlett MD, et al. Hip flexion contractures: a comparison of measurement methods. *Arch Phys Med Rehabil.* 1985;66(9):620–625.
15. Owen J, Stephens D, Wright JG. Reliability of hip range of motion using goniometry in pediatric femur shaft fractures. *Can J Surg.* 2007;50(4):251–255.
16. Poulsen E, et al. Reproducibility of range of motion and muscle strength measurements in patients with hip osteoarthritis: an inter-rater study. *BMC Musculoskelet Disord.* 2012;13:242.
17. Sutlive TG, et al. Development of a clinical prediction rule for diagnosing hip osteoarthritis in individuals with unilateral hip pain. *J Orthop Sports Phys Ther.* 2008;38(9):542–550.
18. Currier LL, et al. Development of a clinical prediction rule to identify patients with knee pain and clinical evidence of knee osteoarthritis who demonstrate a favorable short-term response to hip mobilization. *Phys Ther.* 2007;87(9):1106–1119.
19. American Academy of Orthopaedic Surgeons. *Joint Motion: Method of Measuring and Recording.* Chicago: American Academy of Orthopaedic Surgeons; 1965.
20. Glanzman AM, Swenson AE, Kim H. Intrarater range of motion reliability in cerebral palsy: a comparison of assessment methods. *Pediatr Phys Ther.* 2008;20(4):369–372.
21. Ahlbaeck SO, Lindahl O. Sagittal mobility of the hip-joint. *Acta Orthop Scand.* 1964;34:310–322.
22. Boone DC, et al. Reliability of goniometric measurements. *Phys Ther.* 1978;58:1355–1360.
23. Fosang AL, et al. Measures of muscle and joint performance in the lower limb of children with cerebral palsy. *Dev Med Child Neurol.* 2003;45(10):664–670.
24. Herrero P, et al. Reliability of goniometric measurements in children with cerebral palsy: a comparative analysis of universal goniometer and electronic inclinometer. A pilot study. *BMC Musculoskelet Disord.* 2011;12:155.
25. Drews JE, Vraciu JK, Pellino G. Range of motion of the joints of the lower extremities of newborns. *Phys Occup Ther Pediatr.* 1984;4:49–62.
26. McWhirk LB, Glanzman AM. Within-session inter-rater reliability of goniometric measures in patients with spastic cerebral palsy. *Pediatr Phys Ther.* 2006;18(4):262–265.
27. Greene WB, Heckman JD. *The Clinical Measurement of Joint Motion.* Rosemont, IL: American Academy of Orthopaedic Surgeons; 1994.

28. Ellison JB, Rose SJ, Sahrmann SA. Patterns of hip rotation range of motion: a comparison between healthy subjects and patients with low back pain. *Phys Ther.* 1990;70(9):537–541.
29. Gradoz MC, et al. Reliability of hip rotation range of motion in supine and seated positions. *J Sports Rehabil.* 2018;16:1–4.
30. Krause DA, et al. Reliability of hip internal rotation range of motion measurement using a digital inclinometer. *Knee Surg Sports Traumatol Arthrosc.* 2015;23:2562–2567.
31. Simoneau G, et al. Influence of hip position and gender on active hip internal and external rotation. *J Orthop Sports Phys Ther.* 1998;28(3):158–164.
32. Brosseau L, et al. Intratester and intertester reliability and criterion validity of the parallelogram and universal goniometers for active knee flexion in healthy subjects. *Physiother Res Int.* 1997;2(3):150–166.
33. Gogia PP, et al. Reliability and validity of goniometric measurements at the knee. *Phys Ther.* 1987;67(2):192–195.
34. Mitchell WS, Millar J, Sturrock RD. An evaluation of goniometry as an objective parameter for measuring joint motion. *Scott Med J.* 1975;20(2):57–59.
35. Rheault W, et al. Intertester reliability and concurrent validity of fluid-based and universal goniometers for active knee flexion. *Phys Ther.* 1988;68(11):1676–1678.
36. Hancock GE, Hepworth T, Wembridge K. Accuracy and reliability of knee goniometry methods. *J Exp Orthop.* 2018;5:46.
37. Mollinger LA, Steffen TM. Knee flexion contractures in institutionalized elderly: prevalence, severity, stability, and related variables. *Phys Ther.* 1993;73(7):437–446.
38. Pandya S, et al. Reliability of goniometric measurements in patients with Duchenne muscular dystrophy. *Phys Ther.* 1985;65(9):1339–1342.
39. Shamsi MB, Mirzaei M, Khabiri SS. Universal goniometer and electro-goniometer intra-examiner reliability in measuring the knee range of motion during active knee extension test in patients with chronic low back pain with short hamstring muscle. *BMC Sports Sci Med Rehabil.* 2019;11:4.
40. Brosseau L, et al. Intra- and intertester reliability and criterion validity of the parallelogram and universal goniometers for measuring maximum active knee flexion and extension of patients with knee restrictions. *Arch Phys Med Rehabil.* 2001;82(3):396–402.
41. Jakobsen TL, et al. Reliability of knee joint range of motion and circumference measurements after total knee arthroplasty: does tester experience matter? *Physiother Res Int.* 2010;15(3):126–134.
42. Peters PG, et al. Knee range of motion: reliability and agreement of 3 measurement methods. *Am J Orthop (Belle Mead NJ).* 2011;40(12):E249–E252.
43. Rothstein JM, Miller PJ, Roettger RF. Goniometric reliability in a clinical setting. *Elbow and knee measurements Phys Ther.* 1983;63(10):1611–1615.
44. Watkins MA, et al. Reliability of goniometric measurements and visual estimates of knee range of motion obtained in a clinical setting. *Phys Ther.* 1991;71(2):90–97.
45. Verhaegen F, et al. Are clinical photographs appropriate to determine the maximal range of motion of the knee? *Acta Orthop Belg.* 2010;76(6):794–798.
46. Fritz JM, et al. An examination of the selective tissue tension scheme, with evidence for the concept of a capsular pattern of the knee. *Phys Ther.* 1998;78(10):1046–1061.
47. Lenssen AF, et al. Reproducibility of goniometric measurement of the knee in the in-hospital phase following total knee arthroplasty. *BMC Musculoskelet Disord.* 2007;8:83.
48. Phillips A, et al. Reliability of radiographic measurements of knee motion following knee arthroplasty for use in a virtual knee clinic. *Ann R Coll Surg Engl.* 2012;94(7):506–512.
49. Allington NJ, Leroy N, Doneux C. Ankle joint range of motion measurements in spastic cerebral palsy children: intraobserver and interobserver reliability and reproducibility of goniometry and visual estimation. *J Pediatr Orthop B.* 2002;11(3):236–239.
50. Bennell KL, et al. Intra-rater and inter-rater reliability of a weight-bearing lunge measure of ankle dorsiflexion. *Aust J Physiother.* 1998;44(3):175–180.
51. Bohannon RW, Tiberio D, Zito M. Selected measures of ankle dorsiflexion range of motion: differences and intercorrelations. *Foot Ankle.* 1989;10(2):99–103.
52. Cipriani D, et al. A proposed modification to the ankle dorsiflexion lunge measurement in weight bearing: clinical application with reliability and validity. *Orthop Prac.* 2020;32:88–90.

53. Custer L, Cosby N. Reliability of three inclinometer placements for weight bearing dorsiflexion. *Athl Train Sports Health Care.* 2018;10:181–187.

54. Denegar CR, Hertel J, Fonseca J. The effect of lateral ankle sprain on dorsiflexion range of motion, posterior talar glide, and joint laxity. *J Orthop Sports Phys Ther.* 2002;32(4):166–173.

55. Diamond JE, et al. Reliability of a diabetic foot evaluation. *Phys Ther.* 1989;69(10):797–802.

56. Dobija L, Jankowski K. Reliability of the non weight bearing inclinometric measurements of the ankle range of motion in older adults with orthopedic problems. *Top Geriatr Rehabil.* 2015;31:164–169.

57. Elveru RA, Rothstein JM, Lamb RL. Goniometric reliability in a clinical setting. Subtalar and ankle joint measurements. *Phys Ther.* 1988;68(5):672–677.

58. Johnson SR, Gross MT. Intraexaminer reliability, interexaminer reliability, and mean values for nine lower extremity skeletal measures in healthy naval midshipmen. *J Orthop Sports Phys Ther.* 1997;25(4):253–263.

59. Kim PJ, et al. Interrater and intrarater reliability in the measurement of ankle joint dorsiflexion is independent of examiner experience and technique used. *J Am Podiatr Med Assoc.* 2011;101(5):407–414.

60. Konor MM, et al. Reliability of three measures of ankle dorsiflexion range of motion. *Int J Sports Phys Ther.* 2012;7(3):279–287.

61. Krause DA, et al. Measurement of ankle dorsiflexion: a comparison of active and passive techniques in multiple positions. *J Sport Rehabil.* 2011;20(3):333–344.

62. Munteanu SE, et al. A weightbearing technique for the measurement of ankle joint dorsiflexion with the knee extended is reliable. *J Sci Med Sport.* 2009;12(1):54–59.

63. Searle A, Spink MJ, Chuter VH. Weight bearing versus non-weight bearing ankle dorsiflexion measurement in people with diabetes: a cross sectional study. *BMC Musculoskelet Disord.* 2018;19(1):183.

64. van der Worp MP, et al. Reproducibility of and sex differences in common orthopaedic ankle and foot tests in runners. *BMC Musculoskelet Disord.* 2014;15:171.

65. Youdas JW, Bogard CL, Suman VJ. Reliability of goniometric measurements and visual estimates of ankle joint active range of motion obtained in a clinical setting. *Arch Phys Med Rehabil.* 1993;74(10):1113–1118.

66. Ekstrand J, et al. Lower extremity goniometric measurements: a study to determine their reliability. *Arch Phys Med Rehabil.* 1982;63(4):171–175.

67. Hall EA, Docherty CL. Validity of clinical outcome measures to evaluate ankle range of motion during the weight-bearing lunge test. *J Sci Med Sport.* 2017;20:618–621.

68. Menadue C, et al. Reliability of two goniometric methods of measuring active inversion and eversion range of motion at the ankle. *BMC Musculoskelet Disord.* 2006;7:60.

69. Smith-Oricchio K, Harris BA. Interrater reliability of subtalar neutral, calcaneal inversion and eversion. *J Orthop Sports Phys Ther.* 1990;12(1):10–15.

70. Hopson MM, McPoil TG, Cornwall MW. Motion of the first metatarsophalangeal joint. Reliability and validity of four measurement techniques. *J Am Podiatr Med Assoc.* 1995;85(4):198–204.

71. Otter SJ, et al. The reliability of a smartphone goniometer application compared with a traditional goniometer for measuring first metatarsophalangeal joint dorsiflexion. *J Foot Ankle Res.* 2015;8:30.

72. Kwon OY, et al. Reliability and validity of measures of hammer toe deformity angle and tibial torsion. *Foot (Edinb).* 2009;19(3):149–155.

73. Wang SS, et al. Lower extremity muscular flexibility in long distance runners. *J Orthop Sports Phys Ther.* 1993;17(2):102–107.

74. Harvey D. Assessment of the flexibility of elite athletes using the modified Thomas test. *Br J Sports Med.* 1998;32(1):68–70.

75. Godges JJ, MacRae PG, Engelke KA. Effects of exercise on hip range of motion, trunk muscle performance, and gait economy. *Phys Ther.* 1993;73(7):468–477.

76. Winters MV, et al. Passive versus active stretching of hip flexor muscles in subjects with limited hip extension: a randomized clinical trial. *Phys Ther.* 2004;84(9):800–807.

77. Clapis PA, Davis SM, Davis RO. Reliability of inclinometer and goniometric measurements of hip extension flexibility using the modified Thomas test. *Physiother Theory Pract.* 2008;24(2):135–141.

78. Peeler J, Anderson JE. Reliability of the Thomas test for assessing range of motion about the hip. *Phys Ther Sport.* 2007;8:14–21.

79. Wakefield B, et al. Reliability of goniometric and trigonometric techniques for measuring hip-extension range of motion using the modified Thomas test. *J Athl Train.* 2015;50(5):460–466.

80. Peeler JD, Anderson JE. Reliability limits of the modified Thomas test for assessing rectus femoris muscle flexibility about the knee joint. *J Athl Train.* 2008;43(5):470–476.

81. Piva SR, et al. Reliability of measures of impairments associated with patellofemoral pain syndrome. *BMC Musculoskelet Disord.* 2006;7:33.

82. Hsieh CY, Walker JM, Gillis K. Straight-leg-raising test. Comparison of three instruments. *Phys Ther.* 1983;63(9):1429–1433.

83. Rose MJ. The statistical analysis of the intra-observer repeatability of four clinical measurement techniques. *Physiotherapy.* 1991;77:89–91.

84. Hanten WP, Chandler SD. Effects of myofascial release leg pull and sagittal plane isometric contract-relax techniques on passive straight-leg raise angle. *J Orthop Sports Phys Ther.* 1994;20(3):138–144.

85. Gajdosik R, Lusin G. Hamstring muscle tightness. Reliability of an active-knee-extension test. *Phys Ther.* 1983;63(7):1085–1090.

86. Worrell TW, Smith TL, Winegardner J. Effect of hamstring stretching on hamstring muscle performance. *J Orthop Sports Phys Ther.* 1994;20(3):154–159.

87. Webright WG, Randolph BJ, Perrin DH. Comparison of nonballistic active knee extension in neural slump position and static stretch techniques on hamstring flexibility. *J Orthop Sports Phys Ther.* 1997;26(1):7–13.

88. Shepard E, Winter S, Gordon S. Comparing hamstring muscle length measurements of the traditional active knee extension test and a functional hamstring flexibility test. *Physiother Rehabil.* 2017;2(1):125.

89. Rakos DM, et al. Interrater reliability of the active-knee-extension test for hamstring length in school-aged children. *Pediatr Phys Ther.* 2001;13(1):37–41.

90. Fredriksen H, et al. Passive knee extension test to measure hamstring muscle tightness. *Scand J Med Sci Sports.* 1997;7(5):279–282.

91. Gajdosik RL, et al. Comparison of four clinical tests for assessing hamstring muscle length. *J Orthop Sports Phys Ther.* 1993;18(5):614–618.

92. Bandy WD, Irion JM. The effect of time on static stretch on the flexibility of the hamstring muscles. *Phys Ther.* 1994;74(9):845–852.

93. Bandy WD, Irion JM, Briggler M. The effect of time and frequency of static stretching on flexibility of the hamstring muscles. *Phys Ther.* 1997;77:1090–1096.

94. Nelson RT, Bandy WD. Eccentric training and static stretching improve hamstring flexibility of high school males. *J Athl Train.* 2004;39(3):254–258.

95. Sullivan MK, Dejulia JJ, Worrell TW. Effect of pelvic position and stretching method on hamstring muscle flexibility. *Med Sci Sports Exerc.* 1992;24(12):1383–1389.

96. Melchione WE, Sullivan MS. Reliability of measurements obtained by use of an instrument designed to indirectly measure iliotibial band length. *J Orthop Sports Phys Ther.* 1993;18(3):511–515.

97. Reese NB, Bandy WD. Use of an inclinometer to measure flexibility of the iliotibial band using the Ober test and the modified Ober test: differences in magnitude and reliability of measurements. *J Orthop Sports Phys Ther.* 2003;33(6):326–330.

98. Gajdosik RL, Sandler MM, Marr HL. Influence of knee positions and gender on the Ober test for length of the iliotibial band. *Clin Biomech (Bristol, Avon).* 2003;18(1):77–79.

99. Banwell H, Uden H, Marshall N, et al. The iPhone measure app level function as a measuring device for the weight bearing lunge test in adults: a reliability study. *J Foot Ankle Res.* 2019;12.

100. Langarika-Rocafort A, Ignacio Emparanza J, Aramendi J, et al. Intrarater reliability and agreement of various methods of measurement to assess dorsiflexion in the weight bearing dorsiflexion lunge test (WBLT) among female athletes. *Phys Ther Sport.* 2017;23:37–44.

101. Rabin A, Kozol Z. Weightbearing and nonweightbearing ankle dorsiflexion range of motion: are we measuring the same thing? *J Am Podiatr Med Assoc.* 2012;102:406–411.

102. Awatani T, Enoki T, Morikita I. Inter-rater reliability and validity of angle measurements using smartphone applications for weight-bearing ankle dorsiflexion range of motion measurements. *Phys Ther Sport.* 2018;34:113–120.

103. Balsalobre-Fernández C, Romero-Franco N, Jiménez-Reyes P. Concurrent validity and reliability of an iPhone app for the measurement of ankle dorsiflexion and inter-limb asymmetries. *J Sports Sci.* 2019;37:249–253.

16

PEDIATRIC RANGE of MOTION

Charlotte Yates and Leah Lowe

The focus of this chapter is on examining differences in range of motion (ROM) values and techniques for pediatric patients compared with adults. The chapter is organized so that upper extremity ROM is discussed, followed by techniques associated with the upper extremity. Lower extremity ROM then is discussed, followed by techniques associated with the lower extremity. Pediatric cervical range of motion is discussed, followed by techniques associated with measuring cervical range of motion to assess infants with torticollis. The chapter concludes with special tests that are specific to the pediatric population with focus on alignment changes through development.

UPPER EXTREMITY ROM

ROM of many upper extremity joints appears to differ in infants and young children compared with adults (Table 16.1).[1-3] Measurements reported in a study of more than 300 Japanese infants and children from birth to 2 years of age demonstrated an increased range of shoulder extension and lateral rotation, forearm pronation, and wrist flexion, along with a decreased range of elbow extension, in this age group compared with adults.[1] The amount of shoulder lateral rotation present in the neonate appears to decrease as the child ages, with the range of shoulder rotation approaching adult levels by the age of 2 years (Table 16.2).[1] As a child ages, elbow extension ROM also changes to approach adult levels, but more quickly than does the range of shoulder lateral rotation.

Table 16.1 CHANGES IN UPPER EXTREMITY RANGE OF MOTION: BIRTH TO 19 YEARS OF AGE					
SHOULDER	**BIRTH–2 YEAR** **WATANABE ET AL.**	**2–8 YEAR** **SOUCIE ET AL.**	**3–9 YEAR** **MCKAY ET AL.**	**9–19 YEAR** **SOUCIE ET AL.**	**10–19 YEAR** **MCKAY ET AL.**
Flexion	172°–180°	M 177.8° F 178.6°		M 170.9° F 171.8°	
Extension	79°–89°				
Abduction	177°–187°				
Medial rotation	72°–90°		M/F 67°		M 62° F 66°
Lateral rotation	123°		M 98° F 99°		M/F 93°
ELBOW	**BIRTH–2 YEAR**	**2–8 YEAR**	**3–9 YEAR**	**9–19 YEAR**	**10–19 YEAR**
Flexion	148°–158°	M 151.4° F 152.9°	M 146° F 147°	M 148.3° F 149.7°	M 148° F 150°
Extension	− 2° (lacks zero)	M 2.2° F 6.8°	M/F 7°	M 5.3° F 6.4°	M 4° F 7°
FOREARM	**BIRTH–2 YEAR**	**2–8 YEAR**	**3–9 YEAR**	**9–19 YEAR**	**10–19 YEAR**
Pronation	90°–96°	M 79.6° F 84.6°		M 79.8° F 81.2°	
Supination	81°–93°	M 86.4° F 93.7°		M 87.8° F 90.0°	
WRIST	**BIRTH–2 YEAR**	**2–8 YEAR**	**3–9 YEAR**	**9–19 YEAR**	**10–19 YEAR**
Flexion	88°–96°				
Extension	82°–89°				

Data from Watanabe H, Ogata K, Amano T, Okabe TL. The range of joint motions of the extremities in healthy Japanese people: The difference according to age. Cited in Walker JM: Musculoskeletal development: A review. *Phys Ther*. 1991;71:878; Soucie JM, Wang C, Forsyth A, et al. Range of motion measurements: reference values and a database for comparison studies. *Hemophilia*. 2011;17(3):500–507; McKay MJ, Baldwin JN, Ferreira P, et al. Normative reference values for strength and flexibility of 1000 children and adults. *Neurology*. 2017;88(1):36–43.

Table 16.2   UPPER EXTREMITY MOTIONS DEMONSTRATING SIGNIFICANT CHANGE IN AMPLITUDE DURING THE FIRST 2 YEARS

AGE	SHOULDER LATERAL ROTATION	ELBOW EXTENSION
Birth ($n=62$)	134°	− 14°
2–4 Weeks ($n=57$)	126°	− 6°
4–8 Months ($n=54$)	120°	0°
8–12 Months ($n=45$)	124°	1°
1 Year ($n=64$)	116°	3°
2 Years ($n=57$)	118°	5°

Data from Watanabe H, Ogata K, Amano T, Okabe TL. The range of joint motions of the extremities in healthy Japanese people: The difference according to age. Cited in Walker JM: Musculoskeletal development: A review. *Phys Ther.* 1991;71:878.

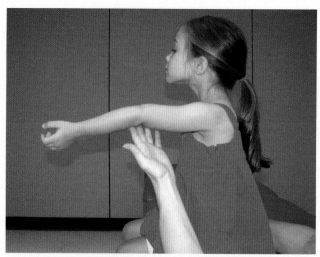

Fig. 16.1   Lateral view of passive hyperextension of the elbow demonstrated by a 3-year-old female.

The limitation in elbow extension seen in the neonate ($M=19.5°$, $SD=2.97$)[4] appears to resolve by the age of 3 to 8 months (see Table 16.2),[1,5] progresses to hyperextension in many children by the age of 2 to 3 years[1,6,7] (Fig. 16.1), and then gradually resolves to adult levels. Studies examining the elbow in boys and girls have consistently shown greater carrying angles in girls.[8,9] Golden et al. report a clinically observable increase in elbow extension in females compared to males and suggest that this increased elbow extension in females may contribute to the statistically significant increase in female carrying angle.[7] A limitation in shoulder abduction also has been reported in neonates, but by only one investigator on a fairly small sample of subjects.[3] The limitation in shoulder abduction had disappeared in these infants by 3 months of age.

TECHNIQUES OF MEASUREMENT: UPPER EXTREMITY

We have not included techniques for every joint of the upper extremity because the focus of the chapter is to examine changes in the pediatric population compared with adults. The techniques that are included focus on joints with an increased or decreased ROM and alternative positions that are used compared with those used for adults. Please reference the chapters on adults for alternative positioning of joints or movements that have not been included. As in adults, follow standard procedures for measuring ROM that have been outlined in Chapter 1.

Shoulder Flexion

Fig. 16.2 Starting position for measurement of shoulder flexion. Bony landmarks for goniometer alignment (lateral aspect of acromion process, lateral midline of thorax, lateral humeral epicondyle) indicated by red line and dots.

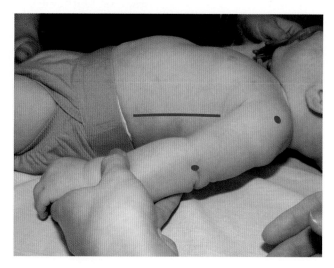

Patient position	Supine with shoulder in 0-degree flexion, elbow fully extended, forearm in neutral rotation with palm facing trunk or pronated (Fig. 16.2).
Stabilization	Proximal to humeral head and distal to elbow (Fig. 16.3).
Examiner action	Flex patient's shoulder through available ROM, avoiding extension of spine. Return limb to starting position. Performing passive movement provides an estimate of ROM (see Fig. 16.3).
Goniometer alignment	Palpate bony landmarks shown in Fig. 16.2 and align goniometer accordingly.
Stationary arm	Lateral midline of thorax.
Axis	Midpoint of lateral aspect of acromion process
Moving arm	Lateral midline of humerus toward lateral humeral epicondyle.
	Read scale of goniometer.

Fig. 16.3 End of shoulder flexion ROM, showing proper hand placement for stabilizing and flexing shoulder. Bony landmarks for goniometer alignment (lateral aspect of acromion process, lateral midline of thorax, lateral humeral epicondyle) indicated by red line and dot.

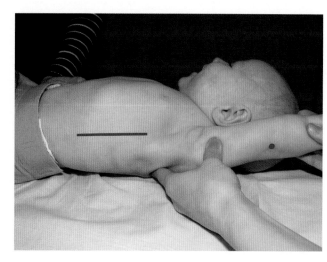

Fig. 16.4 End of shoulder flexion ROM, demonstrating proper alignment of goniometer at end of range.

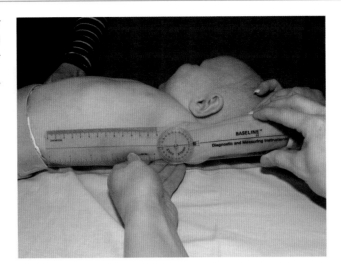

Patient/Examiner action	Perform passive shoulder flexion (Fig. 16.4).
Confirmation of alignment	Repalpate landmarks and confirm proper goniometric alignment at end of ROM, correcting alignment as necessary (see Note). Read scale of goniometer (see Fig. 16.4).
Documentation	Record patient's ROM.
Note	No extension of spine should be allowed during measurement of shoulder flexion to prevent artificial inflation of ROM measurements.
Alternative patient position	Side-lying; goniometer alignment remains the same.
	Because of decreased ability to stabilize the trunk in these positions, great care must be taken to ensure that stationary arm of goniometer remains aligned with lateral midline of thorax and that extension of spine does not occur. Failure to exercise such care will result in errors in measurement.

Shoulder Lateral Rotation

Fig. 16.5 Starting position for measurement of shoulder lateral rotation. Landmarks for goniometer alignment (olecranon and styloid processes of ulna) indicated by red dots.

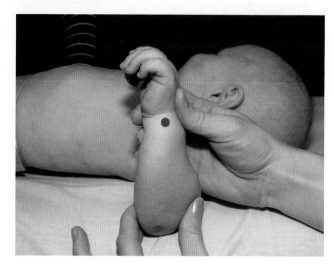

Patient position	Supine with shoulder abducted to 90 degrees, elbow flexed to 90 degrees, forearm pronated, and folded towel under humerus (optional) (Fig. 16.5).
Stabilization	At infant's elbow to maintain alignment (Fig. 16.6).
Examiner action	Laterally rotate patient's shoulder through available ROM. Return limb to starting position. Performing passive movement provides an estimate of ROM (see Fig. 16.6).
Goniometer alignment	Palpate bony landmarks as shown in Fig. 16.5 and align goniometer accordingly (Fig. 16.7).
Stationary arm	Perpendicular to floor.
Axis	Olecranon process of ulna.
Moving arm	Ulnar border of forearm toward ulnar styloid process.
	Read scale of goniometer.

Fig. 16.6 End of shoulder lateral rotation ROM, showing proper hand placement for stabilizing and laterally rotating shoulder. Landmarks for goniometer alignment (olecranon and styloid processes of ulna) indicated by red dots.

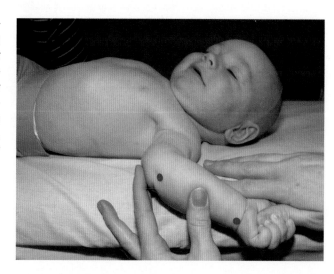

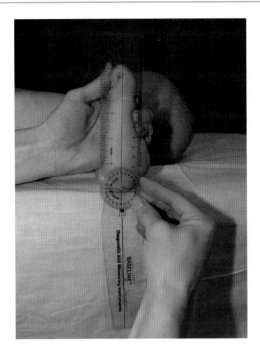

Fig. 16.7 Starting position for measurement of shoulder lateral rotation, demonstrating proper initial alignment of goniometer.

Patient/Examiner action	Perform passive lateral rotation of the shoulder, stopping at the point of elevation of the scapula off the table.
Confirmation of alignment	Repalpate landmarks and confirm proper goniometer alignment at end of ROM, correcting alignment as necessary. Read scale of goniometer (Fig. 16.8).
Documentation	Record patient's ROM.

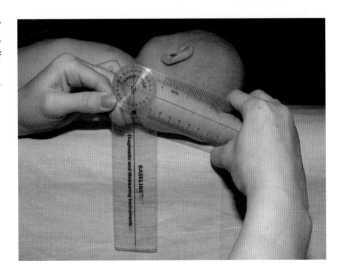

Fig. 16.8 End of shoulder lateral rotation ROM, demonstrating proper alignment of goniometer at end of range.

Elbow Extension

Fig. 16.9 Starting position for measurement of elbow extension. Bony landmarks for goniometer alignment (lateral aspect of acromion process, lateral humeral epicondyle, radial styloid process) indicated by red dots.

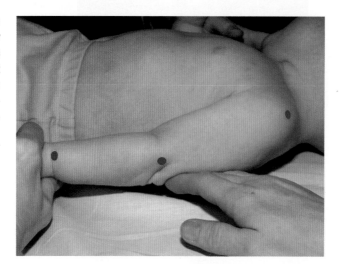

Patient position	Supine with upper extremity in anatomical position (see Note), with elbow extended as far as possible, folded towel under distal humerus, proximal to humeral condyles (optional) (Fig. 16.9).
Stabilization	At the wrist or anterior forearm and posterior humerus.
Examiner action	Determine whether elbow is extended as far as possible, providing pressure across the elbow in the direction of extension (Fig. 16.10).

Fig. 16.10 End of elbow extension ROM, showing proper hand placement for stabilizing humerus and extending elbow. Bony landmarks for goniometer alignment (lateral aspect of acromion process, lateral humeral epicondyle, radial styloid process) indicated by red dots.

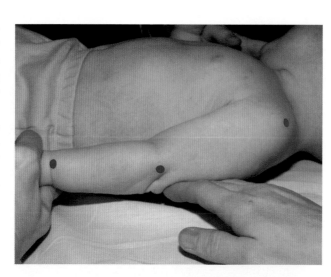

Fig. 16.11 Goniometer alignment for measurement of elbow extension.

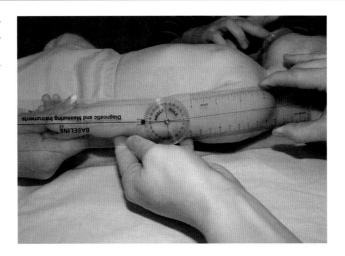

Goniometer alignment	Palpate bony landmarks shown in Fig. 16.9 and align goniometer accordingly (Fig. 16.11).
Stationary arm	Lateral midline of humerus toward acromion process.
Axis	Lateral epicondyle of humerus.
Moving arm	Lateral midline of radius toward radial styloid process (see Note).
	Read scale of goniometer (see Fig. 16.11).
Documentation	Record patient's ROM.
Note	Patient's forearm should be completely supinated at beginning of ROM or beginning reading of goniometer.
Alternative patient position	Seated or side-lying; towel not needed; goniometer alignment remains the same.

Wrist Flexion

Fig. 16.12 Starting position for measurement of wrist flexion using lateral alignment technique. Bony landmarks for goniometer alignment (olecranon process of ulna, triquetrum, lateral midline of fifth metacarpal) indicated by red dots.

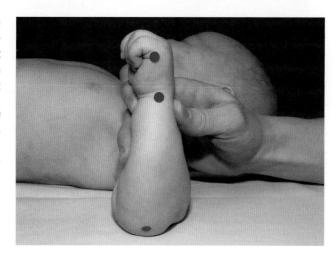

Patient position	Supine with shoulder abducted to 90 degrees, elbow flexed to 90 degrees, forearm pronated (Fig. 16.12).
Stabilization	Over dorsal surface of hand and proximal to the elbow (Fig. 16.13).
Examiner action	Flex patient's wrist through available ROM (see Note). Return wrist to neutral position. Performing passive movement provides an estimate of ROM (see Fig. 16.13).
Goniometer alignment	Palpate bony landmarks shown in Fig. 16.12 and align goniometer accordingly (Fig. 16.14).

Fig. 16.13 End of wrist flexion ROM, showing proper hand placement for stabilizing forearm and flexing wrist. Bony landmarks for goniometer alignment (olecranon process of ulna, triquetrum, lateral midline of fifth metacarpal) indicated by red dots.

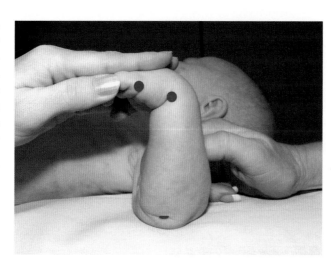

Fig. 16.14 Starting position for measurement of wrist flexion, demonstrating proper initial alignment of goniometer.

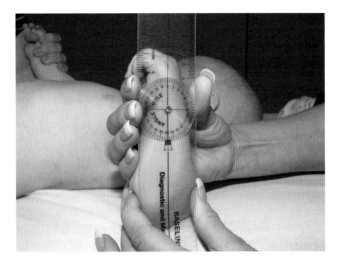

Stationary arm	Lateral midline of ulna toward olecranon process.
Axis	Triquetrum.
Moving arm	Lateral midline of fifth metacarpal.
	Read scale of goniometer.
Patient/Examiner action	Perform passive wrist flexion (Fig. 16.15).
Confirmation of alignment	Repalpate landmarks and confirm proper goniometric alignment at end of ROM, correcting alignment as necessary. Read scale of goniometer (see Fig. 16.15).
Documentation	Record patient's ROM.
Note	Flexion of fingers should be avoided during measurement of wrist flexion to prevent limitation of motion by tension in extrinsic finger extensors.
Alternative patient position	Supportive sitting for lateral alignment. See Chapter 5.

Fig. 16.15 End of wrist flexion ROM, demonstrating proper alignment of goniometer at end of range.

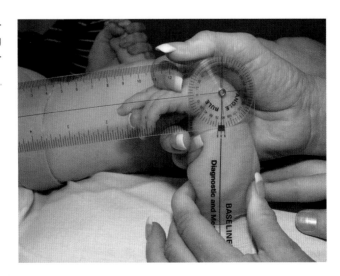

Lower Extremity ROM

Normal ROM in the lower extremity joints is not static but changes across the life span. This chapter examines from birth through adolescence (Tables 16.3 to 16.6)[1–3,10–21] Changes in lower extremity range of motion have been explored by age and sex (Table 16.6).[2,3,19–21] Furthermore, Sankar et al. have reported changes in hip range of motion stratified by age, sex, and race (only Black and White children are reported).[19]

Studies in the pediatric population have demonstrated increased hip flexion, abduction, and rotation ROM in infants and young children compared with the adult population (see Table 16.3).[12–15] Extension of the hip is decreased in neonates, resulting in a hip flexion contracture that appears to resolve by the age of 2 years (see Table 16.5).[1,10,11,16–18] A similar flexion contracture (15° of flexion lacks zero)[13] is seen at the knee of neonates,[1,16] but this contracture appears to resolve fairly quickly, with knee extension approaching adult values by the time the infant reaches 3 to 6 months of age (see Table 16.4)[1,14,15] and progressing to hyperextension in some children by 3 years of age. At birth, Schwarze[13] reports mean knee flexion values in neonates of 150°, and as the knee flexion contracture resolves, male and female children maintain adult-like knee flexion (see Table 16.6).[2,3,19–21] Studies of large groups of children in China, England, and Scotland revealed hyperextension of the knee in young children that disappeared at some point between the ages of 6 and 10 years.[22,23]

	Table 16.3 CHANGES IN HIP RANGE OF MOTION: BIRTH TO 16 YEARS OF AGE							
HIP	**BIRTH SCHWARZE ET AL.**	**4–7 YEARS MUDGE ET AL.**	**5 YEARS RAO ET AL.**	**4–10 YEARS MCDOWELL ET AL.**	**8 YEARS RAO ET AL.**	**8–11 YEARS MUDGE ET AL**	**11–17 YEARS MCDOWELL ET AL**	**12–16 YEARS MUDGE ET AL**
Flexion	140°		146.8° ± 7.8°		139.9° ± 5.2°			
Extension	20° Flexion, lacks zero	15.0° (4.5)	25.6° ± 4.0°		19.4° ± 5.7°	13.0° (6.4)		9.1° (3.4)
Abduction	78°	42.1° (6.5)	79.8° ± 8.5°	48.8° ± 7.4° (46.3–51.0)	62.8° ± 9.4°	36.4° (4.8)	44.5° ± 5.7° (42.2–46.6)	33.6° (6.4)
Adduction	15°		33.1° ± 4.3°		28.4° ± 4.0°			
Medial rotation	58° Prone 58° supine		52.4° ± 11.5°	58.9° ± 11.6° (55.2–62.7)	43.5° ± 8.9°		50.2° ± 10.9° (46.6–54.5)	
Lateral rotation	80° Prone 80° supine		54.7° ± 9.5°	50.2° ± 8.1° (47.6–52.8)	48.4° ± 7.0°		50.1° ± 10.7° (46.2–54.0)	

Data from Schwarze D, Denton J. Normal values of the neonatal lower limbs: An evaluation of 1000 neonates. *J Pediatr Orthop*. 1993;13:758–760; Mudge AJ, et al. Normative reference values for lower limb joint range, bone torsion, and alignment in children aged 4–16 years. *J Pediatr Orthop B*. 2014;23:15–25; Rao KN, Joseph B. Value of measurement of hip movements in childhood hip disorders, *J Pediatr Orthop*. 2001;21:495–501. McDowell BC, et al. Passive range of motion in a population-based sample of children with spastic cerebral palsy who walk, *Phys Occup Ther Pediatr*. 2012;32:139–50.

	BIRTH–2 YEARS		**4–10 YEARS**		**11–17 YEARS**	
KNEE	**WANTANTANABE ET AL.**	**4–7 YEARS MUDGE ET AL.**	**MCDOWELL ET AL.**	**8–11 YEARS MUDGE ET AL.**	**MCDOWELL ET AL.**	**12–16 YEARS MUDGE ET AL.**
Extension	4°(lacks zero)	22.9° (6.1)	3.5° (3.9)	21.9° (4.4)	0.2° (2.2)	18.8° (4.9)

Table 16.4   CHANGES IN KNEE EXTENSION RANGE OF MOTION: BIRTH TO 16 YEARS OF AGE

Data from Watanabe H, Ogata K, Amano T, Okabe, TL. The range of joint motions of the extremities in healthy Japanese people: the difference according to the age. Cited in Walker JM: Musculoskeletal development: a review. *Phys Ther.* 1991:878; Mudge AJ, et al. Normative reference values for lower limb joint range, bone torsion, and alignment in children aged 4–16 years. *J Pediatr Orthop B.* 2014;23:15–25; McDowell BC, Salazar-Torres JJ, Kerr C, Cosgrove AP. Passive range of motion in a population-based sample of children with spastic cerebral palsy who walk. *Phys Occup Ther Pediatr.* 2012;32(2):139–150.

The range of ankle and foot motion in neonates also differs from adult values, with components of pronation and supination showing increased motion compared with adults. Motion of the dorsiflexion and eversion components of pronation, as well as of the inversion component of supination, have been shown to be increased in children birth to 2 years of age.[1,16] The amount of plantarflexion reported in children birth to two years of age has been variable compared with adult values.[1,24]

Table 16.5 CHANGES IN HIP RANGE OF MOTION FROM BIRTH TO 2 YEARS: SELECTED SOURCES					
AGE	**FLEXION**	**EXTENSION**	**ABDUCTION**	**MEDIAL ROTATION**	**LATERAL ROTATION**
Neonates					
Drews et al.		$-28°\pm6°$[*]	$56°\pm10°$[†]	$80°\pm9°$[‡]	$114°\pm10°$[‡]
Forero et al.	$128°\pm5°$	$-30°\pm4°$[§]	$39°\pm5°$[†]	$76°\pm6°$[‡]	$92°\pm3°$[‡]
Haas et al.		$-30°\pm8°$[§]	$76°\pm12°$[‡]	$62°\pm13°$[‡]	$89°\pm14°$[‡]
Watanabe et al. (4–8 months)	120°	−25°	48°	21°	77°
1–13 Months					
Watanabe et al. (4 weeks)	138°	−12°	51°	24°	66°
Coon et al. (6 months)		$-19°\pm6°$[§]	$24°\pm5°$[‖]	$48°\pm11°$	
Coon et al. (3 months)		$-7°\pm4°$[§]	$26°\pm31°$[‖]	$45°\pm5°$[‖]	
4–8 Months					
Coon et al. (6 months)		$-7°\pm4°$	$21°\pm4°$[‖]	$46°\pm5°$[‖]	
Watanabe et al. (4–8 months)	136°	−4°	55°	39°	66°
9–12 Months					
Phelps et al. (9 months)		$-10°\pm3°$[¶]	$59°\pm7°$[†]	$41°\pm8°$[‖]	$56°\pm7°$[‖]
Watanabe et al. (8–12 months)	138°	3°	60°	38°	79°
1 Year					
Phelps et al.		$-9°\pm5°$[¶]	$54°\pm8°$[†]	$44°\pm9°$[‖]	$58°\pm9°$[‖]
Watanabe et al.	141°	15°	66°	49°	74°
2 Years					
Phelps et al.		$-3°\pm3°$[¶]	$60°\pm7°$[†]	$52°\pm10°$[‖]	$47°\pm9°$[‖]
Watanabe et al.	143°	21°	63°	59°	58°

[*]Measured with subject side-lying, contralateral hip flexed.
[†]Measured with subject supine, hip and knee extended.
[‡]Measured with subject supine, hips, and knees flexed to 90°.
[§]Measured with subject supine, contralateral hip flexed.
[‖]Measured with subject prone, hip extended, knee flexed to 90°.
[¶]Measured with subject prone, both hips flexed over end of table.

Table 16.6 NORMATIVE LOWER EXTREMITY RANGE-OF-MOTION DATA BY AGE AND SEX

MALES

	2–5 YEARS SANKAR ET AL.	2–8 YEARS SOUCIE ET AL.	3–9 YEARS MCKAY ET AL.	6–10 YEARS SANKAR ET AL.	11–17 YEARS SANKAR ET AL.	10–19 YEARS MCKAY ET AL.
Hip						
Abduction	51° (11)			43° (12)	34° (10)	
Adduction	17° (5)			15° (5)	14° (5)	
Flexion	118° (12)	131.1°	133° (9.1)	118° (9)	113° (12)	120° (9.9)
Extension	21° (5)	28.3°		19° (4)	15° (5)	
Internal rotation	47° (9)		40° (8.4)	42° (10)	36° (11)	37° (9.3)
External rotation	47° (10)		32° (8.1)	42° (12)	39° (11)	31° (6.4)
Knee						
Flexion		147.8°	145° (5.5)			140° (6.7)
Extension (reported as degrees of hyperextension)		1.6°	4° (3.3)			2° (2.6)

FEMALES

	2–5 YEARS SANKAR ET AL.	2–8 YEARS SOUCIE ET AL.	3–9 YEARS MCKAY ET AL.	6–10 YEARS SANKAR ET AL.	11–17 YEARS SANKAR ET AL.	10–19 YEARS MCKAY ET AL.
Hip						
Abduction	53° (15)			51° (12)	44° (14)	
Adduction	18° (5)			18° (6)	17° (5)	
Flexion	121° (10)	140.8	133° (9.8)	122° (13)	120° (8)	124° (10.2)
Extension	51° (9)	26.2		47° (11)	42° (9)	
Internal rotation	51° (9)		43° (9.1)	47° (11)	42° (9)	39° (7.7)
External rotation	50° (12)		32° (9.2)	45° (12)	44° (8)	31° (9.1)
Knee						
Flexion		152.6°	144° (5.7)			142° (6.6)
Extension (reported as degrees of hyperextension)		5.4°	4° (3.9)			2° (2.6)

ANKLE

	2–8 YEARS SOUCIE ET AL.	3–9 YEARS MCKAY ET AL.	7–14 YEARS ALANEN ET AL.	14–16 YEARS GRIMSTON ET AL.	10–19 YEARS MCKAY ET AL.
Dorsiflexion	24.8°	31° (5.7)	25° (7.2)	26.3 (1.3)	31° (7.1)
Plantarflexion	67.1°	63° (9.2)	57° (6.8)	46.6 (1.3)	63° (7.3)
Inversion			33° (6.1)	27.2 (1.9)	
Eversion			12° (5.3)	12.4 (1.2)	

*MEAN DEG. (SD).

Data from Soucie JM, Wang C, Forsyth A, et al. Range of motion measurements: reference values and a database for comparison studies. *Hemophilia.* 2011;17(3):500–507; McKay MJ, Baldwin JN, Ferreira P, et al. Normative reference values for strength and flexibility of 1000 children and adults. *Neurology.* 2017;88(1):36–43; Sankar WN, Laird CT, Baldwin KD. Hip range of motion in children: what is the norm? *J Pediatr Orthop.* 2012; 32(4):399–405; Alanen JT, Levola JV, Helenius HY, Kvist MH. Ankle joint complex mobility of children 7 to 14 years old. *J Pediatr Orthop.* 2001; 21(6):731–737; Grimston SK, Nigg BM, Hanley DA, Engsberg JR. Differences in ankle joint complex range of motion as a function of age. *Foot Ankle.* 1993; 14(4):215–222.

Hip Flexion

Fig. 16.16 Starting position for measurement of hip
flexion. Bony landmarks for
goniometer alignment (lateral midline of pelvis/trunk,
greater trochanter, lateral
femoral epicondyle) indicated
by red lines and dot.

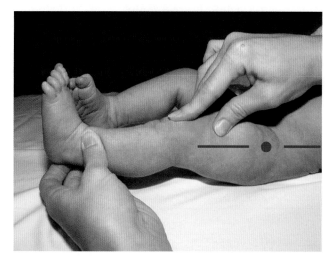

Patient position	Supine, with lower extremities in anatomical position (Fig. 16.16).
Stabilization	Over anterior aspect of ipsilateral tibia and contralateral femur (Fig. 16.17).
Examiner action	Stabilize contralateral femur while flexing patient's ipsilateral hip through available ROM. Ipsilateral knee should be allowed to flex as well. Hip should not be flexed past the point at which pelvic motion is detected. Return limb to starting position. Performing passive movement provides an estimate of the ROM (see Hip Flexion in Adult, Chapter 11) (see Fig. 16.17).
Goniometer alignment	Palpate bony landmarks and align goniometer accordingly as shown in Fig. 16.16.
Stationary arm	Lateral midline of pelvis and trunk.
Axis	Greater trochanter of femur.

Fig. 16.17 End of hip flexion
ROM, showing proper hand
placement for stabilizing contralateral LE and flexing ipsilateral hip. Bony landmarks
for goniometer alignment
(lateral midline of pelvis/
trunk, greater trochanter, lateral femoral epicondyle) indicated by red lines and dot.

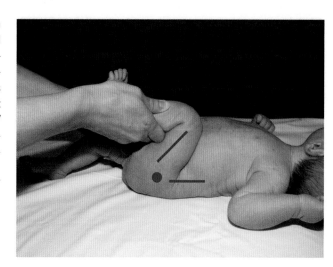

Fig. 16.18 End of hip flexion ROM, demonstrating proper alignment of goniometer at end of range.

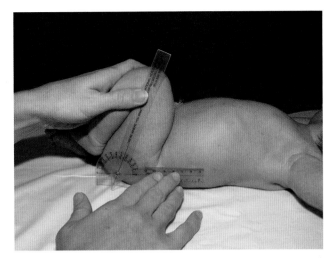

Moving arm	Lateral midline of femur toward lateral femoral epicondyle.
	Read scale of goniometer.
Patient/Examiner action	Perform passive hip flexion. Hip flexion should not be allowed to continue past the point at which pelvic motion is detected.
Confirmation of alignment	Repalpate landmarks and confirm proper goniometric alignment at end of ROM, correcting alignment as necessary (Fig. 16.18). Read scale of goniometer.
Documentation	Record patient's ROM.
Precaution	Should hip be allowed to flex past point at which pelvic motion begins to occur, motion measured will include hip and lumbar flexion. To isolate hip flexion, pelvic motion must not be permitted.
Alternative patient position	Side-lying; stabilization of pelvis more difficult with patient in this position. Goniometer alignment remains the same.

Hip Extension

Fig. 16.19 Starting position for measurement of hip extension. Bony landmarks for goniometer alignment (lateral midline of pelvis/trunk, greater trochanter, lateral femoral epicondyle) indicated by red lines and dot.

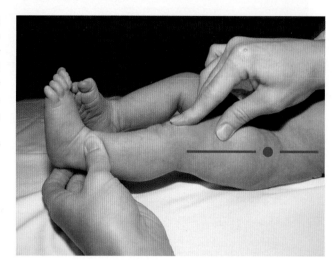

Patient position	Supine, with lower extremities in anatomical position (Fig. 16.19).
Stabilization	Over ipsilateral femur (Fig. 16.20).
Examiner action	Extend patient's hip through available ROM while extending ipsilateral knee. Return limb to starting position. Performing passive movement provides an estimate of the ROM.
Goniometer alignment	Palpate bony landmarks and align goniometer accordingly as shown in Fig. 16.19.
Stationary arm	Lateral midline of pelvis and trunk.
Axis	Greater trochanter of femur.

Fig. 16.20 End of hip extension ROM, demonstrating proper alignment of goniometer at end of range.

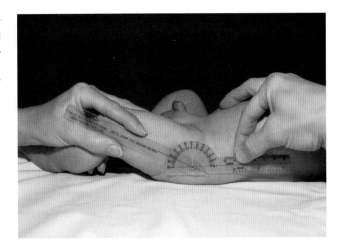

Moving arm	Lateral midline of femur toward lateral femoral epicondyle.
	Read scale of goniometer.
Patient/Examiner action	Perform passive hip extension (see Fig. 16.19).
Confirmation of alignment	Repalpate landmarks and confirm proper goniometric alignment at end of ROM, correcting alignment as necessary (see Fig. 16.20). Read scale of goniometer.
Documentation	Record patient's ROM.
Alternative patient position	Side-lying; stabilization of pelvis more difficult with patient in this position. Goniometer alignment remains the same.

Hip Abduction

Fig. 16.21 End of hip abduction ROM, showing proper hand placement for stabilizing and abducting LE. Bony landmarks for goniometer alignment (ipsilateral ASIS, contralateral ASIS, midline of patella) indicated by red lines and dot.

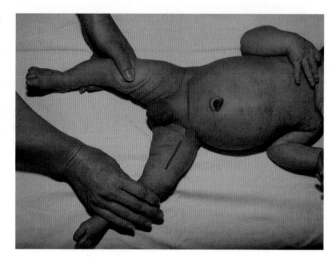

Patient position	Supine, with lower extremities in anatomical position.
Stabilization	Over anterior aspect of contralateral patella (Fig. 16.21).
Examiner action	Abduct patient's hip through available ROM, avoiding hip rotation. Return limb to starting position. Performing passive movement provides an estimate of the ROM (see Fig. 16.21).
Goniometer alignment	Palpate bony landmarks shown in Fig. 16.21 and align goniometer accordingly.
Stationary arm	Toward contralateral ASIS.
Axis	Ipsilateral ASIS.

Fig. 16.22 End of hip ab-
duction ROM, demonstrating
proper alignment of goniometer at end of range.

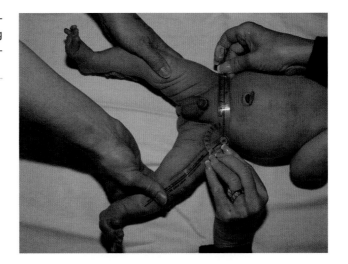

Moving arm	Anterior midline of ipsilateral femur, using midline of patella as reference.
	Read scale of goniometer
Patient/Examiner action	Perform passive hip abduction (see Fig. 16.21).
Confirmation of alignment	Repalpate landmarks and confirm proper goniometric alignment at end of ROM, correcting alignment as necessary (Fig. 16.22). Read scale of goniometer.
Documentation	Record patient's ROM.
Note	Confirmation of alignment of stationary arm is critical.

Hip Lateral Rotation

Fig. 16.23 Starting position for measurement of hip lateral rotation. Bony landmarks for goniometer alignment (tibial tuberosity, tibial crest) indicated by red dot and line.

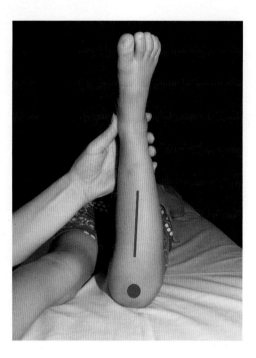

Patient position	Prone, hip extended, knee flexed to 90 degrees (Fig. 16.23).
Stabilization	Ipsilateral posterior femur (Fig. 16.24).
Examiner action	Laterally rotate patient's hip through available ROM by keeping the thigh stationary and moving the leg, foot, and ankle medially. Return limb to starting position. Performing passive movement provides an estimate of the ROM (see Fig. 16.24).
Goniometer alignment	Palpate bony landmarks shown in Fig. 16.23 and align the goniometer accordingly (Fig. 16.25).
Stationary arm	Perpendicular to floor.
Axis	Tibial tubercle.

Fig. 16.24 End of hip lateral rotation ROM. Examiner's hand stabilizes thigh to maintain alignment. Bony landmarks for goniometer alignment (tibial tuberosity, tibial crest) indicated by red dot and line.

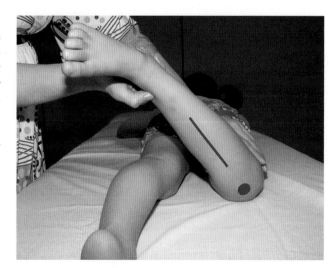

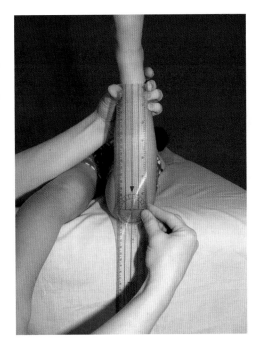

Fig. 16.25 Starting position for measurement of hip lateral rotation, demonstrating proper initial alignment of goniometer.

Moving arm	Anterior midline of tibia, along tibial crest.
	Read scale of goniometer.
Patient/Examiner action	Perform passive hip lateral rotation. Patient should be monitored to maintain equal weight on bilateral ASIS and monitored to maintain alignment of femur (see Fig. 16.25).
Confirmation of alignment	Repalpate landmarks and confirm proper goniometric alignment at end of ROM, correcting alignment as necessary (Fig. 16.26). Read scale of goniometer.
Documentation	Record patient's ROM.
Alternative patient position	Seated with hip and knee flexed to 90 degrees. See test for hip lateral rotation (see Chapter 11). Alignment of rest of goniometer remains the same.

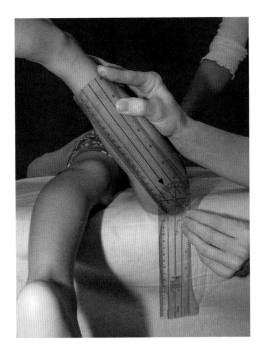

Fig. 16.26 End of hip lateral rotation ROM, demonstrating proper alignment of goniometer at end of range.

Hip Medial Rotation

Fig. 16.27 Starting position for measurement of hip medial rotation. Bony landmarks for goniometer alignment (tibial tuberosity, tibial crest) indicated by red dot and line.

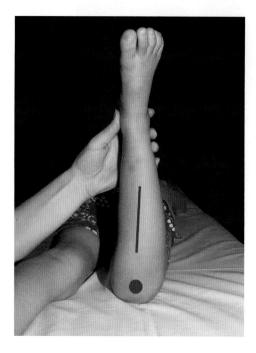

Patient position	Prone, hip extended, knee flexed to 90 degrees (Fig. 16.27).
Stabilization	Ipsilateral posterior femur (Fig. 16.28).
Examiner action	Medially rotate patient's hip through available ROM by keeping the thigh stationary and moving the leg, foot, and ankle laterally. Return limb to starting position. Performing passive movement provides an estimate of the ROM.
Goniometer alignment	Palpate bony landmarks shown in Fig. 16.27 and align goniometer accordingly (Fig. 16.29).
Stationary arm	Perpendicular to floor.
Axis	Tibial tubercle.

Fig. 16.28 End of hip medial rotation ROM. Examiner's hand stabilizes knee alignment. Bony landmarks for goniometer alignment (tibial tuberosity, tibial crest) indicated by red dot and line.

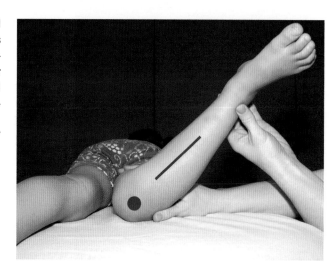

Fig. 16.29 Starting position for measurement of hip medial rotation, demonstrating proper initial alignment of goniometer.

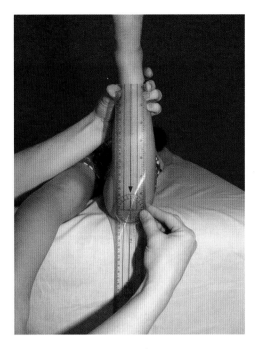

Moving arm	Anterior midline of tibia, along tibial crest.
	Read scale of goniometer.
Patient/Examiner action	Perform passive hip medial rotation. Patient should be monitored to maintain equal weight on bilateral ASIS and monitored to maintain alignment of femur (see Fig. 16.29).
Confirmation of alignment	Repalpate landmarks and confirm proper goniometric alignment at end of ROM, correcting alignment as necessary (Fig. 16.30). Read scale of goniometer.
Documentation	Record patient's ROM.
Precaution	Do not allow patient to laterally flex trunk to contralateral side or lift ipsilateral hip from table during measurement, as doing so will result in a falsely increased ROM.
Alternative patient position	Seated with hip and knee flexed to 90 degrees. See test for hip medial rotation in Chapter 11.

Fig. 16.30 End of hip medial rotation ROM, demonstrating proper alignment of goniometer at end of range.

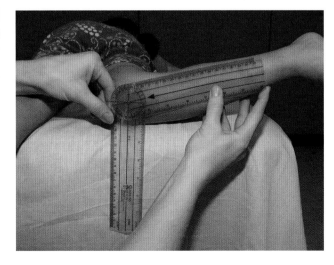

Knee Extension

Fig. 16.31 Starting position for measurement of knee extension. Bony landmarks for goniometer alignment (greater trochanter, lateral femoral epicondyle, lateral malleolus) indicated by red lines and dot.

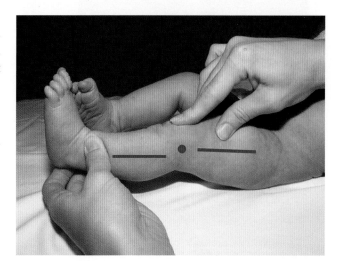

Patient position	Supine, with knee extended as far as possible (Fig. 16.31).
Stabilization	Over anterior ipsilateral patella and posterior ankle (see Fig. 16.31).
Examiner action	Provide passive extension by providing passive pressure on the knee in the direction of extension (see Fig. 16.31).

Fig. 16.32 Measurement of knee extension demonstrating proper alignment of goniometer.

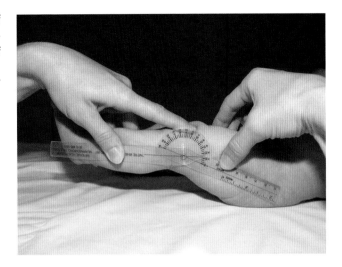

Goniometer alignment	Palpate bony landmarks shown in Fig. 16.31 and align goniometer accordingly (Fig. 16.32).
Stationary arm	Lateral midline of femur toward greater trochanter.
Axis	Lateral epicondyle of femur.
Moving arm	Lateral midline of fibula, in line with fibular head and lateral malleolus.
	Read scale of goniometer.
Documentation	Record patient's ROM.
Alternative patient position	Side-lying; in side-lying, goniometer alignment remains the same.

Ankle Pronation: Dorsiflexion Component

Fig. 16.33 Starting position for measurement of ankle pronation: dorsiflexion component. Bony landmarks for goniometer alignment (fibular head, lateral malleolus, lateral midline of fifth metatarsal) indicated by red lines and dot.

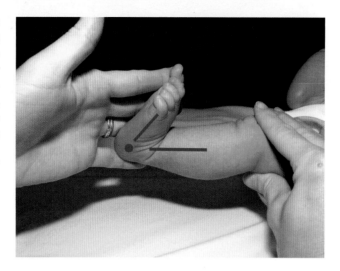

Patient position	Supine with knee flexed approximately 10 degrees, ankle in anatomical position (Fig. 16.33).
Stabilization	Over anterior and posterior femur (see Fig. 16.33).
Examiner action	Dorsiflex patient's ankle through available ROM. Return to starting position. Performing passive movement provides an estimate of the ROM (see Fig. 16.33).
Goniometer alignment	Palpate bony landmarks shown in Fig. 16.33 and align goniometer accordingly.
Stationary arm	Lateral midline of fibula, in line with fibular head.
Axis	Distal to but in line with lateral malleolus, at intersection of lines through lateral midline of fibula and lateral midline of fifth metatarsal.

Fig. 16.34 End of ankle pronation: dorsiflexion component ROM, demonstrating proper alignment of goniometer at end of range.

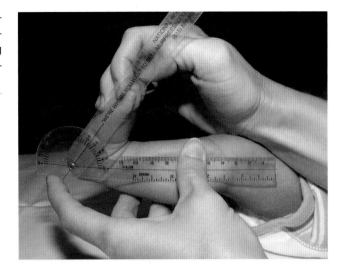

Moving arm	Lateral midline of fifth metatarsal.
	Read scale of goniometer.
Patient/Examiner action	Perform passive ankle dorsiflexion (see Fig. 16.33).
Confirmation of alignment	Repalpate landmarks and confirm proper goniometric alignment at end of ROM, correcting alignment as necessary. Read scale of goniometer (Fig. 16.34).
Documentation	Record patient's ROM.
Note	Excessive dorsiflexion is normal in the infant (see Table 16.6).
Alternative patient position	Side-lying; goniometer alignment remains the same. Motion also can be measured with knee fully extended, providing an estimation of gastrocnemius tightness (see Chapter 14).

Ankle/Foot Supination: Inversion Component

Fig. 16.35 Starting position for measurement of combined ankle/foot supination: inversion component.

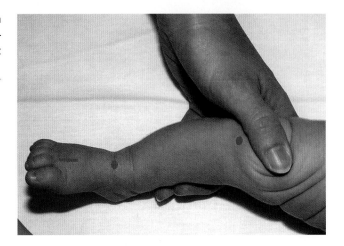

Patient position	Supine, with ankle in anatomical position (Fig. 16.35).
Stabilization	Thumb stabilizes anterior tibia and fingers over posterior aspect of distal leg (see Fig. 16.36).
Examiner action	Invert patient's foot/ankle through available ROM. Return to starting position. Performing passive movement provides an estimate of the ROM (Fig. 16.36).
Goniometer alignment	Palpate bony landmarks shown in Fig. 16.36 and align goniometer accordingly.
Stationary arm	Anterior midline of tibia, in line with tibial crest.
Axis	Anterior aspect of talocrural joint, midway between medial and lateral malleoli.

Fig. 16.36 End of combined ankle/foot supination: inversion component showing proper hand placement for stabilizing tibia and inverting ankle/foot. Bony landmarks for goniometer alignment (tibial crest, anterior midline of talocrural joint, anterior midline of second metatarsal) indicated by red lines and dot. Note: Photo shows alignment of third metatarsal.

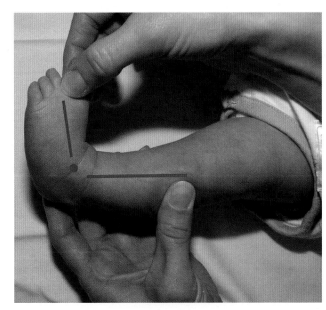

Fig. 16.37 End of ankle/foot supination: inversion component ROM, demonstrating proper alignment of goniometer at end of range.

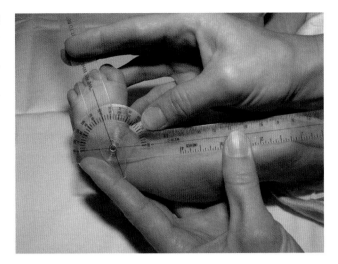

Moving arm	Anterior midline of second metatarsal.
	Read scale of goniometer.
Patient/Examiner action	Perform passive ankle/foot inversion (see Fig. 16.36).
Confirmation of alignment	Repalpate landmarks and confirm proper goniometric alignment at end of ROM, correcting alignment as necessary. Read scale of goniometer (Fig. 16.37).
Documentation	Record patient's ROM.
Alternative patient position	Seated, supported in parent's lap; goniometer alignment remains the same.

Ankle/Foot Pronation: Eversion Component

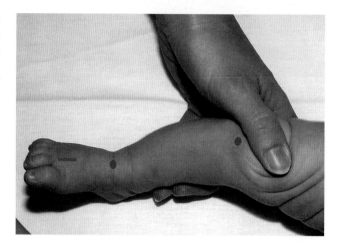

Fig. 16.38 Starting position for measurement of combined ankle/foot pronation: eversion component.

Patient position	Supine, with ankle in anatomical position (Fig. 16.38).
Stabilization	Thumb stabilizes anterior tibia and fingers over posterior aspect of distal leg (Fig. 16.39).
Examiner action	Evert patient's foot/ankle through available ROM. Return to starting position. Performing passive movement provides an estimate of the ROM (see Fig. 16.39).
Goniometer alignment	Palpate bony landmarks shown in Fig. 16.39 and align goniometer accordingly.
Stationary arm	Anterior midline of tibia, in line with tibial crest.
Axis	Anterior aspect of talocrural joint, midway between medial and lateral malleoli.
Moving arm	Anterior midline of second metatarsal.
	Read scale of goniometer.

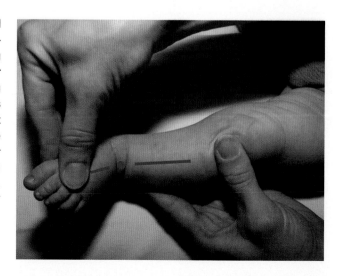

Fig. 16.39 End of combined ankle/foot pronation: eversion component showing proper hand placement for stabilizing tibia and everting ankle/foot. Bony landmarks for goniometer alignment (tibial crest, anterior midline of talcrural joint, anterior midline of second metatarsal) indicated by red lines and dot.

Fig. 16.40 End of ankle/foot pronation: eversion component ROM, demonstrating proper alignment of goniometer at end of range.

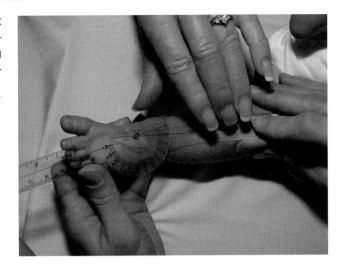

Patient/Examiner action	Perform passive ankle/foot eversion (see Fig. 16.39).
Confirmation of alignment	Repalpate landmarks and confirm proper goniometric alignment at end of ROM, correcting alignment as necessary. Read scale of goniometer (Fig. 16.40).
Documentation	Record patient's ROM.
Alternative patient position	Seated, supported in parent's lap with ankle in anatomical position; goniometer alignment remains the same.

Cervical ROM

Cervical range of motion in older children may be measured utilizing the techniques previously described in Chapter 9 of this text. For infants and children younger than 5 years of age, methods for measuring cervical rotation and lateral flexion have been explored using an arthrodial protractor as well as a variety of AROM techniques including the valid and reliable Muscle Function Scale.[25–27] For this age group (0–5 years), congenital muscular torticollis (CMT) is a common diagnosis requiring careful examination of cervical ROM, and the techniques recommended in the clinical practice guidelines on the management of CMT will be emphasized here.[28,29]

Ohman and Beckung have reported values for passive cervical rotation and lateral flexion ROM in infants from two to 10 months of age.[25] In that study, using an arthrodial protractor, the authors reported the mean value was 110° for passive cervical rotation and 70° for lateral flexion.[25] The techniques for obtaining these passive ROM measures in infants are described in Figs. 16.41 and 16.42. Values in 3.5 to 5-year-old children using these same techniques show that, on average, cervical ROM values decrease by 10°, while lateral flexion values remain the same (Table 16.7).[26] The pediatric spine is similar to an adult's by eight years of age. Authors have suggested that cervical range of motion values in both rotation and lateral flexion decrease by approximately 3° every 10 years of life in both males and females.[25,30]

Active ROM assessment techniques are also described below in Figs. 16.43–16.47. While two of these clinical assessments provide qualitative data the examiner may incorporate into the evaluation, the Muscle Function Scale allows the examiner to assign a score on an ordinal scale as described by Ohman and Beckung.[27] The previously mentioned clinical practice guidelines on the management of CMT also recommend assessments stratified by age.[28,29]

Table 16.7 MEAN PASSIVE CERVICAL RANGE OF MOTION IN DEGREES BY AGE					
	2 MONTHS	**4 MONTHS**	**6 MONTHS**	**10 MONTHS**	**3.5–5 YEARS**
Rotation	105.2°	111.8°	112.4°	111.7°	100° (7.7)
Lateral Flexion	68.1°	69.5°	69.2°	70°	69° (3.4)

Values in parentheses represent standard deviations.

Data from Ohman AM, Beckung ERE. Reference values for range of motion and muscle function of the neck in infants. *Pediatr Phys Ther.* 2008;20:53–58; Ohman AM, Beckung ERE. A pilot study on changes in passive range of motion in the cervical spine, for children aged 0–5. *Physiother Theory Pract.* 2013;29(6):457–460.

Passive Rotation—Cervical Spine: Arthrodial Protractor Technique

Fig. 16.41 End position of left passive rotation of the cervical spine using the arthrodial protractor technique.

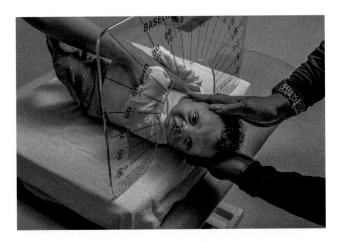

Patient Position

Supine with caregiver or assistant stabilizing the trunk and the vertically placed protractor (may require two assistants). The patient nose is aligned with the 90-degree reference on the protractor. The infant is positioned with the head off the support surface but supported by the examiner.

Examiner Action

Examiner passively rotates the cervical spine through the available ROM. Examiner reads angle on the arthrodial protractor at the end of rotation ROM. See Fig. 16.41.

Passive Lateral Flexion—Cervical Spine: Arthrodial Protractor Technique

Fig. 16.42 End position of left passive lateral flexion of the cervical spine using the arthrodial protractor technique.

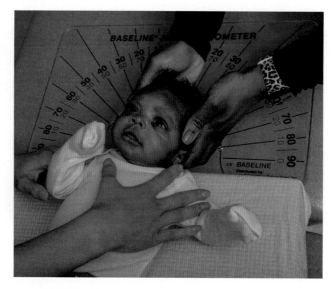

Patient Position

Supine with caregiver or assistant stabilizing the trunk. The infant is positioned with the head off the support surface but supported by the examiner and over the horizontally placed protractor. The patient nose is aligned with the 90-degree reference on the protractor.

Examiner Action

The examiner passively, laterally flexes (side bends) the cervical spine through the available ROM. Examiner reads angle on the arthrodial protractor at the end of the lateral flexion ROM. See Fig. 16.42.

Active Rotation—Cervical Spine: Supine Position (Infants 0–3 months)

Fig. 16.43 Right active rotation of the cervical spine with rattle stimulus.

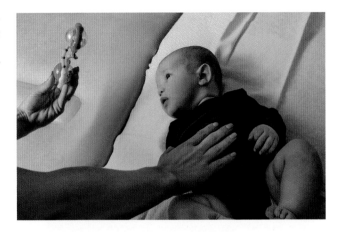

Patient Position

Supine on a mat (cueing may be required to limit shoulder elevation and rotation).

Examiner Action

Examiner utilizes visual and auditory stimuli to entice the infant to rotate the cervical spine in desired direction. Examiner notes position of the chin in relation to the ipsilateral shoulder at the end of the rotation ROM. Fig. 16.43.

Active Rotation—Cervical Spine: Rotating Stool Test (Infants ≥3 months)

Fig. 16.44 Start position of right active rotation of the cervical spine using the rotating stool test.

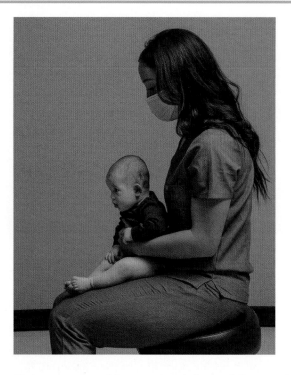

Patient Position   Sitting supported in examiner's lap, while examiner is seated on a rotating stool.

Examiner Action   Examiner utilizes visual and auditory stimuli to entice the infant to rotate the cervical spine in desired direction. Visual and auditory attention to caregiver or parent may be helpful. Examiner notes position of the chin in relation to the ipsilateral shoulder at the end of the rotation ROM. Figs. 16.44–16.46.

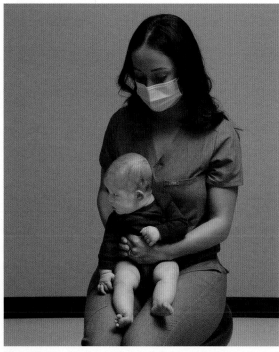

Fig. 16.45 End position of right active rotation of the cervical spine using the rotating stool test.

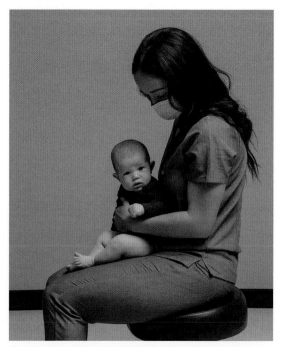

Fig. 16.46 End position of left active rotation of the cervical spine using the rotating stool test from the parent/guardian perspective.

Active Lateral Flexion—Cervical Spine: Muscle Function Scale (Infants ≥2 months)

Fig. 16.47 Therapist performing the muscle function scale with supportive hand holds.

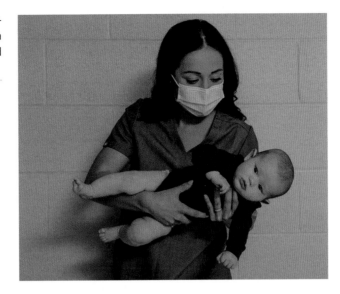

Patient Position	Patient is held by the examiner.
Examiner Action	Examiner holds the infant and stands in front of a mirror. Examiner tilts the patient from vertical to horizontal (90 degrees) and observes the activation of the lateral flexors of the neck in a righting response. Fig. 16.47 Examiner scores the head righting position with a score of 0–5. Scoring instructions are outlined in the 2009 article by Ohman et al.[27]

Special Tests: Muscle Length—Passive Knee Extension Test

Fig. 16.48 End of ROM for passive knee extension test. Bony landmarks for goniometer alignment (greater trochanter, lateral femoral epicondyle, lateral malleolus) indicated by red lines and dots.

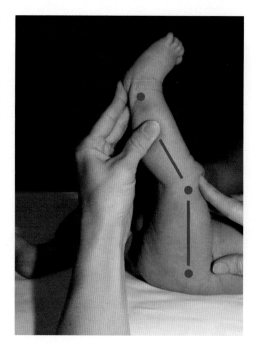

Patient position	Supine with hip flexed to 90 degrees. Contralateral lower extremity should be stabilized with knee in available extension as possible. It is imperative that the contralateral lower extremity be maintained in this position throughout testing (Fig. 16.48).
Examiner action	Extend patient's knee through full available ROM while maintaining hip in 90 degrees of flexion. This passive movement allows an estimate of available ROM (see Fig. 16.48).
Goniometer alignment	Palpate bony landmarks shown in Fig. 16.48 and align goniometer accordingly.
Stationary arm	Greater trochanter of femur.
Axis	Lateral epicondyle of femur.
Moving arm	Lateral malleolus.
	Maintaining proper goniometer alignment, read scale of goniometer.

Thigh-Foot Angle

The thigh-foot angle is a special test that allows for examination of the alignment of the lower leg in the pediatric patient (Table 16.8).

Patient position

Prone, with hip extended and knee flexed to 90 degrees and the foot allowed to assume a natural resting position.

Stabilization

At ankle to allow patient to maintain position, but examiner should not realign the foot.

Examiner action

The angle is formed from the bisection of the axis of the thigh and the axis of the foot through the second metatarsal (see Fig. 16.49). In-toeing angles were given negative values and out-toeing angles positive values.

Table 16.8 CHANGES IN THIGH-FOOT ANGLE DURING DEVELOPMENT	
AGE	**THIGH-FOOT ANGLE MEAN VALUE**
Birth	−14°
1 Year	−5°
2 Years	4°
3–4 Years	5°
5–7 Years	10°
9 Years	7°
11 Years	10°
15–19 Years	7°

From Staheli LT, et al. Lower-extremity rotational problems in children. Normal values to guide management. *J Bone Joint Surg Am.* 1985;67:39–47.

Transmalleolar Axis

Fig. 16.49 Allow patient to assume a normal foot position and draw lines according to bony landmarks. Bony landmarks for lines include bisection of the thigh and bisection of the foot through the second metatarsal.

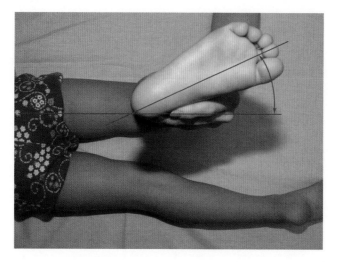

The transmalleolar axis is a special test that is described as one component used to assess rotation of the distal tibia (Table 16.9). This test has been previously described by Staheli et al.[31] This method may limit the effects of hindfoot varus/valgus as well as foot adduction/abduction on the values obtained.[32]

Patient position

Prone, with hip extended and knee flexed to 90 degrees and the foot stabilized in a natural resting position (Fig. 16.49).

Table 16.9 CHANGES IN TRANSMALLEOLAR AXIS DURING DEVELOPMENT	
AGE	**THIGH-FOOT ANGLE MEAN VALUE**
Birth	− 8°
1 Year	0°
2–3 Years	8°
4 Years	14°
5–7 Years	18°
8 Years	20°
9 Years	16°
10–14 Years	18°–22°

From Staheli LT, et al. Lower-extremity rotational problems in children. Normal values to guide management. *J Bone Joint Surg Am.* 1985;67:39–47.

Fig. 16.50 Allow patient to assume a normal foot position, and draw lines according to bony landmarks. Bony landmarks for lines include bisection of the thigh and formation of a line perpendicular to the line drawn between the medial and lateral malleoli.

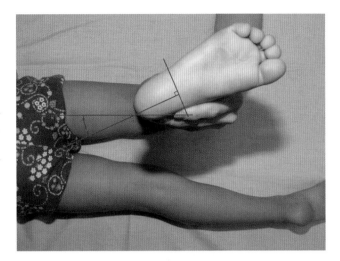

Stabilization

At ankle to allow patient to maintain position, but examiner should not realign the foot (see Fig. 16.49).

Examiner action

The angle is formed from the bisection of the axis of the thigh and the line obtained from a perpendicular line to the line formed between the lateral and medial malleoli (Fig. 16.50).

Special Test: Standing Alignment During Development

Fig. 16.51 A 5 month old
with minimal genu varum
compared to a newborn
infant.

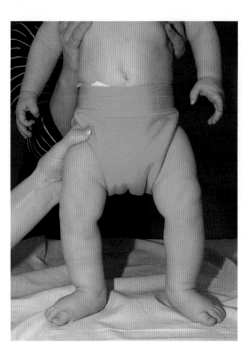

Fig. 16.51 A 5 month old with minimal genu varum compared to a newborn infant.

Genu varum and genu valgus changes are observed in typical development. Cheng et al.[33] described the technique of measuring the clinical tibiofemoral angle. The patient is positioned in standing. The superior iliac spines, the midline of the patella, and the midpoint of the ankle joint were bony landmarks used to form the angle.

Children commonly present with genu varum through the age of 18 months.[34] Children 18 months and older often present with genu valgum, which normalizes to expected values in an adult (7–8 degrees of valgus) by the age of 7 years.[35–37] See Figs. 16.51–16.53 to observe alignment changes from age 5 months to 4 years.

Fig. 16.52 A 2-year, 3-month-old with genu valgus.

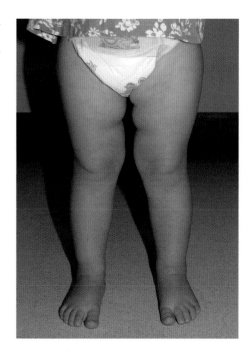

Fig. 16.52 A 2-year, 3-month-old with genu valgus.

Fig. 16.53   A 4-year-old with normal alignment.

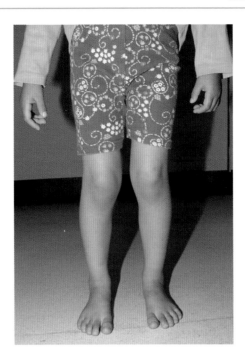

References

1. Watanabe H, Ogata K, Amano T, Okabe TL. The range of joint motions of the extremities in healthy Japanese people: the difference according to the age. Cited in Walker JM: musculoskeletal development: a review. *Phys Ther.* 1991;878.
2. Soucie JM, Wang C, Forsyth A, et al. Range of motion measurements: reference values and a database for comparison studies. *Haemophilia.* 2011;17(3):500–507.
3. McKay MJ, Baldwin JN, Ferreira P, et al. Normative reference values for strength and flexibility of 1,000 children and adults. *Neurology.* 2017;88(1):36–43.
4. Vidhi S, Parmar L, Khandare S, Palekar T. Measurement of elbow range of motion in full term neonates. *Int J Sci Res Edu.* 2017;5(11):7721–7731.
5. Hoffer MM. Joint motion limitation in newborns. *Clin Orthop Relat Res.* 1980;94–96.
6. Cheng JC, Chan PS, Hui PW. Joint laxity in children. *J Pediatr Orthop.* 1991;11:752–756.
7. Golden DW, Jhee JT, Gilpin SP, Sawyer JR. Elbow range of motion and clinical carrying angle in a healthy pediatric population. *J Pediatr Orthop B.* 2007;16:144–149.
8. Balasubramanian P, Madhuri V, Muliyil J. Carrying angle in children: a normative study. *J Pediatr Orthop B.* 2006;15:37–40.
9. Yilmaz E, Karakurt L, Belhan O, et al. Variation of carrying angle with age, sex, and special reference to side. *Orthopedics.* 2005;28:1360–1363.
10. Haas SS, Epps CH, Adams JP. Normal ranges of hip motion in the newborn. *Clin Orthop Relat Res.* 1973;114–118.
11. Coon V, Donato G, Houser C, Bleck EE. Normal ranges of hip motion in infants six weeks, three months and six months of age. *Clin Orthop Relat Res.* 1975;110:256–260.
12. Rao KN, Joseph B. Value of measurement of hip movements in childhood hip disorders. *J Pediatr Orthop.* 2001;21:495–501.
13. Schwarze D, Denton J. Normal values of the neonatal lower limbs: an evaluation of 1,000 neonates. *J Pediatr Orthop.* 1993;13:758–760.
14. Mudge AJ, et al. Normative reference values for lower limb joint range, bone torsion, and alignment in children aged 4-16 years. *J Pediatr Orthop B.* 2014;23:15–25.
15. McDowell BC, Salazar-Torres JJ, Kerr C, Cosgrove AP. Passive range of motion in a population-based sample of children with spastic cerebral palsy who walk. *Phys Occup Ther Pediatr.* 2012;32(2):139–150.
16. Drews JE, Vraciu JK, Pellino G. Range of motion of the joints of the lower extremities of newborns. *Phys Occup Ther Pediatr.* 1984;4:49–62.
17. Forero N, Okamura LA, Larson MA. Normal ranges of hip motion in neonates. *J Pediatr Orthop.* 1989;9:391–395.
18. Phelps E, Smith LJ, Hallum A. Normal ranges of hip motion of infants between nine and 24 months of age. *Dev Med Child Neurol.* 1985;27:785–792.
19. Sankar WN, Laird CT, Baldwin KD. Hip range of motion in children: what is the norm? *J Pediatr Orthop.* 2012;32:399–405.
20. Alanen JT, Levola JV, Helenius HY, Kvist MH. Ankle joint complex mobility of children 7 to 14 years old. *J Pediatr Orthop.* 2001;21(6):731–737.
21. Grimston SK, Nigg BM, Hanley DA, Engsberg JR. Differences in ankle joint complex range of motion as a function of age. *Foot Ankle.* 1993;14(4):215–222.
22. Silverman S, Constine L, Harvey W, Grahame R. Survey of joint mobility and in vivo skin elasticity in London schoolchildren. *Ann Rheum Dis.* 1975;34(2):177–180.
23. Wynne-Davies R. Acetabular dysplasia and familial joint laxity: two etiological factors in congenital dislocation of the hip. A review of 589 patients and their families. *J Bone Joint Surg Br.* 1970;52:704–716.
24. Williams M, Green D, Eyzaguirre M, Tanikawa D. The newborn musculoskeletal examination: Assessment of lower extremity range of motion. *Medicine.* 2007;268–273.
25. Ohman AM, Beckung ERE. Reference values for range of motion and muscle function of the neck in infants. *Pediatr Phys Ther.* 2008;20:53–58.
26. Ohman AM, Beckung ERE. A pilot study on changes in passive range of motion in the cervical spine, for children aged 0-5. *Physiother Theory Pract.* 2013;29(6):457–460.
27. Ohman AM, Nilsson S, Beckung ERE. Validity and reliability of the muscle function scale, aimed to assess the lateral flexors of the neck in infants. *Physiother Theory Pract.* 2009;25(2):129–137.
28. Kaplan SL, Coulter C, Fetters L. Physical therapy management of congenital muscular torticollis: an evidence-based clinical practice guideline from the section on pediatrics of the American Physical Therapy Association. *Pediatr Phys Ther.* 2013;25:348–394.
29. Kaplan SL, Coulter C, Sargent B. Physical therapy management of congenital muscular torticollis: a 2018 evidence-based clinical practice guideline from the American Physical Therapy Association academy of pediatric physical therapy. *Pediatr Phys Ther.* 2018;30(4):240–290.
30. Youdas JW, Garett TR, Suman VJ, et al. Normal range of motion of the cervical spine: an initial goniometric study. *Phys Ther.* 1992;72:770–780.
31. Staheli LT, Corbett M, Wyss C, King H. Lower-extremity rotational problems in children. Normal values to guide management. *J Bone Joint Surg Am.* 1985;67(1):39–47.
32. Jacquemier M, Glard Y, Pomero V, et al. Rotational profile of the lower limb in 1319 healthy children. *Gait Posture.* 2008;28(2):187–193.
33. Cheng JC, Chan PS, Chiang SC, Hui PW. Angular and rotational profile of the lower limb in 2,630 Chinese children. *J Pediatr Orthop.* 1991;11:154–161.
34. Salenius P, Vankka E. The development of the tibiofemoral angle in children. *J Bone Joint Surg Am.* 1975;57:259–261.
35. Sabharwal S, Zhao C, Edgar M. Lower limb alignment in children: reference values based on a full-length standing radiograph. *J Pediatr Orthop.* 2008;28:740–746.
36. Staheli LT. Rotational problems in children. *J Bone Joint Surg Am.* 1993;75:939–949.
37. Yeo A. Normal lower limb variants in children. *Br Med J.* 2015;8016:27–31.

SAMPLE DATA RECORDING FORMS

JOINT RANGE OF MOTION						
			Patient: _____			
			Age: _____			
			Indicate:			
			AROM _____			
			PROM _____			

LEFT				RIGHT		
			Date/Examiner's Initials			
			Shoulder			
			Flexion			
			Extension			
			Abduction			
			Medial Rotation			
			Lateral Rotation			
			Elbow/Forearm			
			Flexion			
			Extension			
			Supination			
			Pronation			
			Wrist/Fingers			
			Wrist Flexion			
			Wrist Extension			
			Wrist Abduction			
			Wrist Adduction			
			CMC Flexion			
			CMC Extension			
			CMC Abduction			
			MCP Flexion			
			MCP Extension			
			IP Flexion (indicate digit and whether IP, PIP, or DIP)			

Fig. A.1

JOINT RANGE OF MOTION				Patient: _____ Age: _____ Indicate: AROM _____ PROM _____		
LEFT				**RIGHT**		
			Date/Examiner's Initials			
			Hip			
			Flexion			
			Extension			
			Abduction			
			Adduction			
			Medial Rotation			
			Lateral Rotation			
			Knee			
			Flexion			
			Extension			
			Foot/Ankle			
			Dorsiflexion			
			Plantarflexion			
			Inversion			
			Eversion			
			1st MTP Flexion			
			1st MTP Extension			
			MTP Flexion: Digits 2–5			
			MTP Extension: Digits 2–5			
			IP Flexion (indicate digit and whether IP, PIP, or DIP)			
			IP Extension (indicate digit and whether IP, PIP, or DIP)			

Fig. A.2

JOINT RANGE OF MOTION	Patient:_____
	Age:_____
	Measurement Device Used:
	_____

Date/Examiner's Initials			
Lumbar			
Flexion			
Extension			
Lateral Flexion - Right			
Lateral Flexion - Left			
Rotation - Right			
Rotation - Left			
Thoracolumbar			
Flexion			
Extension			
Lateral Flexion - Right			
Lateral Flexion - Left			
Rotation - Right			
Rotation - Left			

Fig. A.3

JOINT RANGE OF MOTION

Patient:_____

Age:_____

Measurement Device Used:

_____

Date/Examiner's Initials			
Cervical			
Flexion			
Extension			
Lateral Flexion - Right			
Lateral Flexion - Left			
Rotation - Right			
Rotation - Left			
Temporomandibular Joint			
Mandibular depression (opening)			
Protrusion			
Lateral Deviation - Right			
Lateral Deviation - Left			

Fig. A.4

MUSCLE LENGTH

Patient: _____
Age: _____
Indicate:
AROM _____
PROM _____

		LEFT		RIGHT		
			Date/Examiner's Initials			
			Latissimus Dorsi			
			Pectoralis Major - General			
			Pectoralis Major - Clavicular			
			Pectoralis Minor			
			Triceps			
			Biceps			
			Forearm Flexor Muscles			
			Forearm Extensor Muscles			

Fig. A.5

JOINT RANGE OF MOTION

Patient: _____
Age: _____
Indicate:
AROM _____
PROM _____

		LEFT		RIGHT		
			Date/Examiner's Initials			
			Iliopsoas (indicate test used)			
			Rectus Femoris			
			Quadriceps			
			Hamstrings (indicate test used)			
			Iliotibial Band (indicate test used)			
			Gastrocnemius			
			Soleus (indicate position)			

Fig. A.6

NORMATIVE RANGE of MOTION of the EXTREMITIES and SPINE in ADULTS

Table B.1 SUGGESTED VALUES FOR NORMAL ROM FOR JOINTS OF THE UPPER EXTREMITY IN ADULTS BASED ON ANALYSIS OF EXISTING DATA

JOINT	ROM
Shoulder	
Flexion	0°–160°
Extension	0°–60°
Abduction	0°–165°
Medial rotation	0°–70°
Lateral rotation	0°–90°
Elbow	
Flexion	0°–140°
Extension	0°
Forearm	
Pronation	0°–80°
Supination	0°–80°
Wrist	
Flexion	0°–80°
Extension	0°–70°
Abduction (radial deviation)	0°–20°
Adduction (ulnar deviation)	0°–30°
First Carpometacarpal joint	
Flexion	0°–15°
Extension	0°–20°
Abduction	0°–70°
Metacarpophalangeal joints	
Flexion	
Thumb	0°–50°
Fingers	0°–90°
Extension	
Thumb	0°
Fingers	0°–20°
Interphalangeal joints	
Flexion	
IP joint (thumb)	0°–65°
PIP joint (fingers)	0°–100°
DIP joint (fingers)	0°–70°
Extension	
IP joint (thumb)	0°–10° to 20°
PIP joint (fingers)	0°
DIP joint (fingers)	0°

DIP, Distal interphalangeal; *IP*, interphalangeal; *PIP*, proximal interphalangeal.

Table B.2 TRADITIONALLY QUOTED VALUES FOR NORMAL ROM FOR JOINTS OF THE UPPER EXTREMITY IN ADULTS

JOINT	AMERICAN ACADEMY OF ORTHOPAEDIC SURGEONS[1]	AMERICAN MEDICAL ASSOCIATION[2]
Shoulder		
Flexion	0°–180°	0°–180°
Extension	0°–60°	0°–50°
Abduction	0°–180°	0°–180°
Medial rotation	0°–70°	0°–90°
Lateral rotation		0°–90°
Elbow		
Flexion	0°–150°	0°–140°
Extension	0°	
Forearm		
Pronation	0°–80°	0°–80°
Supination	0°–80°	0°–80°
Wrist		
Flexion	0°–80°	
Extension	0°–70°	0°–60°
Abduction (radial deviation)	0°–20°	0°–20°
Adduction (ulnar deviation)	0°–30°	0°–30°
First Carpometacarpal joint		
Flexion	0°–15°	
Extension	0°–20°	0°–50°
Abduction		
Metacarpophalangeal joints		
Flexion		
Thumb	0°–50°	0°–60°
Fingers	0°–90°	0°–90°
Extension		
Thumb	0°	0°
Fingers	0°–45°	0°–20°
Interphalangeal joints		
Flexion		
IP joint (thumb)	0°–80°	0°–80°
PIP joint (fingers)	0°–100°	0°–100°
DIP joint (fingers)	0°–90°	0°–70°
Extension		
IP joint (thumb)	0°–20°	0°–10°
PIP joint (fingers)	0°	
DIP joint (fingers)	0°	

DIP, distal interphalangeal; *IP*, interphalangeal; *PIP*, proximal interphalangeal.

Table B.3 SUGGESTED VALUES FOR NORMAL ROM OF THORACIC AND LUMBAR SPINE IN ADULTS BASED ON ANALYSIS OF EXISTING DATA

MOTION	TAPE MEASURE	GONIOMETER	INCLINOMETER	BROM
Flexion	6–7 cm	90°	60°	45°
Extension	—	30°	25°	15°
Lateral flexion	22 cm	35°	30°	35°
Rotation	—	—	6°	8°

BROM, Back range of motion device.

Table B.4 TRADITIONALLY QUOTED VALUES FOR NORMAL ROM OF THORACIC AND LUMBAR SPINE IN ADULTS

MOTION	SCHOBER[*]	GONIOMETER[†]	INCLINOMETER[‡]
Flexion	3–5 cm	90°	60°
Extension	—	30°	25°
Lateral flexion	—	30°	25°
Rotation	—	—	30°

[*]From Rothschild.[3]
[†]Measurement of thoracolumbar spine norms provided by the American Medical Association.
[‡]Measurement of rotation is for thoracic spine; all other measures are lumbar spine. Norms provided by the American Medical Association.[2]

Table B.5 SUGGESTED VALUES FOR NORMAL ROM OF CERVICAL ROM IN ADULTS BASED ON ANALYSIS OF EXISTING DATA

MOTION	TAPE MEASURE[*]	GONIOMETER[†]	INCLINOMETER[‡]	CROM[§]
Flexion	1–4 cm	45°	50°	50°
Extension	20 cm	45°	60°	75°
Lateral flexion	15 cm	45°	45°	45°
Rotation	10 cm	70°	80°	70°

CROM, Cervical range of motion device.
[*]Cervical spine norms derived from data by Balogun et al.[4] and Hsieh and Yeung.[5]
[†]Cervical spine norms provided by the American Medical Association.[6]
[‡]Cervical spine norms provided by the American Medical Association.[2]
[§]Cervical spine norms derived from means of male and female data from ages 20–40 years according to study by Youdas et al.[7]
Note: The American Academy of Orthopedic Surgeons does not provide normative data using a tape measure, inclinometer, or CROM for cervical range of motion.

Table B.6 SUGGESTED VALUES FOR NORMAL ROM FOR JOINTS OF THE LOWER EXTREMITY IN ADULTS BASED ON ANALYSIS OF EXISTING DATA

JOINT	ROM
Hip	
Flexion	0°–120°
Extension	0°–20°
Abduction	0°–40° to 45°
Adduction	0°–25° to 30°
Medial rotation	0°–35° to 40°
Lateral rotation	0°–35° to 40°
Knee	
Flexion	0°–140° to 145°
Extension	0°
Ankle/foot	
Dorsiflexion[*]	0°–15° to 20°
Plantarflexion[†]	0°–40° to 50°
Inversion[†]	0°–30° to 35°
Eversion[†]	0°–20°
First Metatarsophalangeal joint	
Flexion	0°–20°
Extension	0°–80°

[*]Component of pronation. (ROM values apply to foot, not to isolated subtalar joint, motion.)
[†]Component of supination. (ROM values apply to foot, not to isolated subtalar joint, motion.)

Table B.7 TRADITIONALLY QUOTED VALUES FOR NORMAL ROM FOR JOINTS OF THE LOWER EXTREMITY IN ADULTS

JOINT	AMERICAN ACADEMY OF ORTHOPAEDIC SURGEONS[1]	AMERICAN MEDICAL ASSOCIATION[2]
Hip		
Flexion	0°–120°	0°–100°
Extension	0°–30°	0°–30°
Abduction	0°–45°	0°–40°
Adduction	0°–30°	0°–20°
Medial rotation	0°–45°	0°–50°
Lateral rotation	0°–45°	0°–40°
Knee		
Flexion	0°–135°	0°–150°
Extension	0°–10°	0°
Ankle/foot		
Dorsiflexion[*]	0°–20°	0°–20°
Plantarflexion[†]	0°–50°	0°–40°
Inversion[†]	0°–35°	0°–30°
Eversion[*]	0°–15°	0°–20°
First Metatarsophalangeal joint		
Flexion	0°–30°	0°–45°
Extension	0°–70°	0°–50°

[*]Component of pronation.
[†]Component of supination.

Table B.8	INVESTIGATIONS REPORTING DATA FOR SHOULDER FLEXION ROM						
STUDY	**SAMPLE**	**AGES**	**METHOD USED**	**NO. OF EXAMINERS**	**TYPE OF MOTION**	**RELIABILITY COEFFICIENT CALCULATED?**	**ROM**
Aizawa et al.[8]	20 (10 M, 10 F)	18–34 years	Standing using FASTRAK	Not stated	AROM	No	152°±10°
Barnes et al.[9]	140 F	4–70 years	AAOS	1	AROM	No	177°±6° (D) 176°±6° (ND)
Barnes et al.[9]	140 M	4–70 years	AAOS	1	AROM	No	174°±8° (D) 174°±8° (ND)
Barnes et al.[9]	140 F	4–70 years	AAOS	1	PROM	No	179°±4° (D) 178°±4° (ND)
Barnes et al.[9]	140 M	4–70 years	AAOS	1	PROM	No	176°±7° (D) 176°±7° (ND)
Boone and Azen[10]	53 M	1–19 years	AAOS	1	AROM	No	168°±4°
Boone and Azen[10]	56 M	20–54 years	AAOS	1	AROM	No	165°±5°
Conte et al.[11]	50 F	20–29 years	Palmer and Epler	1	PROM	ICC 0.84 (R) ICC 0.94 (L)	167°±8° (R) 168°±7° (L)
Desrosiers et al.[12]	60 M	60–69 years	AAOS	1	AROM	No	161°±10° (R) 161°±11° (L)
Desrosiers et al.[12]	60 M	70–79 years	AAOS	1	AROM	No	155°±11° (R) 156°±12° (L)
Desrosiers et al.[12]	60 M	80–90 years	AAOS	1	AROM	No	146°±14° (R) 147°±14° (L)
Desrosiers et al.[12]	60 F	60–69 years	AAOS	1	AROM	No	162°±10° (R) 163°±10° (L)
Desrosiers et al.[12]	60 F	70–79 years	AAOS	1	AROM	No	159°±11° (R) 161°±11° (L)
Desrosiers et al.[12]	60 F	80–90 years	AAOS	1	AROM	No	151°±12° (R) 153°±13 (L)
Escalante et al.[13]	687*	64–79 years	Supine	4	PROM	ICC 0.42	156°±12° (R) 158°±12° (L)
Fiebert et al.[14]	102 (71 F, 31 M)	61–93 years	AAOS	1	AROM	No	165°±11°
Gill et al.[15]	97 M	20–24 years	Not stated	Not stated	AROM	No	168.6°±13.1° (L) 170.8°±18.2° (R)
Gill et al.[15]	99 F	20–24 years	Not stated	Not stated	AROM	No	166.4°±10.1° (L) 164.7°±11.1° (R)
Gill et a[15]	170 M	25–29 years	Not stated	Not stated	AROM	No	165.0°±10.1° (L) 165.2°±9.8° (R)
Gill et al.[15]	119 F	25–29 years	Not stated	Not stated	AROM	No	164.8°±12.8° (L) 166.0°±13.1° (R)
Gill et al.[15]	146 M	30–34 years	Not stated	Not stated	AROM	No	166.2°±12.9° (L) 167.9°±11.5° (R)
Gill et al.[15]	145 F	30–34 years	Not stated	Not stated	AROM	No	162.9°±12.2° (L) 164.4°±13.1° (R)
Gill et al.[15]	131 M	35–39 years	Not stated	Not stated	AROM	No	162.3°±21.7° (L) 162.8°±24.3° (R)
Gill et al.[15]	122 F	35–39 years	Not stated	Not stated	AROM	No	165.2°±13.3° (L) 166.2°±12.5° (R)
Gill et al.[15]	140 M	40–44 years	Not stated	Not stated	AROM	No	160.9°±14.2° (L) 166.0°±13.1° (R)
Gill et al.[15]	125 F	40–44 years	Not stated	Not stated	AROM	No	160.2°±13.7° (L) 163.7°±14.0° (R)
Gill et al.[15]	113 M	45–49 years	Not stated	Not stated	AROM	No	162.9°±12.4° (L) 164.9°±13.1° (R)
Gill et al.[15]	105 F	45–49 years	Not stated	Not stated	AROM	No	158.0°±13.3° (L) 159.9°±14.0° (R)
Gill et al.[15]	94 M	50–54 years	Not stated	Not stated	AROM	No	163.6°±16.7° (L) 165.0°±18.6° (R)
Gill et al.[15]	89 F	50–54 years	Not stated	Not stated	AROM	No	158.0°±14.5° (L) 160.1°±14.5° (R)
Gill et al.[15]	86 M	55–59 years	Not stated	Not stated	AROM	No	157.3°±15.1° (L) 159.4°±15.6° (R)

Continued

Table B.8 INVESTIGATIONS REPORTING DATA FOR SHOULDER FLEXION ROM—cont'd

STUDY	SAMPLE	AGES	METHOD USED	NO. OF EXAMINERS	TYPE OF MOTION	RELIABILITY COEFFICIENT CALCULATED?	ROM
Gill et al.[15]	86 F	55–59 years	Not stated	Not stated	AROM	No	154.7°±15.5° (L) 157.1°±14.6° (R)
Gill et al.[15]	58 M	60–64 years	Not stated	Not stated	AROM	No	155.9°±15.2° (L) 157.4°±16.5° (R)
Gill et al.[15]	55 F	60–64 years	Not stated	Not stated	AROM	No	146.0°±26.1° (L) 146.5°±27.1° (R)
Gill et al.[15]	62 M	65–69 years	Not stated	Not stated	AROM	No	149.9°±20.1° (L) 152.3°±20.1° (R)
Gill et al.[15]	61 F	65–69 years	Not stated	Not stated	AROM	No	151.6°±18.0° (L) 152.1°±15.7° (R)
Gill et al.[15]	49 M	70–74 years	Not stated	Not stated	AROM	No	143.3°±27.2° (L) 146.8°±19.3° (R)
Gill et al.[15]	54 F	70–74 years	Not stated	Not stated	AROM	No	145.9°±17.9° (L) 144.8°±29.7° (R)
Gill et al.[15]	52 M	75–79 years	Not stated	Not stated	AROM	No	143.0°±18.7° (L) 143.4°±26.1° (R)
Gill et al.[15]	46 F	75–79 years	Not stated	Not stated	AROM	No	138.1°±21.0° (L) 141.9°±21.5° (R)
Gill et al.[15]	31 M	80–84 years	Not stated	Not stated	AROM	No	137.1°±25.2° (L) 140.2°±22.0° (R)
Gill et al.[15]	51 F	80–84 years	Not stated	Not stated	AROM	No	132.1°±25.2° (L) 133.7°±24.3° (R)
Gill et al.[15]	10 M	85+ years	Not stated	Not stated	AROM	No	129.6°±23.2° (L) 127.8°±24.4° (R)
Gill et al.[15]	10 F	85+ years	Not stated	Not stated	AROM	No	129.9°±30.9° (L) 124.1°±39.6° (R)
Vairo et al.[16]	548 M	18.8±1.0 years	Not stated	4	AROM	No	165°±8° (D) 164°±9° (ND)
Vairo et al.[16]	548 M	18.8±1.0 years	Not stated	4	PROM	No	170°±8° (D) 169°±10° (ND)
Vairo et al.[16]	74 F	18.7±0.9 years	Not stated	4	AROM	No	168°±9° (D) 168°±8° (ND)
Vairo et al.[16]	74 F	18.7±0.9 years	Not stated	4	PROM	No	173°±9° (D) 172°±8° (ND)
Gûnal et al.[17]	1,000 M (RHD)	18–22 years	AAOS	2	PROM	No	121°±6° (R) 125°±7° (L)
Kalscheur et al.[18]	61 F	73.1±6.2 years	Supine	Not stated	AROM	No	158°±20° (R) 159°±9° (L)
Kalscheur et al.[18]	25 M	73.3±5.9 years	Supine	Not stated	AROM	No	152°±17° (R) 153°±16° (L)
Kolber et al.[19]	30 (12 M, 18 F)	25.9±3.1 years	Sitting; Digital inclinometer	2	AROM	ICC 0.83	173°±4°
Kolber and Hanney[20]	30 (21 F, 9 M)	26±4.2 years	Sitting; Digital inclinometer	1	AROM	ICC 0.95	164±9°
Kolber and Hanney[20]	30 (21 F, 9 M)	26±4.2 years	Sitting; Universal Goniometer	1	AROM	ICC 0.95	156±9°
Macedo and Magee[21]	30*	18–29 years	Supine	1	PROM	ICC 0.98	147°±14°
Macedo and Magee[21]	20*	30–39 years	Supine	1	PROM	ICC 0.98	138°±14°
Macedo and Magee[21]	20*	40–49 years	Supine	1	PROM	ICC 0.98	139°±15°
Macedo and Magee[21]	20*	50–59 years	Supine	1	PROM	ICC 0.98	141°±14°
Macedo and Magee[21]	90*	18–59 years	Supine	1	PROM	ICC 0.98	173°±4°
McIntosh et al.[22]	20*	50–69 years	Sitting	1	AROM	No	138°±7°
McIntosh et al.[22]	20*	50–69 years	Sitting	1	PROM	No	146°±8°
McIntosh et al.[22]	21*	70+ years	Sitting	1	AROM	No	127°±

Table B.8	INVESTIGATIONS REPORTING DATA FOR SHOULDER FLEXION ROM—cont'd						
STUDY	SAMPLE	AGES	METHOD USED	NO. OF EXAMINERS	TYPE OF MOTION	RELIABILITY COEFFICIENT CALCULATED?	ROM
McIntosh et al.[22]	21*	70+ years	Sitting	1	PROM	No	$144° \pm 10°$
Murray et al.[23]	10 F	25–35 years	AAOS	1	AROM	No	$172° \pm 1°$
Murray et al.[23]	10 M	26–36 years	AAOS	1	AROM	No	$170° \pm 2°$
Murray et al.[23]	10 F	60–64 years	AAOS	1	AROM	No	$170° \pm 1°$
Murray et al.[23]	10 M	56–66 years	AAOS	1	AROM	No	$165° \pm 2°$
Sabari et al.[24]	30*	17–92 years	Supine	1	AROM	ICC 0.95	$160° \pm 12°$
Sabari et al.[24]	30*	17–92 years	Sitting	1	AROM	ICC 0.97	$158° \pm 15°$
Sabari et al.[24]	30*	17–92 years	Supine	1	PROM	ICC 0.94	$163° \pm 13°$
Sabari et al.[24]	30*	17–92 years	Sitting	1	PROM	ICC 0.95	$160° \pm 15°$
Soucie et al.[25]	39 F	2–8 years	Supine	9	PROM	No	178.6°
Soucie et al.[25]	55 M	2–8 years	Supine	9	PROM	No	177.8°
Soucie et al.[25]	56 F	9–19 years	Supine	9	PROM	No	171.8°
Soucie et al.[25]	48 M	9–19 years	Supine	9	PROM	No	170.9°
Soucie et al.[25]	143 F	20–44 years	Supine	9	PROM	No	172°
Soucie et al.[25]	114 M	20–44 years	Supine	9	PROM	No	168.8°
Soucie et al.[25]	123 F	45–69 years	Supine	9	PROM	No	168.1°
Soucie et al.[25]	96 M	45–69 years	Supine	9	PROM	No	164°
Stubbs et al.[26]	55 M	25–54 years	AAOS	1	AROM	No	$178° \pm 11°$ (L) $180° \pm 11°$ (R)
Valentine and Lewis[27]	45 (23F, 22 M)	23–56 years	Standing; Inclinometer	1	AROM	ICC 0.94 ICC 0.91	$169° \pm 10°$ (R) $166° \pm 10°$ (L)
Walker et al.[28]	60 (30 M, 30 F)	60–84 years	AAOS	1	AROM	Pearson's $r >$ 0.81	$165° \pm 10°$
Watanabe et al.[29]	339/Japanese*	Birth to 2 years	Not stated	Not stated	PROM	Unknown	172°–180°

AAOS, American Academy of Orthopaedic Surgeons; *AROM*, active range of motion; *D*, dominant; *F*, females; *ICC*, intraclass correlation; *M*, males; *ND*, nondominant; *PROM*, passive range of motion; R, right; L, left.
*Number of males and females not stated.

				NO. OF	TYPE OF	RELIABILITY COEFFICIENT	
STUDY	**SAMPLE**	**AGES**	**METHOD USED**	**EXAMINERS**	**MOTION**	**CALCULATED?**	**ROM**
Aizawa et al.[7]	20 (10 M, 10 F)	18–34 years	Standing using FASTRAK	Not stated	AROM	No	151°±10°
Barnes et al.[8]	140 F	4–70 years	AAOS	1	AROM	No	188°±16° (D) 189°±15° (ND)
Barnes et al.[8]	140 M	4–70 years	AAOS	1	AROM	No	180°±18° (D) 182°±17° (ND)
Barnes et al.[8]	140 F	4–70 years	AAOS	1	PROM	No	195°±17° (D) 195°±17° (ND)
Barnes et al.[8]	140 M	4–70 years	AAOS	1	PROM	No	187°±19° (D) 189°±18° (ND)
Bassey et al.[30]	207 M	65–74 years	Standing; 45° to coronal plane	10	AROM	Coefficient of variation 5.3%	129°±14°
Bassey et al.[30]	255 F	65–74 years	Standing; 45° to coronal plane	10	AROM	Coefficient of variation 5.3%	129°±19°
Bassey et al.[30]	158 M	75+ years	Standing; 45° to coronal plane	10	AROM	Coefficient of variation 5.3%	121°±19°
Bassey et al.[30]	274 F	75+ years	Standing; 45° to coronal plane	10	AROM	Coefficient of variation 5.3%	114°±22°
Boone and Azen[9]	53 M	1–19 years	AAOS	1	AROM	No	185°±4°
Boone and Azen[9]	56 M	20–54 years	AAOS	1	AROM	No	183°±9°
Conte et al.[10]	50 F	20–29 years	Palmer and Epler	1	PROM	ICC 0.81 (R) ICC 0.80 (L)	171°±5° (R) 172°±5° (L)
Desrosiers et al.[12]	60 M	60–69 years	AAOS	1	AROM	No	167°±10° (R) 165°±10° (L)
Desrosiers et al.[12]	60 M	70–79 years	AAOS	1	AROM	No	159°±12° (R) 158°±14° (L)
Desrosiers et al.[12]	60 M	80–90 years	AAOS	1	AROM	No	155°±15° (R) 151°±16° (L)
Desrosiers et al.[12]	60 F	60–69 years	AAOS	1	AROM	No	162°±12° (R) 161°±11° (L)
Desrosiers et al.[12]	60 F	70–79 years	AAOS	1	AROM	No	163°±11° (R) 162°±13° (L)
Desrosiers et al.[12]	60 F	80–90 years	AAOS	1	AROM	No	159°±13° (R) 155°±15° (L)
Fiebert et al.[14]	102 (71 F, 31 M)	61–93 years	AAOS	1	AROM	No	158°±17°
Gill et al.[15]	97 M	20–24 years	Not stated	Not stated	AROM	No	158.8°±21.7° (L) 158.4°±25.0° (R)
Gill et al.[15]	99 F	20–24 years	Not stated	Not stated	AROM	No	156.0°±13.8° (L) 156.4°±12.1° (R)
Gill et al.[15]	170 M	25–29 years	Not stated	Not stated	AROM	No	153.4°±14.0° (L) 154.1°±13.6° (R)
Gill et al.[15]	119 F	25–29 years	Not stated	Not stated	AROM	No	155.2°±13.3° (L) 157.3°±15.3° (R)
Gill et al.[15]	146 M	30–34 years	Not stated	Not stated	AROM	No	156.1°±14.2° (L) 157.0°±15.7° (R)
Gill et al[15]	145 F	30–34 years	Not stated	Not stated	AROM	No	155.9°±12.9° (L) 156.0°±12.7° (R)
Gill et al[15]	131 M	35–39 years	Not stated	Not stated	AROM	No	153.4°±20.7° (L) 155.1°±21.3° (R)
Gill et al[15]	122 F	35–39 years	Not stated	Not stated	AROM	No	156.4°±13.0° (L) 158.8°±12.3° (R)
Gill et al[15]	140 M	40–44 years	Not stated	Not stated	AROM	No	151.6°±16.2° (L) 154.9°±14.3° (R)
Gill et al.[15]	125 F	40–44 years	Not stated	Not stated	AROM	No	152.5°±15.1° (L) 154.9°±15.4° (R)
Gill et al.[15]	113 M	45–49 years	Not stated	Not stated	AROM	No	152.4°±14.1° (L) 154.5°±14.0° (R)
Gill et al.[15]	105 F	45–49 years	Not stated	Not stated	AROM	No	148.5°±14.5° (L) 151.1°±14.9° (R)
Gill et al.[15]	94 M	50–54 years	Not stated	Not stated	AROM	No	154.6°±16.2° (L) 158.1°±15.9° (R)
Gill et al.[15]	89 F	50–54 years	Not stated	Not stated	AROM	No	149.3°±15.0° (L) 151.4°±16.9° (R)
Gill et al.[15]	86 M	55–59 years	Not stated	Not stated	AROM	No	146.5°±19.2° (L) 148.6°±18.8° (R)

Table B.9	INVESTIGATIONS REPORTING DATA FOR SHOULDER ABDUCTION ROM—cont'd						
STUDY	SAMPLE	AGES	METHOD USED	NO. OF EXAMINERS	TYPE OF MOTION	RELIABILITY COEFFICIENT CALCULATED?	ROM
Gill et al.[15]	86 F	55–59 years	Not stated	Not stated	AROM	No	146.2°±14.7° (L) 149.6°±13.7° (R)
Gill et al.[15]	58 M	60–64 years	Not stated	Not stated	AROM	No	145.0°±18.9° (L) 145.9°±18.1° (R)
Gill et al.[15]	55 F	60–64 years	Not stated	Not stated	AROM	No	138.2°±23.5° (L) 138.8°±26.5° (R)
Gill et al.[15]	62 M	65–69 years	Not stated	Not stated	AROM	No	135.7°±28.4° (L) 137.5°±28.9° (R)
Gill et al.[15]	61 F	65–69 years	Not stated	Not stated	AROM	No	140.5°±19.3° (L) 142.6°±17.7° (R)
Gill et al.[15]	49 M	70–74 years	Not stated	Not stated	AROM	No	134.8°±27.4° (L) 137.2°±21.7° (R)
Gill et al.[15]	54 F	70–74 years	Not stated	Not stated	AROM	No	131.8°±22.9° (L) 132.7°±30.9° (R)
Gill et al.[15]	52 M	75–79 years	Not stated	Not stated	AROM	No	134.2°±17.3° (L) 136.4°±18.1° (R)
Gill et al.[15]	46 F	75–79 years	Not stated	Not stated	AROM	No	127.8°±23.5° (L) 133.3°±26.2° (R)
Gill et al.[15]	31 M	80–84 years	Not stated	Not stated	AROM	No	125.0°±27.1° (L) 130.5°±22.8° (R)
Gill et al.[15]	51 F	80–84 years	Not stated	Not stated	AROM	No	115.0°±28.7° (L) 120.9° ± 26.5° (R)
Gill et al.[15]	10 M	85+ years	Not stated	Not stated	AROM	No	119.7°±22.2° (L) 118.9°±23.4° (R)
Gill et al.[15]	10 F	85+ years	Not stated	Not stated	AROM	No	118.9°±28.8° (L) 119.5°±35.3° (R)
Gûnal et al.[17]	1000 M/ Turkish	18–22 years	AAOS	2	PROM	No	166°±6° (R) 168°±19° (L)
Kalscheur et al.[18]	61 F	65–85 years	Supine	Not stated	AROM	No	155°±21° (R) 150°±22° (L)
Kalscheur et al.[18]	25 M	65–86 years	Supine	Not stated	AROM	No	131°±35° (R) 150°±22° (L)
Kolber et al.[19]	30 (12 M, 18 F)	25.9±3.1 years	Sitting; Digital inclinometer	2	AROM	ICC 0.91	172°±7°
Kolber and Hanney[20]	30 (21 F, 9 M)	26±4.2 years	Sitting; Digital inclinometer	1	AROM	ICC 0.97	162±11°
Kolber and Hanney[20]	30 (21 F, 9 M)	26±4.2 years	Sitting; Universal goniometer	1	AROM	ICC 0.97	161±11°
Macedo and Magee[21]	30*	18–29 years	Supine	1	PROM	ICC 0.84	91°±17°
Macedo and Magee[21]	20*	30–39 years	Supine	1	PROM	ICC 0.84	81°±18°
Macedo and Magee[21]	20*	40–49 years	Supine	1	PROM	ICC 0.84	81°±9°
Macedo and Magee[21]	20*	50–59 years	Supine	1	PROM	ICC 0.84	85°±27°
Macedo and Magee[21]	90*	18–59 years	Supine	1	PROM	ICC 0.84	85°±19°
McIntosh et al.[22]	20*	50–69 years	Sitting	1	AROM	No	151°±9°
McIntosh et al.[22]	20*	50–69 years	Sitting	1	PROM	No	155°±10°
McIntosh et al.[22]	21*	70+ years	Sitting	1	AROM	No	144°±10°
McIntosh et al.[22]	21*	70+ years	Sitting	1	PROM	No	148°±9°
Murray et al.[23]	10 F	25–35 years	AAOS	1	AROM	No	180°±1°
Murray et al.[23]	10 M	26–36 years	AAOS	1	AROM	No	178°±1°
Murray et al.[23]	10 F	60–64 years	AAOS	1	AROM	No	178°±1°
Murray et al.[23]	10 M	56–66 years	AAOS	1	AROM	No	178°±1°
Sabari et al.[24]	30*	17–92 years	Supine	1	AROM	ICC 0.99	162°±19°
Sabari et al.[24]	30*	17–92 years	Sitting	1	AROM	ICC 0.97	156°±17°
Sabari et al.[24]	30*	17–92 years	Supine	1	PROM	ICC 0.98	163°±17°
Sabari et al.[24]	30*	17–92 years	Sitting	1	PROM	ICC 0.95	158°±16°
Stubbs et al.[26]	55 M	25–54 years	AAOS	1	AROM	No	178°±11° (L) 176°±9° (R)
Valentine and Lewis[27]	45 (23 F, 22 M)	23–56 years	Standing; Inclinometer	1	AROM	ICC 0.93 ICC 0.91	167°±10° (R) 165°±10° (L)
Walker et al.[28]	60 (30 M, 30 F)	60–84 years	AAOS	1	AROM	Pearson's r > 0.81	165°±19°
Watanabe et al.[29]	339/Japanese*	Birth to 2 years	Not stated	Not stated	PROM	Unknown	177°–187°

AAOS, American Academy of Orthopaedic Surgeons; *AROM*, active range of motion; *D*, dominant; *F*, females; *ICC*, intraclass correlation; *M*, males; *ND*, nondominant; *PROM*, passive range of motion; *R*, right; *L*, left.
*Number of males and females not stated.

Table B.10 INVESTIGATIONS REPORTING DATA FOR INTERPHALANGEAL FLEXION (THUMB) ROM

STUDY	SAMPLE	AGES	METHOD USED	NO. OF EXAMINERS	TYPE OF MOTION	RELIABILITY COEFFICIENT CALCULATED?	ROM
De Smet et al.[31]	101 (58 M, 43 F)	16–83 years	Dorsal alignment of UG	Not stated	AROM	No	79°±10°
Hume et al.[32]	35 M	26–28 years	Lateral alignment	1	AROM	No	73°
Jenkins et al.[33]	119 (50 M, 69 F)	16–72 years	Elbow flexed to 90°; wrist/forearm neutral	1	AROM	No	67°±11°
Shaw and Morris[34]	348 (199 M, 149 F)	16–86 years	Not stated	Not stated	AROM	No	64°±13° (R) 65°±12° (L)

AROM, Active range of motion; *F*, females; *L*, left; *M*, males; *R*, right.

Table B.11 INVESTIGATIONS REPORTING DATA FOR THORACIC AND LUMBAR FLEXION ROM

STUDY	SAMPLE	AGES	INSTRUMENTATION	METHOD USED	NO. OF EXAMINERS	ROM	RELIABILITY COEFFICIENT CALCULATED?
Einkauf et al.[35]	109 F	20–84 years	Tape measure	Modified Schober	2	5–7±1 cm	Unknown correlation (inter) 0.98
Fitzgerald et al.[36]	172 (168 M, 4 F)	20–82 years	Tape measure	Schober	Not reported	2–4 cm	Pearson's r (inter) 1.0
Haley et al.[37]	282 (140 M, 142 F)	5–9 years	Tape measure	Modified Schober	1	6–7 cm±1 cm	ICC 0.83
Lindell et al.[38]	20 (6 M, 14 F)	22–55 years	Tape measure	Modified Schober	1	7 cm	ICC (intra) 0.87
Moll and Wright[39]	237 (119 M, 118 F)	15–75 years	Tape measure	Modified Schober	Not reported	5–7 cm±1 cm	No
van Adrichem and van der Korst[40]	66 (34 M, 32 F)	15–18 years	Tape measure	Modified Schober	Not reported	6 cm±1 cm	No
Chiarello and Savidge[41]	12 (4 M, 8 F)	23–35 years	Double inclinometer	—	3	59°±5°	ICC (inter) 0.74
Dillard et al.[42]	20 (10 M, 10 F)	20–40 years	Double inclinometer	—	1	63°±11°	Pearson's r 0.79
Mayer et al.[43]	13*	x̄=31 years	Double inclinometer	—	1	55°±9°	No
Ng et al.[44]	35 M	x̄=29.9±7.3 years	Double inclinometer		1	52°±9°	ICC (intra) 0.87
Breum et al.[45]	47 (27 M, 20 F)	18–38 years	BROM	—	1	56°±10°	ICC 0.63
Kachingwe and Phillips[46]	91 (30 M, 61 F)	x̄=28.0 years	BROM		2	33°±7°	ICC (intra) 0.84, 0.79

BROM, Back range of motion device; *F*, females; *ICC*, intraclass correlation; *M*, males.
*Number of males and females not stated.

Table B.12 INVESTIGATIONS REPORTING DATA FOR THORACIC AND LUMBAR EXTENSION ROM

STUDY	SAMPLE	AGES	INSTRUMENTATION	NO. OF EXAMINERS	ROM	RELIABILITY EFFICIENT CALCULATED?
Beattie et al.[47]	100 (63 M, 37 F)	20–76 years	Tape measure	1	.58–2.0 cm±0–1 cm	ICC 0.93
Einkauf et al.[35]	109 F	20–84 years	Goniometer	2	18°–36°	Unknown correlation (inter) 0.93
Fitzgerald et al.[36]	172 (168 M, 4 F)	20–82 years	Goniometer	Not reported	16°–41°	Pearson's r (inter) 0.88
Chiarello and Savidge[41]	12 (4 M, 8 F)	25–35 years	Double inclinometer	3	32°±10°	ICC (inter) 0.65
Dillard et al.[42]	20 (10 M, 10 F)	20–40 years	Double inclinometer	Not reported	29°±8°	Pearson's r 0.28
Mayer et al.[43]	13*	x̄=31 years	Double inclinometer	1	27°±13°	No
Ng et al.[44]	35 M	W=29.9±7.3 years	Double inclinometer	1	19°±9°	ICC (intra) 0.92
Breum et al.[45]	47 (27 M, 20 F)	18–38 years	BROM	1	22°±8°	ICC 0.35
Kachingwe and Phillips[46]	30 M, 61 F	x̄=28.0 years	BROM	2	10°±5°	ICC (intra) 0.60, 0.74

BROM, Back range of motion device; *F*, females; *ICC*, intraclass correlation; *M*, males.
*Number of males and females not stated.

Table B.13   INVESTIGATIONS REPORTING DATA FOR THORACIC AND LUMBAR LATERAL FLEXION ROM

STUDY	SAMPLE	AGES	INSTRUMENTATION	METHOD USED	NO. OF EXAMINERS	ROM	RELIABILITY COEFFICIENT CALCULATED?
Lindell et al.[38]	20 (6 M, 14 F)	22–55 years	Tape measure	Marks at lateral thigh	1	21 cm (R)	ICC 0.99 (R)
Rose[48]	18 (15 M, 3 F)	$\bar{x} = 19 \pm 4.6$ years	Tape measure	Marks at lateral thigh	1	23 cm ± 3 cm (R) 23 cm ± 3 cm (L)	Pearson's r 0.89 (R), 0.78 (L)
Einkauf et al.[35]	109 F	20–84 years	Goniometer	Thoracolumbar	2	24°–36° (R) 20°–33° (L)	Pearson's r (intra) 0.89 (R), 0.78 (L)
Fitzgerald et al.[36]	172 (168 M, 4 F)	20–82 years	Goniometer	Thoracolumbar	Not reported	18°–38° (R) 19°–39° (L)	Pearson's r (inter) 0.76 (R), 0.91 (L)
Dillard et al.[42]	20 (10 M, 10 F)	20–40 years	Single inclinometer	Lumbar	1	37° ± 8° (R) 37° ± 8° (L)	Pearson's r 0.59 (R), 0.62 (L)
Ng et al.[44]	35 M	$\bar{x} = 29.9 \pm 7.3$ years	Double inclinometer		1	31° ± 6° (R) 30° ± 6° (L)	ICC 0.96 (R), 0.92 (L)
Breum et al.[45]	47 (27 M, 20 F)	18–38 years	BROM	Lumbar	1	30° ± 6° (R) 33° ± 6° (L)	ICC 0.89 (R), 0.92 (L)
Kachingwe and Phillips[46]	91 (30 M, 61 F)	$\bar{x} = 28.0$ years	BROM		2	35° ± 7° (R) 35° ± 7° (L)	ICC 0.85, 0.84 (R) 0.83, 0.85 (L)

BROM, Back range of motion device; F, females; ICC, intraclass correlation; L, left; M, males, R, right.

Table B.14   INVESTIGATIONS REPORTING DATA FOR THORACIC AND LUMBAR ROTATION ROM

STUDY	SAMPLE	AGES	INSTRUMENTATION	METHOD USED	NO. OF EXAMINERS	ROM	RELIABILITY COEFFICIENT CALCULATED?
Dillard et al.[42]	20 (10 M, 10 F)	20–40 years	Double inclinometer	Standing	1	28° ± 5° (R) 29° ± 8° (L)	Pearson's r 0.64 (R), 0.40 (L)
Ng et al.[44]	35 M	$\bar{x} = 29.9 \pm 7.3$ years	Double inclinometer	Standing	1	32° ± 9° (R) 33° ± 9° (L)	ICC 0.96 (R), 0.95 (L)
Boline et al.[49]	25 (17 M, 8 F)	$\bar{x} = 33 \pm 4.1$ years	Single inclinometer	Flexed to horizontal and rotate	2	6° ± 3° (R) 6° ± 3° (L)	ICC (inter) 0.73
Breum et al.[45]	47 (27 M, 20 F)	18–38 years	BROM	Sitting	Not reported	8° ± 6° (R) 7° ± 4° (L)	ICC 0.57 (R), 0.56 (L)
Kachingwe and Phillips[46]	91 (30 M, 61 F)	$\bar{x} = 28.0$ years	BROM	Sitting	2	8° ± 4° (R) 7° ± 3° (L)	ICC 0.73 (R), 0.64 (L)

BROM, Back range of motion device; F, females; ICC, intraclass correlation; L, left; M, males; R, right.

Table B.15 INVESTIGATIONS REPORTING DATA FOR CERVICAL FLEXION ROM

STUDY	SAMPLE	AGES	INSTRUMENTATION	NO. OF EXAMINERS	ROM	RELIABILITY COEFFICIENT CALCULATED?
Audette et al.[50]	20 (9 M, 11 F)	$\bar{x}=37\pm15$ years	CROM	1	$40.2°\pm8.1°$	ICC (intra) 0.89
Capuano-Pucci et al.[51]	20 (4 M, 16 F)	$\bar{x}=23.5\pm3$ years	CROM	2	$50°\pm9°$ $53°\pm8°$	Pearson's r (intra) 0.63, 0.91
Fletcher and Bandy[52]	25 (8 M, 17 F)	$\bar{x}=26.0$ years	CROM	1	$53°\pm8°$	ICC (intra) 0.87
Nyland and Johnson[53]	119 M	$\bar{x}=15.7\pm1.4$ years	CROM	3	$56.2°\pm10°$	ICC (inter) 0.87–.96
Nyland and Johnson[53]	70 F	$\bar{x}=19.5\pm1.5$ years	CROM	3	$63.6°\pm13°$	ICC (inter) 0.87–.96
Ordway et al.[54]	20 (9 M, 11 F)	20–49 years	CROM	Not reported	$48°\pm13°$	No
Prushansky et al.[55]	30 (15 M, 15 F)	$\bar{x}=24.2\pm2.4$ years	CROM	1	$57.8°\pm8.6°$	ICC (intra) 0.91
Tousignant et al.[56]	20 (9 M, 11 F)	20–49 years	CROM	Not reported	$48°\pm13°$	No
Youdas et al.[7]	337 (166 M, 177 F)	11–97 years	CROM	5	$36°–64°\pm8°–11°$	ICC (intra) 0.23–.88
Balogun et al.[4]	21 (15 M, 6 F)	18–26 years	Tape measure	3	$4\,cm\pm2\,cm$	Pearson's r (intra) 0.26, 0.49, 0.48
Hsieh and Yeung[5]	34 (27 M, 7 F)	14–31 years	Tape measure	2	$4\,cm\pm2\,cm$	Pearson's r (intra) 0.26, 0.49, 0.48
Pringle et al.[57]	27 (19 M, 8 F)	$\bar{x}=27.6$ years	Goniometer	1	$39°\pm11°$	ICC (intra) 0.90
Pringle et al.[57]	27	$\bar{x}=27.6$ years	Inclinometer	1	$49°\pm12°$	ICC (intra) 0.87

CROM, Cervical; F, females; ICC, intraclass correlation; M, males.

Table B.16 INVESTIGATIONS REPORTING DATA FOR CERVICAL EXTENSION ROM

STUDY	SAMPLE	AGES	INSTRUMENTATION	NO. OF EXAMINERS	ROM	RELIABILITY COEFFICIENT CALCULATED?
Audette et al.[50]	20 (9 M, 11 F)	$\bar{x}=37\pm15$ years	CROM	1	$68.5°\pm14.5°$	ICC (intra) 0.91
Capuano-Pucci et al.[51]	20 (4 M, 16 F)	$\bar{x}=23.5\pm3$ years	CROM	2	$71°\pm9°$	Pearson's r (intra) 0.90, 0.82
Fletcher and Bandy[52]	25 (8 M, 17 F)	$\bar{x}=26.0$ years	CROM	1	$79°\pm13°$	ICC (intra) 0.90
Nyland and Johnson[53]	119 M	$\bar{x}=15.7\pm1.4$ years	CROM	3	$65.2°\pm11°$	ICC (inter) 0.92–.98
Nyland and Johnson[53]	70 F	$\bar{x}=19.5\pm1.5$ years	CROM	3	$70.7°\pm13°$	ICC (inter) 0.92–.98
Ordway et al.[54]	20 (9 M, 11 F)	20–49 years	CROM	Not reported	$79°\pm18°$	No
Prushansky et al.[55]	30 (15 M, 15 F)	$\bar{x}=24.2\pm2.4$ years	CROM	1	$69.6°\pm10.0°$	ICC (intra) 0.94
Tousignant et al.[56]	55 (21 M, 34 F)	19–85 years	CROM	1	$50.4°\pm14.4°$	No
Youdas et al.[7]	337 (166 M, 177 F)	11–97 years	CROM	5	$52°–86°\pm10°–18°$	ICC (intra) 0.89–.96
Balogun et al.[4]	21 (15 M, 6 F)	18–26 years	Tape measure	3	$19\,cm\pm2\,cm$	Pearson's r (intra) 0.72, 0.87, 0.88
Hsieh and Yeung[5]	34 (27 M, 7 F)	14–31 years	Tape measure	2	$22\,cm\pm2\,cm$	Pearson's r (intra) 0.79, 0.94
Pringle et al.[57]	27*	$\bar{x}=27.6$ years	Goniometer	1	$35°\pm10°$	ICC (intra) 0.90
Pringle et al.[57]	27*	$\bar{x}=27.6$ years	Inclinometer	1	$58°\pm1.5°$	ICC (intra) 0.87

CROM, Cervical range of motion device; F, females; ICC, intraclass correlation; M, males.
*Number of males and females not stated.

Table B.17   INVESTIGATIONS REPORTING DATA FOR CERVICAL LATERAL FLEXION ROM

STUDY	SAMPLE	AGES	INSTRUMENTATION	NO. OF EXAMINERS	ROM	RELIABILITY COEFFICIENT CALCULATED?
Audette et al.[50]	20 (9 M, 11 F)	$\bar{x}=37\pm15$ years	CROM	1	$32.8°\pm9.0°$ (R) $35.8°\pm10.0°$ (L)	ICC (intra) 0.92 ICC (intra) 0.95
Capuano-Pucci et al.[51]	20 (4 M, 16 F)	$\bar{x}=23.5\pm3$ years	CROM	2	$43°\pm7°$ (R) $44°\pm8°$ (L)	Pearson's r (intra) 0.79, 0.90
Fletcher and Bandy[52]	25 (8 M, 17 F)	$\bar{x}=26.0$ years	CROM	1	$42°\pm9°$ (R) $47°\pm9°$ (L)	ICC 0.92 (R) ICC 0.92 (L)
Nyland and Johnson[53]	119 M	$\bar{x}=15.7\pm1.4$ years	CROM	3	$42.6°\pm8°$ (R) $42.3°\pm9°$ (L)	ICC (inter) 0.89–.94
Nyland and Johnson[53]	70 F	$\bar{x}=19.5\pm1.5$ years	CROM	3	$44.7°\pm8°$ (R) $46.8°\pm8°$ (L)	ICC (inter) 0.89–.94
Prushansky et al.[55]	30 (15 M, 15 F)	$\bar{x}=24.2\pm2.4$ years	CROM	1	$43.3°\pm5.9°$ (R) $42.7°\pm5.7°$ (L)	ICC (intra) 0.90 ICC (intra) 0.82
Tousignant et al.[56]	55 (21 M, 34 F)	19–85 years	CROM	1	$30.4°\pm9.1°$ (R) $32.8°\pm8.6°$ (L)	No
Youdas et al.[7]	337 (166 M, 177 F)	11–97 years	CROM	5	$22°–49°$ (R) $22°–47°$ (L)	ICC (intra) 0.60–0.94
Balogun et al.[4]	21 (15 M, 6 F)	18–26 years	Tape measure	3	13 cm $\pm$ 2 cm (R) 13 cm $\pm$ 2 cm (L)	Pearson's r (infra) 0.53, 0.77
Hsieh and Yeung[5]	34 (27 M, 7 F)	14–31 years	Tape measure	2	12 cm $\pm$ 2 cm (R)	Pearson's r (intra) 0.86, 0.91
Pringle et al.[57]	27	$\bar{x}=27.6$ years	Goniometer	1	$42°\pm11°$ (R) $44°\pm11°$ (L)	ICC 0.97 (Combined)
Pringle et al.[57]	27	$\bar{x}=27.6$ years	Inclinometer	1	$47°\pm9°$ (R)	ICC 0.83 (Combined)

CROM, Cervical range of motion device; *F*, females; *ICC*, intraclass correlation; *L*, left; *M*, males; *R*, right.

Table B.18   INVESTIGATIONS REPORTING DATA FOR CERVICAL ROTATION ROM

STUDY	SAMPLE	AGES	INSTRUMENTATION	NO. OF EXAMINERS	ROM	RELIABILITY COEFFICIENT CALCULATED?
Audette et al.[50]	20 (9 M, 11 F)	$\bar{x}=37\pm15$ years	CROM	1	$58.0°\pm9.0°$ (R) $60.2°\pm9.3°$ (L)	ICC (intra) 0.97 ICC (intra) 0.97
Capuano-Pucci et al.[51]	20 (4 M, 16 F)	$\bar{x}=23.5\pm3$ years	CROM	2	$70°\pm7°$ (R) $69°\pm7°$ (L)	Pearson's r (intra) .69 0.62, 0.89
Fletcher and Bandy[52]	25 (8 M, 17 F)	$\bar{x}=26.0$ years	CROM	1	$73°\pm7°$ (R) $75°\pm9°$ (L)	ICC 0.90 (R) ICC 0.94 (L)
Nyland and Johnson[53]	119 M	$\bar{x}=15.7\pm1.4$ years	CROM	3	$67.3°\pm9°$ (R) $66.6°\pm9°$ (L)	ICC (inter) 0.91–0.93
Nyland and Johnson[53]	70 F	$\bar{x}=19.5\pm1.5$ years	CROM	3	$68.5°\pm11°$ (R) $71.8°\pm10°$ (L)	ICC (inter) 0.91–.093
Prushansky et al.[55]	30 (15 M, 15 F)	$\bar{x}=24.2\pm2.4$ years	CROM	1	$76.8°\pm5.6°$ (R) $78.2°\pm4.8°$ (L)	ICC (intra) 0.92 ICC (intra) 0.84
Tousignant et al.[56]	55 (21 M, 34 F)	19–85 years	CROM	1	$55.6°\pm10.3°$ (R) $56.1°\pm11.7°$ (L)	No
Youdas et al.[7]	337 (166 M, 177 F)	11–97 years	CROM	5	$44°–75°$ (R) $45°–72°$ (L)	ICC (intra) 0.58–0.99
Balogun et al.[4]	21 (15 M, 6 F)	18–26 years	Tape measure	3	11 cm $\pm$ 3 cm (R) 11 cm $\pm$ 2 cm (L)	Pearson's r (intra) 0.59–0.86
Hsieh and Yeung[5]	34 (27 M, 7 F)	14–31 years	Tape measure	2	11 cm $\pm$ 2 cm (R) 11 cm $\pm$ 2 cm (L)	Pearson's r (intra) 0.78, 0.88
Pringle et al.[57]	27*	$\bar{x}=27.6$ years	Goniometer	1	$70°\pm19°$ (R) $70°\pm16°$ (L)	ICC 0.97 (Combined)
Pringle et al.[57]	27*	$\bar{x}=27.6$ years	Inclinometer	1	$84°\pm13°$ (R) $84°\pm11°$ (L)	ICC 0.92 (Combined)

CROM, Cervical range of motion device; *F*, females; *ICC*, intraclass correlation; *L*, left; *M*, males; *R*, right.
*Number of males and females not stated.

Table B.19 INVESTIGATIONS REPORTING DATA FOR HIP EXTENSION ROM

STUDY	SAMPLE	AGES	METHOD USED	NO. OF EXAMINERS	TYPE OF MOTION	RELIABILITY COEFFICIENT CALCULATED?	ROM
Ahlberg et al.[58]	50 M/Saudi Arabian	30–40 years	AAOS	1	PROM	No	14°±6°
Boone and Azen[9]	53 M	1–19 years	AAOS	1	AROM	No	7°±7°
Boone and Azen[9]	56 M	20–54 years	AAOS	1	AROM	No	12°±6°
Broughton et al.[59]	57*	Neonates; 1–7 days	Not sufficiently described	1	PROM	No	−34°±6°
Broughton et al.[59]	57*	3 months	Not sufficiently described	1	PROM	No	−19°±6°
Broughton et al.[59]	57*	6 months	Not sufficiently described	1	PROM	No	−8°±6°
Chevillotte et al.[60]	20*	21–87 years	Lateral decubitus position	5	PROM	No	0°±.6°
Coon et al.[61]	44 (25 M, 19 F)	6 weeks	Supine, contralateral hip flexed	1	PROM	No	−19°±6°
Coon et al.[61]	44 (25 M, 19 F)	3 months	Supine, contralateral hip flexed	1	PROM	No	−7°±4°
Coon et al.[61]	40 (19 M, 21 F)	6 months	Supine, contralateral hip flexed	1	PROM	No	−7°±4°
Drews et al.[62]	54 (26 M, 28 F)	12 h–6 days	Sidelying, contralateral hip flexed	2	PROM	Pearson's r (inter) 56 (L) 0.74 (R)	−28°±6°
Forero et al.[63]	60 (34 M, 26 F) (42 Hispanic, 15 white, 3 black)	1–3 days	Supine, contralateral hip flexed	1	PROM	Pearson's r 0.99	−30°±4°
Haas et al.[64]	400 (192 M, 208 F) / (200 white, 200 black)	1 h–3 days	Supine, contralateral hip flexed	2	PROM	No	−30°±8°
Macedo and Magee[21]	30*	18–29 years	Prone	1	PROM	ICC 0.82	14°±5°
Macedo and Magee[21]	20*	30–39 years	Prone	1	PROM	ICC 0.82	14°±4°
Macedo and Magee[21]	20*	40–49 years	Prone	1	PROM	ICC 0.82	13°±5°
Macedo and Magee[21]	20*	50–59 years	Prone	1	PROM	ICC 0.82	13°±4°
Macedo and Magee[21]	90*	18–59 years	Prone	1	PROM	ICC 0.82	13°±5°
Moreside and McGill[65]	77 M	22.8±3.2 years	Modified Thomas test	1	PROM	No	4°
Moreside and McGill[65]	22 M	22.8±3.2 years	Prone	1	PROM	No	−10°
Mudge et al.[66]	53 (15 M, 38 F)	4–16 years	Modified Thomas test using standardized pelvic position	3	PROM	No	13°±5°
Mundale et al.[67]	36 (16 M, 20 F)	20–30 years	Mundale technique	Not stated	PROM	95% within ±4°	−11°
Phelps et al.[68]	25*	9 months	Prone, both hips flexed over end of table	1	PROM	No	−10°±3°
Phelps et al.[68]	25*	12 months	Prone, both hips flexed over end of table	1	PROM	No	−9°±5°
Phelps et al.[68]	18*	18 months	Prone, both hips flexed over end of table	1	PROM	No	−4°±3°
Phelps et al.[68]	18*	24 months	Prone, both hips flexed over end of table	1	PROM	No	−3°±3°
Prather et al.[69]	28 (10 M, 18 F)	18–51 years	Prone	2	PROM	ICC 0.44	16.5°±6°
Roaas and Anderson[70]	105 M (210 hips)/Swedish	30–40 years	AAOS, 1965; contralateral hip flexed	1	PROM	No	9°±5° (R) 10°±5° (L)
Roach and Miles[71]	433 (200 M, 233 F) / (346 white, 87 black)	25–39 years	Prone, with knee extended	1	AROM	"Satisfactory level of reproducibility not achieved."	22°±8°
Roach and Miles[71]	727 (368 M, 359 F) / (565 white, 162 black)	40–59 years	Prone, with knee extended	1	AROM	"Satisfactory level of reproducibility not achieved."	18°±7°

Study	Sample	Age	Position	No.	ROM	Reproducibility	ROM value
Roach and Miles[71]	523 (253 M, 270 F)/(402 white, 121 black)	60–74 years	Prone, with knee extended	1		"Satisfactory level of reproducibility not achieved."	17° ±8°
Sankar et al.[72]	41 M	2–5 years	Prone	2	PROM	ICC 0.81	21° ±5°
Sankar et al.[72]	22 F	2–5 years	Prone	2	PROM	ICC 0.81	21° ±5°
Sankar et al.[72]	67 M	6–10 years	Prone	2	PROM	ICC 0.81	19° ±4°
Sankar et al.[72]	39 F	6–10 years	Prone	2	PROM	ICC 0.81	21° ±5°
Sankar et al.[72]	55 M	11–17 years	Prone	2	PROM	ICC 0.81	15° ±5°
Sankar et al.[72]	28 F	11–17 years	Prone	2	PROM	ICC 0.81	22° ± 3°
Soucie et al.[25]	39 F	2–8 years	Sidelying	9	PROM	No	26.2°
Soucie et al.[25]	55 M	2–8 years	Sidelying	9	PROM	No	28.3°
Soucie et al.[25]	56 F	9–19 years	Sidelying	9	PROM	No	20.5°
Soucie et al.[25]	48 M	9–19 years	Sidelying	9	PROM	No	18.2°
Soucie et al.[25]	143 F	20–44 years	Sidelying	9	PROM	No	18.1°
Soucie et al.[25]	114 M	20–44 years	Sidelying	9	PROM	No	17.4°
Soucie et al.[25]	123 F	45–69 years	Sidelying	9	PROM	No	16.7°
Soucie et al.[25]	96 M	45–69 years	Sidelying	9	PROM	No	13.5°
Svenningsen et al.[73]	103 (51 M, 52 F)	4 years	AAOS	1	PROM	No	29°
Svenningsen et al.[73]	102 (50 M, 52 F)	6 years	AAOS	1	PROM	No	26°
Svenningsen et al.[73]	104 (52 M, 52 F)	8 years	AAOS	1	PROM	No	27°
Svenningsen et al.[73]	134 (65 M, 69 F)	11 years	AAOS	1	PROM	No	25°
Svenningsen et al.[73]	114 (57 M, 57 F)	15 years	AAOS	1	PROM	No	26°
Svenningsen et al.[73]	206 (102 M, 104 F)	Adult; x̄=23 years	AAOS	1	PROM	No	24°
Walker et al.[28]	60 (30 M, 30 F)	60–84 years	AAOS	1	AROM	Pearson's r > .81	−11° ±4°
Watanabe et al.[29]	62/Japanese*	Neonates	Not stated	Not stated	PROM	Unknown	−25°
Watanabe et al.[29]	62/Japanese*	4 weeks	Not stated	Not stated	PROM	Unknown	−12°
Watanabe et al.[29]	54/Japanese*	4–8 months	Not stated	Not stated	PROM	Unknown	−4°
Watanabe et al.[29]	45/Japanese*	8–12 months	Not stated	Not stated	PROM	Unknown	3°
Watanabe et al.[29]	64/Japanese*	1 years	Not stated	Not stated	PROM	Unknown	15°
Watanabe et al.[29]	64/Japanese*	2 years	Not stated	Not stated	PROM	Unknown	21°
Waugh et al.[74]	40 (18 M, 22 F)	9 months	Prone, both hips flexed over end of table	1	PROM	No	−10° ±3°

AAOS, American Academy of Orthopaedic Surgeons; *AROM*, active range of motion; *F*, females; *M*, males; *PROM*, passive range of motion;
*Number of males and females not stated.

Table B.20　INVESTIGATIONS REPORTING DATA FOR HIP LATERAL ROTATION ROM

STUDY	SAMPLE	AGES	METHOD USED	NO. OF EXAMINERS	TYPE OF MOTION	RELIABILITY COEFFICIENT CALCULATED?	ROM
Ahlberg et al.[58]	50 M/Saudi Arabian	30–40 years	AAOS	1	PROM	No	73°±11°
Bennell et al.[75]	40 F	10 years	Supine, knee flexed to 90°; inclinometer	4	AROM	No	37°±10°
Bennell et al.[75]	40 F	11 years	Supine, knee flexed to 90°; inclinometer	4	AROM	No	47°±10°
Boone and Azen[9]	53 M	1–19 years	AAOS-seated	1	AROM	No	51°±6°
Boone and Azen[9]	56 M	20–54 years	AAOS-seated	1	AROM	No	44°±5°
Chevillotte et al.[60]	20*	21–87 years	Supine, with knees flexed 90°	5	PROM	ICC 0.45	34°±10°
Coon et al.[61]	44 (25 M, 19 F)	6 weeks	Prone, hip extended, knee flexed to 90°	1	PROM	No	48°±11°
Coon et al.[61]	44 (25 M, 19 F)	3 months	Prone, hip extended, knee flexed to 90°	1	PROM	No	45°±5°
Drews et al.[62]	54 (26 M, 28 F)	12 h–6 days	Supine, hip and knee flexed to 90°; contralateral hip and knee extended; stationary arm-parallel anterior midline of trunk; moving arm-tibial crest axis-midpatella	2	PROM	Pearson's r (inter) 0.63 (L) 0.79 (R)	114°±10°
Ellison et al.[76]	100 (25 M, 75 F)	20–41 years	Prone, knee flexed to 90°	1	PROM	ICC 0.96	36°±8° (R) 35°±7° (L)
Forero et al.[63]	60 (34 M, 26 F) (42 Hispanic, 15 white, 3 black)	1–3 days	Supine, hip/knee flexed to 90°	1	PROM	Pearson's r 0.99	92°±3°
Giladi et al.[77]	295 males	18–20 years	AAOS, hip flexed to 90°	Not stated	Not stated	No	57°±9°
Haas et al.[64]	400 (192 M, 208 F) / (200 white, 200 black)	1 h–3 days	Supine, hips and knees flexed to 90°	2	PROM	No	89°±14°
Haley[78]	50 F	21–50 years	Seated, hip and knee flexed to 90°	1	AROM	No	33°±5°
Haley[78]	50 F	21–50 years	Seated, hip and knee flexed to 90°	1	PROM	No	45°±5°
Haley[78]	50 F	21–50 years	Supine, hip extended	1	AROM	No	31°±6°
Haley[78]	50 F	21–50 years	Supine, hip extended	1	PROM	No	43°±5°
Hoaglund et al.[79]	211 (112 M, 99 F)/Chinese	55–85+ years	Hip flexed to 90°	1	PROM (according to photo; not stated)	No	62°±13°
Hoaglund et al.[79]	211 (112 M, 99 F)/Chinese	55–85+ years	Hip neutral flexion/extension	1	PROM (according to photo; not stated)	No	53°±9°
Kouyoumdjian et al.[80]	120*	22–60 years	Supine, hip and knee flexed 90°	1	PROM	No	38.5°±8.7°
Kouyoumdjian et al.[80]	120*	22–60 years	Prone, hip and knee flexed 90°	1	PROM	No	41.8°±10.2°
Kouyoumdjian et al.[80]	120*	22–60 years	Seated with knee flexed 90°	1	PROM	No	40.7°±7.6°
Macedo and Magee[21]	30*	18–29 years	Seated, hips and knees flexed 90° with 0° hip abduction	1	PROM	ICC 0.90	38°±7°
Macedo and Magee[21]	20*	30–39 years	Seated, hips and knees flexed 90° with 0° hip abduction	1	PROM	ICC 0.90	36°±6°
Macedo and Magee[21]	20*	40–49 years	Seated, hips and knees flexed 90° with 0° hip abduction	1	PROM	ICC 0.90	33°±7°
Macedo and Magee[21]	20*	50–59 years	Seated, hips and knees flexed 90° with 0° hip abduction	1	PROM	ICC 0.90	32°±6°
Macedo and Magee[21]	90*	18–59 years	Seated, hips and knees flexed 90° with 0° hip abduction	1	PROM	ICC 0.90	35°±7°
McKay et al.[81]	70 M	3–9 years	Not stated	2	AROM	ICC 0.80–99	32°±8.1°
McKay et al.[81]	70 F	3–9 years	Not stated	2	AROM	ICC 0.80–99	32°±9.2°
McKay et al.[81]	80 M	10–19 years	Not stated	2	AROM	ICC 0.80–99	31°±6.4°
McKay et al.[81]	80 F	10–19 years	Not stated	2	AROM	ICC 0.80–99	31°±9.1°
McKay et al.[81]	200 M	20–59 years	Not stated	2	AROM	ICC 0.80–99	30°±8.3°
McKay et al.[81]	200 F	20–59 years	Not stated	2	AROM	ICC 0.80–99	27°±8.3°

Study	Sample	Age	Position/Method	No.	Type	Reliability	Value
McKay et al.[81]	150 M	60+ years	Not stated	2	AROM	ICC 0.80–99	26° ±7.0°
McKay et al.[81]	150 F	60+ years	Not stated	2	AROM	ICC 0.80–99	22° ±6.7°
Moreside and McGill[65]	77 M	22.8 ±3.2 years	Prone with knee flexed 90° using Vicon MX Motion System	1	PROM	No	50°
Moreside and McGill[65]	22 M	22.8 ±3.2 years	Prone with knee flexed 90° using UG	1	PROM	No	44°
Mudge et al.[66]	53 (15 M, 38 F)	4–16 years	Prone with ipsilateral knee flexed to 90°	3	PROM	No	48° ±11°
Phelps et al.[68]	25*	9 months	Prone, hip extended, knee flexed to 90°	1	PROM	No	56° ±7°
Phelps et al.[68]	25*	12 months	Prone, hip extended, knee flexed to 90°	1	PROM	No	58° ±9°
Phelps et al.[68]	18*	18 months	Prone, hip extended, knee flexed to 90°	1	PROM	No	52° ±9°
Phelps et al.[68]	18*	24 months	Prone, hip extended, knee flexed to 90°	1	PROM	No	47° ±9°
Prather et al.[69]	28 (10 M, 18 F)	18–51 years	Prone with knee flexed to 90°	2	PROM	ICC 0.18	39.8° ±9°
Prather et al.[69]	28 (10 M, 18 F)	18–51 years	Supine with knee flexed 90°	2	PROM	ICC 0.63	47.4° ±13°
Roaas and Anderson[70]	105 M (210 hips)/Swedish	30–40 years	AAOS	1	PROM	No	34° ±7°
Roach and Miles[71]	433 (200 M, 233 F)/(346 white, 87 black)	25–39 years	Seated, hip and knee flexed to 90°	1	AROM	"Satisfactory level of reproducibility not achieved"	34° ±8°
Roach and Miles[71]	727 (368 M, 359 F)/(565 white, 162 black)	40–59 years	Seated, hip and knee flexed to 90°	1	AROM	"Satisfactory level of reproducibility not achieved"	32° ±8°
Roach and Miles[71]	523 (253 M, 270 F)/(402 white, 121 black)	60–74 years	Seated, hip and knee flexed to 90°	1	AROM	"Satisfactory level of reproducibility not achieved"	29°
Sankar et al.[72]	41 M	2–5 years	Supine, hip and knee flexed to 90°	2	PROM	ICC 0.81	51° ±11°
Sankar et al.[72]	22 F	2–5 years	Supine, hip and knee flexed to 90°	2	PROM	ICC 0.81	49° ±12°
Sankar et al.[72]	67 M	6–10 years	Supine, hip and knee flexed to 90°	2	PROM	ICC 0.81	44° ±11°
Sankar et al.[72]	39 F	6–10 years	Supine, hip and knee flexed to 90°	2	PROM	ICC 0.81	48° ±5°
Sankar et al.[72]	55 M	11–17 years	Supine, hip and knee flexed to 90°	2	PROM	ICC 0.81	40° ±12°
Sankar et al.[72]	28 F	11–17 years	Supine, hip and knee flexed to 90°	2	PROM	ICC 0.81	46° ±3°
Simoneau et al.[82]	60 (21 M, 39 F)	18–27 years	Seated, hip and knee flexed to 90°	6	AROM	ICC (inter) 0.90	36° ±8°
Simoneau et al.[82]	60 (21 M, 39 F)	18–27 years	Seated, hip and knee flexed to 90°	6	AROM	ICC (inter) 0.93	45° ±11°
Svenningsen et al.[73]	103 (51 M, 52 F)	4 years	AAOS	1	PROM	No	46°
Svenningsen et al.[73]	102 (50 M, 52 F)	6 years	AAOS	1	PROM	No	45°
Svenningsen et al.[73]	104 (52 M, 52 F)	8 years	AAOS	1	PROM	No	43°
Svenningsen et al.[73]	134 (65 M, 69 F)	11 years	AAOS	1	PROM	No	42°
Svenningsen et al.[73]	114 (57 M, 57 F)	15 years	AAOS	1	PROM	No	43°
Svenningsen et al.[73]	206 (102 M, 104 F)	Adult; x̄ = 23 years	AAOS	1	PROM	No	42°
Walker et al.[28]	60 (30 M, 30 F)	60–84 years	AAOS	1	AROM	Pearson's r > .81	32° ±6°
Watanabe et al.[29]	62/Japanese*	Neonates	Not stated	Not stated	PROM	Unknown	77°
Watanabe et al.[29]	62/Japanese*	4 weeks	Not stated	Not stated	PROM	Unknown	66°
Watanabe et al.[29]	54/Japanese*	4–8 months	Not stated	Not stated	PROM	Unknown	66°
Watanabe et al.[29]	45/Japanese*	8–12 months	Not stated	Not stated	PROM	Unknown	79°
Watanabe et al.[29]	64/Japanese*	1 years	Not stated	Not stated	PROM	Unknown	74°
Watanabe et al.[29]	57/Japanese*	2 years	Not stated	Not stated	PROM	Unknown	58°

AAOS, American Academy of Orthopaedic Surgeons; *AROM*, active range of motion; *F*, females; *ICC*, intraclass correlation; *M*, males; *PROM*, passive range of motion.
*Number of males and females not stated.

Table B.21 INVESTIGATIONS REPORTING DATA FOR HIP MEDIAL ROTATION ROM

STUDY	SAMPLE	AGES	METHOD USED	NO. OF EXAMINERS	TYPE OF MOTION	RELIABILITY COEFFICIENT CALCULATED?	ROM
Ahlberg et al.[58]	50 M/Saudi Arabian	30–40 years	AAOS	1	PROM	No	37°±12°
Bennell et al.[75]	40 F	10 years	Supine, knee flexed to 90°; inclinometer	4	AROM	No	36°±9°
Bennell et al.[75]	40 F	11 years	Supine, knee flexed to 90°; inclinometer	4	AROM	No	37°±12°
Boone and Azen[9]	53 M	1–19 years	AAOS-seated	1	AROM	No	50°±6°
Boone and Azen[9]	56 M	20–54 years	AAOS-seated	1	AROM	No	44°±4°
Chevillotte et al.[60]	20*	21–87 years	Supine, with knees flexed 90°	5	PROM	ICC 0.43	19°±9°
Coon et al.[61]	44 (25 M, 19 F)	6 weeks	Prone, hip extended, knee flexed to 90°	1	PROM	No	24°±5°
Coon et al.[61]	44 (25 M, 19 F)	3 months	Prone, hip extended, knee flexed to 90°	1	PROM	No	26°±3°
Coon et al.[61]	40 (19 M, 21 F)	6 months	Prone, hip extended, knee flexed to 90°	1	PROM	No	21°±4°
Drews et al.[62]	54 (26 M, 28 F)	12 h–6 days	Supine, hip and knee flexed to 90°; contralateral hip and knee extended; stationary arm-parallel anterior midline of trunk; moving arm-tibial crest axis-midpatella	2	PROM	Pearson's r (inter) 0.63 (L) 0.79 (R)	80°±9°
Ellison et al.[76]	100 (25 M, 75 F)	20–41 years	Prone, knee flexed to 90°	1	PROM	ICC 0.96	38°±11° (R) 38°±11° (L)
Forero et al.[63]	60 (34 M, 26 F) (42 Hispanic, 15 white, 3 black)	1–3 days	Supine, hip/knee flexed to 90°	1	PROM	Pearson's r 0.99	76°±6°
Giladi et al.[77]	295 males	18–20 years	AAOS, hip flexed to 90°	Not stated	Not stated	No	53°±11°
Haas et al.[64]	400 (192 M, 208 F)/ (200 white, 200 black)	1 h–3 days	Supine, hips and knees flexed to 90°	2	PROM	No	62°±13°
Haley[78]	50 F	21–50 years	Seated, hip and knee flexed to 90°	1	AROM	No	37°±7°
Haley[78]	50 F	21–50 years	Seated, hip and knee flexed to 90°	1	PROM	No	45°±5°
Haley[78]	50 F	21–50 years	Supine, hip extended	1	AROM	No	26°±5°
Haley[78]	50 F	21–50 years	Supine, hip extended	1	PROM	No	38°±6°
Hoaglund et al.[79]	112 M	55–85+ years	Hip flexed to 90°	1	PROM (according to photo; not stated)	No	22°±8°
Hoaglund et al.[79]	99 F	55–85+ years	Hip flexed to 90°	1	PROM (according to photo; not stated)	No	31°±10°
Hoaglund et al.[79]	112 M	55–85+ years	Hip neutral flexion/extension	1	PROM (according to photo; not stated)	No	29°±11°
Hoaglund et al.[79]	99 F	55–85+ years	Hip neutral flexion/extension	1	PROM	No	37°±8°
Kouyoumdjian et al.[80]	120*	22–60 years	Supine, hip and knee flexed 90°	1	PROM	No	29.6°±9°
Kouyoumdjian et al.[80]	120*	22–60 years	Prone, hip and knee flexed 90°	1	AROM	No	35.3°±11.9°
Kouyoumdjian et al.[80]	120*	22–60 years	Seated with knee flexed 90°	1	PROM	No	37.9°±8.4°
Macedo and Magee[21]	30*	18–29 years	Seated, hips and knees flexed 90° with 0° hip abduction	1	PROM	ICC 0.91	43°±7
Macedo and Magee[21]	20*	30–39 years	Seated, hips and knees flexed 90° with 0° hip abduction	1	PROM	ICC 0.91	41°±7
Macedo and Magee[21]	20*	40–49 years	Seated, hips and knees flexed 90° with 0° hip abduction	1	PROM	ICC 0.91	42°±7
Macedo and Magee[21]	20*	50–59 years	Seated, hips and knees flexed 90° with 0° hip abduction	1	PROM	ICC 0.91	41°±7
Macedo and Magee[21]	90*	18–59 years	Seated, hips and knees flexed 90° with 0° hip abduction	1	PROM	ICC 0.91	42°±7
McKay et al.[81]	70 M	3–9 years	Not stated	2	AROM	ICC 0.80–.99	40°±8.4°
McKay et al.[81]	70 F	3–9 years	Not stated	2	AROM	ICC 0.80–.99	43°±9.1°
McKay et al.[81]	80 M	10–19 years	Not stated	2	AROM	ICC 0.80–.99	37°±9.3°

Study	Sample	Age	Testing position	Trials	AROM/PROM	Reliability	Mean ± SD
McKay et al.[81]	80 F	10–19 years	Not stated	2	AROM	ICC 0.80–.99	39° ± 7.7°
McKay et al.[81]	200 M	20–59 years	Not stated	2	AROM	ICC 0.80–.99	36° ± 7.9°
McKay et al.[81]	200 F	20–59 years	Not stated	2	AROM	ICC 0.80–.99	40° ± 8.8°
McKay et al.[81]	150 M	60+ years	Not stated	2	AROM	ICC 0.80–.99	33° ± 8.0°
McKay et al.[81]	150 F	60+ years	Not stated	2	AROM	ICC 0.80–.99	35° ± 8.4°
Moreside and McGill[65]	77 M	22.8 ± 3.2 years	Prone with knee flexed 90° using Vicon MX Motion System	1	PROM	No	42°
Moreside and McGill[65]	22 M	22.8 ± 3.2 years	Prone with knee flexed 90° using UG	1	PROM	No	46°
Mudge et al.[66]	53 (15 M, 38 F)	4–16 years	Prone with ipsilateral knee flexed to 90°	3	PROM	No	41° ± 8°
Phelps et al.[68]	25*	9 months	Prone, hip extended, knee flexed to 90°	1	PROM	No	44° ± 9°
Phelps et al.[68]	25*	12 months	Prone, hip extended, knee flexed to 90°	1	PROM	No	45° ± 8°
Phelps et al.[68]	18*	18 months	Prone, hip extended, knee flexed to 90°	1	PROM	No	52° ± 10°
Phelps et al.[68]	18*	24 months	Prone, hip extended, knee flexed to 90°	1	PROM	No	33° ± 8°
Prather et al.[69]	28 (10 M, 18 F)	18–51 years	Prone with knee flexed to 90°	2	PROM	ICC 0.79	30.6° ± 12°
Prather et al.[69]	28 (10 M, 18 F)	18–51 years	Supine with knee flexed 90°	2	PROM	ICC 0.75	28.2° ± 11°
Roaas and Anderson[70]	105 M (210 hips)/Swedish	30–40 years	AAOS	1	PROM	No	58° ± 12°
Roach and Miles[71]	433 (200 M, 233 F)/(346 white, 87 black)	25–39 years	Seated, hip and knee flexed to 90°	1	AROM	"Satisfactory level of reproducibility not achieved"	33° ± 7°
Roach and Miles[71]	727 (368 M, 359 F) (565 white, 162 black)	40–59 years	Seated, hip and knee flexed to 90°	1	AROM	"Satisfactory level of reproducibility not achieved"	31° ± 8°
Roach and Miles[71]	523 (253 M, 270 F)/(402 white, 121 black)	60–74 years	Seated, hip and knee flexed to 90°	1	AROM	"Satisfactory level of reproducibility not achieved"	30° ± 7°
Sankar et al.[72]	41 M	2–5 years	Supine, hip and knee flexed to 90°	2	PROM	ICC 0.81	45° ± 13°
Sankar et al.[72]	22 F	2–5 years	Supine, hip and knee flexed to 90°	2	PROM	ICC 0.81	47° ± 11°
Sankar et al.[72]	67 M	6–10 years	Supine, hip and knee flexed to 90°	2	PROM	ICC 0.81	40° ± 10°
Sankar et al.[72]	39 F	6–10 years	Supine, hip and knee flexed to 90°	2	PROM	ICC 0.81	41° ± 11°
Sankar et al.[72]	55 M	11–17 years	Supine, hip and knee flexed to 90°	2	PROM	ICC 0.81	35° ± 11°
Sankar et al.[72]	28 F	11–17 years	Supine, hip and knee flexed to 90°	2	PROM	ICC 0.81	35° ± 10°
Simoneau et al.[82]	39 F	18–27 years	Seated, hip and knee flexed to 90°	6	AROM	ICC (inter) 0.91	35° ± 6°
Simoneau et al.[82]	21 M	18–27 years	Seated, hip and knee flexed to 90°	6	AROM	ICC (inter) 0.91	30° ± 7°
Simoneau et al.[82]	39 F	18–27 years	Prone, hip extended, knee flexed to 90°	6	AROM	ICC (inter) 0.94	38° ± 9°
Simoneau et al.[82]	21 M	18–27 years	Prone, hip extended, knee flexed to 90°	6	AROM	ICC (inter) 0.94	32° ± 9°
Svenningsen et al.[73]	103 (51 M, 52 F)	4 years	AAOS	1	PROM	No	56°
Svenningsen et al.[73]	102 (50 M, 52 F)	6 years	AAOS	1	PROM	No	55°
Svenningsen et al.[73]	104 (52 M, 52 F)	8 years	AAOS	1	PROM	No	54°
Svenningsen et al.[73]	134 (65 M, 69 F)	11 years	AAOS	1	PROM	No	48°
Svenningsen et al.[73]	114 (57 M, 57 F)	15 years	AAOS	1	PROM	No	45°
Svenningsen et al.[73]	206 (102 M, 104 F)	Adult; x̄ = 23 years	AAOS	1	PROM	No	45°
Walker et al.[28]	30 M	60–84 years	AAOS	1	AROM	Pearson's r > .81	22° ± 6°
Walker et al.[28]	30 F	60–84 years	AAOS	1	AROM	Pearson's r > .81	36° ± 7°
Watanabe et al.[29]	62/Japanese*	Birth	Not stated	Not stated	PROM	Unknown	21°
Watanabe et al.[29]	62/Japanese*	4 weeks	Not stated	Not stated	PROM	Unknown	24°
Watanabe et al.[29]	54/Japanese*	4–8 months	Not stated	Not stated	PROM	Unknown	39°
Watanabe et al.[29]	45/Japanese*	8–12 months	Not stated	Not stated	PROM	Unknown	38°
Watanabe et al.[29]	64/Japanese*	1 year	Not stated	Not stated	PROM	Unknown	49°
Watanabe et al.[29]	57/Japanese*	2 years	Not stated	Not stated	PROM	Unknown	59°

*Number of males and females not stated.

Table B.22   INVESTIGATIONS REPORTING DATA FOR FIRST MTP EXTENSION

STUDY	SAMPLE	AGES	METHOD USED	NO. OF EXAMINERS	TYPE OF MOTION	RELIABILITY COEFFICIENT CALCULATED?	ROM
Buell et al.[83]	15*	19–30 years	STJN; midtarsal joint fully medial alignment	Not stated	AROM	No	88°
Buell et al.[83]	24*	30–45 years	STJN; midtarsal joint fully medial alignment	Not stated	AROM	No	77°
Buell et al.[83]	11*	Older than 45 years	STJN; midtarsal joint fully medial alignment	Not stated	AROM	No	62°
Buell et al.[83]	15*	19–30 years	STJN; midtarsal joint fully medial alignment	Not stated	PROM	No	95°
Buell et al.[83]	24*	30–45 years	STJN; midtarsal joint fully medial alignment	Not stated	PROM	No	82°
Buell et al.[83]	11*	Older than 45 years	STJN; midtarsal joint fully medial alignment	Not stated	PROM	No	65°
Hopson et al.[84]	20 (10 M, 10 F)	21–43 years	Supine, medial alignment of UG	1	PROM	ICC 0.95	96° ±10°
Hopson et al.[84]	20 (10 M, 10 F)	21–43 years	Supine, medial alignment of UG	1	PROM	ICC 0.91	85° ±11°
Hopson et al.[84]	20 (10 M, 10 F)	21–43 years	Seated, partial weight bearing, medial alignment	1	PROM	ICC 0.95	100° ±6°
Hopson et al.[84]	20 (10 M, 10 F)	21–43 years	Standing, full weight bearing, medial alignment	1	PROM	ICC 0.98	110° ±11°
Joseph[85]	17 M	Younger than 30 years	Angles measured from lateral radiographs	Not stated	AROM	No	54° (R) 56° (L)
Joseph[85]	17 M	30 years	Angles measured from lateral radiographs	Not stated	AROM	No	52° (R) 2° (L)
Joseph[85]	16 M	30–45 years	Angles measured from lateral radiographs	Not stated	PROM	No	46° (R) 44° (L)
Joseph[85]	16 M	Older than 45 years	Angles measured from lateral radiographs	Not stated	PROM	No	78° (R) 77° (L)
Joseph[85]	17 M	Younger than 30 years	Angles measured from lateral radiographs	Not stated	PROM	No	76° (R) 75° (L)
Joseph[85]	16 M	30–45 years	Angles measured from lateral radiographs	Not stated	PROM	No	71° (R) 63° (L)
Otter et al.[86]	26 (11 F, 15 M)	18–21 years	Universal goniometer; medial alignment of UG	8	PROM	ICC 0.69	83° ±12°
Otter et al.[86]	26 (11 F, 15 M)	18–21 years	Dr. G smartphone app, medial alignment of smartphone	8	PROM	ICC 0.71	83° ±11°
Walker et al.[28]	60 (30 M, 30 F)	60–84 years	AAOS	1	AROM	Pearson's r > .81	61° ±13°

AAOS, American Academy of Orthopaedic Surgeons; *AROM*, active range of motion; *F*, females; *ICC*, intraclass correlation; *L*, left; *M*, males; *MTP*, metatarsophalangeal; *PROM*, passive range of motion; *R*, right; *STJN*, subtalar joint neutral; *UG*, universal goniometer.
*Number of males and females not stated.

Table B.23   INVESTIGATIONS REPORTING DATA FOR FIRST MTP FLEXION ROM

STUDY	SAMPLE	AGES	METHOD USED	NO. OF EXAMINERS	TYPE OF MOTION	RELIABILITY COEFFICIENT CALCULATED?	ROM
Buell et al.[83]	15*	19–30 years	STJN; midtarsal joint fully medial alignment	Not stated	PROM	No	20°
Buell et al.[83]	24*	30–45 years	STJN; midtarsal joint fully medial alignment	Not stated	PROM	No	17°
Buell et al.[83]	11*	Older than 45 years	STJN; midtarsal joint fully medial alignment	Not stated	PROM	No	14°
Joseph[85]	17 M	Younger than 30 years	Angles measured from lateral radiographs	Not stated	AROM	No	26° ± 2° (R) 25° ± 2° (L)
Joseph[85]	17 M	30–45 years	Angles measured from lateral radiographs	Not stated	AROM	No	24° ± 2° (R) 23° ± 2° (L)
Joseph[85]	16 M	Older than 45 years	Angles measured from lateral radiographs	Not stated	AROM	No	18° ± 2° (R) 21° ± 2° (L)
Walker et al.[28]	60 (30 M, 30 F)	60–84 years	AAOS	2	AROM	Pearson's $r > .81$	7° ± 12°

AAOS, American Academy of Orthopaedic Surgeons; *AROM*, active range of motion; *F*, females; *L*, left, *M*, males; *MTP*, metatarsophalangeal; *PROM*, passive range of motion; *R*, right; *STJN*, subtalar joint neutral.
*Number of males and females not stated.

Table B.24   HAMSTRING MUSCLE LENGTH STRAIGHT LEG RAISE

STUDY	SAMPLE	AGE	HAMSTRING* (DEGREES)
Gajdosik et al.[87]	30 M	$\bar{x} = 22.8 \pm 5.3$ years	62.0
Girouard and Hurley[88]	31 M	63.0 years	69.0
Hsieh et al.[89]	6 F, 4 M	$\bar{x} = 26$–30 years	53.5
Rose[48]	15 F, 3 M	$\bar{x} = 19.5$ years	74.0
Youdas et al.[90]	20 M	20–29 years	69.4
Youdas et al.[90]	23 F	20–29 years	78.2

F, Female; *M*, male.
*Average of right and left hamstring flexibility

Table B.26   HAMSTRING MUSCLE LENGTH ACTIVE KNEE EXTENSION TEST

STUDY	SAMPLE	AGE	HAMSTRING FLEXIBILITY*
Corkery et al.[92]	25 M	$\bar{x} = 20.72 \pm 1.49$ years	25.9°
Corkery et al.[92]	47 F	$\bar{x} = 20.96 \pm 1.25$ years	37.1°
Gajdosik et al.[87]	30 M	$\bar{x} = 22.8 \pm 5.3$ years	43.0°
Gajdosik and Lusin[93]	15 M	21 years	35.6°

F, Female; *M*, male.
*Average of right and left hamstring flexibility.

Table B.25   HAMSTRING MUSCLE LENGTH PASSIVE KNEE EXTENSION TEST

STUDY	SAMPLE	AGE	HAMSTRING FLEXIBILITY* (DEGREES)
Gajdosik et al.[87]	30 M	$\bar{x} = 22.8 \pm 5.3$ years	31.0
Hartig and Henderson[91]	298 M	$\bar{x} = 20.0$ years	43.8
Youdas et al.[90]	20 M	20–29 years	37.7
Youdas et al.[90]	23 F	20–29 years	25.2

F, Female; *M*, male.
*Average of right and left hamstring flexibility

Table B.27   SUGGESTED NORMATIVE VALUES FOR HAMSTRING FLEXIBILITY BASED ON METHOD OF MEASUREMENT BASED ON ANALYSIS OF EXISTING DATA

MEASUREMENT METHOD	MALE	FEMALE
Passive knee extension	40°	25°
Active knee extension	35°	35°
Straight leg raise	65°–70°	75°

Table B.28   SOLEUS MUSCLE LENGTH—SMARTPHONE AND INCLINOMETER METHODS IN WEIGHT-BEARING LUNGE POSITION (AS DESCRIBED IN FIGS. 14.50 TO 14.57 IN CHAPTER 14)

STUDY	SAMPLE	AGES	METHOD	ROM
Awatani et al.[94]	9 F, 9 M	$\bar{x} = 25.3$ years	Smartphone	30.0° ± 7.0°
Balsalobre-Fernandez et al.[95]	5 F, 7 M	$\bar{x} = 28.6$ years	Smartphone	35.7° ± 3.2°
Balsalobre-Fernandez et al.[95]	5 F, 7 M	$\bar{x} = 28.6$ years	Inclinometer	35.2° ± 3.3°
Konor et al.[96]	13 F, 7 M	$\bar{x} = 24.0$ years	Inclinometer	38.8° ± 5.2°
Langarika-Rocafort et al.[97]	25 F (volleyball players)	$\bar{x} = 15.5$ years	Inclinometer	49.55° ± 6.11°
Rabin et al.[98]	29 F, 14 M	$\bar{x} = 25.5$ years	Inclinometer	49.5° ± 6.4°

F, Female; *M*, male.

References

1. American Academy of Orthopaedic Surgeons. *Joint Motion: Method of Measuring and Recording*. Chicago: American Academy of Orthopaedic Surgeons; 1965.

2. American Medical Association. *Guides to the Evaluation of Permanent Impairment*. xvii. Chicago, Ill: American Medical Association; 1993:339.

3. Rothschild B. *Rheumatology: A Primary Care Approach*. Brooklyn, NY: Yorke Medical Books; 1982.

4. Balogun J, Abereoje O, MO O, Obajuluwa V. Inter- and intratester reliability of measuring neck motions with tape measure and Myrin gravity-reference goniometer. *J Orthop Sports Phys Ther*. 1989;248–253.

5. Hsieh CY, Yeung BW. Active neck motion measurements with a tape measure*. *J Orthop Sports Phys Ther*. 1986;8:88–90.

6. American Medical Association. *Guides to the Evaluation of Permanent Impairment*. Chicago Ill: American Medical Association; 1984.

7. Youdas JW, Garrett TR, Suman VJ, Bogard CL, Hallman HO, Carey JR. Normal range of motion of the cervical spine: an initial goniometric study. *Phys Ther*. 1992;72:770–780.

8. Aizawa J, Masuda T, Hyodo K, et al. Ranges of active joint motion for the shoulder, elbow, and wrist in healthy adults. *Disabil Rehabil*. 2013;35:1342–1349.

9. Barnes CJ, Van Steyn SJ, Fischer RA. The effects of age, sex, and shoulder dominance on range of motion of the shoulder. *J Shoulder Elbow Surg*. 2001;10:242–246.

10. Boone DC, Azen SP. Normal range of motion of joints in male subjects. *J Bone Joint Surg Am*. 1979;61:756–759.

11. Conte AL, Marques AP, Casarotto RA, Amado-João SM. Handedness influences passive shoulder range of motion in nonathlete adult women. *J Manipulative Physiol Ther*. 2009;32:149–153.

12. Desrosiers J, Hebert R, Bravo G, Dutil E. Shoulder range of motion of healthy elderly people: A normative study. *Phys Occup Ther Geriatr*. 1995;13:101–114.

13. Escalante A, Lichtenstein MJ, Hazuda HP. Determinants of shoulder and elbow flexion range: results from the San Antonio Longitudinal Study of Aging. *Arthritis Care Res*. 1999;12:277–286.

14. Fiebert IM, Downey PA, Brown JS. Active shoulder range of motion in persons aged 60 years and older. *Phys Occup Ther Geriatr*. 1995;13:115–128.

15. Gill TK, Shanahan EM, Tucker GR, Buchbinder R, Hill CL. Shoulder range of movement in the general population: age and gender stratified normative data using a community-based cohort. *BMC Musculoskelet Disord*. 2020;21:676.

16. Vairo GL, Duffey ML, Owens BD, Cameron KL. Clinical descriptive measures of shoulder range of motion for healthy, young and physically active cohort. *Sports Medicine, Arthroscopy, Rehabilitation, Therapy & Technology*. 2012;4:33–39.

17. Gûnal I, Köse N, Erdogan O, Göktürk E, Seber S. Normal range of motion of the joints of the upper extremity in male subjects, with special reference to side. *J Bone Joint Surg Am*. 1996;78:1401–1404.

18. Kalscheur MS, Costello PS, Emery LJ. Gender differences in range of motion in older adults. *Phys Occup Ther Geriatr*. 2004;22:77–89.

19. Kolber MJ, Vega F, Widmayer K, Cheng MS. The reliability and minimal detectable change of shoulder mobility measurements using a digital inclinometer. *Physiother Theory Pract*. 2011;27:176–184.

20. Kolber MJ, Hanney WJ. The reliability and concurrent validity of shoulder mobility measurements using a digital inclinometer and goniometer: a technical report. *Int J Sports Phys Ther*. 2012;7:306–313.

21. Macedo LG, Magee DJ. Effects of age on passive range of motion of selected peripheral joints in healthy adult females. *Physiother Theory Pract*. 2009;25:145–164.

22. McIntosh L, McKenna K, Gustafsson L. Active and passive shoulder range of motion in healthy older people. *Br J Occup Ther*. 2003;66:318–324.

23. Murray MP, Gore DR, Gardner GM, Mollinger LA. Shoulder motion and muscle strength of normal men and women in two age groups. *Clin Orthop Relat Res*. 1985;268–273.

24. Sabari JS, Maltzev I, Lubarsky D, Liszkay E, Homel P. Goniometric assessment of shoulder range of motion: comparison of testing in supine and sitting positions. *Arch Phys Med Rehabil*. 1998;79:647–651.

25. Soucie JM, Wang C, Forsyth A, et al. Range of motion measurements: reference values and a database for comparison studies. *Haemophilia*. 2011;17:500–507.

26. Stubbs N, Fernandez J, Glenn W. Normative data on joint ranges of motion of 25- to 54-year-old males. *Int J Ind Ergon*. 1993;12:265–272.

27. Valentine RE, Lewis JS. Intraobserver reliability of 4 physiologic movements of the shoulder in subjects with and without symptoms. *Arch Phys Med Rehabil*. 2006;87:1242–1249.

28. Walker JM, Sue D, Miles-Elkousy N, Ford G, Trevelyan H. Active mobility of the extremities in older subjects. *Phys Ther*. 1984;64:919–923.

29. Watanabe H, Ogata K, Amano T, Okabe T. The range of joint motions of the extremities in healthy Japanese people: the difference according to the age. Cited in Walker JM: Musculoskeletal Development: a review. *Phys Ther*. 1991;878.

30. Bassey EJ, Morgan K, Dallosso HM, Ebrahim SB. Flexibility of the shoulder joint measured as range of abduction in a large representative sample of men and women over 65 years of age. *Eur J Appl Physiol Occup Physiol*. 1989;58:353–360.

31. De Smet L, Urlus M, Spriet A, Fabry G. Metacarpophalangeal and interphalangeal flexion of the thumb: influence of sex and age, relation to ligamentous injury. *Acta Orthop Belg*. 1993;59:357–359.

32. Hume MC, Gellman H, McKellop H, Brumfield RH. Functional range of motion of the joints of the hand. *J Hand Surg Am*. 1990;15:240–243.

33. Jenkins M, Bamberger HB, Black L, Nowinski R. Thumb joint flexion. What is normal? *J Hand Surg Br*. 1998;23:796–797.

34. Shaw SJ, Morris MA. The range of motion of the metacarpophalangeal joint of the thumb and its relationship to injury. *J Hand Surg Br*. 1992;17:164–166.

35. Einkauf DK, Gohdes ML, Jensen GM, Jewell MJ. Changes in spinal mobility with increasing age in women. *Phys Ther*. 1987;67:370–375.

36. Fitzgerald GK, Wynveen KJ, Rheault W, Rothschild B. Objective assessment with establishment of normal values for lumbar spinal range of motion. *Phys Ther*. 1983;63:1776–1781.

37. Haley SM, Tada WL, Carmichael EM. Spinal mobility in young children. A normative study. *Phys Ther*. 1986;66:1697–1703.

38. Lindell O, Eriksson L, Strender LE. The reliability of a 10-test package for patients with prolonged back and neck pain: could an examiner without formal medical education be used without loss of quality? A methodological study. *BMC Musculoskelet Disord*. 2007;8:31.

39. Moll JM, Wright V. Normal range of spinal mobility. An objective clinical study. *Ann Rheum Dis*. 1971;30:381–386.

40. van Adrichem JA, van der Korst JK. Assessment of the flexibility of the lumbar spine. A pilot study in children and adolescents. *Scand J Rheumatol*. 1973;2:87–91.

41. Chiarello CM, Savidge R. Interrater reliability of the Cybex EDI-320 and fluid goniometer in normals and patients with low back pain. *Arch Phys Med Rehabil*. 1993;74:32–37.

42. Dillard J, Trafimow J, Andersson GB, Cronin K. Motion of the lumbar spine. Reliability of two measurement techniques. *Spine (Phila Pa 1976)*. 1991;(16):321–324.

43. Mayer TG, Tencer AF, Kristoferson S, Mooney V. Use of noninvasive techniques for quantification of spinal range-of-motion in normal subjects and chronic low-back dysfunction patients. *Spine (Phila Pa 1976)*. 1984;(9):588–595.

44. Ng JK, Kippers V, Richardson CA, Parnianpour M. Range of motion and lordosis of the lumbar spine: reliability of measurement and normative values. *Spine (Phila Pa 1976)*. 2001;(26):53–60.

45. Breum J, Wiber J, Bolton JE. Reliability and concurrent validity of the BROM II for measuring lumbar motility. *J Manipulative Physiol Ther*. 1995;18:497–502.

46. Kachingwe AF, Phillips BJ. Inter- and intrarater reliability of a back range of motion instrument. *Arch Phys Med Rehabil*. 2005;86:2347–2353.

47. Beattie P, Rothstein JM, Lamb RL. Reliability of the attraction method for measuring lumbar spine backward bending. *Phys Ther*. 1987;67:364–369.

48. Rose MJ. The statistical analysis of the intra-observer repeatability of four clinical measurement techniques. *Physiotherapy*. 1991;77:89–91.

49. Boline PD, Keating JC, Haas M, Anderson AV. Interexaminer reliability and discriminant validity of inclinometric measurement of lumbar rotation in chronic low-back pain patients and subjects without low-back pain. *Spine (Phila Pa 1976)*. 1992;(17):335–338.

50. Audette I, Dumas JP, Côté JN, De Serres SJ. Validity and between-day reliability of the cervical range of motion (CROM) device. *J Orthop Sports Phys Ther*. 2010;40:318–323.

51. Capuano-Pucci D, Rheault W, Aukai J, Bracke M, Day R, Pastrick M. Intratester and intertester reliability of the cervical range of motion device. *Arch Phys Med Rehabil*. 1991;72:338–340.

52. Fletcher JP, Bandy WD. Intrarater reliability of CROM measurement of cervical spine active range of motion in persons with and without neck pain. *J Orthop Sports Phys Ther*. 2008;38:640–645.

53. Nyland J, Johnson D. Collegiate football players display more active cervical spine mobility than high school football players. *J Athl Train.* 2004;39:146–150.

54. Ordway NR, Seymour R, Donelson RG, Hojnowski L, Lee E, Edwards WT. Cervical sagittal range-of-motion analysis using three methods. Cervical range-of-motion device, 3space, and radiography. *Spine (Phila Pa 1976).* 1997;(22):501–508.

55. Prushansky T, Deryi O, Jabarreen B. Reproducibility and validity of digital inclinometry for measuring cervical range of motion in normal subjects. *Physiother Res Int.* 2010;15:42–48.

56. Tousignant M, Smeesters C, Breton AM, Breton E, Corriveau H. Criterion validity study of the cervical range of motion (CROM) device for rotational range of motion on healthy adults. *J Orthop Sports Phys Ther.* 2006;36:242–248.

57. Pringle RK. Intra-instrument reliability of 4 goniometers. *J Chiropr Med.* 2003;2:91–95.

58. Ahlberg A, Moussa M, Al-Nahdi M. On geographical variations in the normal range of joint motion. *Clin Orthop Relat Res.* 1988;229–231.

59. Broughton NS, Wright J, Menelaus MB. Range of knee motion in normal neonates. *J Pediatr Orthop.* 1993;13:263–264.

60. Chevillotte CJ, Ali MH, Trousdale RT, Pagnano MW. Variability in hip range of motion on clinical examination. *J Arthroplasty.* 2009;24:693–697.

61. Coon V, Donato G, Houser C, Bleck EE. Normal ranges of hip motion in infants six weeks, three months and six months of age. *Clin Orthop Relat Res.* 1975;256–260.

62. Drews JE, Vraciu JK, Pellino G. Range of motion of the joints of the lower extremities of newborns. *Phys Occup Ther Pediatr.* 1984;4:49–62.

63. Forero N, Okamura LA, Larson MA. Normal ranges of hip motion in neonates. *J Pediatr Orthop.* 1989;9:391–395.

64. Haas SS, Epps CH, Adams JP. Normal ranges of hip motion in the newborn. *Clin Orthop Relat Res.* 1973;114–118.

65. Moreside JM, McGill SM. Quantifying normal 3D hip ROM in healthy young adult males with clinical and laboratory tools: hip mobility restrictions appear to be plane-specific. *Clin Biomech (Bristol, Avon).* 2011;26:824–829.

66. Mudge AJ, Bau KV, Purcell LN, et al. Normative reference values for lower limb joint range, bone torsion, and alignment in children aged 4-16 years. *J Pediatr Orthop B.* 2014;23:15–25.

67. Mundale MO, Hislop HJ, Rabideau RJ, Kottke FJ. Evaluation of extension of the hip. *Arch Phys Med Rehabil.* 1956;37:75–80.

68. Phelps E, Smith LJ, Hallum A. Normal ranges of hip motion of infants between nine and 24 months of age. *Dev Med Child Neurol.* 1985;27:785–792.

69. Prather H, Harris-Hayes M, Hunt DM, Steger-May K, Mathew V, Clohisy JC. Reliability and agreement of hip range of motion and provocative physical examination tests in asymptomatic volunteers. *PM R.* 2010;2:888–895.

70. Roaas A, Anderson G. Normal range of motion of the hip, knee and ankle joints in male subjects, 30-40 years of age. *Acta Orthop Scand.* 1982;53:205–208.

71. Roach KE, Miles TP. Normal hip and knee active range of motion: the relationship to age. *Phys Ther.* 1991;71:656–665.

72. Sankar WN, Laird CT, Baldwin KD. Hip range of motion in children: what is the norm? *J Pediatr Orthop.* 2012;32:399–405.

73. Svenningsen S, Terjesen T, Auflem M, Berg V. Hip motion related to age and sex. *Acta Orthop Scand.* 1989;60:97–100.

74. Waugh KG, Minkel JL, Parker R, Coon VA. Measurement of selected hip, knee, and ankle joint motions in newborns. *Phys Ther.* 1983;63:1616–1621.

75. Bennell KL, Khan KM, Matthews BL, Singleton C. Changes in hip and ankle range of motion and hip muscle strength in 8-11 year old novice female ballet dancers and controls: a 12 month follow up study. *Br J Sports Med.* 2001;35:54–59.

76. Ellison JB, Rose SJ, Sahrmann SA. Patterns of hip rotation range of motion: a comparison between healthy subjects and patients with low back pain. *Phys Ther.* 1990;70:537–541.

77. Giladi M, Milgrom C, Stein M, et al. External rotation of the hip. A predictor of risk for stress fractures. *Clin Orthop Relat Res.* 1987;131–134.

78. Haley ET. Range of hip rotation and torque of hip rotator muscle groups. *Am J Phys Med.* 1953;32:261–270.

79. Hoaglund FT, Yau AC, Wong WL. Osteoarthritis of the hip and other joints in southern Chinese in Hong Kong. *J Bone Joint Surg Am.* 1973;55:545–557.

80. Kouyoumdjian P, Coulomb R, Sanchez T, Asencio G. Clinical evaluation of hip joint rotation range of motion in adults. *Orthop Traumatol Surg Res.* 2012;98:17–23.

81. McKay MJ, Baldwin JN, Ferreira P, Simic M, Vanicek N, Burns J. Normative reference values for strength and flexibility of 1,000 children and adults. *Neurology.* 2017;88:36–43.

82. Simoneau GG, Hoenig KJ, Lepley JE, Papanek PE. Influence of hip position and gender on active hip internal and external rotation. *J Orthop Sports Phys Ther.* 1998;28:158–164.

83. Buell T, Green DR, Risser J. Measurement of the first metatarsophalangeal joint range of motion. *J Am Podiatr Med Assoc.* 1988;78:439–448.

84. Hopson MM, McPoil TG, Cornwall MW. Motion of the first metatarsophalangeal joint. Reliability and validity of four measurement techniques. *J Am Podiatr Med Assoc.* 1995;85:198–204.

85. Joseph J. Range of movement of the great toe in men. *J Bone Joint Surg.* 1954;450–457.

86. Otter SJ, Agalliu B, Baer N, et al. The reliability of a smartphone goniometer application compared with a traditional goniometer for measuring first metatarsophalangeal joint dorsiflexion. *J Foot Ankle Res.* 2015;8:30.

87. Gajdosik RL, Rieck MA, Sullivan DK, Wightman SE. Comparison of four clinical tests for assessing hamstring muscle length. *J Orthop Sports Phys Ther.* 1993;18:614–618.

88. Girouard CK, Hurley BF. Does strength training inhibit gains in range of motion from flexibility training in older adults? *Med Sci Sports Exerc.* 1995;27:1444–1449.

89. Hsieh CY, Walker JM, Gillis K. Straight-leg-raising test. Comparison of three instruments. *Phys Ther.* 1983;63:1429–1433.

90. Youdas JW, Krause DA, Hollman JH, Harmsen WS, Laskowski E. The influence of gender and age on hamstring muscle length in healthy adults. *J Orthop Sports Phys Ther.* 2005;35:246–252.

91. Hartig DE, Henderson JM. Increasing hamstring flexibility decreases lower extremity overuse injuries in military basic trainees. *Am J Sports Med.* 1999;27:173–176.

92. Corkery M, Briscoe H, Ciccone N. Establishing normal values for lower extremity muscle length in college-age students. *Phys Ther Sport.* 2007;66–74.

93. Gajdosik R, Lusin G. Hamstring muscle tightness. Reliability of an active-knee-extension test. *Phys Ther.* 1983;63:1085–1090.

94. Awatani T, Enoki T, Morikita I. Inter-rater reliability and validity of angle measurements using smartphone applications for weight-bearing ankle dorsiflexion range of motion measurements. *Phys Ther Sport.* 2018;34:113–120.

95. Balsalobre-Fernández C, Romero-Franco N, Jiménez-Reyes P. Concurrent validity and reliability of an iPhone app for the measurement of ankle dorsiflexion and inter-limb asymmetries. *J Sports Sci.* 2019;37:249–253.

96. Konor MM, et al. Reliability of three measures of ankle dorsiflexion range of motion. *Int J Sports Phys Ther.* 2012;7(3):279–287.

97. Langarika-Rocafort A, Ignacio Emparanza J, Aramendi J, et al. Intra-rater reliability and agreement of various methods of measurement to assess dorsiflexion in the weight bearing dorsiflexion lunge test (WBLT) among female athletes. *Phys Ther Sport.* 2017;23:37–44.

98. Rabin A, Kozol Z. Weightbearing and nonweightbearing ankle dorsiflexion range of motion: are we measuring the same thing? *J Am Podiatr Med Assoc.* 2012;102:406–411.

INDEX

Note: Page numbers followed by *f* indicate figures,
t indicate tables, and *b* indicate boxes.